AF762919

ADAPTING COGNITIVE BEHAVIORAL THERAPY FOR INSOMNIA

ADAPTING COGNITIVE BEHAVIORAL THERAPY FOR INSOMNIA

Edited by

SARA NOWAKOWSKI
Baylor College of Medicine Medicine-Health Services Research, Houston, TX, United States

SHEILA N. GARLAND
Department of Psychology, Memorial University, St. John's, NL, Canada

MICHAEL A. GRANDNER
Sleep and Health Research Program, University of Arizona, Tucson, AZ, United States
Behavioral Sleep Medicine Clinic, Banner - University Medical Center Tucson, Tucson, AZ, United States
Department of Psychiatry and Medicine, UA College of Medicine, Tucson, AZ, United States

LEISHA J. CUDDIHY
Sleep Disorders Center, Spectrum Health Medical Group, Grand Rapids, MI, United States

ELSEVIER

ACADEMIC PRESS
An imprint of Elsevier

Academic Press is an imprint of Elsevier
125 London Wall, London EC2Y 5AS, United Kingdom
525 B Street, Suite 1650, San Diego, CA 92101, United States
50 Hampshire Street, 5th Floor, Cambridge, MA 02139, United States
The Boulevard, Langford Lane, Kidlington, Oxford OX5 1GB, United Kingdom

Library of Congress Cataloging-in-Publication Data
A catalog record for this book is available from the Library of Congress

British Library Cataloguing-in-Publication Data
A catalogue record for this book is available from the British Library

ISBN 978-0-12-822872-2

For information on all Academic Press publications
visit our website at https://www.elsevier.com/books-and-journals

Publisher: Nikki Levy
Editorial Project Manager: Barbara Makinster
Production Project Manager: Sreejith Viswanathan
Cover designer: Matthew Limbert

Typeset by STRAIVE, India

Contents

3. CBT-I for patients with phase disorders or insomnia with circadian misalignment

Marissa A. Evans and Brant P. Hasler

4. CBT-I for patients with shift work disorder

Philip Cheng

5. CBT-I for patients with hypersomnia disorders

Jason C. Ong and Matthew D. Schuiling

6. CBT-I for patients with orthosomnia

Kelly Glazer Baron

3

CBT-I in psychiatric disorders

4

CBT-I in medical disorders

5

CBT-I across the lifespan

6

Other special considerations

Contributors

Erin A. Almklov VA San Diego Healthcare System-Center of Excellence for Stress and Mental Health (CESAMH), San Diego, CA, United States

Kelly Glazer Baron Department of Family and Preventive Medicine, University of Utah, Salt Lake City, UT, United States

Gabrielle E. Bowyer Sleep and Circadian Research Laboratory, Department of Psychiatry, University of Michigan, Ann Arbor, MI, United States

Trevor M. Brooks Sleep and Circadian Research Laboratory, Department of Psychiatry, University of Michigan, Ann Arbor, MI, United States

Philip Cheng Department of Internal Medicine, Thomas Roth Sleep Disorders and Research Center, Henry Ford Health System, Detroit, MI, United States

Deirdre A. Conroy Sleep and Circadian Research Laboratory, Department of Psychiatry, University of Michigan, Ann Arbor, MI, United States

Earl Charles Crew Behavioral Health Program, Mental Health Care Line, Michael E. DeBakey Veteran's Affairs Medical Center; Psychology Division, Menninger Department of Psychiatry and Behavioral Sciences, Baylor College of Medicine, Houston, TX, United States

Leisha J. Cuddihy Pediatric Behavioral Health, Spectrum Health Helen DeVos Children's Hospital, Grand Rapids, MI, United States

Darius B. Dawson Department of Medicine, Baylor College of Medicine, Houston, TX, United States

Spencer Dawson Department of Psychological and Brain Sciences, University of Indiana; Better Sleep Bloomington, Bloomington, IN, United States

Denise Rodriguez Esquivel Department of Psychiatry and Medicine, UA College of Medicine; Behavioral Sleep Medicine Clinic, Banner—University Medical Center Tucson, Tucson, AZ, United States

Marissa A. Evans Department of Psychology, University of Pittsburgh, Pittsburgh, PA, United States

Julio Fernandez-Mendoza Sleep Research and Treatment Center, Department of Psychiatry and Behavioral Health, Penn State Health Milton S. Hershey Medical Center, Penn State University College of Medicine, Hershey, PA, United States

Sheila N. Garland Department of Psychology, Faculty of Science; Discipline of Oncology, Faculty of Medicine, Memorial University of Newfoundland, St. John's, NL, Canada

Caitlin E. Gasperetti Department of Psychology, University of California, Berkeley, CA, United States

Philip Gehrman Department of Psychiatry, Perelman School of Medicine of the University of Pennsylvania; Department of Behavioral Health, Corporal Michael J. Crescenz VA Medical Center, Philadelphia, PA, United States

Jennifer Goldschmied Department of Psychiatry, Perelman School of Medicine of the University of Pennsylvania, Philadelphia, PA, United States

Michael A. Grandner Sleep and Health Research Program, University of Arizona; Behavioral Sleep Medicine Clinic, Banner–University Medical Center Tucson; Department of Psychiatry and Medicine, UA College of Medicine, Tucson, AZ, United States

Alison R. Hartman Department of Psychology, Drexel University, Philadelphia, PA, United States

Allison G. Harvey Department of Psychology, University of California, Berkeley, CA, United States

Brant P. Hasler Department of Psychiatry, University of Pittsburgh, Pittsburgh, PA, United States

Jaime M. Hughes Department of Population Health Sciences, School of Medicine, Duke University, Health Services Research & Development, Durham VA Healthcare System, Durham, NC, United States

Anna L. MacKinnon Department of Psychology, University of Calgary, Calgary, AB, Canada

Rachel Manber Department of Psychiatry & Behavioral Sciences, Stanford University, Palo Alto, CA, United States

Jennifer L. Martin Geriatric Research, Education, and Clinical Center, VA Greater Los Angeles Healthcare System, David Geffen School of Medicine at the University of California Los Angeles, Los Angeles, CA, United States

Jessica M. Meers Department of Medicine, Baylor College of Medicine; Department of Medicine—Health Services Research, Center for Innovations in Quality, Effectiveness, and Safety, Michael E. DeBakey VA Medical Center; South Central Mental Illness Research Education Clinical, Centers of Excellence (MIRECC), Michael E. DeBakey VA Medical Center; Department of Psychology, University of Houston, Houston, TX, United States

Melisa E. Moore Department of Child and Adolescent Psychiatry and Behavioral Sciences, Children's Hospital of Philadelphia, Philadelphia, PA, United States

Alexandria Muench Behavioral Sleep Medicine Program, Department of Psychiatry; Chronobiology & Sleep Institute, Department of Medicine, University of Pennsylvania, Philadelphia, PA, United States

Sara Nowakowski Department of Medicine, Baylor College of Medicine; Department of Medicine—Health Services Research, Center for Innovations in Quality, Effectiveness, and Safety; South Central Mental Illness Research Education Clinical, Centers of Excellence (MIRECC), Michael E DeBakey VA Medical Center, Houston, TX, United States

Jason C. Ong Department of Neurology, Center for Circadian and Sleep Medicine, Northwestern University Feinberg School of Medicine, Chicago, IL, United States

Henry Orff VA San Diego Healthcare System-Center of Excellence for Stress and Mental Health (CESAMH); Clinical Health Sciences, Department of Psychiatry, UCSD, San Diego, CA, United States

Michael L. Perlis Behavioral Sleep Medicine Program, Department of Psychiatry; School of Nursing; Chronobiology & Sleep Institute, Department of Medicine, University of Pennsylvania, Philadelphia, PA, United States

Donn Posner Department of Psychiatry & Behavioral Sciences, Stanford University School of Medicine, Stanford, CA, United States

Guadalupe L. Rivera VA San Diego Healthcare System, San Diego, CA, United States

Matthew D. Schuiling Department of Neurology, Center for Circadian and Sleep Medicine, Northwestern University Feinberg School of Medicine, Chicago, IL, United States

Ivan D. Sedov Alberta Health Services, Calgary, AB, Canada

Norah Simpson Department of Psychiatry & Behavioral Sciences, Stanford University, Palo Alto, CA, United States

Michael T. Smith Psychiatry and Behavioral Sciences, Johns Hopkins University, Baltimore, MD, United States

Lianne M. Tomfohr-Madsen Department of Psychology, University of Calgary, Calgary, AB, Canada

Andrew Scott Tubbs Sleep and Health Research Program, Department of Psychiatry, The University of Arizona College of Medicine – Tucson, Tucson, AZ, United States

Ivan Vargas Department of Psychological Science, University of Arkansas, Fayetteville, AR, United States

Preface

Insomnia has been classified as a public health crisis (Kraus & Rabin, 2012). Roughly 30% of the general population will face occasional insomnia and for 10% of the population, insomnia will become a chronic problem (NIH, 2005). The prevalence of insomnia can skyrocket to greater than 50% when considering groups of people with other sleep, medical, and/or psychological disorders, who are at greater risk for the development and maintenance of insomnia. The full range and scope of the impact of insomnia are hard to fully appreciate and quantify, but it is safe to say that insomnia comes at a great cost for the individual and society, in terms of health, safety, and productivity. Insomnia has been linked to an array of physical health conditions including diabetes (Ogilvie & Patel, 2018), cardiovascular disease (Grimaldi, Goldstein, & Carter, 2019), cancer (Samuelsson et al., 2018), and neurodegenerative diseases (Shamim et al., 2019). In addition, insomnia is known to precipitate the development (Scott et al., 2021) or worsen the severity of several psychological disorders, not limited to mood (Riemann et al., 2020), anxiety (Cox & Olatunji, 2020), and substance use disorders (Koob & Colrain, 2020). Insomnia can not only impact one's ability to go to work but also how effective they are while at work, with financial implications for the individual and society (Kessler et al., 2011). Fortunately, we know a great deal about how to address insomnia using a combination of cognitive and behavioral techniques.

The techniques that eventually became incorporated into Cognitive Behavioral Therapy for Insomnia (CBT-I) have their roots in the pioneering work on relaxation that occurred in the early part of the 20th century. Decades later, these techniques would be refined and applied to improving sleep. In the 1970s and 1980s, the core elements of CBT-I emerged as unique therapies for what eventually came to be known as psychophysiological insomnia. Throughout this period, Richard Bootzin, Arthur Spielman, Peter Hauri, and others further developed stimulus control, sleep restriction therapy, sleep hygiene, and the increasingly cohesive multicomponent therapy that CBT-I eventually became.

Over time, CBT-I has been developed, refined, tested, and proven. As the scientific understanding around the clinical etiology, pathophysiology, presentation, and treatment of insomnia grew, the versatile, multicomponent CBT-I consistently demonstrated efficacy and effectiveness in the presence of increasingly heterogeneous and divergent forms of insomnia. CBT-I has shown, repeatedly, that it works. It does so across age groups, in both men and women, and the presence of medical and psychological comorbidities. In short, there is a preponderance of the evidence that CBT-I is an effective treatment for insomnia. The weight of evidence supporting CBT-I, summarized in several metaanalyses (Morin, Culbert, & Schwartz, 1994; Murtagh & Greenwood, 1995; Smith et al., 2002), led to its recognition as a first-line treatment for insomnia by the NIH Consensus Statement (NIH, 2005), and organizations such as the American College of Physicians (Qaseem et al., 2016). Improvements following CBT-I are equivalent to those achieved during acute treatment with hypnotic medications at 4–8 weeks (Edinger et al., 2001; Morin et al., 1999) and its effects are more durable after treatment discontinuation (Mitchell et al., 2012; Morin et al., 1999).

Despite the empirical evidence and fact that clinical trials for CBT-I generally enroll carefully selected samples of individuals with no comorbidities, the basic application of CBT-I in populations with sleep, medical, and/or psychological comorbidities produces results that are in line with trials of patients with insomnia as an independent disorder (Geiger-Brown et al., 2015; Wu et al., 2015). Using CBT-I to treat insomnia comorbid with sleep, medical, and psychological conditions can improve sleep and sometimes improve symptoms of the comorbid condition (Geiger-Brown et al., 2015; Manber et al., 2008, 2011, 2016; Nowakowski et al., 2017; Taylor et al., 2007; Vitiello et al., 2013, 2014). Although many patients improve quickly, the question remains as to whether can we further improve CBT-I to optimize treatment gains by accounting for other symptoms and comorbid conditions. While the evidence shows that the application of standard CBT-I is generally effective across groups, it does not mean that CBT-I cannot be adapted or optimized to better address the needs of different groups, especially in the areas of treatment engagement and adherence.

Given these advances, it is now time to make available a manual for clinicians on how to adapt CBT-I for insomnia in the context of different demographic groups and a variety of comorbid conditions. This book is intended to provide a thorough overview of contexts, symptoms, or conditions that may interfere with the implementation of, or adherence to, standard application of CBT-I. Also, this book will provide a description of how to adapt CBT-I or add adjunctive therapeutic components to achieve optimal therapeutic results from a patient-centered perspective. Thus, treatment can be tailored based on patient history and case conceptualization to target factors that may have originally accompanied the onset of insomnia but are ongoing (i.e., ongoing precipitating factors) and now also serve as maintaining or perpetuating factors of insomnia. This book was shaped by researchers and clinicians with expertise in insomnia and various other conditions. It is shaped by their experience and clinical insights from success and failures delivering CBT-I to various patient populations.

This book is appropriate for the advanced clinician with prior experience delivering standard CBT-I who is looking to expand their skill set to tailor CBT-I to patients with various comorbid conditions, such as sleep, psychiatric, or medical disorders, patients at various stages across their lifespan, and special considerations (e.g., hypnotic use, patients who have "failed" CBT-I). This book has six parts.

The first part of the book will provide an overview of the standard application of CBT-I. It will also provide a rationale against jumping head-first into modifying CBT-I for any patient with a more complex insomnia picture. The next three parts address the application of CBT-I in the context of other sleep disorders, psychiatric disorders, and medical disorders. In the part on sleep disorders, chapters will address strategies for treating insomnia in the context of sleep apnea, circadian rhythm disorders, shift work sleep disorder, hypersomnia disorders, and orthosomnia. In the part on comorbid psychiatric conditions, chapters will address the treatment of insomnia in the context of depression, schizophrenia and other psychotic disorders, bipolar disorder, and alcohol use and other substance use disorders. In the part on medical disorders, the chapters address the implementation of CBT-I with patients who suffer from chronic pain, are cancer survivors, and have experienced traumatic brain injuries. The fifth part addresses issues across the lifespan. It includes chapters on treating insomnia in adolescents, insomnia that arises during pregnancy, insomnia that emerges during menopause and postmenopause, and insomnia that occurs in older adults. The final part addresses the treatment of insomnia in other special groups. These include short sleepers, people who have participated in CBT-I in the past but have not benefitted from it, and chronic users of hypnotic medications.

Each chapter will be accompanied by a table that describes standard CBT-I components and how those components are adapted for different conditions. This will provide the reader with a quick reference and summary on recommendations of how to adapt CBT-I.

For the reader that is a novice to CBT-I, it is important to understand the rationale behind CBT-I recommendations. The absence of such understanding hinders the delivery of treatment, impacts patients' buy-in, compromises adherence, and ultimately leads to poorer therapeutic outcomes. A basic understanding of the rationale behind CBT-I and comfort in delivering standard CBT-I to routine patients is recommended before attempting to include more complex presentations into case conceptualization. We strongly recommend that this book is used when accompanied by an apprenticeship model and supervised/mentored clinical experiences. Although individualizing therapy is an attractive notion, clinicians with minimal prior exposure to CBT-I may initially find adapting CBT-I and maintaining a flexible approach to tailoring CBT-I to be challenging. We would encourage the reader new to CBT-I to begin with a more thorough review of the standard application of CBT-I, such as Cognitive Behavioral Therapy for Insomnia: A Session-by-Session Guide by Perlis, Jungquist, Smith, and Posner; Insomnia: A Clinician's Guide to Assessment and Treatment by Morin; and Treatment Plans and Interventions for Insomnia: A Case Formulation Approach by Manber and Carney.

This book is intended as a companion to other CBT-I manuals available for those interested in learning more about what encompasses Behavioral Sleep Medicine expanding beyond the standard application of CBT-I. We ultimately believe that specific adaptations of CBT-I components will maximize the clinical relevance of the book and will be a useful guide to the more seasoned clinician. We hope that this book—which started as a conversation at the annual SLEEP meeting among a group of friends—provides a useful resource to the growing community of clinicians and researchers incorporating behavioral sleep medicine approaches to the treatment of insomnia.

Sara Nowakowski
Sheila N. Garland
Michael A. Grandner
Leisha J. Cuddihy

References

Cox, R. C., & Olatunji, B. O. (2020). Sleep in the anxiety-related disorders: A meta-analysis of subjective and objective research. *Sleep Medicine Reviews, 51*, 101282.

Edinger, J. D., et al. (2001). Cognitive behavioral therapy for treatment of chronic primary insomnia: A randomized controlled trial. *JAMA, 285*(14), 1856–1864.

Geiger-Brown, J. M., et al. (2015). Cognitive behavioral therapy in persons with comorbid insomnia: A meta-analysis. *Sleep Medicine Reviews, 23*, 54–67.

Grimaldi, D., Goldstein, M. R., & Carter, J. R. (2019). Insomnia and cardiovascular autonomic control. *Autonomic Neuroscience, 220*, 102551.

Kessler, R. C., et al. (2011). Insomnia and the performance of US workers: Results from the America insomnia survey. *Sleep, 34*(9), 1161–1171.

Koob, G. F., & Colrain, I. M. (2020). Alcohol use disorder and sleep disturbances: A feed-forward allostatic framework. *Neuropsychopharmacology, 45*(1), 141–165.

Kraus, S. S., & Rabin, L. A. (2012). Sleep America: Managing the crisis of adult chronic insomnia and associated conditions. *Journal of Affective Disorders, 138*(3), 192–212.

Manber, R., et al. (2008). Cognitive behavioral therapy for insomnia enhances depression outcome in patients with comorbid major depressive disorder and insomnia. *Sleep, 31*(4), 489–495.

Manber, R., et al. (2011). CBT for insomnia in patients with high and low depressive symptom severity: Adherence and clinical outcomes. *Journal of Clinical Sleep Medicine, 7*(6), 645–652.

Manber, R., et al. (2016). Efficacy of cognitive-behavioral therapy for insomnia combined with antidepressant pharmacotherapy in patients with comorbid depression and insomnia: A randomized controlled trial. *The Journal of Clinical Psychiatry, 77*(10), e1316–e1323.

Mitchell, M. D., et al. (2012). Comparative effectiveness of cognitive behavioral therapy for insomnia: A systematic review. *BMC Family Practice, 13*, 40.

Morin, C. M., Culbert, J. P., & Schwartz, S. M. (1994). Nonpharmacological interventions for insomnia: A meta-analysis of treatment efficacy. *The American Journal of Psychiatry, 151*(8), 1172–1180.

Morin, C. M., et al. (1999). Behavioral and pharmacological therapies for late-life insomnia: A randomized controlled trial. *JAMA, 281*(11), 991–999.

Murtagh, D. R., & Greenwood, K. M. (1995). Identifying effective psychological treatments for insomnia: A meta-analysis. *Journal of Consulting and Clinical Psychology, 63*(1), 79–89.

NIH. (2005). National institutes of health state of the science conference statement on manifestations and management of chronic insomnia in adults, June 13-15, 2005. *Sleep, 28*(9), 1049–1057.

Nowakowski, S., Heimbach, E., Manber, R., Sadruddin, S. M., Hayman, J. M., Stout-Aguilar, J., et al. (2017). Effects of cognitive behavioral therapy for menopausal insomnia on depressive symptoms. *Menopause, 24*(12), 1428–1429.

Ogilvie, R. P., & Patel, S. R. (2018). The epidemiology of sleep and diabetes. *Current Diabetes Reports, 18*(10), 82.

Qaseem, A., et al. (2016). Management of chronic insomnia disorder in adults: A clinical practice guideline from the American College of Physicians. *Annals of Internal Medicine, 165*(2), 125–133.

Riemann, D., et al. (2020). Sleep, insomnia, and depression. *Neuropsychopharmacology, 45*(1), 74–89.

Samuelsson, L. B., et al. (2018). Sleep and circadian disruption and incident breast cancer risk: An evidence-based and theoretical review. *Neuroscience and Biobehavioral Reviews, 84*, 35–48.

Scott, J., et al. (2021). Sleep disturbances and first onset of major mental disorders in adolescence and early adulthood: A systematic review and meta-analysis. *Sleep Medicine Reviews, 57*, 101429.

Shamim, S. A., et al. (2019). Insomnia: Risk factor for neurodegenerative diseases. *Cureus, 11* (10), e6004.

Smith, M. T., et al. (2002). Comparative meta-analysis of pharmacotherapy and behavior therapy for persistent insomnia. *The American Journal of Psychiatry, 159*(1), 5–11.

Taylor, D. J., et al. (2007). A pilot study of cognitive-behavioral therapy of insomnia in people with mild depression. *Behavior Therapy, 38*(1), 49–57.

Vitiello, M. V., et al. (2013). Cognitive-behavioral treatment for comorbid insomnia and osteoarthritis pain in primary care: The lifestyles randomized controlled trial. *Journal of the American Geriatrics Society, 61*(6), 947–956.

Vitiello, M. V., et al. (2014). Short-term improvement in insomnia symptoms predicts long-term improvements in sleep, pain, and fatigue in older adults with comorbid osteoarthritis and insomnia. *Pain, 155*(8), 1547–1554.

Wu, J. Q., et al. (2015). Cognitive behavioral therapy for insomnia comorbid with psychiatric and medical conditions: A meta-analysis. *JAMA Internal Medicine, 175*(9), 1461–1472.

Acknowledgments

This book represents the culmination of a process that required hard work and dedication from a lot of people at a time when the world and the lives of everyone in it were in a state of upheaval due to a global pandemic. First and foremost, we would like to thank all of the colleagues and friends who were generous with their time and efforts and contributed excellent chapters. The value and utility of this volume depend almost entirely on the amazing contributions that all of the contributors made, and we wish to thank them for their efforts. Writing an academic book chapter is often a thankless job, and we did not want this to be the case. In particular, we especially wish to thank the many contributors who took lead roles in drafting chapters. In alphabetical order, this includes (but are not limited to): Kelly Baron, Marissa Bowman, Dierdre Conroy, Chuck Crew, Phil Cheng, Julio Fernandez-Mendoza, Phil Gehrman, Jen Goldschmied, Allison Harvey, Brant Hasler, Jamie Hughes, Rachel Manber, Jennifer Martin, Melisa Moore, Jason Ong, Henry Orff, Michael Perlis, Donn Posner, Norah Simpson, Michael Smith, Lianne Tomfohr-Madsen, Andrew Tubbs, and Ivan Vargas.

We also wish to thank our mentors, who taught us CBT-I for use in our clinical practice. This training built the foundations upon which all of our work is built. First and foremost, we wish to thank Michael Perlis, whose mentorship connects the four of us over many years. Not only has he been a key mentor for all of us, but his leadership in the area of insomnia diagnosis and treatment has separately inspired us to work in this area. In addition, we would like to thank our other CBT-I mentors, including Sonia Ancoli-Israel, Dick Bootzin, Phil Gehrman, Rachel Manber, Donn Posner, and J. Todd Arnedt.

Throughout this whole process, we were really fortunate to have the help of Chloe Wills from the Arizona Sleep and Health Research Program who served as a project manager for this book. She always made sure that the authors knew what was going on, she answered questions, and kept the whole process on track and moving forward. Also, the team at Elsevier has done an excellent job in helping us take what was the germination of an idea into a final volume that is very well put together. In particular, Barbara Makinster was a consistent force forward, as she helped shepherd the book from draft proposal to finished product.

Most importantly, we wish to thank each other for being willing to share the load of an important but time-consuming project, and our families, who give our work meaning and support us as we do what we can to help the world sleep a little better.

PART 1

Traditional CBT-I components and delivery

CHAPTER

1

Standard cognitive behavioral therapy for insomnia (CBT-I)

When is the adaptation of CBT-I warranted?

Alexandria Muench[a,d], *Ivan Vargas*[b], *Donn Posner*[e], *and Michael L. Perlis*[a,c,d]

[a]Behavioral Sleep Medicine Program, Department of Psychiatry, University of Pennsylvania, Philadelphia, PA, United States, [b]Department of Psychological Science, University of Arkansas, Fayetteville, AR, United States, [c]School of Nursing, University of Pennsylvania, Philadelphia, PA, United States, [d]Chronobiology & Sleep Institute, Department of Medicine, University of Pennsylvania, Philadelphia, PA, United States, [e]Department of Psychiatry & Behavioral Sciences, Stanford University School of Medicine, Stanford, CA, United States

Introduction

Cognitive Behavioral Therapy for insomnia (CBT-I) is a multicomponent treatment that specifically targets sleep continuity disturbance[a] (difficulties initiating and/or maintaining sleep). CBT-I is typically comprised of

[a]Sleep continuity refers to the class or set of variables that represent "sleep performance." That is, it is a class term (vs. sleep architecture or sleep microarchitecture) for variables that represent latency to, and duration and efficiency of, the sleep that occurs during the sleep period, including Sleep Latency (SL), Number of Awakenings (NWAK), Wake After Sleep Onset (WASO), Early Morning Awakening (EMA), Total Sleep Time (TST), and Sleep efficiency (SE%). When one or more of these variables are pathologic, this may be referred to as *sleep continuity disturbance*. More, the use of this class term promotes a level of specificity that is unconfounded with the many denotations and connotations of the vernacular term "insomnia."

https://doi.org/10.1016/B978-0-12-822872-2.00012-8

Sleep Restriction Therapy, Stimulus Control procedures, and Sleep Hygiene instructions. Classical CBT-I included some form of relaxation training, though this is less true of contemporary protocols. With respect to the acronym "CBT-I," this was adopted (the hyphenated or "rodomized" form of the acronym) to elicit the response "I know what CBT is, but what the heck is CBT-I?!" (i.e., the abbreviation was and is used so that patients and clinicians may distinguish the insomnia form of CBT from other modalities [e.g., CBT-D, CBT-A, etc.]). The purpose of this chapter is to review the components of standard CBT-I, discuss its efficacy and effectiveness as a multicomponent therapy, and review common alternative approaches, rules, and therapies. The chapter closes with a discussion about the need to adapt CBT-I for specific clinical conditions or demographic groups.

Components of therapy

Standard CBT-I is delivered over the course of six to eight sessions (session length may vary between 15 and 90min) (Perlis, Jungquist, Smith, & Posner, 2006). Each session typically has a specific agenda (e.g., evaluation, rationale, and Rx delivery of single therapies; adherence management; relapse prevention; etc.) (Perlis et al., 2006). Sessions most often occur in person on a weekly or biweekly schedule as individual or group encounters (Bastien, Morin, Ouellet, Blais, & Bouchard, 2004; Perlis et al., 2006; Verbeek, Konings, Aldenkamp, Declerck, & Klip, 2006; Yamadera et al., 2013; Zwart & Lisman, 1979a). Which prescriptive components are thought to be essential or to account for the most clinical outcome variance is a matter of debate and continues to be a subject of empirical evaluation (Epstein, Sidani, Bootzin, & Belyea, 2012; Harvey et al., 2014). Absent definitive data, most treatment protocols, and/or published treatment manuals focus on Sleep Restriction and Stimulus Control as the core therapies (Edinger & Carney, 2014; Manber & Carney, 2015; Morin & Espie, 2007; Perlis et al., 2006). More, the two treatment modalities are often used (and explained to patients) as complementary therapies. SRT's primary indication is to induce sleep quickly and to allow for consolidated sleep (Spielman, Saskin, & Thorpy, 1987). SCT's primary indication is to manage nocturnal wakefulness (Bootzin & Perlis, 2011). In the instances where these treatments are applied without specific cognitive therapy exercises (i.e., to debunk dysfunctional beliefs or to address catastrophization), treatment still includes a fair amount of cognitive work in the form of psychoeducation, the delivery of paradoxical instructions (i.e., stay awake longer and when awake at night get out of bed and be awake), and the management of nonadherence.

Sleep restriction therapy (SRT)

According to the Behavioral model of insomnia, the most important perpetuating factor for chronic insomnia is sleep extension. Sleep extension is the tendency for individuals to compensate for sleep loss by extending their time in bed, either by going to sleep earlier or waking up later (or by napping) (Spielman et al., 1987). A consequence of sleep extension, however, is the mismatch between sleep opportunity (i.e., how much time the patient spends in bed) and sleep ability (i.e., how much time the person actually sleeps). Therefore, the primary goal of SRT is to address this mismatch by limiting the amount of time a patient spends in bed to the amount of time that they are actually sleeping. SRT is thought to be effective owing to its effects on "Process S" (sleep restriction increases the homeostatic pressure for sleep and consequently reduces the time taken to fall asleep (SL) and/or the amount of time spent awake at night (WASO).

While the procedures for SRT vary from investigation to investigation (Kyle et al., 2015) and from treatment manual to manual (see Table 1), the following represents the original formulation (Spielman et al., 1987). The first step is to determine the patient's basal sleep ability in terms of average total sleep time (TST [as assessed with daily sleep diaries gathered over a period of two weeks]). Note that TST may be based on self-reported TST or by a derived measure of TST (TST-C = TIB + [SL + WASO + EMA]). The latter has the value of being internally valid. The next step is to determine a morning wake-up time that the patient can closely adhere to on a daily basis. Given these data, the clinician then sets the prescribed time in bed (PTIB, i.e., the patients' sleep window). This is done by subtracting PTIB from the desired wake-up time. For example, if a patient has a 6-h sleep ability and chooses to get up at 7:00 am every morning, their designated bedtime is 1:00 am. This sleep schedule is maintained or altered based upon how consolidated the individual's sleep is, as assessed with sleep efficiency SE% [sleep time/time in bed × 100]) once every 7 days. If SE% is less than 85%, PTIB is reduced by 15 min. If SE% is between 85% and 90%, PTIB is remains as prescribed. If SE% is greater than 90%, PTIB is increased by 15 min. Adjustments to the sleep schedule are usually accomplished by delaying, advancing, or leaving unchanged the individual's time to bed (TTB).

In theory, this titration process continues for as long as needed to recover or exceed baseline TST. In practice, titration is limited by the number of sessions allowed by the protocol (or third-party payers). It should be noted that most patients do not recover baseline TST within 8 sessions (83% based on one study (Perlis et al., 2019; Scott et al., 2021)). This has prompted some researchers and clinicians to modify SRT to use: (1) PTIB's that are in excess of average total sleep times; (2) shorter assessment

TABLE 1 Sleep restriction therapy (SRT) rules based on the first four published treatment manuals.

		Manual			
SRT elements/rules	Issue	Morin and Espie (2007)	Perlis et al. (2006)	Edinger and Carney (2014)	Manber and Carney (2015)
Session for SRT Rx	When is SRT implemented ?	Session 2 or 3	Session 2	Session 2	Session 2 (1)
# days baseline	How much baseline data is required ?	14 days	7–14 days	At least 14 days	14 days (2)
PTIB calculation	How is the TIB Rx calculated ?	Mean TST; PTIB = mean TST (1)	Mean TST; PTIB = mean TST (1)	Mean TST +30 min (1)	Mean TST; PTIB = Mean TST
PTIB minimum	What is the minimum allowable PTIB ?	5 h	4.5 h (2)	Not specified (2)	5 h
Initial Rx for PTIB	How is the sleep schedule set ? (1)	PTIB from earliest TOB (2)	PTIB from earliest TOB	PTIB from earliest TOB	PTIB from earliest TOB
Point of titration	What time point is used for SSE ? (2)	TTB or TOB	TTB (titrate back toward baseline)	Not specified	TTB or TOB (3)
Number of sessions	How many sessions are recommended ?	6–10 sessions	8 sessions	4 sessions (3)	6 sessions
Cycle length	How many days are required between RXs ?	7 days	7 days	Not specified (4)	7–14 days
Titration rule	What is the threshold for change in PTIB ?	> 90% (increase)	< 85 (decrease) 85–90 (stick) > 90 (increase) (3)	< 80 (decrease) 80–85 (stick) > 85 (increase) (5)	< 80 (decrease) 80–85 (stick) > 85 (increase) (4)
Titration increment	How much time is added/substracted from PTIB ?	15 min	15 min	15 min	15 or 30 (5)

TIB, time in bed; *PTIB*, prescribed time in bed; *SSE*, systematic sleep extension; *TST*, total sleep time; *TTB*, time in bed; *TOB*, time out of bed

	(1) Given PTIB, the procedure for setting the sleep schedule or sleep window? For example, if PTIB is 6 hours and the desired TOB is 7am, then TTB = 1am.	(1) 10 day sample of 14 is allowed. This may be to accommodate extreme values. For example, the first 4 days after d/c medication.	(1) It is curently reccomended that TST-C be used in liu of TST where TST-C = (TIB + [SL+WASO+EMA])	(1) The rationale for this accomodation is that +30 accounts for normal duration SL, WASO, and/or EMA and for subjective overestimates in these parameters	(1) Six biweekly sessions are reccomended. But less or more sessions are allowed based on patint needs
	(2) Systematic sleep extension (sleep period or sleep window expansion or time in bed expansion). This rule pertains to where time is added or subtracted during titration (e.g., TTB or TOB)	(2) The selection of TOB is generally based on patient preference, but is biased toward whatever time is earlest.	(2) 4.5 h is based on the orginal Speilman formulation. Less experienced clinicians should not go below 5 h	(2) (Personal Communication). PTIB is generally not set to less than 6 h	(2) 14 days is reccomended with the caveat that more may be needed with patients with highly variable sleep schedules
			(3) Using a lower threshold (e.g., 85% [increase]) may allow for more opportunities for increased TST and exposure opportunities for setbacks.	(3) Two sessions are clearly delineated but there appears to be an allowence for more sessions as needed.	(3) Rounded to the nearest quarter hour
				(4) (Personal Communication). The initial Rx is fixed for 1 month.	(4) This element is not specified in the text (delination of the procedures) but examples are given for both TTB and TOB
				(5) (Personal Communication). Generally acccomplished using SE% (< 85 (decrease) 85–90 (stick) > 90 (increase)). But this may vary by patient.	(5) 30 min is allowed based on elevated ESS scores.

intervals; (3) lower SE% criteria; and/or (4) greater than 15 min increases when conducting upward titration (e.g., see Table 1). Finally, please bear in mind that the above-described procedures are only half of what it takes to deliver SRT. The other half pertains to how the prescription is delivered (i.e., how it is explained to the patient to garner their buy-in). The metaphors, examples, exercises, and dialogs are what make the delivery vehicle as important as the prescription itself. For examples of therapist "deliveries," the reader is referred to the various treatment manuals (Edinger & Carney, 2014; Manber & Carney, 2015; Morin & Espie, 2007; Perlis et al., 2006).

Stimulus control therapy (SCT)

Stimulus Control procedures, while a standard behavioral method, were first applied to the problem of insomnia by Richard Bootzin in 1972 (Bootzin, 1972). The goal of the treatment is to reverse the patient's tendency to stay in bed and "rest" and/or to engage in nonsleep behaviors in the bedroom or during the sleep period. Such practices are thought to lead to stimulus dyscontrol (the reduced probability that sleep will occur when and where the patient wants). Put differently, SCT is based on learning principles and the idea that one stimulus may elicit a variety of responses depending on the conditioning history. In good sleepers, the environmental stimuli typically associated with sleep (e.g., bed, bedroom, etc.) are paired with the response of sleep. In patients with insomnia, sleep-related stimuli become paired with activities other than sleep, such as reading, watching television, and most importantly, lying awake in bed. Engaging in these other behaviors while in bed contributes to maladaptive conditioning and further strengthens the association between one's bed and *wakefulness*. In other words, the bed and the bedroom become cues for wakefulness and frustration (which likely exacerbates sleep onset and maintenance problems). Accordingly, the treatment is to limit the time spent awake and the activities engaged in when the individual is awake at night. This is done by following a simple set of rules (as below).

1. Lie down intending to go to sleep only when you are *sleepy*.
2. Do not read or watch television in the bedroom.
3. If you find yourself unable to fall asleep, get up and go into another room. Stay up *as long as you wish* and then return to the bedroom to sleep.
4. If you still cannot fall asleep, repeat Step 3. Do this as often as is necessary throughout the night. The above rules were to form the basis for the development of permanent sleeping habits. Thus, the same rules were to be observed even after success was achieved.

Please note the above rules are the original version of Stimulus Control instructions. As with SRT, these rules have been modified over time. The rationale for such modifications, while not based on evidentiary criteria, have been altered based on logistical and/or theoretical considerations. Logistically speaking, Rule 1, in the context of CBT-I (vs. SCT as a monotherapy) is no longer relevant because *Time to Bed* (TTB) is a prescribed element of SRT. Theoretically speaking, the admonishments to (1) adopt a 15-min rule for when to implement SCT and (2) self-monitor for "sleepiness" as a que for when to return to bed may be less than optimal approaches. The former may prompt "clock-watching," and this may be anxiogenic. The latter may fuel sleep effort and cause the patient to "under dose" SCT. Finally, it has been suggested that SCT, while unquestionably efficacious, may work via mechanisms not related to, but compatible with, correcting stimulus dyscontrol. One alternative explanation is that SCT prevents microsleeping (sleep episodes that are not perceived as sleep but when they occur diminish sleep pressure) and enforces full wakefulness at a time of day where this may result in "twice the prime" for subsequent sleep (Klerman et al., 2019). These perspectives have led some to formulate versions of SCT that do not counsel the patient to engage in sedentary/nonactivating activities while practicing SCT.

Finally, while it is clear that the mechanism of action for, and the delivery of, SCT is more nuanced than one might expect, it remains the case that sharing the rules with the patient is only half of what constitutes good treatment. The other half pertains to how the prescription is delivered (i.e., what problem is addressed by SCT, how this applies to the specific patient, how it is to be implemented, what problems the patient is likely to encounter, etc.). As above, the metaphors, examples, exercises, and dialogs are what make the delivery vehicle as important as the prescription itself (i.e., the pill capsule is as important as the medication it contains). For examples of therapist "deliveries," the reader is referred to the various treatment manuals (Edinger & Carney, 2014; Manber & Carney, 2015; Morin & Espie, 2007; Perlis et al., 2006).

Cognitive therapy (CT)

Cognitive therapy for insomnia includes at least three specific exercise-based procedures, including the disputation of dysfunctional beliefs, decatastrophization, and "behavioral experiments" (Perlis, Aloia, & Kuhn, 2010). These are briefly described below.

Disputing dysfunctional beliefs is a psychoeducational procedure where faulty beliefs are identified and addressed. For example, "everyone needs 8h of sleep and if one fails to achieve this, their next day function will be significantly compromised." Using this form of CT, one would share what is known empirically to make the points that "how much sleep one needs and how one functions given that they don't meet their sleep need" varies dramatically from person-to-person (e.g., the normative range for sleep duration ranges from 7 to 9 h and there are many people who suffer no next-day effects with 5–6 h of sleep).

Decatastrophization is a dyadic exercise for dealing with the projected extreme consequences of dysfunctional beliefs. For example, "if I don't sleep 8 h tonight, I will [*suffer some terrible thing*] tomorrow." The exercise requires that the therapist and the patient (1) review how long the patient has had insomnia (and tabulate how many affected days); (2) identify the catastrophic thoughts that come to mind for the patient when they are sleepless (e.g., I will wreck my car, lose my job, strike someone in anger, have a heart attack, etc.); (3) assign a value to how certain they are that such an outcome will occur when they are sleepless and "think the thought"; (4) determine the actual frequency of occurrence of the anticipated "catastrophes"; and (5) calculate the frequency rate that corresponds to the certainty estimate. These data are used to show the patient that there is a huge mismatch between the patient's level of certainty regarding negative outcomes and their actual occurrence. This ultimately allows for a discussion of how it is that one is prone to such overestimates and what to do when such intrusive thoughts come to mind.

Behavioral Experiments are conducted to gather the data needed to challenge dysfunctional beliefs and/or catastrophic thoughts. Thus, the method may be behavioral, but the intent is cognitively focused (address anxiogenic sleep preventing thoughts). For example, if the patient believes and/or has the recurrent thought "when I don't sleep, I look dreadful, and the change in my appearance will be obvious to everyone." One possible behavioral experiment is to gather daily photographs (standardizing the time of day and conditions for the photograph). The photographs (which should be day and time-stamped) then can be reviewed at the next session where the therapist asks the patient to identify which picture was taken following their worst nights' sleep. Typically, most people cannot choose a specific photo (because they all look similar) or they choose a photo that does not correspond to the morning following their worst sleep (Harvey & Talbot, 2010; Harvey, Tang, & Browning, 2005).

Sleep hygiene (SH)

The earliest mention of sleep hygiene was by Nathaniel Kleitman in 1939, where he presented and reviewed the evidence regarding sleep satiety, body position, bedtime rituals, sleep surface, and ambient temperature (Kleitman, 1939). His work, however, does not resemble the "Do's and Don'ts" of contemporary SH instructions. In fact, it was not until

1977 that Peter Hauri formally codified this intervention (Hauri, 1977). Hauri expanded on the ideas of Kleitman by suggesting that SH should include information on lifestyle behaviors, relaxation, and environmental factors. The Hauri formulation was intended to offer rules to follow that would ameliorate sleep initiation and maintenance problems.

SH usually includes a one-page handout that outlines various methods to decrease the risk of having "a bad night's sleep" (e.g., limit caffeine and alcohol use, napping, and exercise before bed, etc.). SH is thought to be most useful when it is explained in full, where the patient's understanding is reflected to the therapist and a specific and agreed-upon plan is put into place. Ideally, within the context of CBT-I, SH should focus solely on sleep hygiene issues as opposed to adopting proxy rules for SRT and SCT. The following 10 rules (imperatives and rationales) are offered as optimal (see Table 2).

Please note, it is generally held that sleep hygiene is not effective as monotherapy. This common belief may be a bit of overgeneralization from the existing facts that are more consistent with the 2006 AASM Standards of Practice Committee's conclusion that there is "insufficient evidence to recommend sleep hygiene as a single therapy" (p. 221) (Morin, Culbert, & Schwartz, 1994). In sum, the most reasonable conclusion about sleep hygiene is this: it is a useful addition to CBT-I in that engaging in improved sleep hygiene may enhance outcomes or at least remove obstacles to progress.

Efficacy and effectiveness of CBT-I

There is an overwhelming preponderance of the evidence that in-person CBT-I is effective (Irwin, Cole, & Nicassio, 2006; Koffel, Koffel, & Gehrman, 2015; Miller et al., 2014; Montgomery & Dennis, 2003; Murtagh & Greenwood, 1995; Okajima, Komada, & Inoue, 2011; Pallesen, Nordhus, & Kvale, 1998; Perlis et al., 2006; van Straten et al., 2018), as effective as sedative-hypnotics during acute treatment (4–8 weeks), and is more effective than sedative-hypnotics in the long term (e.g., 3+ months following treatment) (Rios et al., 2019; Smith et al., 2002). This overall profile, along with CBT-I's low propensity for side effects or harm, is likely what prompted the American College of Physicians to recommend that CBT-I be considered the first-line treatment for chronic insomnia (Qaseem, Kansagara, Forciea, Cooke, & Denberg, 2016).

Pre-to-Post Treatment Change (Overall). In terms of symptom reduction (pre-post treatment change), subjective sleep latency (SL) and wake after sleep onset (WASO) times are reduced from baseline averages of about 60 min to 35 minutes at treatment end. These absolute changes corresponded to average treatment effects of about 50% reductions in symptom

TABLE 2 Sleep hygiene.

1. Exercise in the early evening.
Rationale: There is evidence to suggest that exercise in the early evening allows one to fall asleep more quickly, stay asleep for longer and to sleep more deeply.
2. Do not take naps during the day.
Rationale: Napping during the day decreases one's overall "pressure" to sleep at bedtime, and therefore, the overall chance that one will fall and/or stay asleep [at bedtime]. There are caveats for "safety naps" and those with medical illness (e.g., cancer), and in those situations, the patient should be instructed to nap in bed, with an alarm, and for a maximum of 30 min
3. Eat a light snack before bedtime.
Rationale: Eating a light carbohydrate snack one hour before bedtime (e.g., crackers or fruit) may help improve sleep quality.
4. Avoid liquids before bedtime.
Rationale: Increased liquids before bedtime may increase the chance that one has to wake-up to use the restroom.
5. Avoid caffeinated products ~6 h before bedtime.
Rationale: Although stimulants, like caffeine, don't have to be entirely discouraged and may even improve the chances that one functions better during the day, caffeine's biological half-life is on average about 6 h and therefore consuming caffeine within 6 h of bedtime may increase sleep latency and/or wake after sleep onset problems.
6. Avoid nicotine.
Rationale: Like caffeine, nicotine's stimulant properties may impede sleep continuity.
7. Use ear plugs and/or white noise to mitigate outside noise.
Rationale: Outside noise can be disruptive to sleep, using earplugs may improve the chances that one falls and/or stays asleep.
8. Avoid co-sleeping with pets.
Rationale: Co-sleeping can be disruptive to sleep, thus removing pets from the bed at night may be helpful in the long term.
9. Make sure the sleep environment is conducive to sleep (e.g., bedding, temperature, light).
Rationale: A comfortable bed, temperature and minimal light has been shown to be important for adequate sleep. Thus, assessing these items with the patient will be helpful to better understand whether these factors may be contributing to their sleep problems.
10. Keep a regular sleep schedule (e.g., set an alarm).
Rationale: Keeping a regular sleep schedule decreases the chance for sleep extension and increases the chance for a match between sleep ability and opportunity, which is a core component of CBT-I.

severity and pre-to-post effect sizes of about 1.0 (Murtagh & Greenwood, 1995; Smith et al., 2002). Please note, Early Morning Awakenings (EMA) are generally collapsed into WASO measures, and therefore, little is known about the effects of CBT-I on EMA. In the context of acute treatment, total sleep time (TST) is minimally affected during 6–8 session CBT-I with only about 45% of patients exceeding baseline TST at treatment end (Perlis et al., 2019). Such outcomes generally correspond to mean changes of <30 min and <10% pre-post change with within-subject effect sizes of < 0.5. When assessed in terms of pre-post insomnia severity (e.g., the Insomnia Severity Index (Bastien, Vallières, & Morin, 2001)), the within-subject and between-subject effect sizes are reliably larger than single measures of sleep continuity effects, with within-subject effects sizes of around 2.0 (Smith et al., 2002). This is not surprising as the ISI not only assesses illness severity (magnitude of sleep continuity disturbance) but also the degree of insomnia-related daytime impairment/complaint. When evaluated in terms of the percent of patients who exhibit treatment responses (variably defined), between 70 and 80% of patients achieve a therapeutic response during acute treatment (Beaulieu-Bonneau, Ivers, Guay, & Morin, 2017; Morin & Benca, 2012; Morin, Colecchi, Stone, Sood, & Brink, 1999).

Durability of CBT-I Effects Over Time. In what are perhaps the first long-term RCTs of CBT-I, it was found that SL and WASO effects are remarkably stable over time periods of up to 24 months (Beaulieu-Bonneau et al., 2017; Morin et al., 1999; Morin et al., 2009; Morin & Benca, 2012). This is to say that clinical gains are maintained for months and years *after treatment is discontinued*. Interestingly, TST effects (which are initially marginal) appear to accrue with time. That is, when followed longitudinally, patients exhibit an average increase in TST of about 50 min. These gains do not appear to be related to additional improvements in SL and WASO, but instead are likely to be related to increased time in bed while maintaining good sleep efficiency. When evaluated in terms of percent of patients who exhibit remission, 50%–60% of treatment responders achieve remission in the 6–12 months that follow therapy. Similar findings were recently presented for a large-scale clinical case series study (Castronovo et al., 2018). In this study, mean ISI values from end-of-treatment (T1) to follow-up (T2 [4–10 years]) were found to be remarkably stable (baseline ISI 17.1 ± 4.5, $T_1 = 9.7 \pm 4.6$, and $T_2 = 9.9 \pm 6.3$). In contrast to these studies, a recent meta-analysis on the durability of CBT-I showed that CBT-I continues to be effective at 3, 6, and 12 months as compared to nonactive controls, but that the clinical gains in the active treatment group appeared to decline over time (van der Zweerde, Bisdounis, Kyle, Lancee, & van Straten, 2019). While these differences in claims remain to be reconciled, it may be the case that the meta-analytic findings differ owing to between-study differences in the application of CBT-I. If protocol differences yield different long-term outcomes, and the individual studies summarized here used the most robust methodologies, then the durability outcomes in the meta-analysis may represent the inclusion of studies with small magnitude outcomes and/or greater variability in the effect size estimates. Given the absence of end of treatment effect sizes in the meta-analysis, one cannot be sure if such data were comparable to the single studies summarized here or other meta-analytic studies regarding the acute effects of CBT-I.

1. Traditional CBT-I components and delivery

The Efficacy of "Real World" CBT-I (RCTs vs. Clinical Case Series Studies). The conclusions that can be drawn from RCTs are often subject to some skepticism as the most that can be said is that RCT outcomes represent the best-case scenario. This perspective is rooted in the reasonable belief that RCTs are populated by exceptionally healthy patients (individuals that have the illness of interest but little else in the way of comorbidity) while in-clinic patients often have complex medical, psychiatric, and psychosocial profiles and therefore may be (understandably) less responsive to targeted treatments. In perhaps the first evaluation of this idea, clinical case series data were obtained on 47 subjects (Perlis et al., 2000). In this analysis, it was found that, on average, subjects who completed at least a minimum dose of CBT-I ($\geq$4 sessions) experienced about a 23-min decrease in SL ($d=1.00$), a 39-min decrease in WASO ($d=1.09$), and a 20-min increase in TST ($d=0.36$) (Perlis, Sharpe, Smith, Greenblatt, & Giles, 2001). Note, while it stands to reason that the sum of SL+WASO (i.e., total wake time or TWT) decreases should equal TST gains, this is often not true, and for two reasons. First, with sleep restriction, the change in TIB limits potential gains in TST. Second, patients rarely calculate TST but instead provide their impression of how much sleep was obtained. That is, given TIB and SL, WASO, and EMA, it is possible to estimate TST in a manner that is not a "guesstimate", but instead may be arithmetically calculated, and in a manner that is internally valid (i.e., TST = TIB − [SL+WASO+EMA]). Given these two considerations, it is rarely the case that the decrease in TWT equals the increase in TST. With this caveat in mind, these data are clearly comparable to the "meta-analytic norms", if not significantly better. In sum, it may indeed be the case that "real world" patients benefit from CBT-I to the same extent as subjects in clinical trials, perhaps more. This surprising result may be ascribable to a variety of factors including better outcomes due to professional therapists, the tailoring of the clinical treatment regimen to the individual case, and/or a variety of other nonspecific factors such as cognitive dissonance (e.g., paying for treatment vs. no payment or being paid to be treated).

Efficacy of CBT-I in "Secondary Insomnia" (Comorbid Insomnia). By and large, the effects summarized above are from foundational RCTs that were undertaken from 1990 until the early 2000s. The overwhelming majority of these trials were conducted in subjects with "Primary Insomnia" (i.e., individuals without comorbid illness that includes insomnia as a symptom). This was the case because insomnia was construed as both a symptom and a disorder, and it was believed that so-called secondary insomnia could only be effectively treated with therapies for the primary disorder (Zorick & Walsh, 2000). For example, insomnia occurring in the context of chronic pain would only be ameliorated to the extent that the analgesic therapy was successful. Implicit in this perspective was that direct treatment of "secondary insomnia" with CBT-I (i.e., by targeting behavioral factors) would yield little to no positive effects, as pain (not sleep extension) was considered to be the perpetuating factor for that form of chronic insomnia. In the last two decades, literally dozens of CBT-I RCTs have been conducted in patients with "secondary insomnia" (including but not limited to patients with depression (Carney et al., 2017; Cunningham & Shapiro, 2018), bipolar disorder (Harvey et al., 2015), PTSD (Simon et al., 2019), generalized anxiety disorder (Ye et al., 2015), schizophrenia (Hwang, Nam, & Lee, 2019), cancer (Ma et al., 2020), heart failure (Redeker et al., 2018), chronic pain (McCrae et al., 2019), Alzheimer's disease (Siengsukon et al., 2020), multiple sclerosis (Siengsukon, Alshehri, Williams, Drerup, & Lynch, 2020), alcoholism (Chakravorty et al., 2019), chronic obstructive pulmonary disease (Kapella et al., 2011), obstructive sleep apnea (Ong et al., 2020), period limb movement disorder (Edinger et al., 1996), etc. To our knowledge, all of these studies found that CBT-I was effective. Most studies found that the treatment outcomes were similar to those observed in patients with primary insomnia, and several studies found superior treatment outcomes (Carney et al., 2017; Chakravorty et al., 2019; Cunningham & Shapiro, 2018; Edinger et al., 1996; Harvey et al., 2015; Hwang et al., 2019; Kapella et al., 2011; Ma et al., 2020; McCrae et al., 2019; Ong et al., 2020; Redeker et al., 2018; Siengsukon, Alshehri, et al., 2020; Siengsukon, Nelson, et al., 2020; Simon et al., 2019; Ye et al., 2015). At least one clinical case series study (Perlis et al., 2000) was conducted on this topic and there have been several meta-analyses. Geiger-Brown and colleagues (Geiger-Brown et al., 2015) summarized 37 studies (1379 subjects), where SL decreased by 26 min ($d=0.85$), WASO decreased by 36 min ($d=0.92$), and TST increased by 29 min ($d=0.43$). Moreover, there was a 13-point improvement in SE ($d=1.20$) and about a 10-point decrease in ISI ($d=2.1$). These treatment effects were found to be durable for up to 18 months post-treatment. Not only do these data demonstrate the efficacy of CBT-I with insomnia in the context of other comorbidities, but there is now an accumulating evidence base to show that treating insomnia with CBT-I has a beneficial "halo" effect on other medical and behavioral health disorders. For example, CBT-I as an augmenting strategy to the medical management of depression has been found to double antidepressant treatment response and to reduce suicidality by half (Manber et al., 2008; Trockel, Karlin, Taylor, Brown, & Manber, 2015). A similar set of outcomes were found for iCBT-I as compared to iCBT-D (Blom, Jernelöv, Rück, Lindefors, & Kaldo, 2017), where only insomnia treatment produced positive insomnia outcomes, but both forms of iCBT produced positive depression outcomes. Despite secondary insomnia data showing changes in sleep continuity that are comparable to those found in primary insomnia, the effect sizes tend to be smaller. The reason for this may be, as mentioned above, that the meta-analyses contain studies that are not "best in class" (studies conducted by established experts with best methods and/or professional therapists). This issue aside, it may be that there are fewer treatment responders but the response itself is of equal magnitude to those found in primary insomnia. This may speak to issues of adherence in patients with other comorbidities (e.g., those diagnosed with cancer may focus on cancer and not insomnia as the primary issue). In other words, it may be harder to garner adherence day-to-day and week-to-week in patients who have other significant areas of concern. This may, in turn, account for lower treatment responder rates. Note: These data support the notion that standard CBT-I should be adapted in order to enhance treatment responder rates in specific clinical populations. Which populations require this and what adaptations should be made remains to be empirically determined.

Common alternative rules & therapies

Common alternative rules

Sleep Restriction. In a recent and seminal work by Kyle and colleagues (Kyle et al., 2015), it was shown (in the context of RCTs) that SRT is rarely delineated component-by-component in the methods sections of such investigations; and when details are provided they often vary from study to study.

Stimulus Control. There are a variety of ways that SCT has been modified, relative to its core components. In the absence of a formal study of its variants, a cursory review of the rules as they are presented in three treatment manuals suggests that the application of SCT is also highly variable.

In Tables 1 and 3, the rules for SRT and SCT are listed from the four published treatment manuals. It is interesting to note for SRT, there is no particular rule for which there is unanimous agreement.

Alternative variants or adjuvants to SRT and SCT

Counter-Control. This particular variant of SCT was originally developed as a comparator condition for the empirical evaluation of the mechanism of action for stimulus control. More specifically, it was developed to be a "counter control"; the exact opposite of SCT instructions. If the central element of SCT is to be awake somewhere other than the bed and bedroom, the counter condition is to intentionally be awake in the bed and bedroom (both during the sleep period and for 30 min a day when not intending to sleep). In what is now a classic study by Zwart and Lisman (1979b), it was shown that SCT did not significantly differ from the counter control condition (i.e., both conditions worked about equally well to ameliorate sleep onset problems) (Zwart & Lisman, 1979b). Given

TABLE 3 Stimulus control therapy (SCT) rules based on the first four published treatment manuals.

	Manual			
Issue	**Morin and Espie (2007)**	**Perlis et al. (2006)**	**Edinger and Carney (2014)**	**Manber and Carney (2015)**
When to get out of bed?	After 15 min of wakefulness (1)	After 15 min of wakefulness (1)	After 20 min of wakefulness	When feeling alert (1)
Where to go?	Out of bedroom	Out of the bedroom	Out of the bedroom	Out of bed
What to do when out of bed?	Not specified (2)	Anything enjoyable (2)	Not specified (1)	Things that are not activating (2)
When to return to bed?	When sleepy	When sleepy (3)	When sleepy	When sleepy
	(1) The 15 min rule is to be applied to both SL and WASO. In regards to WASO, the manual suggests that patient's go back to bed "when sleepy again" but to wait no longer than 15 min to try to go back to sleep. (2) While no rule of thumb or potential lists are given, it is clear from the dialogs that a plan should be enacted with each patient.	(1) The 15 min rule is acknoweldged as the standard but it is reccomended that, in an effort to prevent "clock watching" behavior, patients should leave the bedroom as soon as they feel "clearly awake" or are annoyed at being awake. (2) A later development to this protocol was the stipulation that the behavior must be something that can be done during the day (i.e., not a prohibited behavior) or a behavior that reinforces wakefulness. (3) A later development to this protocol was a modifcation to this instruction to have the patient simply pick a time frame to be awake (30, 60, or 120 min) and then to return to bed, sleepy or not.		(1) In order to discourage clock watching, it is recommended that patients use their own sensation of alertness, to determine when they should get out of bed or go back to the bedroom. (2) In addition to the list of activites provided in the manual, it is recommended that the therapist and the patient work to collaboratively make a list of things to do when out of the bedroom.

these findings, Davies and colleagues evaluated counter control as a therapeutic intervention for individuals with sleep maintenance problems, with an end goal of producing a more practical therapy for older adults (Davies, Lacks, Storandt, & Bertelson, 1986). While they did not find a "by age" effect for efficacy, counter control was again found to be effective, producing about a 30% improvement at the end of treatment, with gradual improvement continuing through a 4-week follow-up period.

Many understood these results to be a substantial challenge to the belief that SCT works via instrumental conditioning or by increasing the associational strength between sleep-related stimuli and sleep. While still a controversial issue, the manipulation may be successful owing to the instruction to "sit up and do something (other than trying to sleep)". This instruction still encourages a separation between sleep stimuli and sleep based on body position and the prescription has within it a component that derails sleep effort. In the final analysis, and irrespective of whether SCT works based on good stimulus control, the success of counter control instructions has prompted clinicians to adopt this strategy in patients that (1) cannot, or cannot safely, get up and out of bed at night or (2) live in dwellings, or under circumstances, that do not allow them to leave the bedroom and to be awake elsewhere.

Sleep Compression. Perhaps one of the first and most innovative adaptations to CBT-I came with the proposal to substitute sleep compression for sleep restriction. While the alternative therapy was explicitly proffered for patients with sleep continuity disturbance *without daytime sequelae* (i.e., short sleep patients with normal to high sleep opportunity and low sleep need and ability), it has become common (at least in clinical practice) to use this procedure for patients that are resistant to (and/or nonadherent with) sleep restriction. The method is comparable to sleep restriction in that sleep opportunity is matched to sleep ability (i.e., step 1 of therapy is to match average TIB to average TST). Unlike sleep restriction, where the "reset" is accomplished on night one, during sleep compression the reset is achieved over a series of weeks. In the original formulation of this treatment, therapy was discontinued when one reached the target SE%. There was no need for systematic sleep extension because it was assumed that the participant had achieved their true sleep need. In more recent iterations, as applied to patients with insomnia disorder, sleep extension remains a component of this treatment regimen. Lichstein and colleagues first demonstration of this method was in a sample of 74 older adults (59 years or older) (Lichstein, Riedel, Wilson, Lester, & Aguillard, 2001). Subjects were randomized into three groups, relaxation ($n=27$), sleep compression ($n=24$), or placebo desensitization ($n=23$). The sleep compression condition fared better than placebo, where SL decreased by about 12 min ($d=0.48$), WASO by about 24 min ($d=0.75$), SE increased by about 8 points ($d=0.55$), and TST decreased by about 14 min ($d=0.20$). This study provides preliminary evidence that sleep compression is effective for short sleepers who have low levels of daytime impairment.

Mindfulness. It can be argued that the single most influential change to CBT-I in the last two decades has been the adoption of mindfulness training. Mindfulness was first introduced, in the context of insomnia, by Ong, Shapiro, and Manber (2008). The stated goal for the adjuvant therapy was to better address sleep-related cognitive arousal. The approach, however, substantially differs from traditional cognitive therapy in that it is not focused on disputing, derailing, or disengaging worry or intrusive negative thoughts. Instead, mindfulness is focused on the nonjudgmental observation of one's cognitions, with the desired goal of changing one's relationship to their thoughts as opposed to fighting with them. In this way, the process encourages "acceptance." Ong et al. (2008) conducted a treatment-development study (using a simple pre-post design) to evaluate the effectiveness of mindfulness meditation as an adjuvant to six-session in-person CBT-I ($n=30$). Significant pre-post-treatment reductions were found in the study's primary outcome variable, total wake time (TWT [SL+WASO+EMA]). The corresponding pre-post effect size for this variable was -1.17. Significant reductions were also found in secondary analyses of the single component measures, including an 18-min decrease in SL ($d=-0.84$), 25-min decrease in WASO ($d=-0.62$), and a 5-min decrease in TST ($d=-0.11$). Improvements were also found in SE and the ISI, where SE improved by approximately 9 points ($d=-1.1$) and the ISI decreased by 5 points ($d=-1.32$). A follow-up study showed that these sleep-related benefits were maintained over a 12-months post-treatment (Ong, Shapiro, & Manber, 2009).

Dual Therapy with Medication. There have been a variety of RCTs that evaluate how treatment outcomes vary when sedatives (e.g., temazepam or zolpidem) are prescribed in conjunction with CBT-I (Beaulieu-Bonneau et al., 2017; Morin, 2006; Morin et al., 2009; Morin et al., 2014). Combined treatment and monotherapy with CBT-I have been found to produce equivalent gains in the short term (during acute treatment), that is, similar gains with respect to sleep initiation and maintenance (diary measures of SL, WASO, and TST), similar gains on multifactorial measures of insomnia severity (ISI), and similar percentages with respect to the subjects that achieve treatment responses. In contrast, there is some evidence that long-term durability of CBT-I may be attenuated in patients cotreated with hypnotics and/or they tend not to exhibit the increases in total sleep time that occur with CBT-I following treatment discontinuation (Perlis et al., 2001). Given this profile, one might wonder under what circumstances combined treatment might ever be indicated? The possibilities include: (1) when the time to a treatment response needs to be accelerated (Morin et al., 2014) and/or (2) when the short-term iatrogenic effects of CBT-I need to be blocked or attenuated (Perlis & Smith, 2008). Some have argued that one or both of these considerations can be better managed with the short-term use of stimulants (e.g., modafinil qam or bid along with CBT-I [1st four sessions of SRT]) (Cheung, Bartlett, Armour, Laba, & Saini, 2018; Perlis et al., 2004). While there is some data to suggest that this strategy blocks iatrogenic sleepiness[77], there is no evidence that cotreatment with stimulants speeds the latency to treatment response or maintains the long-term benefits of monotherapy with CBT-I. Clinically, both strategies seem to be reasonable alternative approaches for the management of insomnia, when indicated.

Conclusion

In the absence of data regarding which clinical populations or demographic groups *require modified CBT-I*, it seems premature to recommend that standard CBT-I be altered. In an ideal world, this issue would be addressed systematically.

> First, demonstrate a need (i.e., standard CBT-I is not as effective for whom), conduct research into likely causes (factors associated with reduced efficacy or treatment nonresponse), and then develop and test adapted versions of CBT-I that address the factors for whether or not they produce superior outcomes as compared to standard CBT-I.

Given that such work is not fundable in the present climate, perhaps the next best approach is to develop alternative rules and therapies that can be adopted by clinicians on an as-needed basis. In this case, clinicians could decide to adopt nonstandard therapy a priori by asking and answering the question "Is there anything about the comorbid conditions or life circumstances of a given patient that would interfere with, or be worsened by, the conduct of CBT-I?"(Smith & Perlis, 2006). While one should be conservative about the need to adapt standard CBT-I, "interference" may be managed by using alternative forms of CBT-I, forms that are more compatible with the patients' status. For example, if the patient is immobile or has limited mobility, one may opt to go forward with treatment but to use "counter control" instructions (Davies et al., 1986; Zwart & Lisman, 1979b) rather than usual stimulus control instructions. "Worsening" (CBT-I may aggravate one or more of the comorbid conditions) is a more serious consideration, but perhaps less so than many think. On the one hand, there is the legitimate concern that (for example) sleep deprivation may trigger certain conditions such as parasomnias, manic episodes, and/or seizures in patients predisposed to, or diagnosed with, such problems. The counterpoint to this is that (1) sleep restriction is not sleep deprivation, and it is the latter that is the known risk factor for such adverse events (note: sleep restriction usually entails between 1 and 2 hours' sleep loss while sleep deprivation entails between 4 and 8h sleep loss); (2) if the comorbid disorder is stable owing to ongoing treatment, it is not a given that even sleep deprivation can trigger adverse events in such cases; and (3) CBT-I is a short duration intervention (usually 4–8 weeks), and thus, the window of vulnerability is narrow. If the risks of potential sleep loss in CBT-I are of concern, one may opt to not conduct CBT-I, to conduct CBT-I without the sleep restriction component, or to use sleep compression. Ultimately, the following chapters in this book can serve as a menu for the options that might be engaged, if the clinician is certain that standard CBT-I needs to be adopted for a given patient. The trick, or the art of assessment, will be to know when such adaptations are necessary versus when such adaptations are unwarranted or premature and may only serve to delay or attenuate therapeutic gains.

References

Bastien, C. H., Morin, C. M., Ouellet, M. C., Blais, F. C., & Bouchard, S. (2004). Cognitive-behavioral therapy for insomnia: Comparison of individual therapy, group therapy, and telephone consultations. *Journal of Consulting and Clinical Psychology, 72*(4), 653.

Bastien, C. H., Vallières, A., & Morin, C. M. (2001). Validation of the Insomnia Severity Index as an outcome measure for insomnia research. *Sleep Medicine, 2*(4), 297–307.

Beaulieu-Bonneau, S., Ivers, H., Guay, B., & Morin, C. M. (2017). Long-term maintenance of therapeutic gains associated with cognitive-behavioral therapy for insomnia delivered alone or combined with zolpidem. *Sleep, 40*(3).

Blom, K., Jernelöv, S., Rück, C., Lindefors, N., & Kaldo, V. (2017). Three-year follow-up comparing cognitive behavioral therapy for depression to cognitive behavioral therapy for insomnia, for patients with both diagnoses. *Sleep, 40*(8).

Bootzin, R. R. (1972). Stimulus control treatment for insomnia. *Proceedings of the American/Psychological Association, 7*, 395–396.

Bootzin, R. R., & Perlis, M. L. (2011). Stimulus control therapy. In *Behavioral treatments for sleep disorders* (pp. 21–30). Academic Press.

Carney, C. E., Edinger, J. D., Kuchibhatla, M., Lachowski, A. M., Bogouslavsky, O., Krystal, A. D., et al. (2017). Cognitive behavioral insomnia therapy for those with insomnia and depression: A randomized controlled clinical trial. *Sleep, 40*(4), zsx019.

Castronovo, V., Galbiati, A., Sforza, M., Poletti, M., Giarolli, L., Kuo, T., et al. (2018). Long-term clinical effect of group cognitive behavioral therapy for insomnia: A case series study. *Sleep Medicine, 47*, 54–59.

Chakravorty, S., Morales, K. H., Arnedt, J. T., Perlis, M. L., Oslin, D. W., Findley, J. C., et al. (2019). Cognitive behavioral therapy for insomnia in alcohol-dependent veterans: A randomized, controlled pilot study. *Alcoholism: Clinical and Experimental Research, 43*(6), 1244–1253.

Cheung, J. M., Bartlett, D. J., Armour, C. L., Laba, T. L., & Saini, B. (2018). To drug or not to drug: A qualitative study of patients' decision-making processes for managing insomnia. *Behavioral Sleep Medicine, 16*(1), 1–26.

Cunningham, J. E., & Shapiro, C. M. (2018). Cognitive behavioural therapy for insomnia (CBT-I) to treat depression: A systematic review. *Journal of Psychosomatic Research, 106*, 1–12.

Davies, R., Lacks, P., Storandt, M., & Bertelson, A. D. (1986). Countercontrol treatment of sleep-maintenance insomnia in relation to age. *Psychology and Aging, 1*(3), 233.

Edinger, J. D., & Carney, C. E. (2014). *Overcoming insomnia: A cognitive-behavioral therapy approach, therapist guide*. Oxford University Press.

Edinger, J. D., Fins, A. I., Sullivan, R. J., Marsh, G. R., Dailey, D. S., & Young, M. (1996). Comparison of cognitive-behavioral therapy and clonazepam for treating periodic limb movement disorder. *Sleep, 19*(5), 442–444.

Epstein, D. R., Sidani, S., Bootzin, R. R., & Belyea, M. J. (2012). Dismantling multicomponent behavioral treatment for insomnia in older adults: A randomized controlled trial. *Sleep, 35*(6), 797–805.

Geiger-Brown, J. M., Rogers, V. E., Liu, W., Ludeman, E. M., Downton, K. D., & Diaz-Abad, M. (2015). Cognitive behavioral therapy in persons with comorbid insomnia: A meta-analysis. *Sleep Medicine Reviews, 23*, 54–67.

Harvey, A. G., & Talbot, L. (2010). Intervention to reduce misperception. In *Behavioral treatments for sleep disorders* (pp. 91–95). Amsterdam: Academic Press.

Harvey, A. G., Tang, N. K., & Browning, L. (2005). Cognitive approaches to insomnia. *Clinical Psychology Review, 25*(5).

Harvey, A. G., Bélanger, L., Talbot, L., Eidelman, P., Beaulieu-Bonneau, S., Fortier-Brochu, É., et al. (2014). Comparative efficacy of behavior therapy, cognitive therapy, and cognitive behavior therapy for chronic insomnia: A randomized controlled trial. *Journal of Consulting and Clinical Psychology, 82*(4), 670.

Harvey, A. G., Soehner, A. M., Kaplan, K. A., Hein, K., Lee, J., Kanady, J., et al. (2015). Treating insomnia improves mood state, sleep, and functioning in bipolar disorder: A pilot randomized controlled trial. *Journal of Consulting and Clinical Psychology, 83*(3), 564.

Hauri, P. (1977). *The sleep disorders*. Upjohn.

Hwang, D. K., Nam, M., & Lee, Y. J. G. (2019). The effect of cognitive behavioral therapy for insomnia in schizophrenia patients with sleep disturbance: A non-randomized, assessor-blind trial. *Psychiatry Research, 274*, 182–188.

Irwin, M. R., Cole, J. C., & Nicassio, P. M. (2006). Comparative meta-analysis of behavioral interventions for insomnia and their efficacy in middle-aged adults and in older adults 55+ years of age. *Health Psychology, 25*(1), 3.

Kapella, M. C., Herdegen, J. J., Perlis, M. L., Shaver, J. L., Larson, J. L., Law, J. A., et al. (2011). Cognitive behavioral therapy for insomnia comorbid with COPD is feasible with preliminary evidence of positive sleep and fatigue effects. *International Journal of Chronic Obstructive Pulmonary Disease, 6*, 625.

Kleitman, N. (1939). Sleep and wakefulness as alternating phases in the cycle of existence. *JAMA, 113*.

Klerman, E., St. Hilaire, M., Perlis, M., Hilditch, C., McHill, A., Rahman, S., et al. (2019). *Effect of time-of-day and prior wake on electroencephalographic Delta and Beta Power in 10-min naps during 30 continuous hours of 90-minute "days" EBRS 2019 poster P-53*.

Koffel, E. A., Koffel, J. B., & Gehrman, P. R. (2015). A meta-analysis of group cognitive behavioral therapy for insomnia. *Sleep Medicine Reviews, 19*, 6–16.

Kyle, S. D., Aquino, M. R. J., Miller, C. B., Henry, A. L., Crawford, M. R., Espie, C. A., et al. (2015). Towards standardisation and improved understanding of sleep restriction therapy for insomnia disorder: A systematic examination of CBT-I trial content. *Sleep Medicine Reviews, 23*, 83–88.

Lichstein, K. L., Riedel, B. W., Wilson, N. M., Lester, K. W., & Aguillard, R. N. (2001). Relaxation and sleep compression for late-life insomnia: A placebo-controlled trial. *Journal of Consulting and Clinical Psychology, 69*(2), 227.

Ma, Y., Hall, D. L., Ngo, L. H., Liu, Q., Bain, P. A., & Yeh, G. Y. (2020). Efficacy of cognitive behavioral therapy for insomnia in breast cancer: A meta-analysis. *Sleep Medicine Reviews, 101376*.

Manber, R., & Carney, C. E. (2015). *Treatment plans and interventions for insomnia: A case formulation approach*. Guilford Publications.

Manber, R., Edinger, J. D., Gress, J. L., Pedro-Salcedo, M. G. S., Kuo, T. F., & Kalista, T. (2008). Cognitive behavioral therapy for insomnia enhances depression outcome in patients with comorbid major depressive disorder and insomnia. *Sleep*, *31*(4), 489–495.

McCrae, C. S., Williams, J., Roditi, D., Anderson, R., Mundt, J. M., Miller, M. B., et al. (2019). Cognitive behavioral treatments for insomnia and pain in adults with comorbid chronic insomnia and fibromyalgia: Clinical outcomes from the SPIN randomized controlled trial. *Sleep*, *42*(3), zsy234.

Miller, C. B., Espie, C. A., Epstein, D. R., Friedman, L., Morin, C. M., Pigeon, W. R., et al. (2014). The evidence base of sleep restriction therapy for treating insomnia disorder. *Sleep Medicine Reviews*, *18*(5), 415–424.

Montgomery, P., & Dennis, J. A. (2003). Cognitive behavioral interventions for sleep problems in adults aged 60+. *Cochrane Database of Systematic Reviews, 1*.

Morin, C. M. (2006). Combined therapeutics for insomnia: Should our first approach be behavioral or pharmacological? *Sleep Medicine*, *7*, S15–S19.

Morin, C. M., Beaulieu-Bonneau, S., Ivers, H., Vallières, A., Guay, B., Savard, J., et al. (2014). Speed and trajectory of changes of insomnia symptoms during acute treatment with cognitive–behavioral therapy, singly and combined with medication. *Sleep Medicine*, *15*(6), 701–707.

Morin, C. M., & Benca, R. (2012). Chronic insomnia. *The Lancet*, *379*(9821), 1129–1141.

Morin, C. M., Colecchi, C., Stone, J., Sood, R., & Brink, D. (1999). Behavioral and pharmacological therapies for late-life insomnia: A randomized controlled trial. *JAMA*, *281*(11), 991–999.

Morin, C. M., Culbert, J. P., & Schwartz, S. M. (1994). Nonpharmacological interventions for insomnia: A meta-analysis of treatment efficacy. *The American Journal of Psychiatry*, *151*(8), 1172–1180.

Morin, C. M., & Espie, C. A. (2007). *Insomnia: A clinical guide to assessment and treatment*. Springer Science & Business Media.

Morin, C. M., Vallières, A., Guay, B., Ivers, H., Savard, J., Mérette, C., et al. (2009). Cognitive behavioral therapy, singly and combined with medication, for persistent insomnia: A randomized controlled trial. *JAMA*, *301*(19), 2005–2015.

Murtagh, D. R., & Greenwood, K. M. (1995). Identifying effective psychological treatments for insomnia: A meta-analysis. *Journal of Consulting and Clinical Psychology*, *63*(1), 79.3.

Okajima, I., Komada, Y., & Inoue, Y. (2011). A meta-analysis on the treatment effectiveness of cognitive behavioral therapy for primary insomnia. *Sleep and Biological Rhythms*, *9*(1), 24–34.

Ong, J. C., Crawford, M. R., Dawson, S. C., Fogg, L. F., Turner, A. D., Wyatt, J. K., et al. (2020). A randomized controlled trial of CBT-I and PAP for obstructive sleep apnea and comorbid insomnia: Main outcomes from the MATRICS study. *Sleep, 43*.

Ong, J. C., Shapiro, S. L., & Manber, R. (2008). Combining mindfulness meditation with cognitive-behavior therapy for insomnia: A treatment-development study. *Behavior Therapy*, *39*(2), 171–182.

Ong, J. C., Shapiro, S. L., & Manber, R. (2009). Mindfulness meditation and cognitive behavioral therapy for insomnia: A naturalistic 12-month follow-up. *Explorer*, *5*(1), 30–36.

Pallesen, S., Nordhus, I. H., & Kvale, G. (1998). Nonpharmacological interventions for insomnia in older adults: A meta-analysis of treatment efficacy. *Psychotherapy: Theory, Research, Practice, Training*, *35*(4), 472.

Perlis, M. L., Aloia, M., & Kuhn, B. (Eds.). (2010). Behavioral experiments. In *Behavioral treatments for sleep disorders: A comprehensive primer of behavioral sleep medicine interventions* Academic Press.

Perlis, M., Aloia, M., Millikan, A., Boehmler, J., Smith, M., Greenblatt, D., et al. (2000). Behavioral treatment of insomnia: A clinical case series study. *Journal of Behavioral Medicine*, *23*(2), 149–161.

Perlis, M. L., Jungquist, C., Smith, M. T., & Posner, D. (2006). *Cognitive behavioral treatment of insomnia: A session-by-session guide. Vol. 1*. Springer Science & Business Media.

Perlis, M. L., Morin, C. M., Ivers, H., Muench, A., Posner, D., & Grandner, M. (2019). 0380 Does TST appreciably change during or after CBT-I? *Sleep, 42*, A154–A155.

Perlis, M. L., Sharpe, M., Smith, M. T., Greenblatt, D., & Giles, D. (2001). Behavioral treatment of insomnia: Treatment outcome and the relevance of medical and psychiatric morbidity. *Journal of Behavioral Medicine, 24*(3), 281–296.

Perlis, M. L., & Smith, M. T. (2008). How can we make CBT-I and other BSM services widely available? *Journal of Clinical Sleep Medicine, 4*.

Perlis, M. L., Smith, M. T., Orff, H., Enright, T., Nowakowski, S., Jungquist, C., et al. (2004). The effects of modafinil and cognitive behavior therapy on sleep continuity in patients with primary insomnia. *Sleep, 27*(4), 715–725.

Qaseem, A., Kansagara, D., Forciea, M. A., Cooke, M., & Denberg, T. D. (2016). Management of chronic insomnia disorder in adults: A clinical practice guideline from the American College of Physicians. *Annals of Internal Medicine, 165*(2), 125–133.

Redeker, N. S., Conley, S., Anderson, G., Cline, J., Andrews, L., Mohsenin, V., et al. (2018). Effects of cognitive behavioral therapy for insomnia on sleep, symptoms, stress, and autonomic function among patients with heart failure. *Behavioral Sleep Medicine*, 1–13.

Rios, P., Cardoso, R., Morra, D., Nincic, V., Goodarzi, Z., Farah, B., et al. (2019). Comparative effectiveness and safety of pharmacological and non-pharmacological interventions for insomnia: An overview of reviews. *Systematic Reviews, 8*(1), 281.

Scott, H., Cheung, J., Muench, A., Hans, I., Grandner, M. A., Lack, L., et al. (2021). *Does total sleep time substantially increase after CBT-I?*. Manuscript submitted for publication.

Siengsukon, C. F., Alshehri, M., Williams, C., Drerup, M., & Lynch, S. (2020). Feasibility and treatment effect of cognitive behavioral therapy for insomnia in individuals with multiple sclerosis: A pilot randomized controlled trial. *Multiple Sclerosis and Related Disorders, 40*, 101958.

Siengsukon, C. F., Nelson, E., Williams-Cooke, C., Ludwig, R., Beck, E. S., Jr., Vidoni, E. D., et al. (2020). Cognitive behavioral therapy for insomnia to enhance cognitive function and reduce the rate of Aβ deposition in older adults with symptoms of insomnia: A single-site randomized pilot clinical trial protocol. *Contemporary Clinical Trials, 99*, 106190.

Simon, N., McGillivray, L., Roberts, N. P., Barawi, K., Lewis, C. E., & Bisson, J. I. (2019). Acceptability of internet-based cognitive behavioural therapy (i-CBT) for post-traumatic stress disorder (PTSD): A systematic review. *European Journal of Psychotraumatology, 10*(1), 1646092.

Smith, M. T., & Perlis, M. L. (2006). Who is a candidate for cognitive-behavioral therapy for insomnia? *Health Psychology, 25*(1), 15.

Smith, M. T., Perlis, M. L., Park, A., Smith, M. S., Pennington, J., Giles, D. E., et al. (2002). Comparative meta-analysis of pharmacotherapy and behavior therapy for persistent insomnia. *American Journal of Psychiatry, 159*(1), 5–11.

Spielman, A. J., Saskin, P., & Thorpy, M. J. (1987). Treatment of chronic insomnia by restriction of time in bed. *Sleep, 10*(1), 45–56.

Trockel, M., Karlin, B. E., Taylor, C. B., Brown, G. K., & Manber, R. (2015). Effects of cognitive behavioral therapy for insomnia on suicidal ideation in veterans. *Sleep, 38*(2), 259–265.

van der Zweerde, T., Bisdounis, L., Kyle, S. D., Lancee, J., & van Straten, A. (2019). Cognitive behavioral therapy for insomnia: A meta-analysis of long-term effects in controlled studies. *Sleep Medicine Reviews, 48*, 101208.

van Straten, A., van der Zweerde, T., Kleiboer, A., Cuijpers, P., Morin, C. M., & Lancee, J. (2018). Cognitive and behavioral therapies in the treatment of insomnia: A meta-analysis. *Sleep Medicine Reviews, 38*, 3–16.

Verbeek, I. H., Konings, G. M., Aldenkamp, A. P., Declerck, A. C., & Klip, E. C. (2006). Cognitive behavioral treatment in clinically referred chronic insomniacs: Group versus individual treatment. *Behavioral Sleep Medicine, 4*(3), 135–151.
Yamadera, W., Sato, M., Harada, D., Iwashita, M., Aoki, R., Obuchi, K., et al. (2013). Comparisons of short-term efficacy between individual and group cognitive behavioral therapy for primary insomnia. *Sleep and Biological Rhythms, 11*(3), 176–184.
Ye, Y. Y., Zhang, Y. F., Chen, J., Liu, J., Li, X. J., Liu, Y. Z., et al. (2015). Internet-cognitive behavioral therapy for insomnia (ICBT-i) improves comorbid anxiety and depression—A meta-analysis of randomized controlled trials. *PLoS One, 10*(11), e0142258.
Zorick, F. J., & Walsh, J. K. (2000). Evaluation and management of insomnia: An overview. In *Principles and practice of sleep medicine* (3rd ed., pp. 615–623). Philadelphia: Saunders.
Zwart, C. A., & Lisman, S. A. (1979a). Analysis of stimulus control treatment of sleep-onset insomnia. *Journal of Consulting and Clinical Psychology, 47*(1), 113.
Zwart, C. A., & Lisman, S. A. (1979b). Analysis of stimulus control treatment of sleep-onset insomnia. *Journal of Consulting and Clinical Psychology, 47*(1), 113.

PART 2

CBT-I in other sleep disorders

CHAPTER

2

CBT-I in patients with obstructive sleep apnea

Earl Charles Crew[a,b]

[a]Behavioral Health Program, Mental Health Care Line, Michael E. DeBakey Veteran's Affairs Medical Center, Houston, TX, United States, [b]Psychology Division, Menninger Department of Psychiatry and Behavioral Sciences, Baylor College of Medicine, Houston, TX, United States

Introduction

In obstructive sleep apnea (OSA), the pharyngeal airway collapses during sleep, contributing to snoring and incidents of partial (hypopneic) or complete (apneic) cessation of breathing, which produces recurrent hypoxemia, autonomic arousal, and fragmentation of the sleep episode (Strollo & Rogers, 1996). Diagnosis of OSA is typically accomplished by observing a patients' nighttime sleep using polysomnography, a comprehensive "sleep study" test performed in the laboratory while monitoring their brain electrical activity, eye movements, muscle activity, heart rate, respiration, snoring, and blood oxygen levels (Kapur et al., 2017). The apnea/hypopnea index (AHI)—a calculation of the number of apneic and hypopneic breathing events occurring per hour of sleep—is often used to characterize the severity of OSA. Clinically significant OSA is typically defined as (1) an AHI $\geq$5 (mild OSA) in the presence of one or more associated consequences (e.g., insomnia, sleepiness, fatigue, snoring, hypertension, atrial fibrillation, congestive heart failure) or (2) an AHI $\geq$15 (moderate OSA). An AHI $\geq$30 corresponds with a designation of severe OSA (American Academy of Sleep Medicine, 2014). The prevalence of OSA in the general adult population ranges from 9% to 39% (Senaratna et al., 2017). Risk factors for developing OSA include increasing age, higher body mass index, and male gender (Young, Skatrud, & Peppard, 2004).

https://doi.org/10.1016/B978-0-12-822872-2.00001-3

Effective management of OSA is imperative given the immediate (e.g., daytime sleepiness, cognitive deficits) and longer-term sequelae (e.g., the risk for motor vehicle accidents, hypertension, MI, stroke, major depression, and dementia; Osman, Carter, Carberry, & Eckert, 2018). Positive airway pressure (PAP; Sullivan, Berthon-Jones, Issa, & Eves, 1981) is the most commonly recommended treatment for OSA. PAP therapy uses pressurized air as a "splint" within the upper airway to prevent collapse during sleep (Calik, 2016). PAP is widely considered to be the "gold standard" of treatment for OSA given its long-term cost-effectiveness (Ayas et al., 2006; Guest, Helter, Morga, & Stradling, 2008) and efficacy in managing the range of OSA severities (Patel, White, Malhotra, Stanchina, & Ayas, 2003) relative to more-invasive treatment options with higher risk for adverse side-effects (Franklin et al., 2009). Alternative treatment options for OSA include surgeries (e.g., uvulopalatopharyngoplasty [UPPP], maxillomandibular advancement), hypoglossal nerve stimulation, oral appliances (e.g., mandibular advancement devices), pharmacotherapy, positional therapy, weight loss, nasal expiratory positive airway pressure, and oral pressure therapy (Calik, 2016).

Despite its overwhelming benefits, PAP is poorly tolerated by many patients with OSA. Up to 50% of patients initially refuse PAP therapy, while an additional 12%–25% have discontinued PAP use by 3 years (Engleman & Wild, 2003). Adherence to CPAP therapy is defined by the Centers for Medicare and Medicaid Services (CMS) as 4+ hours of use per night on 70% of nights during any consecutive 30 day period (Centers for Medicare & Medicaid Services, 2016). Suboptimal adherence with CPAP therapy is estimated in 30%–60% of those diagnosed with OSA (Sawyer et al., 2011). The efficacy of PAP therapy is dependent on patient adherence, with a dose–response relationship for benefits to primary consequences of OSA including daytime sleepiness, cognition, and blood pressure when nightly use exceeds 5h (Antic et al., 2011; Barbé et al., 2010; Weaver et al., 2007). The range of treatment-related factors affecting adherence can include discomfort (e.g., with the mask and/or hose interface), sleep disruptions due to noise/pressure changes, development of side effects (e.g., rashes, congestion), social factors (e.g., embarrassment), and psychological factors (e.g., feeling "claustrophobic," insomnia; Means, Edinger, & Husain, 2004).

Rationale for CBT-I in OSA

A growing appreciation of the prevalence of comorbid insomnia and OSA (COMISA) has amassed within the past 20 years (Krakow et al., 2001; Lichstein, Riedel, Lester, & Aguillard, 1999). A recent systematic review and meta-analysis of 37 investigations reported a pooled prevalence estimate of 38% for patients with OSA who meet criteria for insomnia, with difficulties maintaining sleep (42%) being more common than difficulties falling asleep (18%) or early morning awakenings (21%; Zhang et al., 2019). Additionally, the authors reported that 35% of patients diagnosed with insomnia have an AHI $\geq$5, and 29% of patients with insomnia have an AHI $\geq$15. This analysis excluded studies with patient samples consisting of military personnel, veterans, or patients reporting a history of trauma, where some estimates of comorbid insomnia symptoms and OSA are much higher than the general population (up to 81%–88%; Mysliwiec et al., 2014; Wallace, Vargas, Schwartz, Aloia, & Shafazand, 2013).

There is evidence that patients with comorbid insomnia and OSA experience the negative nighttime symptoms of both disorders cumulatively and report more severe sleep disruption than when either disorder occurs independently (Sweetman et al., 2017). This has been observed with polysomnography (PSG), whereby patients with COMISA experience more frequent arousals and decreased time spent in deep sleep compared to patients with insomnia alone (Bianchi, Williams, Mckinney, & Ellenbogen, 2013; Li et al., 2015) and exhibit shorter total sleep time, longer sleep latencies, and more wake after sleep onset than patients with OSA without clinical insomnia (Krakow et al., 2001). Sleep deprivation has been demonstrated to decrease upper airway muscle activity and increase the frequency and severity of apneic events (Guilleminault, 1981; Persson & Svanborg, 1996), possibly explaining one mechanism by which insomnia can exacerbate OSA. The use of psychotropic/hypnotic medications and other sleep aids is greater in patients with comorbid insomnia and OSA relative to the use of these in OSA alone (Krakow et al., 2001; Ye et al., 2014). This is concerning since hypnotic use can potentially worsen the frequency/severity of breathing events by reducing upper airway muscle tone, impairing respiratory drive control, and possibly increasing the risk of acute respiratory failure (Guilleminault, 1990; Wang et al., 2019).

The compounding nature of these clinical disorders co-occurring is also linked to greater daytime impairments due to neurocognitive decrements (Philip et al., 2017), psychiatric symptoms (e.g., anxiety, depression, posttraumatic stress disorder; Hayley et al., 2015; Mysliwiec et al., 2014), and lower overall quality of life (Tasbakan, Gunduz, Pirildar, & Basoglu, 2018) compared to OSA or insomnia presenting alone. Increased sleep-related distress among patients with COMISA is also evidenced by their endorsement of more dysfunctional beliefs and attitudes about sleep (e.g., perceptions of loss of control and unpredictability of sleep, misconceptions about sleep-promoting habits; Espie, Inglis, Harvey, & Tessier, 2000) relative to patients with OSA without insomnia (Smith et al., 2004; Yang, Liao, Lin, Chou, & Wang, 2011). Excessive daytime sleepiness and complaints of unrefreshing sleep in OSA may be greater when comorbid insomnia is present (Gooneratne et al., 2006; Kapur, Baldwin, Resnick, Gottlieb, & Nieto, 2005). Reports of daytime sleepiness may vary based on the severity of OSA, the severity of insomnia symptoms, or the type of insomnia complaints. More severe OSA is linked with increased daytime sleepiness and fewer insomnia complaints (Bjorvatn et al., 2015), while sleep onset insomnia (but not sleep maintenance issues) and lower AHI have been linked to lower levels of daytime sleepiness (Chung, 2005), suggesting that manifestations of hyperarousal in insomnia may become more apparent in patients with milder OSA symptoms.

There are several possible explanations for why OSA might promote the development of insomnia. Fragmentation from apneic events—manifesting in cortical arousals—has been considered the primary pathway which promotes difficulties with sleep maintenance (Krakow et al., 2001). To this end, increasing OSA severity would be expected to account for a greater prevalence of sleep maintenance complaints. However, when taking into account both objective (e.g., PSG) and subjective characteristics (e.g., self-report), the severity of OSA has not been found to predict the co-occurrence of insomnia, while the incidence of both sleep onset and sleep maintenance complaints are both common among patients with chronic insomnia with or without OSA (Lichstein, Thomas, Woosley, & Geyer, 2013). A similar assumption would be that subsequent treatment of OSA to eliminate breathing events would be expected to improve symptoms of both disorders. However, Glidewell, Renn, Roby, and Orr (2014) reported that less than half of patients with OSA and comorbid insomnia that initiated and were adherent with PAP therapy also experienced significant reductions in insomnia symptoms. Taken together, these findings suggest that insomnia that occurs in the context of OSA is an independent, self-sustaining disorder likely deserving of disease-specific intervention.

Finally, there is also considerable evidence that patients with OSA and comorbid insomnia exhibit lower rates of acceptance and poorer longer-term adherence than patients with OSA alone (Eysteinsdottir et al., 2017; Pieh et al., 2013; Wallace et al., 2013; Wallace, Sawyer, & Shafazand, 2018; Wickwire, Smith, Birnbaum, & Collop, 2010). It has been proposed that the presence of clinical insomnia poses a risk for lower adherence to PAP due to the mask/air pressure producing physical discomfort, which becomes more of an issue as individuals lay awake for extended periods attending to these sensations (Krakow et al., 2001). Therefore, more time and effort are required to achieve tolerance, which may prevent acceptance and precipitate early discontinuation. This is particularly impactful since early PAP use predicts longer-term adherence (Budhiraja et al., 2007), so anything that might create a negative first impression can reduce the incentive to work through these initial discomforts. When queried about the interference that insomnia poses to PAP adherence, patients have shared that difficulties adhering to PAP are due to perceptions that PAP is not beneficial because they are unable to sleep (i.e., lying awake in bed) or that residual insomnia actually "knocks off" the effectiveness of PAP by replacing sleep disruption from breathing events with increased/prolonged interruptions due to the PAP itself (Ong et al., 2017).

Evidence for the effectiveness of CBT-I in comorbid OSA

An obvious concern might be whether CBT-I can be effectively implemented in patients with OSA and promote the same short-term and sustained improvements to subjective sleep complaints and daytime functioning as seen with non-OSA samples with insomnia.

Early work investigating the benefits of addressing insomnia before targeted treatments for OSA revealed encouraging results. For instance, one small pilot study found that the combination of participation in a CBT-I program followed by OSA treatment using PAP, oral appliance, or turbinectomy was the most optimal sequence to improve symptoms of insomnia and daytime functioning (relative to medical treatment of OSA only; Krakow et al., 2004). More recent pilot investigations and randomized controlled trials (RCTs) have confirmed that clinical improvements in insomnia symptoms can be achieved when proceeding with CBT-I before targeting OSA symptoms. Fung and colleagues found no significant differences in sleep outcomes between older veterans with insomnia and either no or mild OSA symptoms who completed a five-session protocol of CBT-I, as compared to a sleep education control condition (Fung et al., 2016). Another recent, retrospective study compared insomnia-related outcomes assessed during and 3-months post-treatment (e.g., difficulties falling/staying asleep, sleep efficiency, scores on standardized measures of insomnia severity), which concluded that patients equally benefitted from 4 to 6 sessions of individual CBT-I regardless of whether they were diagnosed with COMISA or insomnia only (Sweetman, Lack, Lambert, Gradisar, & Harris, 2017).

Findings from recent RCTs (Ong et al., 2020; Sweetman et al., 2019; Sweetman et al., 2020) provide the most promising evidence yet that manualized CBT-I protocols can be effective for managing insomnia in patients with comorbid OSA (treated or untreated). While this literature is relatively limited, currently available results do not identify any absolute contraindications for use of CBT-I protocols which include the same standardized set of components as typically utilized with chronic primary insomnia (Edinger, Wohlgemuth, Radtke, Marsh, & Quillian, 2001). Ong et al. (2020) attempted to disentangle the effects of sequencing CBT-I before, or concurrent with, PAP therapy, as compared to a control condition where only PAP was offered. Among their findings, the authors observed that a four-week sequence of CBT-I—delivered before starting PAP—was superior to PAP alone to address insomnia symptoms in patients with COMISA (Ong et al., 2020). Expectedly, CBT-I started concurrently with PAP was superior to PAP therapy only, while there were no significant differences between CBT-I groups with regard to outcomes for insomnia (e.g., reduction in symptoms, % of remitters), PAP adherence, or improvements in daytime functioning. This suggests that either treatment sequence would be expected to promote similar improvements in insomnia symptoms, with either sequence that includes CBT-I being superior to PAP alone.

Given risks of nonadherence to first-line OSA therapies like PAP when insomnia is untreated, starting CBT-I before initiating PAP therapy may be an effective and efficient path when available. Sweetman et al. (2019) observed that a four-session protocol of CBT-I before starting PAP (a) significantly reduced symptoms of insomnia, (b) improved subsequent acceptance of PAP, and (c) increased long-term PAP use by 1 h per night (assessed after 6 months) compared to treatment with PAP alone. This sequence may also be appropriate in clinical contexts when OSA is suspected but there may be delays when referring for further evaluation (e.g., diagnostic and/or titration study). Additionally, CBT-I sequence (initial vs concurrent with PAP) has not been found to significantly improve adherence with PAP (Ong et al., 2020), though concurrent interventions may be helpful to increase initial acceptance and adherence when OSA and PAP-related information (e.g., education, discussion of challenges/benefits, troubleshooting tips) is integrated into treatment together (as observed in: Alessi et al., 2020). Patients with a clinical presentation that includes more severe OSA (Glidewell et al., 2014), primarily sleep maintenance insomnia (Bjornsdottir et al., 2013), and without other significant psychological and/or sleep-related comorbidities (Mendes & dos Santos, 2015) may still benefit from starting PAP or other OSA treatments if CBT-I is not available.

Addressing concerns about CBT-I in comorbid OSA

While these results seem to suggest that CBT-I in COMISA can be as effective to treat insomnia in patients without OSA, there are some notable characteristics of CBT-I and patients with COMISA, which might give some clinicians pause about whether starting with behavioral therapy is an ideal initial treatment option for some patients.

With the expected lag in treatment response (up to 3–4 weeks when attempting to increase sleep efficiency)—and likely augmentation of daytime sleepiness with time-in-bed restriction—it is understandable to be concerned that sleep restriction might be poorly tolerated, promote nonadherence, or even increase the risk for adverse events in patients with higher baseline daytime sleepiness (Kyle et al., 2014; Vincent, Lewycky, & Finnegan, 2008). Sweetman, McEvoy, Smith, Catcheside, et al. (2020) conducted a secondary analysis of their RCT in which 145 patients with untreated OSA (moderate-to-severe) and comorbid insomnia participated in either a four-week trial of CBT-I or a no-treatment control group. They observed that daytime sleepiness, assessed with the Epworth Sleepiness Scale (ESS; Johns, 1991) increased significantly (by 15%) in the CBT-I group after the first week of time-in-bed restriction (average = 6.2 h; minimum = 5.5 h), but then returned to or fell below pretreatment levels during successive weeks. This initial increase in reported daytime sleepiness was accompanied by a nonsignificant (8%) decrease in total sleep time. Higher pretreatment ESS scores were associated with a greater reduction in subjective sleepiness during CBT-I, while the severity of OSA (based on AHI) was not associated with patterns of change in ESS scores during the course of treatment (Sweetman, McEvoy, Smith, Catcheside, et al., 2020). Although complaints of sleepiness, fatigue, and cognitive difficulties were noted, significant adverse events were not reported during this trial, nor were these observed in the RCT conducted by Ong et al. (2020) in which participants in one of the treatment arms completed CBT-I before starting PAP. Collectively, these preliminary findings reinforce that sleepiness should be monitored closely during CBT-I in patients with COMISA, but suggest that this concern would not absolutely contraindicate the use of sleep restriction or other standard treatment components of CBT-I.

Another concern is the risk for nonadherence given the tendency for COMISA patients to endorse higher levels of associated daytime impairments, including greater psychiatric symptoms and dysfunctional beliefs and attitudes about sleep—both of which have been found to predict suboptimal compliance with key components of CBT-I like sleep restriction and maintaining a consistent rise time (Cvengros, Crawford, Manber, & Ong, 2015; Manber et al., 2014). In their RCT, Sweetman et al. (2019) found that, compared to treatment-as-usual, the patients with COMISA who participated in CBT-I did not experience any improvements in anxiety, depression, stress, daytime sleepiness, or fatigue from baseline to six months. Furthermore, a secondary analysis supported that—while roughly half of the total sample endorsed mild symptoms of depression, anxiety, and stress—whether patients' insomnia symptoms improved during treatment was not moderated by the severity of these symptoms (Sweetman et al., 2020). However, notable changes (a 30% reduction) in endorsement of dysfunctional beliefs and attitudes about sleep were identified, suggesting that intervention components like sleep education, time in bed restriction, and monitoring sleep-wake patterns can support adapting more enduring and realistic expectations about sleep and related daytime functions (Espie et al., 2000; Sweetman, McEvoy, Smith, Catcheside, et al., 2020).

Given the primary contribution of OSA-related breathing events to promote cortical arousals, it also seems warranted to ask whether patients with severe OSA—which may contribute to more sleep fragmentation when untreated—would impede efforts to behaviorally improve sleep consolidation in patients with sleep maintenance insomnia. Evidence suggests that improvements in wake after sleep onset after CBT-I are comparable between patients with or without OSA of any severity level (Fung et al., 2016; Sweetman, Lack, Lambert, et al., 2017). Furthermore, among patients who do not show any improvement in insomnia symptoms during CBT-I (sometimes termed as having "treatment-resistant insomnia"), this is not associated with the severity of OSA based on AHI (Sweetman, Lack, Lambert, et al., 2017).

Finally, there is some evidence that CBT-I can improve symptoms of OSA as well. Secondary analysis of PSG data from Sweetman and colleagues' RCT (2020) support that PAP-naïve patients with COMISA who complete CBT-I experience significant reductions in AHI (by ~16%), number of awakenings, wake after sleep onset, and time spent in light (nonrapid eye movement stage 1 or N1) sleep. While anatomical features (e.g., upper airway "crowding") are among the primary contributors to the etiology of OSA affecting severity, nonanatomical factors including low respiratory arousal threshold, pharyngeal muscle responsiveness, and oversensitive ventilatory control also play a substantial role in many patients (Eckert, White, Jordan, Malhotra, & Wellman, 2013). These findings of improved OSA symptoms with CBT-I are notable, as they demonstrate (1) one mechanism by which insomnia may exacerbate OSA, and (2) CBT-I can improve symptoms of OSA even before patients start on a targeted intervention such as PAP (Sweetman et al., 2020).

Adapting CBT-I in patients with comorbid OSA

Although the current body of literature on treating adult patients with COMISA supports that a standard CBT-I protocol—which does not include information about OSA—would be effective to treat insomnia symptoms in the context of comorbid OSA, a more personalized course of treatment that incorporates the unique clinical presentation of these patients can be formulated to better suit the individual needs of each patient.

The recommendations below have been devised to accommodate many of the most common clinical characteristics of adult COMISA patients, which may differ from primary insomnia. In many instances, these recommendations correspond to possible modifications when encountering concerns about patient's acceptance, tolerance, resistance to change, or safety. A majority of these recommendations were generated from the research findings for COMISA characteristics and interventions discussed in the sections above. There are notable limitations of the evidence base for these recommendations as there are only a handful of large randomized controlled trials of CBT-I in patients with COMISA and the most common intervention for OSA (PAP therapy). Some of the proposed modifications are based on anecdotal evidence or assumed effectiveness to accommodate a particular challenge based on application in similar patient populations or clinical contexts. To this extent, clinical judgment is always encouraged when considering any modification of standard CBT-I or decision-making around the sequencing of this treatment with interventions for OSA (e.g., PAP therapy). When not explicitly described herein, it should be assumed that components of CBT-I as typically applied in patients with primary insomnia could also be appropriate among patients with COMISA.

Considerations for assessment of insomnia in patients with suspected OSA

Commensurate with standard practice guidelines for the diagnostic assessment of insomnia (Buysse, Ancoli-Israel, Edinger, Lichstein, & Morin, 2006; Qaseem, Kansagara, Forciea, Cooke, & Denberg, 2016; Schutte-Rodin, Broch, Buysse, Dorsey, & Sateia, 2008), clinicians should conduct a structured or semistructured clinical interview with the patient in conjunction with having them complete validated questionnaires and daily sleep diaries for 7–14 days. Because screening for the presence of other occult sleep disorders and potential contributions to insomnia should already be included in the initial assessment, specific modification to these procedures would only be required in situations where patients carry a confirmed diagnosis of OSA and/or have been prescribed PAP therapy.

Assessing PAP Adherence. When inquiring about adherence to PAP, it may be helpful to ask patients about the following: (a) how many nights they use their device per week, (b) if PAP is used during the entire sleep episode, (c) if they ever remove the mask during the night, (d) do they experience any discomfort or sleep-interference during use, (e) do they experience any issues with equipment or the hose/mask interface, (f) what are their perceived benefits to sleep/daytime function after PAP use, and (g) whether PAP is used during daytime naps? Given significant discrepancies in device-recorded PAP use versus patients' self-report (Kribbs et al., 1993), obtaining a download of their usage data may be warranted (from the SD card or remotely via synchronous telehealth). Typically, this will generate a report of usage during the past 30–90 days. Pertinent details from these reports include (i) average minutes/hours of use per day, (ii) percentage of daily use $\geq$4 h, (iii) residual AHI during use, and (iv) percentage or duration of time spent in a "large leak" (i.e., when [oro]nasal seal is compromised and air escapes out of the sides of the mask interface). Some of this information may be available within a smartphone app synched with the patient's PAP, which has been designed to increase patient adherence by delivering feedback on usage and trigger intervention for any technical issues that arise (Hwang, 2016). Understanding any barriers to PAP adherence and/or treatment efficacy can be helpful to understand whether the most salient issues are primarily behavioral or equipment-related. This will inevitably inform the best approach needed to manage the patients' insomnia (discussed in more detail below).

Insomnia symptoms. The Insomnia Severity Index (ISI) has been found to have high diagnostic accuracy to detect insomnia and monitor changes during the course of CBT-I (Bastien, Vallières, & Morin, 2001; Chiu, Chang, Hsieh, & Tsai, 2016). However, concerns have been raised about the use of the ISI in patients with suspected/confirmed OSA given the substantial symptom overlap with insomnia, particularly regarding daytime consequences (e.g., sleep dissatisfaction, interference with daily functioning, noticeability of impairment, degree of distress about sleep problem). A recent analysis observed that a subset of patients with OSA exhibit elevated ISI total scores without clinically confirmed symptoms of insomnia (i.e., a "false positive"; Wallace & Wohlgemuth, 2019). As a solution, these authors recommend splitting up the ISI into separate subscales for nocturnal (ISI items 1–3) and daytime symptoms (ISI items 4–7) of insomnia in patients with comorbid OSA, with cut-off scores (sum of items 1–3 $\geq$6) to distinguish moderate from subclinical symptoms of nocturnal sleep disturbance (Wallace et al., 2018). These subscales and cut-off scores would be recommended when using the ISI to monitor treatment progress during CBT-I to disentangle the potential confound of improved insomnia severity despite recurrent symptoms of daytime impairment attributable to OSA.

Sleep diaries. In addition to the standard sleep diary items (Carney et al., 2012), the format of the sleep diary for use in treating comorbid sleep apnea can be modified to include a) the frequency, timing, duration, and location of naps (e.g., bedroom versus recliner in the living room); and b) whether PAP was used and for how long (duration or percentage of time asleep). When implementing interventions to reduce daytime napping, clinicians may also recommend scheduling activities around higher propensity napping times. To support this, diaries can also be modified to include items where patients can list the timing and completion of planned activities. In patients with excessive daytime napping, which might impede therapy, clinicians can also consider including a diary item that pertains to sleepiness. The Stanford Sleepiness Scale (SSS) is a single-item measure that asks the rater to select one of seven statements best representing their current level of perceived sleepiness (Hoddes,

Zarcone, Smyth, Phillips, & Dement, 1973). Possible instructions might include having patients complete the SSS upon waking or at other times throughout the day which may correspond with patients' typical napping/dozing times. These can be used during baseline assessment, or during active treatment to monitor changes in subjective sleepiness at various points during the day.

Treatment planning before initiating CBT-I

Given the notable benefits of CBT-I for the management of chronic insomnia, adult patients with OSA who also meet the criteria for this diagnosis based on the intake evaluation would most likely benefit from this therapy. The following guide may therefore be helpful for clinicians to identify an appropriate treatment plan for patients referred for management of insomnia, which includes standard components of CBT-I plus additional steps to address their individual needs:

1. Patients with suspected OSA, pending formal evaluation and/or intervention, should be offered CBT-I with appropriate modifications based on the recommendations discussed elsewhere in this chapter (e.g., for excessive daytime sleepiness).
2. Patients with newly diagnosed OSA, that are recommended PAP therapy, should be offered CBT-I. This can be commenced before or concurrent with starting PAP therapy based on clinical availability; timing of treatment should prioritize patients' preference for sequencing when possible. Modifications to the CBT-I protocol may incorporate education about OSA and PAP, motivational enhancement, or systematic desensitization (see below), as deemed necessary.
3. Patients with OSA who are nonadherent with PAP should be offered CBT-I. Clinicians may also consider modifiable contributors to nonadherence and implement appropriate interventions before proceeding with CBT-I, such as:
   a. If nonadherence is due to poor treatment efficacy or intolerance of PAP at current therapy settings (pressure, mask, modality; e.g., leaks), consult with respiratory therapy and sleep medicine to identify solutions.
   b. If nonadherence is attributable to low motivation or importance to treat OSA, consider proceeding with motivational enhancement before components of CBT-I.
   c. If nonadherence is attributed to significant discomfort or claustrophobic/anxiety reactions, consider proceeding with motivational enhancement and systematic desensitization before components of CBT-I (Table 1).

TABLE 1 Adaptation of cognitive behavioral therapy for insomnia (CBT-I) for obstructive sleep apnea (OSA).

CBT-I components	Standard practice	CBT-I Adaptations for OSA
Sleep education	3-P model, 2-process model of sleep regulation, sleep stages	– Emphasize how napping and variable bed/wake schedules can affect sleep drive and circadian entrainment – Educate about OSA physiology, causes of sleep disruption (e.g., fragmentation, nocturia), safety (i.e., sleepiness when driving), and health risks associated with sleeping too much (≥9 h) – Education on short- and long-term sequelae when untreated, therapy options, and benefits of treatment adherence (e.g., PAP)
Sleep restriction	Improve sleep efficiency by limiting time in bed to the amount of time sleeping then expanding slowly as long as sleep efficiency is preserved	– Prioritize discussion of SRT risks and safety planning – Assess sleepiness at each session – Base initial TIB window on nocturnal TST plus average duration of daytime napping – Consider sleep compression to initially restrict time in bed gradually by 15–30 min each week until target sleep efficiency (e.g., ≥85%) is reached
Stimulus control	Associate bed/bedroom solely as a cue for sleep by eliminating nonsleep activities from the bedroom. Instruction to get out of bed at night if awake >15 min	– Do not sleep outside of the bedroom – Avoid remaining in bed after terminal awakening (i.e., if awaken feeling "unrefreshed") – Plan wake-promoting activities around scheduled rise time (e.g., showering, social commitments, exercise) – Can disconnect PAP mask from those and wear during bathroom trips or during sleep-promoting activities outside of the bedroom
Napping/ daytime sleep	Discontinue or restrict daytime napping to 30 min	– Avoid unintentional napping – Daytime sleep only occurs in bed, always with PAP, and limited to 30–45 min – Consolidate all daytime naps into one scheduled nap during the middle of the day

TABLE 1 Adaptation of cognitive behavioral therapy for insomnia (CBT-I) for obstructive sleep apnea (OSA)—cont'd

CBT-I components	Standard practice	CBT-I Adaptations for OSA
		– Implement nap compression (gradually reduce nap duration by 15–30min each week) concurrent with sleep extension
Sleep hygiene education	Address daytime habits and sleep environment interfering with sleep	– Encourage activity scheduling and use of other proactive countermeasures during patients' "high risk" nap times (early morning, middle of the day) – For specific pharmacologic countermeasures (e.g., caffeine, nicotine), assist patients to reduce intake and optimize the timing of use/discontinuation to prevent effects on nighttime sleep
Cognitive therapy	Challenge patient's dysfunctional beliefs interfering with sleep and misconceptions about sleep. Replace/restructure to more helpful and realistic thoughts about sleep	– Provide information on expected therapeutic changes with CBT-I and sleep symptoms that may persist (e.g., daytime sleepiness) – Discuss other causes of daytime sleepiness (e.g., low energy due to hunger, hydration, mood) and challenge dysfunctional attributions of daytime impairments to sleep – Utilize monitoring and behavioral experiments to track daytime functioning with increased nightly PAP use or increased daytime activity
Relapse prevention	Discuss practicing less rigid sleep plan over time and what do to prevent sleep disturbance from turning into another episode of insomnia in the future	– Identify routine PAP care plan (e.g., cleaning schedule), follow-up schedule (when to request mask replacement, check device pressures/efficacy), and proactive strategies to motivate adherence (e.g., support person who will check-in on nightly use) – Emphasizes OSA as chronic and requiring life-long treatment

Continued

TABLE 1 Adaptation of cognitive behavioral therapy for insomnia (CBT-I) for obstructive sleep apnea (OSA)—cont'd

CBT-I components	Standard practice	CBT-I Adaptations for OSA
Sleep diaries	Establish baseline sleep patterns, track progress, reinforce appropriate behavior change, problem solve obstacles to adherence	– Include columns for (1) napping (time and duration), (2) completion of planned daily activities, (3) PAP use each night (hours of use or % worn during sleep) – May add an item for assessing sleepiness at various points during the day (e.g., with the Stanford Sleepiness Scale)

Sleep education

As a component of CBT-I, the goals of sleep education are to provide the patient with foundational information to better understand the etiology of their condition, factors that have maintained their symptoms over time, and to provide a rationale for the other components of therapy. Adaptation of sleep education in CBT-I for patients with comorbid OSA is best accomplished by providing an overview of each standard concept (e.g., 3-P model, sleep hygiene, etc.), and then integrating a brief discussion of how the clinical symptoms and/or sequelae of OSA might also impact or modify the experience of each phenomenon (detailed below). Additionally, a brief overview of OSA physiology, consequences to health/functioning, available treatments, and interactions with insomnia can be included (see the Introduction to this chapter for talking points that might be covered).

OSA and sleep stage fragmentation. An important distinction when discussing typical sleep architecture in someone with OSA is fragmentation occurring secondary to apneic events that repeatedly interrupt the natural ebb and flow through REM and non-REM stages of sleep. This is akin to being constantly interrupted while completing an important task so that it takes much longer to accomplish the same amount of work (i.e., more time spent asleep is required to feel rested). This can explain why many individuals with sleep apnea feel unrefreshed after sleep, and often require naps or doze unintentionally during the day.

OSA and the 3-P model. With regard to the etiology of insomnia, OSA can serve as a predisposing, precipitating, or perpetuating factor. Some of the anatomical features that contribute to the pathophysiology of OSA are hereditary, increasing the risk to experience disrupted sleep when symptoms emerge during development. The onset of OSA symptoms can be insidious in the context of gradual weight gain or advancing age, but can precipitate sleep disruptions with prolonged difficulties returning to sleep (e.g., cortical arousals with sympathetic activation following a breathing event, nocturia requiring bathroom trips during awakenings), which may contribute to a patient meeting criteria for acute insomnia. Insomnia symptoms that were precipitated by respiratory events or other factors may become more impairing as patients attempt to compensate for frequently interrupted and/or nonrestorative sleep by increasing time in bed, napping during the day, and engaging in other sleep-incompatible behaviors (e.g., excessive caffeine consumption), which maintain insomnia over time until this pattern becomes chronic.

Effects of OSA on sleep regulation. Education on the homeostatic sleep drive—and mechanisms by which OSA negatively affects this system and can contribute to insomnia—should include (a) how OSA reduces recovery from wakefulness by fragmenting sleep and (b) napping and excessive time in bed weaken the sleep drive by reducing sleep need without sufficient time/energy expenditure before attempting sleep again. Additionally, education on the ways in which OSA and daytime sequelae can affect circadian regulation should include (a) how OSA might interfere with entrainment by increasing sedentary activities and reduced sunlight exposure, (b) how attenuations in circadian alertness increase sleep urge in the middle of the day and at night (precipitating naps), and (c) how the timing of sleep initiation is important for sleep maintenance and satisfaction (i.e., feeling refreshed upon waking). These concepts are typically discussed when reviewing circadian regulation in patients with primary insomnia. Therefore, the extent to which additional discussion is needed for patients with OSA would depend on whether their daytime activities can be characterized by low levels of physical activity or sunlight exposure, frequent napping, highly variable bed and rise times, and excessive time spent in bed.

Sleep hygiene education. Adaptation of sleep hygiene education might vary somewhat depending on whether patients have been provided treatment for OSA or are awaiting formal evaluation/initiation of treatment. All patients should be provided information about how napping can impact the sleep drive, as well as how certain substances used to promote wakefulness/combat sleepiness (e.g., caffeine, nicotine) can both a) impair sleep if ingested close to bedtime, and b) may contribute to transient worsening of sleepiness during the day as a symptom of acute withdrawal. Additionally, patients with insomnia and comorbid insomnia who consume alcohol or use hypnotic sleep aids should be informed about the potential role these play in worsening the severity/frequency of breathing events (by relaxing muscles that control the upper airway). Finally, patients should be informed about the role of mood and sedentary activities on worsening insomnia and increased daytime sleepiness and encouraged to enhance behavioral activation during the day via scheduling of activities. The timing of these activities can be adjusted so they correspond with "high risk" (i.e., high propensity) times when patients might doze unintentionally (e.g., early morning, after meals, or during the midday circadian "dip").

Time in bed restriction

When adapting time in bed (TIB) restriction in patients with comorbid OSA, the most pertinent consideration is whether to do so traditionally (via sleep restriction therapy; SRT) or more gradually with a modified approach. While recent RCT investigations of CBT-I in COMISA used standard protocols of SRT with good effect and no significant adverse events (Ong et al., 2020; Sweetman et al., 2019), application of this within a less-controlled clinical setting warrants additional consideration of the potential risks and benefits before proceeding. That said, there do not appear to be any absolute contraindications to implementation of SRT in COMISA aside from patients with other medical comorbidities (e.g., history of seizures, bipolar disorder, some parasomnias) where sleep deprivation may produce significant negative effects (Smith, Huang, & Manber, 2005).

The determination for whether to utilize SRT or another treatment component (e.g., sleep compression) should always be made with the target outcome in mind, which is to consolidate the nocturnal sleep episode by decreasing wakefulness after sleep onset (Spielman, Saskin, & Thorpy, 1987). The effectiveness of TIB restriction is dependent upon patient adherence, so what approach is best-suited should also incorporate what patients can tolerate and implement. In the application of SRT in patients with primary insomnia, it is typically recommended that the initial TIB window be equivalent to the patient's nocturnal total sleep time (TST; based on sleep diary) beginning around the 1st or 2nd session of active treatment. In patients with COMISA, this approach would also be expected to be effective, while some patients may prefer and/or better tolerate SRT with slight modification.

In all situations where SRT is applied to treat insomnia, it is critically important to discuss potential risks and/or adverse reactions and identify a plan for how patients can navigate these situations safely. This safety planning should be prioritized in patients with comorbid OSA—especially those with untreated OSA or who evidence excessive daytime sleepiness (EDS)—before proceeding with the active therapy components of CBT-I. While instructions for SRT often include avoiding naps or remaining in bed and sleeping longer than the scheduled rise time—even following a night with "poor sleep" (e.g., later bedtime, longer sleep latency, more frequent awakenings)—the therapist and patient should discuss conditions where relaxing the restrictions of treatment would be warranted. Situational examples include when resultant daytime sleepiness becomes severely excessive and impairs the patients' ability to fulfill daily responsibilities safely or effectively. Patients should be encouraged to monitor for the acute onset of drowsiness/unintentional dozing in response to treatment, such as before driving or operating heavy machinery, while providing care for young children/infants, or which begins to impair occupational functioning (e.g., napping at work). For patients with concerns about the potential impact of worsening daytime sleepiness/impaired vigilance on work and other responsibilities, conversations may also involve recommending to delay the start of treatment to coincide with planned breaks or vacations. Providers should discuss indicators of excessive sleepiness (e.g., may adopt the late William Dement's warning that "drowsiness is red alert!"; Dement, 2001) and appropriate safety precautions (e.g., allowing for an intentional 15–30 min nap in the bed), which can best mitigate the risk of adverse events and avoid drastically disrupting progress with CBT-I. Providers should also consider that some patients may be engaging in daily behaviors that promote feeling recurrently, subjectively sleepy (e.g., sedentary activities in front of the computer or television), so discussing modifiable reasons for situational sleepiness/feeling "low energy" (e.g., hunger, mood, dehydration, limited physical activity/sunlight exposure) and behavioral countermeasures (e.g., keep snacks available, schedule daily outdoor activities, take a quick shower) should also be discussed.

Before implementing SRT, the following may also be taken into account when considering adaptations: (1) OSA treatment status (treated vs suboptimal adherence vs untreated), (2) evidence of severe excessive daytime sleepiness (e.g., ESS scores $\geq$16), (3) duration of time between follow-up appointments, and (4) average daily napping frequency/duration.

Patients with untreated OSA due to nonadherence may benefit from initial interventions to increase adherence before implementing SRT (e.g., motivational enhancement, desensitization), while treatment-naïve patients may prefer to begin with other components of CBT-I (e.g., sleep hygiene, stimulus control) before SRT. While EDS has not been found to contraindicate or significantly interfere with the effectiveness of SRT, it is a frequent complaint attributed as an adverse side effect that may impede tolerability of the intervention. These patients may benefit from a more gradual approach to limiting TIB (e.g., sleep compression, in which TIB is gradually reduced by 15–30 min each week until a target sleep efficiency is achieved; Lichstein, 1988). Given the relatively higher risk of worsening sleepiness in the initial treatment phase (Kyle et al., 2014; Sweetman,

McEvoy, Smith, Catcheside, et al., 2020), providers should ensure that they can meet with patients frequently (e.g., weekly) to evaluate for any negative treatment effects, assess sleepiness (e.g., using the ESS), and adjust treatment as deemed necessary to ensure prioritization of safety.

Finally, when setting an initial TIB window for patients as part of SRT, providers are encouraged to adhere to the most common practice and not recommend restricting the TIB window below 5.0h (Kyle et al., 2015). When setting the TIB window, providers might take into account nocturnal TST but also the average frequency and duration of any naps. Ideally, patients would be recommended to attempt to avoid daytime napping while treatment focuses on consolidating nocturnal sleep, so an initial TIB window that accounts for all sleep occurring in a 24-h period would better reflect homeostatic sleep need and likely augment patient adherence to treatment. Avoidance of naps is initially encouraged as these can become habitual and worsen daytime sleepiness (Ancoli-Israel & Martin, 2006). If it is observed that patients cannot tolerate avoidance of napping during the day, providers can permit modification to include a scheduled nap opportunity of 30–45min at a prearranged time during the middle of the day (e.g., 6–8h after waking). With regard to napping, it is imperative to stipulate that these (1) are taken intentionally (versus unintentionally dozing), (2) always occur in the patient's bed, and (3) are accompanied by use of PAP, if prescribed. As patients' sleep begins to increasingly consolidate at night, nap compression (i.e., gradually reducing nap duration by 15–30min each day) can be pursued in conjunction with sleep extension (when 15–30min is added to their nocturnal TIB window each week).

Stimulus control

The overarching goals of stimulus control therapy (SCT) as a core component of CBT-I are to target the conditioned (i.e., learned) aspects of insomnia—developing from the repeated experience of sleeplessness, distress, and engagement in nonsleep activities in the bed/bedroom—and to "re-learn" that the bed is a place for naturally occurring sleep and reassociate this with compatible expectations (e.g., dissociate going to bed as stressful/frustrating, reduce the effort to sleep; Bootzin, 1972). Some recent RCTs of brief CBT-I (Sweetman et al., 2019) did not include SCT components but still observed significant improvements in insomnia symptoms by applying other core strategies (e.g., TIB restriction). Therefore, whether to even focus on SCT components as part of CBT-I with comorbid OSA will be case-dependent and should take into account the perceived degree of stimulus dyscontrol (e.g., symptoms of conditioned hyperarousal, engagement in frequent nonsleep activities in the bedroom).

In general, SCT can be implemented without modification to a standard approach for use in patients with comorbid OSA. However, clinicians will want to emphasize the need to have all sleep (naps and nighttime sleep) occur within the bedroom given the tendency for patients to present with patterns of dozing in other locations (e.g., their favorite chair in front of the television). Additionally, patients with untreated OSA or suboptimal adherence to PAP may be increasingly more likely to report nonrestorative sleep and awakening feeling tired and unrefreshed (possibly due to poor sleep quality or normative "sleep inertia"), so will remain in the bed "snoozing" or attempting to fall back to sleep for extensive periods. Education about this is warranted—particularly to normalize the feeling of subjective sleep dissatisfaction upon waking from deeper stages of sleep (i.e., sleep inertia; Hilditch & McHill, 2019)—and to encourage patients to get out of bed when unable to return to sleep (to promote stimulus control) and always around the same time each day (to promote feeling more awake/alert on future mornings once patients have entrained to this schedule). One proactive strategy to enhance adherence is to help patients generate a list of activities that they may schedule shortly after their designated rise time (e.g., exercise, time with family, preparing a favorite breakfast) to provide some additional motivation to implement a consistent morning routine regardless of how sleepy they initially feel around this time.

There is evidence to suggest that patients with insomnia and comorbid OSA more accurately estimate durations of wakefulness compared to patients with primary insomnia (Bianchi et al., 2013). Alternatively, some patients with more fragmented sleep (due to more severe, untreated OSA) may perceive recurrent, proximal awakenings as one long episode of wakefulness (Sweetman, Lack, Catcheside, et al., 2017). In the context of insomnia, the experience of more interrupted, unconsolidated sleep is occurring due to attenuated homeostatic drive, so strategies to increase consolidation would be warranted. Indeed, completion of CBT-I has been shown to reduce AHI and frequency of cortical awakenings in patients with untreated OSA (Sweetman, Lack, McEvoy, Antic, et al., 2020). Therefore, when delivering SCT instructions to patients, an appropriate modification might be stipulate a) getting out of bed after 15–20 min of continual wakefulness or b) during periods of notable restlessness where the patient may be alternating between wake and light sleep interrupted by breathing events (i.e., there is not a continuous 15–20 min of wakefulness nor a continuous period of sleep). Additionally, when providing SCT instructions for patients on PAP therapy, recommend to them that they detach the mask from the hose connected to their device (instead of completely removing the mask) and continue to wear the mask while engaging in stimulus control activities in another room. This will eliminate the need to fumble around to refit the mask in the dark when returning to bed once sleepiness returns.

Cognitive therapy

Interventions to address maladaptive cognitions might follow similar approaches as used in primary insomnia, while the need to consider the inclusion of these strategies for patients with comorbid insomnia and OSA may be increased given the observation that they tend to endorse more dysfunctional beliefs and attitudes about sleep. Completion of standardized questionnaires (Espie et al., 2000) can inform the need to consider cognitive therapy strategies as part of the treatment plan. However, it is likely that some patients' insomnia-perpetuating beliefs could abate following the implementation of other treatment components such as SRT (Sweetman et al., 2019). It is also likely that the complicated interactions between insomnia and OSA can contribute to the development of these dysfunctional beliefs which would improve with sleep education (particularly when this involves thorough discussion of the physiology of OSA). Therefore, assessing for residual evidence of maladaptive sleep-related attitudes/beliefs after initial education and behavioral components have been initiated can inform the need to target other cognitions that are more engrained.

Among patients with OSA, common insomnia-perpetuating beliefs might include (1) expectations that they should always feel rested/refreshed upon waking, (2) expectations that waking up during the night is abnormal, or (3) attributions that sleepiness during the day is entirely dependent on quality/duration of sleep the previous night. In these instances, daytime functioning is intimately entangled with sleep quality, which can worsen insomnia due to heightened distress about the next-day consequences of a poor nights' sleep (e.g., when they experience difficulties falling asleep or awaken spontaneously during the night). Some patients with OSA that are participating in therapy for insomnia may also perseverate on the need to avoid napping as a source of their sleep issues. These patients may then become increasingly concerned if they doze unintentionally during the day, and may be more sensitive to becoming frustrated/distressed if they experience insomnia on the night after a nap. In these examples, concerns are primarily focused on the perceived impact of poor sleep on next-day function. To address this, monitoring daytime variables (e.g., of activities, sleepiness, napping) and reviewing this data in session can be effective. For instance, patients may become more accepting of a nap that slightly affects their nighttime sleep if their data collection supports that this has a little tangible effect on their daytime functioning the following day (e.g., sleepiness or another unintentional nap). To best facilitate this, the sleep diary may be modified to include items corresponding to these daytime variables.

Relapse prevention

The final module typically covered during CBT-I is a review of all of the components covered during the course of treatment, what the patient found most helpful, and generating a relapse prevention plan which outlines (a) key strategies that the patient should attempt to implement each day to support consistent sleep-wake patterns and prevent the return of insomnia, and (b) strategies that they might need to implement on an as-needed basis, should insomnia return, to avoid this from perpetuating into a chronic issue. Additional components to include with the discussion of relapse prevention for patients with COMISA should emphasize that OSA is a chronic condition that will likely require lifelong management for most individuals. However, the treatments that are available (e.g., PAP) are incredibly effective, to the extent that the short- and long-term consequences of OSA can be prevented with regular adherence to therapy.

Additionally, there is evidence that most individuals, over time, start to use their PAP less and less (Rotenberg, Murariu, & Pang, 2016), so identifying strategies to promote adherence in the long term is critical. Examples of long-term motivational strategies might include: leaving reminders around the house, scheduling routine follow-up appointments with their sleep medicine provider, social support (e.g., ask their spouse to remind them if they miss a night, find a friend who is also on PAP and schedule a phone call to check-in on PAP to use a few times per year), setting goals to maintain a streak of continuous use (and then identify rewards when you break a new personal record), and developing a rigid daily routine cleaning up and/or putting away the device (e.g., just like making your bed or taking a shower) that becomes so habitual it might seem strange not to do it each day. Additionally, providers might consider implementing some of the motivational enhancement strategies described in the next paragraphs which target intrinsic motivational factors.

Additional components to consider when managing OSA in comorbid OSA

Given the goals of CBT-I to improve the overall sleep and daytime functioning of the patient, treating insomnia while recommended therapies for OSA like PAP are unutilized potentially limits the maximal benefits of therapy. With some patients, complementing CBT-I with interventions to address sources of PAP nonadherence—delivered before or following the core components targeting insomnia—may offer a practical adaptation with the most far-reaching impact in minimizing nocturnal sleep disruption and optimizing the quality of life.

Motivational enhancement

A primary assumption of motivational interviewing is that many individuals who engage in behaviors with adverse health consequences (e.g., tobacco use, alcohol consumption) often do not receive initial consultation in a state of readiness to begin changing their behavioral patterns (Miller & Rollnick, 2013). The benefits of behavioral change are often balanced by aspects of unhealthy behaviors that are reinforcing or viewed positively, which can create resistance that often disposes these individuals to be insensitive or even defensive when provided straightforward advice. Strategies in motivational interviewing take a different route to motivate behavioral change and are focused on helping patients negotiate ambivalence and articulate for themselves the reasons for concern and their arguments for increasing health-promoting behaviors. Dialogues in motivational interviewing strive to increase the importance of change from the patients' perspective while the consultant (e.g., behavioral health or medical provider) maintains an empathic, supportive, and nonjudgmental demeanor.

Brief applications of motivational interviewing, also referred to as motivational enhancement, are designed for use in medical settings with more time-sensitive contexts (e.g., primary care) while still targeting the key components of behavior change: (1) readiness to change, (2) perceived importance of changing or not changing (decisional balance), and (3) confidence in one's ability to change (self-efficacy; Miller & Rollnick, 2013). Motivational enhancement has been demonstrated to be an effective approach to reduce many health-incompatible behaviors including adolescent tobacco use (Colby et al., 1998) and alcohol use in individuals with a legal history of driving while impaired (Brown et al., 2010). Similarly, among patients with chronic diseases (e.g., asthma, HIV), motivational enhancement can be an effective strategy to increase engagement with treatment regimens (Borrelli, Riekert, Weinstein, & Rathier, 2007; Scharer et al., 2019). Motivational enhancement has been extensively studied as an intervention to increase adherence with PAP therapy, and found to be superior to standard care approaches (e.g., brief education groups) to increase PAP adherence (Aloia et al., 2001; Aloia, Arnedt, Strand, Millman, & Borrelli, 2013; Bakker et al., 2016).

Many patients may be referred for CBT-I who have been prescribed PAP but have discontinued use or demonstrate suboptimal adherence (use <4h/night, <5 nights/week). Among patients who endorse high levels of motivation to use PAP each night, insomnia symptoms have been identified as a primary barrier to regular use and perceived benefit (Ong et al., 2017). Among patients with COMISA who are starting on PAP at the same time they commence treatment for insomnia, motivational enhancement strategies have been successfully integrated with the components of

CBT-I to produce significant improvements in insomnia symptoms with greater adherence relative to PAP alone (Alessi et al., 2020). This seems to support that, in patients with OSA that are nonadherent with PAP, adapting CBT-I with content from motivational enhancement would be of benefit regardless of whether insomnia is the primary barrier to use or not.

Table 2 provides an example of the components to address during a brief (~45 min) motivational enhancement session adapted to facilitate

TABLE 2 Components of Motivational Enhancement to address suboptimal PAP adherence.

Component of motivational enhancement[a]	Example Strategy to Facilitate Intervention
Assessment and exploration	– Patient completes initial self-rating scales (0–10; 0 = none, 10 = very) regarding their: – *Motivation* to increase adherence (readiness to change) – *Knowledge* about OSA and PAP – *Importance* of treating OSA (decisional balance) – *Confidence* that they can use PAP during sleep (self-efficacy) – Therapist inquires about the reason for selecting each value
Information exchange	– Watch a short youtube.com video about OSA featuring a patient being evaluated, receiving their PAP, and discussing their perceived benefits. Solicit impressions (e.g., "Can you relate to the patient in the video?") – Elicit patients' symptoms of OSA and how this impacts them – If available, review and provide feedback on the patient's diagnostic PSG report (AHI severity, # of awakenings) – Dialogue with patient to enhance understanding of the physiology of OSA, risk factors, short- and long-term consequences, and available treatments (including PAP)
Enhance understanding of perceived benefits	– Elicit patient views on the disadvantages of treatment with PAP – Elicit patient views on advantages of treatment with PAP – Provide feedback about added benefits of increasing PAP use (i.e., with regard to sleep, health, daytime functioning)
(SMART) Goal setting	– Elicit long-term goals related to their PAP use (e.g., "100% PAP use during sleep after 6 weeks") – Elicit current barriers to achieving long-term goals (e.g., mask discomfort, uncertain how to use the humidifier, forgetfulness)

Continued

TABLE 2 Components of Motivational Enhancement to address suboptimal PAP adherence—cont'd

Component of motivational enhancement[a]	Example Strategy to Facilitate Intervention
	– Dialog to identify an "action plan" with short-term goals (e.g., will practice in vivo exposures daily, will refer to a sleep clinic for information on the device, will inform their spouse of adherence goals to help give reminders) that will support their progress *en route* to the long-term goal
Identify rewards	– Elicit from the patient the specific benefits they expect will result from increasing PAP adherence (i.e., for putting in the hard work; e.g., have more energy, improved relationship with bed partner)
Align with values	– Elicit patient perceptions of their current health and whether they have any goals for their future health (e.g., how they feel, their level of activity, etc.) – Provide feedback to highlight any discrepancies between current behavior and personal values regarding health (e.g., "do you feel that how much you are using the PAP right now gets in the way of your goal to be more active?") – Elicit from patient how increasing adherence to PAP will support their health goals

[a] *Aloia et al. (2013);* OSA, *obstructive sleep apnea;* PAP, *positive airway pressure;* PSG, *polysomnography;* AHI, *apnea/hypopnea index;* SMART, *specific, measurable, achievable, realistic, time-based (Locke & Latham, 1990).*

intrinsic motivation for behavior change (i.e., increase PAP use) based on theories that provide the framework and rationale for motivational interviewing (Miller & Rollnick, 2013). This is designed to be implemented as an adjunctive treatment component in patients with OSA that are referred for CBT-I with suboptimal adherence to PAP therapy. Selection of these six components (Assessment, Information Exchange, Enhancement of Perceived Benefits, Goal Setting, Identification of Rewards, Align with Values) is based on their inclusion in previous RCTs, whereby implementation across multiple sessions with a provider was observed to increase PAP use in patients with OSA (Aloia et al., 2001; Aloia et al., 2013; Bakker et al., 2016). Published effectiveness in patients with comorbid insomnia is not available, although similar modules (e.g., education, discussion of challenges/benefit) have been integrated with CBT-I in a recent trial with patients who received their PAP device after the second session (Alessi et al., 2020). The content is intended to be delivered during the first session of CBT-I in conjunction with a review of baseline sleep diaries and orientation to the goals and expected outcomes of CBT-I, where a natural transition can be made to discussing potential barriers to maximally benefitting from treatment (e.g., untreated OSA and effects on daytime functioning). However, integration at any point during the course of treatment should not be contraindicated, particularly if patients are adamant that they do not want to use PAP or would initially benefit from other components of CBT-I to address insomnia which impedes tolerance of PAP.

A detailed description of the process of motivational interviewing is beyond the scope of this chapter; readers are therefore recommended to review Miller and Rollnick (2013) for additional information as these techniques can be highly advantageous to optimize adherence with the components of CBT-I as well. Briefly, the first step of motivational enhancement is to gauge patients' readiness for change (i.e., motivation), knowledge about OSA and PAP, the perceived importance of treating their OSA at this time (i.e., decisional balance), and how confident they are that they can use PAP nightly during sleep (self-efficacy). The therapist then inquires as to why each rating was not higher (soliciting information on perceived barriers) or lower (soliciting information on perceived benefits), which will be integrated into dialogues with the successive modules. The remainder of the session is formatted as a series of feedback dialogues in which the therapist—maintaining a neutral, nonjudgmental tone—asks open-ended questions ("elicits"), shares information ("provides"), and follows-up with additional open-ended questions about the patient's reaction to the supplemented information (so the dynamic of the feedback dialogue is "Elicit-Provide-Elicit"; Miller & Rollnick, 2013). The remaining components are designed to enhance motivation (i.e., readiness to change) to increase PAP adherence, while the tangible outcome is the development of an "action plan" that the patient can use to start implementing toward their stated long-term goal for PAP use. For additional information on the application of motivational enhancement to increase PAP use, readers would benefit from reviewing the seminal description of this process by Aloia, Arnedt, Riggs, Hecht, and Borrelli (2004).

Systematic desensitization

Claustrophobia is a common form of specific phobia characterized by a marked, persistent, excessive, or unreasonable fear of restriction and/or fear of suffocation, which is expressed as extreme anxiety and panic in situations where an individual feels closed in or entrapped (Rachman & Taylor, 1993). A subsample of patients who inevitably reject PAP therapy attribute this to panic or claustrophobic reactions in response to wearing the mask and the delivery of pressurized air. Rates of PAP rejection attributable to claustrophobia from the first trial night up to 3 months range from 33% to 63% (Chasens, Pack, Maislin, Dinges, & Weaver, 2005; Edmonds et al., 2015). A handful of published RCTs of behavioral interventions using in vivo exposure (i.e., directly confronting a feared stimulus or situation) support this as an effective intervention to reduce symptoms of claustrophobia (Wiederhold & Bouchard, 2014).

In the implementation of a personalized action plan to increase PAP use for patients who have discontinued this therapy, some may require targeted strategies to reduce avoidance, enhance comfort, and promote tolerance and/or adaptive coping if they experience claustrophobia while using the device. Protocols have been adapted for the use of in vivo exposure in adults to reduce anxiety reactions to PAP and "decondition" patients to the sensations that are initially experienced as aversive, contained within a series of case reports (Edinger & Radtke, 1993; McCrae & Ingmundson, 2006) and larger case series (Means & Edinger, 2007). These protocols demonstrate that the use of graded in vivo exposures (i.e., gradually increasing exposure to the feared stimulus in successive approximations, beginning with less anxiety-inducing situations and proceeding iteratively through a personalized fear and avoidance hierarchy) can be effective in helping patients who experience claustrophobia/anxiety more gradually acclimate to the PAP to support nightly use. Systematic desensitization is an application of exposure therapy, which begins with relaxation training before the implementation of graded in vivo exposures to gradually counter-condition the association of anxiety with the feared stimulus (i.e., the PAP; Davison, 1968).

The use of graded exposure strategies following relaxation training is recommended to provide patients with an improved capacity to self-regulate any anxiety that is experienced in anticipation of, or when directly interacting with, the PAP device. Systematic desensitization should also include education (e.g., on behavioral models of anxiety, how avoidance of feared situations reinforces more avoidance and maintains anxiety over time by reducing tolerance to feared stimuli, the fight-or-flight response, and rationale for graded in vivo exposure to promote desensitization) to best facilitate acceptance of the premise of treatment given the paradoxical nature of intentionally placing oneself in stressful situations.

While there is not a standard protocol used to facilitate desensitization to PAP, a basic sequence might include (1) education, (2) relaxation skills training, (3) identifying the individual steps of the patient's graded exposure hierarchy, (4) goal setting, (5) at home practice, and (6) follow-up support (as a portion of successive CBT-I sessions). Integration of systematic desensitization with the components of motivational enhancement is recommended. However, given that heightened anxiety is incompatible with sleep, the need to implement systematic desensitization should be considered when organizing the treatment plan. Notably, relaxation training (e.g., diaphragmatic breathing) is often included as a supplementary component of CBT-I (to address hyperarousal). For patients who commence the core components of CBT-I before proceeding with motivational enhancement/desensitization in later sessions, an intuitive sequence may include the components of desensitization provided within the same session as would typically spend reviewing strategies to promote relaxation.

Table 3 provides a sample form with a list of possible graded in vivo exposures that might be used to develop patients' individualized fear and avoidance hierarchies. When introducing this, patients should be oriented to the Subjective Units of Discomfort Scale (SUDS; Wolpe & Lazarus, 1966) used to rate their anticipated level of anxiety for each

TABLE 3 Example fear and avoidance hierarchy of in vivo exposures used with systematic desensitization to address PAP-related claustrophobia

SUDS rating	Situation
________	1. Thinking about my PAP device
________	2. Imagining myself using the PAP device with the mask on
________	3. Looking at my PAP device
________	4. Sitting beside my PAP device while relaxing outside of the bedroom (e.g., watching television, reading)
________	5. Wearing just the mask while relaxing outside of the bedroom (e.g., watching television, reading)
________	6. Wearing the mask with the PAP device turned on while relaxing outside of the bedroom (e.g., watching television, reading)
________	7. Wearing just the mask with the PAP device turned off, relaxing in the bedroom
________	8. Wearing just the mask with the PAP device turned on, relaxing in the bedroom
________	9. Wearing the mask attached to the PAP device turned on, relaxing in the bedroom
________	10. Sleeping with the PAP device in the bedroom, turned on
________	11. Sleeping with the PAP device in the bedroom and turned on, mask and hose beside the pillow
________	12. Sleeping with the PAP device in the bedroom and turned on, wearing just the mask (unconnected)
________	13. Sleeping with the mask attached to the PAP, the device turned on

SUDS: Subjective units of discomfort (0–100; 100 = highest level of anxiety ever experienced).

situation (0–100; 100=highest level of anxiety ever experienced). Initial steps may contain exposure situations that involve little-to-no interaction with the PAP (e.g., sitting beside the PAP device while watching television), but may still produce anxiety for patients based on negative associations they have with the device (e.g., guilt about not using the device), or in anticipation of discomfort once they begin interacting with the PAP. Additionally, integration of imaginal (i.e., *in vitro*) exposures may also be incorporated in the initial steps of practice. When initiating at-home practice, patients are encouraged to start with a step rated at moderate anxiety (i.e., SUDS=40–60) and move through the hierarchy at their own pace, with instructions to spend at least 30–45 min each day practicing exposures. During each practice session, patients would remain in the same situation for 30–45 min or until anxiety in that situation decreases by at least 50%, when they can move to the next step in their fear and avoidance hierarchy for the remaining duration of practice.

To avoid reconditioning of bed with heightened anxiety, patients should be cautioned against introducing (or reintroducing) the PAP into the bed/bedroom until the use of the device promotes minimal sustained anxiety reaction in these situations. Given that multiple, brief sessions may be required to check-in on daily practice, it is recommended that an initial session be dedicated to facilitating steps 1–4 of the outline above, while portions of successive sessions in the CBT-I protocol be set aside to check in on progress with daily practice, troubleshoot any issues to implementation, and provide supportive encouragement.

Conclusion

The co-occurrence of insomnia and OSA is pervasive, and therefore commonly observed in patients referred for CBT-I. In the decades since the effectiveness of CBT-I was first demonstrated, clinicians have inevitably provided this treatment to manage insomnia in patients with comorbid OSA despite having limited, evidence-based guidance on expected treatment outcomes and other pertinent considerations. In many instances, concerns about adverse reactions to treatment (e.g., worsening daytime sleepiness, the risk for accidents) have informed recommendations to avoid CBT-I altogether, or forgo essential treatment components (e.g., SRT)—decisions that might have the effect of slowing treatment progress or attenuate the maximal benefits achievable from therapy. It is therefore exciting that emerging evidence from recent clinical trials is now available to inform clinical practice for the implementation of CBT-I within this subpopulation of patients with insomnia.

The current body of literature supports that CBT-I can be effectively and safely implemented in patients with insomnia and comorbid OSA.

However, an abundance of caution should always guide clinical judgments regarding potential risks and tolerability of the components selected for each patient. When providing CBT-I in patients with COMISA, clinicians are encouraged to prioritize patients' individual preferences for sequencing treatment components in conjunction with other interventions (e.g., PAP), particularly given that this has not been found to profoundly impact overall outcomes regarding insomnia. The degree to which treatment is adapted from what is considered a "standard" protocol of CBT-I may depend on whether patients' OSA is being effectively managed by medical therapies such as PAP, and how much adherence to these therapies is impeded by the presence of insomnia. In many instances, augmenting treatment-as-usual with additional OSA/PAP education, motivational enhancement, or systematic desensitization strategies—delivered before proceeding with other CBT-I components or integrated throughout the course of therapy—may provide the most comprehensive approach to optimally manage the symptoms and sequelae of both conditions.

References

Alessi, C. A., Fung, C. H., Dzierzewski, J. M., Fiorentino, L., Stepnowsky, C., Rodriguez Tapia, J. C., et al. (2020). Randomized controlled trial of an integrated approach to treating insomnia and improving use of positive airway pressure therapy in veterans with comorbid insomnia disorder and obstructive sleep apnea. *Sleep*, zsaa235.

Aloia, M. S., Arnedt, J. T., Riggs, R. L., Hecht, J., & Borrelli, B. (2004). Clinical management of poor adherence to CPAP: Motivational enhancement. *Behavioral Sleep Medicine, 2*(4), 205–222.

Aloia, M. S., Arnedt, J. T., Strand, M., Millman, R. P., & Borrelli, B. (2013). Motivational enhancement to improve adherence to positive airway pressure in patients with obstructive sleep apnea: A randomized controlled trial. *Sleep, 36*(11), 1655–1662.

Aloia, M. S., Di Dio, L., Ilniczky, N., Perlis, M. L., Greenblatt, D. W., & Giles, D. E. (2001). Improving compliance with nasal CPAP and vigilance in older adults with OSAHS. *Sleep & Breathing, 5*(1), 13–21.

American Academy of Sleep Medicine. (2014). *The International Classification of Sleep Disorders* (3rd Edition (ICSD-3). Dairen, IL: American Academy of Sleep Medicine.

Ancoli-Israel, S., & Martin, J. L. (2006). Insomnia and daytime napping in older adults. *Journal of Clinical Sleep Medicine, 2*(03), 333–342.

Antic, N. A., Catcheside, P., Buchan, C., Hensley, M., Naughton, M. T., Rowland, S., et al. (2011). The effect of CPAP in normalizing daytime sleepiness, quality of life, and neurocognitive function in patients with moderate to severe OSA. *Sleep, 34*(1), 111–119.

Ayas, N. T., Fitzgerald, J. M., Fleetham, J. A., White, D. P., Schulzer, M., Ryan, C. F., et al. (2006). Cost-effectiveness of continuous positive airway pressure therapy for moderate to severe obstructive sleep apnea/hypopnea. *Archives of Internal Medicine, 166*(9), 977–984.

Bakker, J. P., Wang, R., Weng, J., Aloia, M. S., Toth, C., Morrical, M. G., et al. (2016). Motivational enhancement for increasing adherence to CPAP: A randomized controlled trial. *Chest, 150*(2), 337–345.

Barbé, F., Durán-Cantolla, J., Capote, F., de la Peña, M., Chiner, E., Masa, J. F., et al. (2010). Long-term effect of continuous positive airway pressure in hypertensive patients with sleep apnea. *American Journal of Respiratory and Critical Care Medicine, 181*(7), 718–726.

Bastien, C. H., Vallières, A., & Morin, C. M. (2001). Validation of the Insomnia Severity Index as an outcome measure for insomnia research. *Sleep Medicine, 2*(4), 297–307.

Bianchi, M. T., Williams, K. L., Mckinney, S., & Ellenbogen, J. M. (2013). The subjective–objective mismatch in sleep perception among those with insomnia and sleep apnea. *Journal of Sleep Research, 22*(5), 557–568.

Bjornsdottir, E., Janson, C., Sigurdsson, J. F., Gehrman, P., Perlis, M., Juliusson, S., et al. (2013). Symptoms of insomnia among patients with obstructive sleep apnea before and after two years of positive airway treatment. *Sleep, 36*(12), 1901–1909.

Bjorvatn, B., Lehmann, S., Gulati, S., Aurlien, H., Pallesen, S., & Saxvig, I. W. (2015). Prevalence of excessive sleepiness is higher whereas insomnia is lower with greater severity of obstructive sleep apnea. *Sleep & Breathing, 19*(4), 1387–1393.

Bootzin, R. R. (1972). Stimulus control treatment for insomnia. *Proceedings of the American Psychological Association, 7*, 395–396.

Borrelli, B., Riekert, K. A., Weinstein, A., & Rathier, L. (2007). Brief motivational interviewing as a clinical strategy to promote asthma medication adherence. *Journal of Allergy and Clinical Immunology, 120*(5), 1023–1030.

Brown, T. G., Dongier, M., Ouimet, M. C., Tremblay, J., Chanut, F., Legault, L., et al. (2010). Brief motivational interviewing for DWI recidivists who abuse alcohol and are not participating in DWI intervention: A randomized controlled trial. *Alcoholism: Clinical and Experimental Research, 34*(2), 292–301.

Budhiraja, R., Parthasarathy, S., Drake, C. L., Roth, T., Sharief, I., Budhiraja, P., et al. (2007). Early CPAP use identifies subsequent adherence to CPAP therapy. *Sleep, 30*(3), 320–324.

Buysse, D. J., Ancoli-Israel, S., Edinger, J. D., Lichstein, K. L., & Morin, C. M. (2006). Recommendations for a standard research assessment of insomnia. *Sleep, 29*(9), 1155–1173.

Calik, M. W. (2016). Treatments for obstructive sleep apnea. *Journal of Clinical Outcomes Management, 23*(4), 181.

Carney, C. E., Buysse, D. J., Ancoli-Israel, S., Edinger, J. D., Krystal, A. D., Lichstein, K. L., et al. (2012). The consensus sleep diary: Standardizing prospective sleep self-monitoring. *Sleep, 35*(2), 287–302.

Centers for Medicare & Medicaid Services. (2016). *Positive Airway Pressure (PAP) devices: Complying with documentation and coverage requirements.* Baltimore, MD: U.S. Centers for Medicare & Medicaid Services. Medicare Learning Network Retrieved from: https://www.cms.gov/Outreach-and-Education/Medicare-Learning-Network-MLN/MLNProducts/Downloads/PAP-DocCvg-FactSheet-ICN905064-TextOnly.pdf.

Chasens, E. R., Pack, A. I., Maislin, G., Dinges, D. F., & Weaver, T. E. (2005). Claustrophobia and adherence to CPAP treatment. *Western Journal of Nursing Research, 27*(3), 307–321.

Chiu, H.-Y., Chang, L.-Y., Hsieh, Y.-J., & Tsai, P.-S. (2016). A meta-analysis of diagnostic accuracy of three screening tools for insomnia. *Journal of Psychosomatic Research, 87*, 85–92.

Chung, K. F. (2005). Insomnia subtypes and their relationships to daytime sleepiness in patients with obstructive sleep apnea. *Respiration, 72*(5), 460–465.

Colby, S. M., Monti, P. M., Barnett, N. P., Rohsenow, D. J., Weissman, K., Spirito, A., et al. (1998). Brief motivational interviewing in a hospital setting for adolescent smoking: A preliminary study. *Journal of Consulting and Clinical Psychology, 66*(3), 574.

Cvengros, J. A., Crawford, M. R., Manber, R., & Ong, J. C. (2015). The relationship between beliefs about sleep and adherence to behavioral treatment combined with meditation for insomnia. *Behavioral Sleep Medicine, 13*(1), 52–63.

Davison, G. C. (1968). Systematic desensitization as a counterconditioning process. *Journal of Abnormal Psychology, 73*(2), 91–99.

Dement, W. C. (2001). Reducing America's Sleep Debt. *Sleep Review, 2*, 10–15.

Eckert, D. J., White, D. P., Jordan, A. S., Malhotra, A., & Wellman, A. (2013). Defining phenotypic causes of obstructive sleep apnea: Identification of novel therapeutic targets. *American Journal of Respiratory and Critical Care Medicine, 188*(8), 996–1004.

Edinger, J. D., & Radtke, R. A. (1993). Use of in vivo desensitization to treat a patient's claustrophobic response to nasal CPAP. *Sleep, 16*(7), 678–680.

Edinger, J. D., Wohlgemuth, W. K., Radtke, R. A., Marsh, G. R., & Quillian, R. E. (2001). Cognitive behavioral therapy for treatment of chronic primary insomnia: A randomized controlled trial. *Journal of the American Medical Association, 285*(14), 1856–1864.

Edmonds, J. C., Yang, H., King, T. S., Sawyer, D. A., Rizzo, A., & Sawyer, A. M. (2015). Claustrophobic tendencies and continuous positive airway pressure therapy non-adherence in adults with obstructive sleep apnea. *Heart & Lung, 44*(2), 100–106.

Engleman, H. M., & Wild, M. R. (2003). Improving CPAP use by patients with the sleep apnoea/hypopnoea syndrome (SAHS). *Sleep Medicine Reviews, 7*(1), 81–99.

Espie, C. A., Inglis, S. J., Harvey, L., & Tessier, S. (2000). Insomniacs' attributions: Psychometric properties of the dysfunctional beliefs and attitudes about sleep scale and the sleep disturbance questionnaire. *Journal of Psychosomatic Research, 48*(2), 141–148.

Eysteinsdottir, B., Gislason, T., Pack, A. I., Benediktsdottir, B., Arnardottir, E. S., Kuna, S. T., et al. (2017). Insomnia complaints in lean patients with obstructive sleep apnea negatively affect positive airway pressure treatment adherence. *Journal of Sleep Research, 26*(2), 159–165.

Franklin, K. A., Anttila, H., Axelsson, S., Gislason, T., Maasilta, P., Myhre, K. I., et al. (2009). Effects and side-effects of surgery for snoring and obstructive sleep apnea: A systematic review. *Sleep, 32*(1), 27–36.

Fung, C. H., Martin, J. L., Josephson, K., Fiorentino, L., Dzierzewski, J. M., Jouldjian, S., et al. (2016). Efficacy of cognitive behavioral therapy for insomnia in older adults with occult sleep-disordered breathing. *Psychosomatic Medicine, 78*(5), 629.

Glidewell, R. N., Renn, B. N., Roby, E., & Orr, W. C. (2014). Predictors and patterns of insomnia symptoms in OSA before and after PAP therapy. *Sleep Medicine, 15*(8), 899–905.

Gooneratne, N. S., Gehrman, P. R., Nkwuo, J. E., Bellamy, S. L., Schutte-Rodin, S., Dinges, D. F., et al. (2006). Consequences of comorbid insomnia symptoms and sleep-related breathing disorder in elderly subjects. *Archives of Internal Medicine, 166*(16), 1732–1738.

Guest, J. F., Helter, M. T., Morga, A., & Stradling, J. R. (2008). Cost-effectiveness of using continuous positive airways pressure in the treatment of severe obstructive sleep apnoea/hypopnoea syndrome in the UK. *Thorax, 63*(10), 860–865.

Guilleminault, C. (1981). The arousal threshold: Sleep deprivation, sleep fragmentation, and obstructive sleep apnea syndrome. *Clinical Respiratory Physiology, 17*(3), 341–349.

Guilleminault, C. (1990). Benzodiazepines, breathing, and sleep. *The American Journal of Medicine, 88*(3), S25–S28.

Hayley, A. C., Williams, L. J., Venugopal, K., Kennedy, G. A., Berk, M., & Pasco, J. A. (2015). The relationships between insomnia, sleep apnoea and depression: Findings from the American National Health and Nutrition Examination Survey, 2005–2008. *The Australian and New Zealand Journal of Psychiatry, 49*(2), 156–170.

Hilditch, C. J., & McHill, A. W. (2019). Sleep inertia: Current insights. *Nature and Science of Sleep, 11*, 155.

Hoddes, E., Zarcone, V., Smyth, H., Phillips, R., & Dement, W. C. (1973). Quantification of sleepiness: A new approach. *Psychophysiology, 10*(4), 431–436.

Hwang, D. (2016). Monitoring progress and adherence with positive airway pressure therapy for obstructive sleep apnea: The roles of telemedicine and mobile health applications. *Sleep Medicine Clinics, 11*(2), 161–171.

Johns, M. W. (1991). A new method for measuring daytime sleepiness: The Epworth Sleepiness Scale. *Sleep, 14*(6), 540–545.

Kapur, V. K., Auckley, D. H., Chowdhuri, S., Kuhlmann, D. C., Mehra, R., Ramar, K., & Harrod, C. G. (2017). Clinical practice guideline for diagnostic testing for adult obstructive sleep apnea: An American Academy of Sleep Medicine clinical practice guideline. *Journal of Clinical Sleep Medicine, 13*(3), 479–504.

Kapur, V. K., Baldwin, C. M., Resnick, H. E., Gottlieb, D. J., & Nieto, F. J. (2005). Sleepiness in patients with moderate to severe sleep-disordered breathing. *Sleep, 28*(4), 472–478.

Krakow, B., Melendrez, D., Ferreira, E., Clark, J., Warner, T. D., Sisley, B., et al. (2001). Prevalence of insomnia symptoms in patients with sleep-disordered breathing. *Chest, 120*(6), 1923–1929.

Krakow, B., Melendrez, D., Lee, S. A., Warner, T. D., Clark, J. O., & Sklar, D. (2004). Refractory insomnia and sleep-disordered breathing: A pilot study. *Sleep & Breathing, 8*(1), 15–29.

Kribbs, N. B., Pack, A. I., Kline, L. R., Smith, P. L., Schwartz, A. R., Schubert, N. M., et al. (1993). Objective measurement of patterns of nasal CPAP use by patients with obstructive sleep apnea. *The American Review of Respiratory Disease, 147*(4), 887–895.

Kyle, S. D., Aquino, M. R. J., Miller, C. B., Henry, A. L., Crawford, M. R., Espie, C. A., et al. (2015). Towards standardisation and improved understanding of sleep restriction therapy for insomnia disorder: A systematic examination of CBT-I trial content. *Sleep Medicine Reviews, 23*, 83–88.

Kyle, S. D., Miller, C. B., Rogers, Z., Siriwardena, A. N., MacMahon, K. M., & Espie, C. A. (2014). Sleep restriction therapy for insomnia is associated with reduced objective total sleep time, increased daytime somnolence, and objectively impaired vigilance: Implications for the clinical management of insomnia disorder. *Sleep, 37*(2), 229–237.

Li, Z., Li, Y., Yang, L., Li, T., Lei, F., Vgontzas, A. N., et al. (2015). Characterization of obstructive sleep apnea in patients with insomnia across gender and age. *Sleep & Breathing, 19*(2), 723–727.

Lichstein, K. L. (1988). Sleep compression treatment of an insomnoid. *Behavior Therapy, 19*(4), 625–632.

Lichstein, K. L., Riedel, B. W., Lester, K. W., & Aguillard, R. N. (1999). Occult sleep apnea in a recruited sample of older adults with insomnia. *Journal of Consulting and Clinical Psychology, 67*(3), 405–410.

Lichstein, K. L., Thomas, S. J., Woosley, J. A., & Geyer, J. D. (2013). Co-occurring insomnia and obstructive sleep apnea. *Sleep Medicine, 14*(9), 824–829.

Locke, E. A., & Latham, G. P. (1990). *A theory of goal setting & task performance*. Englewood Cliffs, NJ, US: Prentice-Hall, Inc.

Manber, R., Bernert, R. A., Suh, S., Nowakowski, S., Siebern, A. T., & Ong, J. C. (2014). CBT for insomnia in patients with high and low depressive symptom severity: Adherence and clinical outcomes. *Focus, 12*(1), 90–98.

McCrae, C. S., & Ingmundson, P. T. (2006). Using graduated in vivo exposure to treat a claustrophobic response to nasal continuous positive airway pressure: Hispanic male veteran associates nasal mask with gas masks worn during combat. *Clinical Case Studies, 5*(1), 71–82.

Means, M. K., & Edinger, J. D. (2007). Graded exposure therapy for addressing claustrophobic reactions to continuous positive airway pressure: A case series report. *Behavioral Sleep Medicine, 5*(2), 105–116.

Means, M. K., Edinger, J. D., & Husain, A. M. (2004). CPAP compliance in sleep apnea patients with and without laboratory CPAP titration. *Sleep & Breathing, 8*(1), 7–14.

Mendes, M. S., & dos Santos, J. M. (2015). Insomnia as an expression of obstructive sleep apnea syndrome: The effect of treatment with nocturnal ventilatory support. *Revista Portuguesa de Pneumologia, 21*(4), 203–208.

Miller, W. R., & Rollnick, S. (2013). *Motivational interviewing: Helping people change* (3rd ed.). New York: Guilford Press.

Mysliwiec, V., Matsangas, P., Baxter, T., McGraw, L., Bothwell, N. E., & Roth, B. J. (2014). Comorbid insomnia and obstructive sleep apnea in military personnel: Correlation with polysomnographic variables. *Military Medicine, 179*(3), 294–300.

Ong, J. C., Crawford, M. R., Dawson, S. C., Fogg, L. F., Turner, A. D., Wyatt, J. K., et al. (2020). A randomized controlled trial of CBT-I and PAP for obstructive sleep apnea and comorbid insomnia: Main outcomes from the MATRICS study. *Sleep*, 1–10.

Ong, J. C., Crawford, M. R., Kong, A., Park, M., Cvengros, J. A., Crisostomo, M. I., et al. (2017). Management of obstructive sleep apnea and comorbid insomnia: A mixed-methods evaluation. *Behavioral Sleep Medicine*, *15*(3), 180–197.

Osman, A. M., Carter, S. G., Carberry, J. C., & Eckert, D. J. (2018). Obstructive sleep apnea: Current perspectives. *Nature and Science of Sleep*, *10*, 21–34.

Patel, S. R., White, D. P., Malhotra, A., Stanchina, M. L., & Ayas, N. T. (2003). Continuous positive airway pressure therapy for treating sleepiness in a diverse population with obstructive sleep apnea: Results of a meta-analysis. *Archives of Internal Medicine*, *163*(5), 565–571.

Persson, H. E., & Svanborg, E. (1996). Sleep deprivation worsens obstructive sleep apnea: Comparison between diurnal and nocturnal polysomnography. *Chest*, *109*(3), 645–650.

Philip, R., Catcheside, P., Stevens, D., Lovato, N., McEvoy, D., & Vakulin, A. (2017). Comorbid insomnia and sleep apnoea is associated with greater neurocognitive impairment compared with OSA alone. *Sleep Medicine*, *40*, e260.

Pieh, C., Bach, M., Popp, R., Jara, C., Crönlein, T., Hajak, G., et al. (2013). Insomnia symptoms influence CPAP compliance. *Sleep & Breathing*, *17*(1), 99–104.

Qaseem, A., Kansagara, D., Forciea, M. A., Cooke, M., & Denberg, T. D. (2016). Management of chronic insomnia disorder in adults: A clinical practice guideline from the American College of Physicians. *Annals of Internal Medicne*, *165*(2), 125–133.

Rachman, S., & Taylor, S. (1993). Analyses of claustrophobia. *Journal of Anxiety Disorders*, *7*(4), 281–291.

Rotenberg, B. W., Murariu, D., & Pang, K. P. (2016). Trends in CPAP adherence over twenty years of data collection: A flattened curve. *Journal of Otolaryngology - Head & Neck Surgery*, *45*(1), 1–9.

Sawyer, A. M., Gooneratne, N. S., Marcus, C. L., Ofer, D., Richards, K. C., & Weaver, T. E. (2011). A systematic review of CPAP adherence across age groups: Clinical and empiric insights for developing CPAP adherence interventions. *Sleep Medicine Reviews*, *15*(6), 343–356.

Scharer, J., Arnold, R., Wald, R., Nichols, J., Medoff, D., Himelhoch, S., et al. (2019). Personal approach to treatment choices for HIV (PATCH): Randomized controlled trial of a brief motivational enhancement intervention to improve medication adherence in persons with HIV. *AIDS and Behavior*, 1–10.

Schutte-Rodin, S., Broch, L., Buysse, D., Dorsey, C., & Sateia, M. (2008). Clinical guideline for the evaluation and management of chronic insomnia in adults. *Journal of Clinical Sleep Medicine*, *4*(5), 487–504.

Senaratna, C. V., Perret, J. L., Lodge, C. J., Lowe, A. J., Campbell, B. E., Matheson, M. C., … Dharmage, S. C. (2017). Prevalence of obstructive sleep apnea in the general population: A systematic review. *Sleep Medicine reviews*, *34*, 70–81.

Smith, M. T., Huang, M. I., & Manber, R. (2005). Cognitive behavior therapy for chronic insomnia occurring within the context of medical and psychiatric disorders. *Clinical Psychology Review*, *25*(5), 559–592.

Smith, S., Sullivan, K., Hopkins, W., & Douglas, J. (2004). Frequency of insomnia report in patients with obstructive sleep apnoea hypopnea syndrome (OSAHS). *Sleep Medicine*, *5*(5), 449–456.

Spielman, A. J., Saskin, P., & Thorpy, M. J. (1987). Treatment of chronic insomnia by restriction of time in bed. *Sleep*, *10*(1), 45–56.

Strollo, P. J., & Rogers, R. M. (1996). Obstructive sleep apnea. *New England Journal of Medicine*, *334*(2), 99–104.

Sullivan, C., Berthon-Jones, M., Issa, F., & Eves, L. (1981). Reversal of obstructive sleep apnoea by continuous positive airway pressure applied through the nares. *The Lancet*, *317*(8225), 862–865.

Sweetman, A., Lack, L. C., Catcheside, P. G., Antic, N. A., Chai-Coetzer, C. L., Smith, S. S., et al. (2017). Developing a successful treatment for co-morbid insomnia and sleep apnoea. *Sleep Medicine Reviews*, *33*, 28–38.

Sweetman, A., Lack, L., Catcheside, P. G., Antic, N. A., Smith, S., Chai-Coetzer, C. L., et al. (2019). Cognitive and behavioral therapy for insomnia increases the use of continuous positive airway pressure therapy in obstructive sleep apnea participants with comorbid insomnia: A randomized clinical trial. *Sleep*, *42*(12), 1–12.

Sweetman, A., Lack, L., Lambert, S., Gradisar, M., & Harris, J. (2017). Does comorbid obstructive sleep apnea impair the effectiveness of cognitive and behavioral therapy for insomnia? *Sleep Medicine*, *39*, 38–46.

Sweetman, A., Lack, L., McEvoy, R. D., Antic, N. A., Smith, S., Chai-Coetzer, C. L., et al. (2020). Cognitive behavioural therapy for insomnia reduces sleep apnoea severity: A randomised controlled trial. *ERJ Open Research*, *6*(2), 1–9.

Sweetman, A., Lack, L., McEvoy, R. D., Catcheside, P. G., Antic, N. A., Chai-Coetzer, C. L., et al. (2020). Effect of depression, anxiety, and stress symptoms on response to cognitive behavioral therapy for insomnia in patients with comorbid insomnia and sleep apnea: A randomized controlled trial. *Journal of Clinical Sleep Medicine*, 8944.

Sweetman, A., McEvoy, R. D., Smith, S., Catcheside, P. G., Antic, N. A., Chai-Coetzer, C. L., et al. (2020). The effect of cognitive and behavioral therapy for insomnia on week-to-week changes in sleepiness and sleep parameters in patients with comorbid insomnia and sleep apnea: A randomized controlled trial. *Sleep*, *43*(7), 1–13.

Tasbakan, M. S., Gunduz, C., Pirildar, S., & Basoglu, O. K. (2018). Quality of life in obstructive sleep apnea is related to female gender and comorbid insomnia. *Sleep & Breathing*, *22*(4), 1013–1020.

Vincent, N., Lewycky, S., & Finnegan, H. (2008). Barriers to engagement in sleep restriction and stimulus control in chronic insomnia. *Journal of Consulting and Clinical Psychology*, *76*(5), 820–828.

Wallace, D. M., Sawyer, A. M., & Shafazand, S. (2018). Comorbid insomnia symptoms predict lower 6-month adherence to CPAP in US veterans with obstructive sleep apnea. *Sleep & Breathing*, *22*(1), 5–15.

Wallace, D. M., Vargas, S. S., Schwartz, S. J., Aloia, M. S., & Shafazand, S. (2013). Determinants of continuous positive airway pressure adherence in a sleep clinic cohort of South Florida Hispanic veterans. *Sleep & Breathing*, *17*(1), 351–363.

Wallace, D. M., & Wohlgemuth, W. K. (2019). Predictors of Insomnia Severity Index profiles in United States veterans with obstructive sleep apnea. *Journal of Clinical Sleep Medicine*, *15*(12), 1827–1837.

Wang, S.-H., Chen, W.-S., Tang, S.-E., Lin, H.-C., Peng, C.-K., Chu, H.-T., et al. (2019). Benzodiazepines associated with acute respiratory failure in patients with obstructive sleep apnea. *Frontiers in Pharmacology*, *9*, 1–9.

Weaver, T. E., Maislin, G., Dinges, D. F., Bloxham, T., George, C. F. P., Greenberg, H., et al. (2007). Relationship between hours of CPAP use and achieving normal levels of sleepiness and daily functioning. *Sleep*, *30*(6), 711–719.

Wickwire, E. M., Smith, M. T., Birnbaum, S., & Collop, N. A. (2010). Sleep maintenance insomnia complaints predict poor CPAP adherence: A clinical case series. *Sleep Medicine*, *11*(8), 772–776.

Wiederhold, B. K., & Bouchard, S. (2014). Claustrophobia: Efficacy and treatment protocols. In *Advances in virtual reality and anxiety disorders* (pp. 145–162). San Diego, California, US: Springer.

Wolpe, J., & Lazarus, A. A. (1966). *Behavior therapy techniques*. New York: Pergamon.

Yang, C.-M., Liao, Y.-S., Lin, C.-M., Chou, S.-L., & Wang, E.-N. (2011). Psychological and behavioral factors in patients with comorbid obstructive sleep apnea and insomnia. *Journal of Psychosomatic Research*, *70*(4), 355–361.

Ye, L., Pien, G. W., Ratcliffe, S. J., Björnsdottir, E., Arnardottir, E. S., Pack, A. I., et al. (2014). The different clinical faces of obstructive sleep apnoea: A cluster analysis. *European Respiratory Journal*, *44*(6), 1600–1607.

Young, T., Skatrud, J., & Peppard, P. E. (2004). Risk factors for obstructive sleep apnea in adults. *Journal of the American Medical Association*, *291*(16), 2013–2016.

Zhang, Y., Ren, R., Lei, F., Zhou, J., Zhang, J., Wing, Y.-K., et al. (2019). Worldwide and regional prevalence rates of co-occurrence of insomnia and insomnia symptoms with obstructive sleep apnea: A systematic review and meta-analysis. *Sleep Medicine Reviews*, *45*, 1–17.

CHAPTER

3

CBT-I for patients with phase disorders or insomnia with circadian misalignment

Marissa A. Evans[a] *and Brant P. Hasler*[b]

[a]Department of Psychology, University of Pittsburgh, Pittsburgh, PA, United States, [b]Department of Psychiatry, University of Pittsburgh, Pittsburgh, PA, United States

Case study

Jeff is a 30-year-old male who sought services from our sleep clinic for his long-standing difficulties with initiating and maintaining sleep. He believes these symptoms have been present his entire life but became more apparent when he had to wake up earlier than he preferred to during high school and college. Jeff expresses a wistful desire to be a morning person but reports a history consistent with being a night owl. Beginning in high school, he found it difficult to get up on time for classes, achieved insufficient sleep, and felt very sleepy during the day. Jeff described falling asleep as a "lonely experience" and a "battle." As a result, he often watches videos or reads blog posts on his laptop in bed for hours before he is "ready to put the effort" into going to sleep. Jeff reports that it is particularly difficult to fall asleep when he goes to bed before midnight. Even when he goes to bed after 2:30 am and he feels "super sleepy," Jeff still struggles to fall asleep in less than 1–2h, noting that his sleepiness dissipates and his "mind starts wandering" upon turning off his laptop. Jeff also reports difficulty getting up in time for work during the week, and he sometimes goes back to bed after his first meeting at 9:30 am. On weekends, Jeff sleeps in until noon or later to catch up on sleep loss from the work week. Jeff endorses anxiety and depressive symptoms, which are

https://doi.org/10.1016/B978-0-12-822872-2.00004-9

especially apparent to him when trying to fall asleep. Jeff has tried sleep medications with adverse effects (e.g., feeling "very hazy" in the morning).

Jeff is not currently taking any medications and has no other medical conditions. He denies the use of caffeine, but reports smoking ~7 cigarettes per day, and that he regularly drinks alcohol on weekends, typically 5–6 drinks per night. Jeff reports that the alcohol does not help him to fall asleep.

Jeff's symptom presentation indicated to us that we should evaluate him for a possible circadian phase disorder or insomnia with circadian misalignment.

Introduction

Circadian rhythms are cyclic physiological changes that occur in the brain and body across a 24-h period and are observable in core body temperature, blood pressure, and sleep-wake timing rhythms. Although our endogenous circadian rhythms are approximately 24.2h (Czeisler & Gooley, 2007), we entrain to the 24-h light-dark cycle each day, resulting in a daily resetting of the endogenous rhythms to align with external schedules. Misalignment between endogenous sleep-wake rhythms and exogenous demands on sleep-wake rhythms (due to work, school, or social calendars) can result in circadian rhythm sleep-wake disorders (CRSWD; American Academy of Sleep Medicine, 2014). Individuals with misaligned sleep-wake timing experience impairments in functioning at work (Folkard & Tucker, 2003) and school (Gaultney, 2010), and misalignment is associated with depression (Abe et al., 2011), substance use (Hasler et al., 2017), cardiovascular events (Vyas et al., 2012), and premature mortality (Knutson & von Schantz, 2018). Therefore, it is critical to identify treatments for individuals with misaligned sleep-wake timing to improve their daily functioning, as well as their morbidity and mortality risk.

Cognitive-behavioral therapy for insomnia (CBT-I) is a frontline, evidence-based treatment for patients with insomnia (Qaseem et al., 2016). Although CBT-I includes consideration of circadian factors, the core CBT-I instructions are aimed at behavioral modification of sleep timing rather than directly targeting circadian rhythms; thus, it may be appropriate to modify and adapt CBT-I for individuals with circadian misalignment. This chapter provides an overview of how this might be accomplished.

The first section of this chapter discusses the assessment of phase disorders in the clinic, including diagnostic criteria, differential diagnosis, and clinical assessment. The second section introduces modifications (chronotherapeutics: bright light therapy, exogenous melatonin, and blue-filtering glasses) and adaptations to CBT-I and brief behavioral treatment of insomnia (BBT-I, Troxel, Germain, & Buysse, 2012) for individuals who evidence circadian misalignment, whether or not they meet criteria for a full-blown circadian rhythm sleep-wake disorder (CRSWD).

This chapter is based on the extant literature and our clinical experiences, which are necessarily more anecdotal. Our goal for this chapter is to be useful for clinicians who work with these patients, as well as researchers who may test these questions. We hope that increased attention to circadian rhythm issues in both clinical and research contexts will lead to needed advances in our understanding of the etiology, pathophysiology, proper assessment, and effective treatment of circadian rhythm sleep-wake problems.

Assessment of phase disorders

According to the International Classification of Sleep Disorders-Third Edition (ICSD-3), there are seven CRSWDs, which are characterized by (a) a chronic or recurrent pattern of sleep-wake disruption due primarily to an alteration of the circadian timing system or a misalignment between internal circadian rhythm and the sleep-wake schedule required by the physical environment or work schedule; (b) the circadian rhythm disruption leads to excessive sleepiness, insomnia symptoms, or both; (c) the sleep-wake cycle disturbances cause significant distress or impairment (American Academy of Sleep Medicine, 2014).

In this chapter, we focus on the assessment and treatment of phase disorders: delayed sleep-wake phase disorder (DSWPD) and advanced sleep-wake phase disorder (ASWPD). We will use the term "phase disorder" to refer to an individual who meets full diagnostic criteria for DSWPD or ASWPD, and the terms "phase issues" or "circadian misalignment" to refer to an individual who may not meet full diagnostic criteria for a phase disorder but reports symptoms that are suggestive of a discrepancy between exogenous and endogenous rhythms. Although we acknowledge that most or all CRSWDs may benefit from attending to cognitive-behavioral factors, individuals with phase issues stand out for their prevalence among patients reporting insomnia complaints (Kim, Lee, & Duffy, 2013; Magee, Marbas, Wright, Rajaratnam, & Broussard, 2016) and arguably, appropriateness for treatment within the CBT-I/BBT-I model. We will briefly discuss treatment considerations for other CRSWDS at the end of this chapter.

Diagnostic criteria for DSWPD and ASWPD

Diagnostic assessment of DSWPD and ASWPD is warranted when there is a delay or advance in the phase of the major sleep period in relation to the desired/required sleep time with symptoms present for at least 3 months, symptoms are observed for at least seven days (and preferably 14 days) using a sleep log or actigraphy, and cannot be better explained by any other sleep, psychiatric, or medical disorder (American Academy of Sleep Medicine, 2014).

Phase disorders are assumed to be driven by a mismatch between the desired/required sleep schedule and the central circadian clock. However, inadequate access to clinically feasible and/or sufficiently robust circadian biomarkers (Dijk & Duffy, 2020; Duffy et al., 2021) has led to the present emphasis of the diagnostic criteria on sleep timing and symptoms, requiring the clinician to extrapolate from the observed patient presentation to identify the phase disorder. Moreover, some evidence suggests that half of the individuals who meet the criteria for DSWPD based on a clinical interview do not have a delayed *circadian* phase (Micic, Lovato, Ferguson, Burgess, & Lack, 2020; Murray et al., 2017; Rahman, Kayumov, Tchmoutina, & Shapiro, 2009), and therefore, the tendency toward late sleep-wake timing may be driven by behavior and/or altered homeostatic sleep drive. Thus, there is an increasing realization that current assessment guidance is insufficient, due to poorly understood etiology and pathophysiology, infrequent assessment of circadian phase for diagnosis of phase disorders, and inconsistent operationalization of phase disorders across clinics and research groups (Duffy et al., 2021).

An estimated 10% of adult and 16% of adolescent patients who visit the sleep disorder clinic may meet the criteria for a CRSWD (Kim et al., 2013). Using self-reported bedtimes, waketimes, chronotype, and desire to change sleep schedule to infer prevalence of phase disorders, one study of adults reported that the prevalence of ASWPD ranged from 0.25% to 7.13% and the prevalence of DSWPD ranged from 1.51 to 8.90% depending on the definition (Paine, Fink, Gander, & Warman, 2014). Notably, this survey provides a general estimate of prevalence but was not based on rigorous clinical interviews. Moreover, it may be that the prevalence of ASWPD is underestimated because an advanced sleep schedule is less likely to interfere with obligations or be associated with clinical distress (Duffy et al., 2021). Taken as a whole, however, the extant data suggest that phase disorders affect a substantial proportion of the general population, and more specifically the patient population visiting a sleep disorder clinic.

Although the ICSD-3 provides helpful diagnostic information, it is critical to recognize that phase disorders, like other diagnostic categories of psychopathology (Haslam, Holland, & Kuppens, 2012), may be better characterized along dimensions. The criteria for phase disorders do not provide strict temporal cut-offs for what constitutes "advanced" and "delayed" sleep-wake patterns, but rather that "habitual sleep-wake timing is advanced [or delayed], usually by more than 2h, relative to conventional or socially acceptable sleep timing" (American Academy of Sleep Medicine, 2014), which requires the clinician to determine "convention." Thus, the phase disorders may represent continuous dimensions rather than having natural clinical cut-offs. Future research might test the benefits of varying clinical cut-offs and how that affects treatment course or health outcomes to improve specificity. For now, clinicians should keep this dimensionality in mind, and consider the diagnosis and treatment of a phase disorder in patients who broadly meet criteria and report significant clinical impairment or distress. We consider chronotherapeutic approaches in any patients reporting insomnia with circadian misalignment, regardless of whether they meet full criteria for a phase disorder.

Defining "conventional" sleep-wake timing may vary across age groups. Epidemiological (Roenneberg et al., 2007) and meta-analytic (Evans et al., 2021) studies have shown that a preference for evening chronotype and later sleep timing are more common during adolescence and young adulthood, whereas a preference for morning chronotype and earlier sleep timing is more common during adulthood. These lifespan changes are also supported by experimental studies of biological rhythms shifting later during adolescence (Carskadon, Vieira, & Acebo, 1993) and earlier in older adulthood (Carrier, Paquet, Morettini, & Touchette, 2002; Dijk & Duffy, 1999). Clinicians should be aware of these developmentally normative patterns, and evaluate for circadian misalignment among those individuals whose sleep-wake patterns cause clinically significant distress or impairment.

Differential diagnosis

There is substantial symptom overlap between insomnia and phase disorders. This overlap exists because insomnia is a diagnostic criterion of phase disorders (American Academy of Sleep Medicine, 2014), and insomnia-related processes (conditioned arousal) may develop secondary to phase disorders. Additionally, individuals diagnosed with DSWPD based on behavioral sleep-wake patterns may not demonstrate a delayed circadian phase (Murray et al., 2017; Rahman et al., 2009), and individuals with insomnia may show evidence of circadian misalignment but do not meet the full criteria for a phase disorder (Lack, Lovato, & Micic, 2017; Lack & Wright, 2007). We assert that it is therefore important to assess for circadian misalignment in every patient presenting with insomnia symptoms.

Differential diagnosis, to the extent that it is possible given symptom overlap, is important under the assumption that different pathologies may respond better to different treatments. One potentially useful distinguishing feature from insomnia is that when an individual with a phase disorder sleeps during their preferred sleep-wake window, symptoms are improved (American Academy of Sleep Medicine, 2014), though may not be fully relieved. Thus, asking about how a patient sleeps during periods without external demands (e.g., vacation) may be helpful.

Another potentially useful differential is that excessive daytime sleepiness is more prominent in the morning for DSWPD (Gradisar, Smits, & Bjorvatn, 2014) and the evening for ASWPD (Barion & Zee, 2007), whereas among insomnia patients there should be a less robust circadian pattern to daytime sleepiness. Moreover, individuals with phase disorders frequently report excessive daytime sleepiness (Gradisar et al., 2011), whereas many patients with insomnia deny significant daytime sleepiness (but instead report prominent daytime fatigue; Riedel & Lichstein, 2000).

Individuals with DSWPD may experience difficulty falling asleep (homeostatic sleep drive not yet sufficiently high and the biological clock is signaling wakefulness) and waking up (homeostatic sleep drive remains high and the clock is signaling sleep), with less difficulty maintaining sleep. However, individuals with DSWPD may also develop sleep maintenance issues due to a long-standing history of disregarding phase preferences—going to bed before the individual is sleepy, staying in bed when unable to sleep, and feeling frustrated and/or anxious, and thereby developing conditioned arousal. Likewise, while the prototypical symptom profile for individuals with ASWPD includes substantial difficulty staying awake until the desired bedtime (biological clock is signaling sleep) and with early morning awakenings (sleep drive is low and the clock is signaling wakefulness), sleep maintenance problems can be further exacerbated by staying in bed later than the clock's signal for wakefulness, and thereby developing conditioned arousal.

Returning to the case presented at the beginning of the chapter, Jeff reports that it typically takes him a minimum of 60–120 min to fall asleep (even when retiring well after midnight) and describes that he drifts in and out of sleep for the first half of the night. Jeff reports that after 6 am, he sleeps more soundly (at least on nondrinking nights). Based on his intake interview, these sleep maintenance issues appear to have emerged over time, plausibly developing as a consequence of a long-standing (i.e., over 20 years) history of anxiety and frustration surrounding his sleep experience. Thus, Jeff presents with both phase issues (sleeps better when he goes to bed later) as well as conditioned arousal (his sleepiness appears to dissipate once he retires to bed and/or he turns off his laptop to go to sleep).

In addition to the effects of delayed phase and conditioned arousal, Jeff's difficulty initiating sleep may be in part due to insufficient homeostatic sleep drive at bedtime. Attending to the other end of the sleep bout can help disentangle these contributing factors. Jeff reports that upon awakening, he typically feels sleepy, depressed, anxious, and has low energy, and notes that this can persist for 1–2h after arising. Notably, Jeff reports that his alertness generally improves later in the day and that he functions best in the late evening and night. Taken together, this pattern suggests delayed circadian rhythms of sleep and alertness, although homeostatic factors remain plausible (and likely).

We have reviewed the defining clinical features of phase disorders. We have also summarized both research evidence and clinical experience supporting the notion that it can be challenging for a clinician to determine an appropriate clinical cut-off and to distinguish these disorders from insomnia. Thus, again we assert that circadian misalignment should be evaluated among all insomnia patients.

Assessment tools

There are several assessment tools that can supplement the clinical interview to evaluate phase disorders or circadian misalignment which include sleep diary, measures of chronotype, wrist actigraphy, and, for some clinics, salivary melatonin.

Sleep diary

The ICSD-3 recommends a minimum of seven, preferably 14 days, of sleep diary data for the diagnosis of CRSWDs (American Academy of Sleep Medicine, 2014). In our clinic, we generally endeavor to get at least 14 days of sleep diary data to capture at least two weekends (in case one weekend is atypical for the patient). Sleep diaries have the advantage of a prospective collection of sleep behavior, including not only timing and regularity but also whether patients' difficulty with sleep initiation and wake-up times occurs only on nights with earlier/later sleep timing.

For the assessment of circadian phase issues, we often employ a visual sleep log that includes 14 rows for each 24-h day/night and columns that are blocks of time in 30-min increments. Patients are instructed to use a down arrow for when they go to bed, a solid horizontal line for when they are asleep, a dashed horizontal line for when they experience fragmented sleep, no horizontal line for when they are awake, and an up arrow to indicate when they get out of bed. This sleep log design allows the clinician to easily observe shifts in sleep timing, along with any concomitant changes in duration or continuity, over a 14-day timeframe.

Sleep timing from sleep diaries may be useful for estimating the circadian phase; diary-based sleep timing predicts circadian phase based on dim light melatonin onset (DLMO) to within 1 hr in the majority (74%–80%) of individuals (Burgess & Eastman, 2005; Crowley, Acebo, Fallone, & Carskadon, 2006). Sleep diaries are more strongly correlated with DLMO when individuals are sleeping on their desired sleep schedule (Burgess & Eastman, 2005), which among adolescents manifests in stronger associations between diary and DLMO during the summer compared to during the school year (Crowley et al., 2006). Thus, it may be useful for patients to complete sleep diaries when they can select their sleep-wake schedule for a more accurate derivation of DLMO while being mindful that symptoms for individuals with potential phase disorders may improve during this time.

Chronotype

The ICSD-3 also recommends, though does not require, the use of global measures of chronotype (typically based on the self-report of sleep timing on days unconstrained by other schedule obligations) or morningness-eveningness (which assess preference for the relative timing of sleep and activity). Patients with extreme scores on these questionnaires may alert the clinician to a possible phase disorder, which can then be evaluated further. Widely used measures for adults include the Munich Chronotype Questionnaire (MCTQ; Roenneberg et al., 2007; Roenneberg, Wirz-Justice, & Merrow, 2003), Morningness-Eveningness Questionnaire (MEQ; Horne & Östberg, 1976), and Composite Scale of Morningness (CSM; Smith, Reilly, & Midkiff, 1989). Each measure has adaptations for children (Morningness-Eveningness Scale for Children, Carskadon et al., 1993; MCTQ for Children, Roenneberg, 2015; Children's Chronotype Questionnaire, Werner, Lebourgeois, Geiger, & Jenni, 2009). In our clinic, we prefer administering the CSM, as 14 days of sleep diaries largely supplants the MCTQ, and our anecdotal experience is that the CSM is quicker and easier to complete than the MEQ.

Chronotype scores are only roughly predictive of circadian phase (within a 4-h range of DLMO; Kantermann, Sung, & Burgess, 2015) and thus should be used with caution when developing precise timing recommendations for chronotherapeutics. Other limitations of these chronotype measures are that they may be biased by recent shifts in behaviors, and/or they may reflect social desirability. For example, Jeff reported symptoms consistent with a delayed sleep schedule but he insisted that he was a morning person because he preferred to wake up early and he viewed morningness as being in line with societal mores.

Chronotype measures are easy, inexpensive, and informative for the clinician and represent a low burden for the patient. They can provide insight into patients' timing preferences or tendencies that may be obscured when patients have obligations that influence their sleep-wake schedules on both weekdays and weekends. Furthermore, there is some evidence that changes to chronotype may be clinically meaningful. In a study of BBT-I, individuals who increased their preference for morningness per the CSM experienced a decrease in depressive symptoms and an increase in sleep quality and positive affect (Hasler, Buysse, & Germain, 2016).

Given the current evidence, we would recommend these questionnaires be used as a necessary but not sufficient diagnostic tool. If a full chronotype/morningness-eveningness questionnaire is not available, we find it useful to ask patients about their history (particularly starting in high school) of being more of a morning lark or night owl.

Actigraphy

The ICSD-3 recommends the use of actigraphy "whenever possible" (American Academy of Sleep Medicine, 2014), and AASM clinical practice guidelines states that actigraphy is *suggested* (Smith et al., 2018) for the assessment of phase disorders. Actigraphy provides a behavioral assessment of sleep-wake patterns via analysis of wrist movements. Actigraphy is reliable and ecologically valid, as the assessment occurs in the patient's naturalistic environment and is not entirely reliant on reported experience. Actigraphy assessment of sleep midpoint, waketime (Burgess et al., 2003), or ambulatory light levels in conjunction with activity (Stone et al., 2019; Woelders, Beersma, Gordijn, Hut, & Wams, 2017) can be used to predict DLMO values to within ~1 hr. A newly available open-access website (www.predictDLMO.com) allows clinicians and researchers to upload activity and light data from actigraphs to calculate a predicted DLMO based on the Kronauer algorithm (Cheng et al., 2021).

The AASM clinical guidelines state that while actigraphy may be more objective and a lower burden than sleep diaries, the research evidence is limited, with only six studies comparing actigraphy to polysomnography or sleep diaries for assessment and treatment of CRSWDs (Smith et al., 2018). Therefore, actigraphy may be a particularly useful assessment tool of CRSWDs for patients who have difficulty completing a daily sleep diary.

When research-grade actigraphs are not available, patients' commercial sleep trackers may be of value. While the accuracy of such devices remains questionable in some models (Kubala et al., 2020), the technology is fast improving, increasingly rivaling research-grade actigraphs (e.g., Chinoy et al., 2021; Hamill et al., 2020). Regardless of the accuracy of assessing sleep continuity or sleep stages, our anecdotal experience is that commercial sleep trackers can be useful for monitoring sleep timing and regularity. Although concerns about "orthosomnia" (Baron, Abbott, Jao, Manalo, & Mullen, 2017) should not be overlooked, consistent with the

CBT-I goal of giving patients the tools to manage their sleep, commercial sleep trackers provide an objective means for patients to monitor their sleep (ideally in combination with sleep logs) long after they have completed active treatment in the clinic.

Dim light melatonin onset (DLMO)

DLMO is generally considered the gold standard for measuring the circadian phase in humans (Dijk & Duffy, 2020). DLMO can be assessed using saliva sampling every 30–60 min starting in the evening and continuing until an hour or two after habitual bedtime. Although DLMO occurs, on average, 2–3 h before habitual bedtime, the alignment to bedtime can vary widely (Burgess & Fogg, 2008), particularly in individuals with DSPWD (Murray et al., 2017), and can occur after habitual bedtime in some individuals. Assessing melatonin is encouraged by the ICSD-3 but is not necessary for the diagnosis of a CRSWD (American Academy of Sleep Medicine, 2014).

Obtaining an accurate estimate of DLMO can be challenging among individuals with DSWPD because they experience greater night-to-night variability in sleep-wake timing resulting in larger shifts in DLMO relative to controls (Burgess, Park, Wyatt, Rizvydeen, & Fogg, 2017). Moreover, as noted above, only about half of DSWPD patients demonstrate a relative delay in DLMO (Micic et al., 2020; Murray et al., 2017; Rahman et al., 2009). This heterogeneity may suggest differential treatment strategies, as the individuals with DSWPD without circadian delay may not benefit from chronotherapeutics designed to shift the clock. Treatment studies for DSWPD have not examined whether there is differential response as a function of the DLMO group.

DLMO can be difficult to assess in the clinic. To our knowledge, two clinics in the United States—Northwestern Center for Circadian Sleep Medicine and Brigham and Women's Hospital Circadian Disorders Clinic—are assessing DLMO in patients with suspected phase disorders. The clinic provides instructions and a collection kit for the patient to collect saliva samples at-home, which is feasible and reliable (Pullman, Roepke, & Duffy, 2012), particularly when the collection kit is enhanced with tools to monitor adherence to sample timing instructions (Burgess, Park, Wyatt, & Fogg, 2016). Then, the patient sends their collection kit directly to the assaying lab and pays for the cost of assessment out of pocket. Assessing DLMO can clarify the underlying mechanism of the observed phase disorder (circadian delay or not), and, importantly, provide precise phase information for the timing of chronotherapeutics. When using DLMO for diagnosis and/or treatment timing, we recommend consideration of the day of the week when collecting DLMO, as weekday-weekend shifts can be substantive even outside the context of DSWPD patients (e.g., up to 3 h in a sample of 18- to 22-year-old drinkers;

Hasler, Bruce, Scharf, Ngari, & Clark, 2019) and thus may be mistimed if initiating treatment on a different day of the week than when the phase was assessed.

An emerging option for assaying biological rhythms is via blood samples, using machine learning to identify circadian phase biomarkers that are predictive of external or biological (DLMO) clock time. One to two blood samples (collected up to 12h apart) have been shown to match within 1 (Wittenbrink, Kunz, & Kramer, 2018) to 2h (Braun et al., 2018; Laing et al., 2017) of DLMO or external clock time. While a promising area, the precision of these methods in populations experiencing circadian misalignment remains uncertain (Dijk & Duffy, 2020), blood draws 12h apart may not be clinically feasible, and thus the extent to which these assessments will be useful for informing the diagnosis of a CRSWD remains to be evaluated.

We have reviewed various assessment methods for diagnosing phase disorders and/or subthreshold circadian misalignment, each with its advantages and disadvantages. While these assessment tools are informative, in isolation none is necessary or sufficient to diagnose phase disorders; these tools need to be used in conjunction with a clinical interview and a clinician's expertise to determine if the individual meets the criteria for diagnosis of a phase disorder or subthreshold circadian misalignment.

Clinical interview

As the clinician, there are some key observations that suggest a phase issue may be present: (1) difficulties with falling asleep, waking up, or staying awake are time-dependent; (2) on free days, the patient shifts to a particularly later (or earlier) sleep schedule and experiences some symptom improvement; (3) patient has a pattern of insufficient sleep duration on work/free days and extended sleep bouts on free days, has difficulty getting up in the morning and/or excessive daytime sleepiness, and referring providers may describe as "hypersomnia" (this latter symptom is specific to patients with DSWPD). On occasion, referred patients initially have a primary complaint of hypersomnia but are later more appropriately diagnosed with DSWPD. Our impression across multiple cases is that patients (and nonsleep providers) focus on the salient features of having extended sleep once or twice per week, difficulty waking up even with multiple alarms, and substantial daytime sleepiness, but are less attentive to the fact that their average total sleep time across the week is often within the normal range, and their daytime sleepiness tends to dissipate later in the evening.

For Jeff, his difficulty falling asleep is time-dependent, and his difficulty with waking up seems to be a combination of homeostatic sleep drive (excess sleep debt) and circadian (preference for later wake times) factors. Jeff sleeps better on nights when he goes to bed and wakes up later. Jeff demonstrates extended sleep bouts on the weekends when he does not set an alarm and can sleep past 12 pm. Based on this pattern of symptoms, we diagnosed Jeff with DSWPD, even though he reports sleep maintenance problems and shows evidence of the conditioned arousal more typically associated with insomnia disorder. For individuals like Jeff who are diagnosed with a phase disorder or insomnia with circadian misalignment at a sleep clinic, the next step is to identify what treatment strategies might be effective for them.

Modifications to CBT-I/BBT-I for patients with circadian rhythm disorders

In this section, we introduce three chronotherapeutic options that may be added to CBT-I/BBT-I for patients with a CRSWD (with a focus on individuals with a phase disorder): bright light therapy, exogenous melatonin, and blue-filtering glasses. We then discuss modifications to CBT-I/BBT-I itself. These chronotherapeutic tools may be used in isolation, but are often used in combination with each other to maximize phase shifts (Burke et al., 2013; Paul et al., 2011) as well as other therapeutic approaches (e.g., cognitive-behavioral treatment, parental involvement, motivational enhancement) to improve adherence (Bonnar et al., 2015; Danielsson, Jansson-Fröjmark, Broman, & Markström, 2016; Gradisar et al., 2011). Some experts suggest that the introduction of bright light therapy and melatonin should be considered only after stabilization of the patient's light/dark schedule does not lead to symptom remission (Emens & Burgess, 2015). We will provide an overview of chronotherapeutic tools as informed by research and our clinical experiences, but we encourage readers to read Emens and Burgess (2015) for a cogent and more in-depth review of light and melatonin therapy.

Light therapy

The light-dark cycle is the strongest entrainer of endogenous circadian rhythms (known as a zeitgeber, German for "time giver"; Yan, 2009). Light therapy is effective for improving sleep and circadian factors for individuals with sleep problems, insomnia, and CRSWDs (van Maanen, Meijer, van der Heijden, & Oort, 2016). Individuals with phase disorders may experience limited exposure to light during the biological day due to late wake-up times or early bedtimes, as well as possibly altered light sensitivity (Duffy et al., 2021). The 2015 AASM clinical guidelines for the treatment of CRSWDs reported that though there were only two trials of evening light for ASWPD and two trials of postawakening light for

DSWPD, light therapy was recommended due to the promising evidence, the minimal side effect profile, and patients generally liking light therapy (Auger et al., 2015). Since 2015, three more studies have suggested that light therapy is effective for advancing sleep-wake rhythms among individuals with DSWPD (Danielsson et al., 2016; Danielsson, Jansson-Fröjmark, Broman, & Markström, 2018; Richardson et al., 2018). Limiting stronger recommendations for the use of light therapy in the treatment of phase disorders is the relatively small literature, and heterogeneity across studies in the operationalization of phase disorders, treatment components, and outcomes.

Beyond shifting the biological clock, light therapy can be acutely alerting and can improve mood (Emens & Burgess, 2015), particularly among individuals with depression and seasonal affective disorder (Al-Karawi & Jubair, 2016). This latter finding may be particularly important, given evidence of the high risk for depressive symptoms among individuals with DSWPD and insomnia (Abe et al., 2011; Baglioni et al., 2011; Duffy et al., 2021).

Aiding your patient in the selection of a light therapy device that is both therapeutic (e.g., provides an adequate dose), and integrates with the patient's lifestyle, is essential. There are over 300 light box options and at least five brands of light glasses (worn like eyeglasses) on the market in 2020. Light glasses have a smaller, but promising, evidence base for shifting circadian phase (Hasler, Buysse, Ngari, & Franzen, 2019; Lau, Lovato, & Lack, 2018; Lovato & Lack, 2016), as well as emerging evidence for improving mood and reducing symptoms of other mental and physical health problems that often are comorbid with insomnia (Swanson, Burgess, Zollars, & Arnedt, 2018; Zalta, Bravo, Valdespino-Hayden, Pollack, & Burgess, 2019). Because the light therapy device market is large and unregulated, it is important to guide your patient to options that are more likely to be therapeutic. Specifically, you want to ensure that the device provides an adequate dose (i.e., 2500–10,000 lux in a tabletop white light box, Emens & Burgess, 2015). Light boxes using blue light or light glasses (blue or green LEDs) require lower brightness given the sensitivity of the circadian system to light in the blue-green spectrum (Wahl, Engelhardt, Schaupp, Lappe, & Ivanov, 2019), and the proximity to the eyes, respectively. In terms of lifestyle match, the patient will not benefit from light therapy if they do not use their device! In our experience, some patients, especially adolescents, would rather use light glasses so that they can accomplish their morning routine in a time-restricted window. Other patients may be comfortable setting aside the time to sit in front of the light box while pursuing sedentary activities (e.g., eating, reading, checking emails).

Most clinics recommend patients use light therapy for 30–60 min. This duration can phase advance DLMO (Crowley & Eastman, 2015) and is associated with better compliance than a longer duration of light presentation (Emens & Burgess, 2015). Typically, the human circadian system can advance by approximately 1h per day, and bright light can facilitate this advancement (Burgess, Crowley, Gazda, Fogg, & Eastman, 2003; Crowley & Eastman, 2015). In our experience, once patients are using the light therapy regularly, 30min of light exposure can be sufficient to further advance and/or maintain an earlier sleep-wake schedule.

The proper timing of light exposure depends on the desired direction of circadian shift and estimates of the patient's circadian timing (Emens & Burgess, 2015). The clock time of light exposure may change during treatment to accommodate the shifting of the sleep-wake schedule. Light therapy is used in the maintenance phase of treatment to counteract the patient's naturally delayed/advanced tendencies, as well as perhaps an unusually long circadian period length (e.g., 25 h instead of 24 h).

To *advance* the circadian phase, we recommend using the light device within the first hour of wake-up time. However, if the patients are exposed to bright light too early in the morning, the light exposure may fall into the phase-delaying rather than a phase-advancing portion of the phase response curve (PRC; Emens & Burgess, 2015). We, therefore, recommend that patients sleep until their spontaneous wake-up time on the first day of light therapy to avoid administering light at too early a circadian time (which would unintentionally delay the clock). Because this recommendation often precludes initiating treatment on a school/work day, light therapy in our clinic usually starts on a Saturday for individuals with typical Monday-Friday work/school obligations. Sometimes delayed phase patients' typical Saturday rise time is more than 3h later than their weekday rise time. In such cases, we ask them to set their alarm at 3h past their weekday rise time and to use the light device for 60min on Saturday morning. We then ask them to target a somewhat (30–60min) earlier bedtime on Saturday night (while still waiting until sleepy before retiring) and to get up 90min earlier on Sunday for another 60-min light session. We ask them to attempt to move their bedtime another 30–60min earlier for Sunday night. The goal is to sufficiently advance their circadian timing by Monday morning so that there is no risk of delivering light during the phase delay portion of the PRC.

To *delay* the circadian phase, we recommend the use of light therapy in the evening before bedtime. Initially, we recommend that light therapy exposure ends 1–3h before the patient's habitual bedtime (e.g., when they are usually falling asleep on the couch). Then, in parallel with shifts in their sleep schedule, we suggest moving the light therapy presentation later, until the light therapy is occurring 1–3h before the desired bedtime.

Although light therapy has limited side effects, there are a few safety considerations. First, light therapy may be contraindicated for those with an existing eye disease, migraines elicited by light, and phototoxic medication use (Emens & Burgess, 2015). For individuals who have bipolar I or bipolar II disorder, some studies suggest that the initial dose of light therapy be 15 min to reduce the risk of switching to hypomania or mania (Wirz-Justice, Benedetti, & Terman, 2009). Although a more recent review of the literature suggests that the rate of switching due to morning light therapy is no higher than placebo (Benedetti, 2018), ongoing debate in the literature (e.g., Sit, Terman, & Wisner, 2018) suggests continued caution is warranted.

Exogenous melatonin use

We have discussed endogenous melatonin in the context of DLMO as a marker of circadian rhythms. Exogenous melatonin mimics the properties of endogenous melatonin and has been shown to have both a zeitgeber as well as a hypnotic effect (Wirz-Justice et al., 2009). However, the hypnotic benefits are limited on average, and confined to speeding the initial onset of sleep (and thereby extending total sleep time) but with no apparent benefit for sleep maintenance (Auld, Maschauer, Morrison, Skene, & Riha, 2017; Ferracioli-Oda, Qawasmi, & Bloch, 2013). There are currently three prescription melatonin receptor agonists available on the market (ramelteon, agomelatine, and tasimelteon). Ramelteon is marketed toward patients with sleep-onset insomnia, agomelatine is marketed as an antidepressant and is not currently available in the United States, and tasimelteon is marketed for individuals with non-24-h sleep-wake rhythm disorder (Williams III, McLin III, Dressman, & Neubauer, 2016). Melatonin is also widely available as an over-the-counter supplement, and we will focus here on these supplements given their pervasiveness among patients with sleep problems.

Research evidence has shown that exogenous melatonin may be an effective treatment for phase disorders or issues, but like light therapy, more work is needed to identify how to optimize the use of melatonin. A meta-analysis of randomized trials comparing exogenous melatonin to placebo among individuals with DSWPD or sleep-onset insomnia suggested that DLMO and sleep onset time were advanced by ~1.2 h and 40 min, respectively (Van Geijlswijk, Korzilius, & Smits, 2010). The 2015 AASM treatment guidelines for CRSWDs reported that four studies supported the treatment of DSWPD with strategically timed melatonin, but there were no research studies to support the use of melatonin as a treatment for ASWPD (Auger et al., 2015). Morning administration of melatonin is not often used as a treatment for ASWPD or insomnia with an advanced circadian misalignment, perhaps because these individuals are typically older adults and any lingering sleepiness may increase fall risk (cf. Amstrup, Sikjaer, Mosekilde, & Rejnmark, 2015).

Instructions on melatonin supplements' labels typically suggest that it be taken 30–60 min before bed, a time that may be later than optimal for chronotherapeutic benefit. It is therefore worth discussing with the patient the limited benefits of melatonin for sleep initiation and lack of benefit to sleep maintenance (Auld et al., 2017; Ferracioli-Oda et al., 2013). Instead, we explain to patients that melatonin can be a powerful zeitgeber when administered 3–4 h before bedtime to phase advance the clock (Burgess, Crowley, et al., 2003). As with light therapy, the timing of melatonin should shift with changes to the sleep-wake schedule to ensure that the melatonin is shifting the clock in the desired direction (Burgess, Revell, Molina, & Eastman, 2010).

A dose of 0.5 mg of exogenous melatonin produces blood plasma levels that are approximately similar to the levels of endogenous melatonin during biological night (Sack, Hughes, Edgar, & Lewy, 1997), and 0.5 mg is relatively comparable in its phase-advancing properties to 3 mg, at least in adults (Burgess et al., 2010). Thus, 0.5 mg may be preferable, as it is the lowest efficacious dose, less likely to induce sleepiness when taken during the biological day (Arendt, 2006), and it is less likely to remain in the system during the other side of the PRC (thereby unintentionally counteracting the desired phase shift).

Because the United States Federal Drug Administration does not regulate over-the-counter melatonin supplements, the content may range from much less to much more (sometimes over 400% more) melatonin than the label suggests, and other supplements (such as serotonin) may be included (Erland & Saxena, 2017). Additionally, melatonin is a common additive in other sleep supplements, so it is important to review the ingredient list of patients' supplements to determine if melatonin has been included. A newer formulation of melatonin advertises itself as "extended-release," which purports to aid in both sleep initiation and maintenance although the published data only supports benefits for sleep initiation (Wade et al., 2010). However, we caution patients against the use of extended-release melatonin because while some of the melatonin may release during the phase advance period, some of it may release during the phase delay period, resulting in the so-called "spillover effect" (Lewy, Emens, Jackman, & Yuhas, 2006) and thereby compromising the desired effect.

High doses of melatonin (>10 mg) may have adverse effects such as headaches, hyper- or hypotension, or upset stomach among adults (Auger et al., 2015). The long-term consequences of chronic melatonin use in adult and pediatric samples have been understudied. This is of particular concern among pediatric samples, given some evidence from animal models that melatonin can induce changes in pubertal development and reproductive function (Kennaway, 2015). Although pediatric studies have shown that daily 2–10 mg melatonin use was associated with no adverse events at 3-month (Wasdell et al., 2008), 2-year (Malow et al., 2020), or 4-year follow-up (Carr et al., 2007; Hoebert, Van Der Heijden, Van Geijlswijk, & Smits, 2009), these studies have had varying degrees of methodological rigor, have been mostly in populations with neurodevelopmental disorders (limiting generalizability), and, in our opinion, have had an insufficient assessment of melatonin's impact on pubertal development and reproductive function.

Blue light filtering glasses

More recently, the use of blue light filtering glasses has emerged as a potentially useful tool in managing insomnia and CRSWDs. Although the evidence base is small, a recent meta-analysis of studies of mostly adults showed that blue light filtering glasses seem to improve sleep efficiency and total sleep time measured by actigraphy, and sleep quality and total sleep time based on self-report (Shechter, Quispe, Mizhquiri Barbecho, Slater, & Falzon, 2020).

Blue light filtering glasses work primarily by reducing light input to the circadian clock, which can facilitate a phase shift and may also reduce the acute alerting effects of light. For example, selectively filtering evening light can facilitate a phase advance, and filtering morning light can facilitate phase delay. Blue light filtering glasses may also help to reduce alertness in the hours before bed, which may be helpful for managing hyperarousal related to insomnia and encouraging reduced arousal in DSWPD patients who have trouble winding down in anticipation of an earlier bedtime. As with bright light boxes or glasses, there has been a proliferation in the number of blue light filtering glasses available for purchase. When aiding a patient with selecting blue light filtering glasses, it is important to identify models that sufficiently block short wavelengths, defined as ~100% of blue light transmission (in the spectrum of 450–480nm). Effective blue light filtering glasses are color-tinted (amber, brown, or orange), as the clear lenses cannot block as much blue light (Shechter et al., 2020). If the patient does not choose to purchase blue light filtering glasses, it is worthwhile to have a discussion about alternatives to minimizing evening light exposure, such as the use of f.Lux (justgetflux.com) mobile applications or night shift mode on iPhones and iPads (support.apple.com/en-au/HT207570), and lowering the brightness on electronic devices as much as possible.

Modifying CBT-I/BBT-I for phase disorders or circadian misalignment

Beyond the inclusion of chronotherapeutics, there are some aspects of CBT-I/BBT-I that may need to be modified (or emphasized) for individuals with a CRSWD. In our clinic, we primarily use BBT-I and incorporate adjunctive cognitive therapy and relaxation techniques as needed, so we use this model as the basis for our modifications described below and in Table 1. After we introduce BBT-I to patients, we always explore how much they believe the treatment can work, and how much they think they

TABLE 1 Summary of modifications and adaptations to CBT-I/BBT-I for patients with phase disorders or insomnia with circadian misalignment.

CBT-I/BBT-I components	Standard practice	Modifications/adaptions
Sleep education	3-P model, 2-process model of sleep regulation, sleep stages	Discussion of sleep-wake maintenance zone (i.e. forbidden sleep zone). At this time, Process S is high, but Process C is not signaling sleep, so falling asleep will be challenging, counterproductive, and could lead to conditioned arousal
Sleep restriction	Improve sleep efficiency by limiting time in bed to the amount of time sleeping then expanding slowly as long as sleep efficiency is preserved	Develop a wind-down routine for individuals with DSWPD in the evening, and identify motivators for waking up at a consistent time Encourage individuals with ASWPD to engage in stimulating activities in relatively brighter light conditions in the evening to maintain alertness, and if they experience early morning awakenings engage in distracting, relaxing, low light activities
Stimulus control	Associate bed/bedroom solely as a cue for sleep by eliminating nonsleep activities from the bedroom. Instruction to get out of bed at night if awake >15 min	Development of distracting, relaxing, low light activities out of bed is crucial for phase disorders, as there is the risk that getting out of bed and doing something stimulating while experiencing light exposure would signal to the biological clock that this is a time for wakefulness
Napping/daytime sleep	Discontinue or restrict daytime napping to 30 min	A 20–45 min nap in the afternoon to correspond with their typical circadian dip in alertness. This can help individuals with DSWPD to maintain consistent wake-up times on the weekend and individuals with ASWPD to stay up later in the evening. Constraining the nap to the afternoon should minimize any unwanted phase shifts

TABLE 1 Summary of modifications and adaptations to CBT-I/BBT-I for patients with phase disorders or insomnia with circadian misalignment.—cont'd

CBT-I/BBT-I components	Standard practice	Modifications/adaptions
Sleep hygiene education	Address daytime habits and sleep environment interfering with sleep	Individuals with delayed phase and/or DSWPD may be at higher risk for alcohol use disorder and higher caffeine use, so these substances should be reviewed. Alcohol is not a long-term sleep initiation solution, and evening caffeine delays the biological clock
Cognitive therapy	Challenge patient's dysfunctional beliefs interfering with sleep and misconceptions about sleep. Replace/restructure to more helpful and realistic thoughts about sleep	Individuals with phase issues may have the dysfunctional belief that they could never shift their sleep schedule. Psychoeducation about sleep drive and the biological clock will be important. If work/school obligations permit, begin with the goal of regularizing a sleep-wake window at sleep onset and wake-up times that match the individual's apparent biological tendencies. Once the pattern is regularized, slowly begin shifting the window in the desired direction by 30 min every 4–5 days
Relaxation Training		Relaxation exercises, such as diaphragmatic breathing and progressive muscle relaxation, may help to manage nocturnal worry
Relapse Prevention	Discuss practicing less rigid sleep plan over time and what do to prevent sleep disturbance from turning into another episode of insomnia in the future	Relapse prevention is particularly important with patients with phase issues, as their underlying circadian tendencies will make them predisposed to drift in their circadian/sleep-wake timing to what it was pretherapy. Thus, the long-term continued use of chronotherapeutic techniques is often necessary
Sleep diaries	Establish baseline sleep patterns, track progress, reinforce appropriate behavior change, problem-solve obstacles to adherence	Two weeks of sleep diaries are preferred for adequately evaluating sleep patterns among individuals with a phase disorder. Actigraphy is recommended when available

can adhere to the treatment recommendations. We believe that evaluating motivation, and using motivational enhancement techniques as needed, will help to improve adherence to these challenging behavior changes.

Healthy sleep practices

During the discussion of healthy sleep practices (often referred to as sleep hygiene), it may be useful to spend some more time discussing the effects of alcohol on sleep. Individuals with an evening preference appear to be at greater risk for alcohol use (Hasler et al., 2017; Taylor & Hasler, 2018) and may be more likely to use alcohol as a sleep initiation aid. With patients for whom alcohol may be a problem, it is important to review with them the evidence that alcohol may initially help with sleep onset, but tolerance builds rapidly (requiring more alcohol for similar sleep initiation benefits), and alcohol will increase their nocturnal awakenings in the second half of the night (Colrain, Nicholas, & Baker, 2014). In a sample of individuals with insomnia, alcohol improved sleep efficiency and depth of sleep initially, but by the sixth night of drinking alcohol these sleep benefits had dissipated; yet, counterintuitively, a parallel substudy suggested that individuals with insomnia would continue to choose alcohol as a sleep aid even after tolerance emerged (Roehrs & Roth, 2018).

It may also be worthwhile to discuss the effects of caffeine on sleep with patients with circadian misalignment. Patients with DSWPD may also consume more caffeine (Lovato, Gradisar, Short, Dohnt, & Micic, 2013), perhaps because they are feeling sleepy due to shorter sleep duration. However, evening caffeine consumption (the equivalent of two shots of espresso) has been shown to delay the biological clock (Burke et al., 2015). This information is important to convey to patients with DSWPD—the subsequent phase delay not only makes it more difficult to fall asleep at their desired time but also could make it more difficult to get up the following morning. Our rule of thumb for most patients with insomnia is to avoid caffeine after noon; however, in individuals with circadian misalignment, it often makes sense to adjust that cut-off time to match their sleep schedule. For example, if a patient with a relatively delayed phase has a 3 am-noon sleep schedule, their caffeine cut-off may be at 3 pm.

During the first session of BBT-I, the scientific principle of Borbély's two-process model of the interrelation between homeostatic sleep drive (Process S) and the biological clock (Process C) is introduced (Borbély, 1982). Although we always emphasize both processes as relevant to individuals with more prototypical insomnia, we take particular care in describing the role of Process C for patients with circadian misalignment. With this in mind, we find it particularly fruitful to describe the wake maintenance zone (or, "forbidden sleep zone"), which is the period of time at the end of the biological day when Process S might be relatively high but Process C is not yet signaling sleep, and thus trying to fall asleep during this time will be particularly challenging and counterproductive through its contribution to conditioned arousal (Lack & Wright, 2007). In our experience, patients with a delayed phase issue often resonate with this description. These patients often consider the hours in the late evening (sometimes past midnight) as the time that they "get into the zone" and experience difficulty winding down before their desired bedtime; these experiences may be a reflection of circadian signals for alertness.

Behavioral components

Sleep restriction reduces time in bed to improve sleep efficiency. In our clinical experience, sleep restriction for individuals with phase disorders/circadian misalignment is often less severe than in prototypical insomnia cases (e.g., a 7-h sleep window is not unusual), largely because there often fewer sleep maintenance complaints and the sleep initiation difficulties appear to be driven more by the phase misalignment. For individuals with phase issues, identifying the appropriate sleep window is most important during sleep restriction. Ideally, the initial sleep window would be aligned to their typical sleep onset time and desired wake-up time; we prefer to stabilize the patient at the predisposed delayed or advanced phase, and then, if needed, shift their schedule more gradually over weeks rather than days. However, sometimes work/school demands require that we help them to shift their sleep window immediately.

The instruction to "only go to bed if you are sleepy" may be particularly challenging when phase issues are present. At bedtime, individuals with DSWPD may be challenged because they enjoy staying up late and may experience a "second wind", whereas individuals with ASWPD will feel sleepy much earlier in the evening than their desired bedtime. To address this for individuals with DSWPD, introduce a 1-h wind-down routine before bed, which includes activities that we describe as distracting (to take their mind off of the day or their worry about sleep), relaxing (to prepare them for sleep), and done in low light (to minimize acute alerting effects of light and unintentional phase shifts). This wind-down routine will help individuals with DSWPD to better identify when they feel sleepy and minimize the risk of the second wind maintaining a delayed bedtime. For individuals with ASWPD, it may be important to develop evening activities that are active, engaging, and rewarding in relatively brighter light conditions, so that patients can maintain alertness and be motivated to do something other than going to bed.

Maintaining a consistent rise time is another key instruction of CBT-I/BBT-I. Individuals with delayed phase may be challenged to do so, especially on their free days when they desire to sleep in, and individuals with ASWPD may be waking up earlier than their desired wake-up time. For individuals with DSWPD, develop creative ways to motivate wake-up times, such as a scheduled coffee meeting or workout with a family member or friend. The use of dawn simulators or a light box on a timer can also facilitate consistent rise times. We find it useful to provide education on sleep inertia, as many individuals with DSWPD seem to make the decision to turn off the alarm or press the snooze button based on their subjective level of sleepiness at the moment the alarm goes off, which they interpret as indicating they have not achieved sufficient sleep. We explain that the transition to wakefulness is a gradual, not instantaneous, process and that their degree of sleep inertia depends in part on their stage of sleep when the alarm goes off (Trotti, 2017). Thus, we encourage them to make the judgment about whether their night of sleep was sufficiently restorative after 15–30 min of being out of bed. For individuals with ASWPD, we instruct them that if they get out of bed before their desired wake-up time, it is critical that they only engage in nonstimulating activities (distracting, relaxing, and in low light). Rewarding activities and light exposure at this time would be counterproductive, as this could stimulate alertness and send the inaccurate signal to the biological clock that this is a time for wakefulness.

Stimulus control aims to associate the bed with a place for sleep (or sex) only, and not a place for anxiety or frustration. Some clinicians will instruct the patient to get out of bed after 15–30 min of wakefulness, though be sure that this suggestion does not lead to increased clock-watching by the patient. We often encourage patients with a tendency for clock-watching to determine whether they are "moving toward sleep" or starting to feel frustrated, anxious, and/or more alert, and to use that as the cue to get out of bed. For individuals with delayed phase, this is more likely to occur at the beginning of the night, while for individuals with advanced phase, it is more likely to occur in the morning. However, phase issues do not preclude maintenance issues at any time of night, especially as conditioned arousal may have developed over time. In all instances, encourage the patient to get out of bed and engage in something distracting, relaxing, and in low light. The patient should not engage in any activities that would be too stimulating or in bright light. All that said, in our experience, simply realigning the bedtime (for delayed phase) or rise time (for advanced phase) to a time more consistent with the time the patient is actually falling asleep or waking up, respectively, often obviates the need for leaving the bed per stimulus control instructions.

Patients often ask about whether they can take naps during the day, especially when they learn about their sleep restriction sleep window. Although daytime naps can compromise sleep drive, thereby exacerbating sleep initiation difficulties, they can have their place in cases where patients have insomnia complicated by significant daytime sleepiness and/or circadian misalignment. We recommend patients take a strategically timed nap, meaning that the nap will occur in the afternoon, ideally corresponding with their typical circadian dip. We recommend that the patient set a timer for a nap of sufficiently short duration (20–45 min) so that it does not lead to significant sleep inertia, overly reduce accumulating sleep drive (Takahashi, 2003), and does not induce any phase shifts (Buxton, L'Hermite-Balériaux, Turek, & Van Cauter, 2000). Individuals with a delayed sleep phase may use an afternoon nap to maintain a regular wake-up time on weekends (they will be able to "catch up" on sleep), whereas an afternoon nap for individuals with an advanced sleep phase can help them to stay up later in the evening.

Cognitive components

Cognitive therapy techniques seek to resolve unhelpful beliefs about sleep, behaviors that may support these beliefs, and worry or rumination. Harvey (2005) developed a cognitive therapy for insomnia (CT-I) that focuses on these cognitive components. More recently, Harvey and Buysse (2017) published a transdiagnostic approach to treating sleep problems, which includes treatment modules for correcting unhelpful sleep-related beliefs and reducing sleep-related worry and vigilance. These cognitive techniques may prove helpful in the treatment of individuals with a phase disorder or insomnia with circadian misalignment. For example, these individuals may have the unhelpful belief that they cannot possibly change their current sleep schedule and be able to function the next day. This belief can then become maintained by inconsistent sleep-wake timing. To address this, we return to a discussion of Borbely's two-process model and explain that sleep restriction will help to build sleep drive, and consistent wake-up times will serve to stabilize the biological clock.

In our clinic, we address worry and physiological anxiety with the use of relaxation exercises. Specifically, we frequently employ diaphragmatic breathing (Chen, Huang, Chien, & Cheng, 2017), progressive muscle relaxation (Manzoni, Pagnini, Castelnuovo, & Molinari, 2008), and constructive worry (Jansson-Fröjmark, Lind, & Sunnhed, 2012). We teach diaphragmatic breathing by asking the patient to sit comfortably, place one hand on their stomach and other hand on their chest, and breathe slowly (perhaps counting the inhales and exhales) so that the hand on the stomach but not the chest moves. We introduce progressive muscle relaxation by walking the patient through how to tense and then release one muscle group at a time and suggest that they use a mobile application or online video to guide their practice. We teach a scheduled/constructive worry exercise in a manner closely aligning to the approach developed by Carney and Waters (2006). We encourage patients to view these techniques as skills to develop and to practice them during the day before implementing them at night.

We have found that these cognitive therapy techniques can reduce nocturnal worries and physiological anxiety, perhaps particularly so in individuals with phase delay who commonly have comorbid psychiatric concerns (Abe et al., 2011). CBT-I is effective in individuals with comorbid psychiatric diagnoses (Wu, Appleman, Salazar, & Ong, 2015) and can improve depressive symptoms (Gebara et al., 2018). However, it is worth noting that in some cases cognitive-behavioral therapies to directly address these comorbidities may be necessary to improve adherence to CBT-I/BBT-I (Matthews, Arnedt, McCarthy, Cuddihy, & Aloia, 2013) or to make a sufficient impact on the comorbid symptoms if they are more severe.

Relapse prevention

Once patients have achieved their goals for improving sleep continuity, achieving sufficient sleep duration, and stabilizing sleep timing, we discuss relapse prevention. This traditionally includes a discussion of relaxing the rigidity of the sleep schedule over time, and if another sleep disturbance occurs in the future, returning to the principles of stimulus control and sleep restriction. Relapse prevention is particularly important with patients with phase issues, as their underlying circadian tendencies will always make them predisposed to experience a slow drift in their sleep-wake timing to their pretherapy pattern (Dodson & Zee, 2010). Thus, the continued use of chronotherapeutic techniques is often necessary for maintenance. Clinicians should emphasize both the inherent challenge and the importance of long-term behavior change, empathetically explain that these "slips" can happen and are even likely and that the patient should re-emphasize strict CBT-I principles in combination with chronotherapuetic techniques to regularize sleep-wake patterns and initiate a slow shift in the desired direction.

Cognitive-behavioral therapy + chronotherapeutics

There are only two studies testing the benefits of CBT in combination with chronotherapeutics for the treatment of individuals with phase disorders, and no studies that specifically include CBT-I/BBT-I. These two studies suggested that while CBT in combination with light therapy among individuals with DSWPD reduces sleep onset and advances bedtimes, CBT plus light therapy did not outperform light therapy alone (Danielsson et al., 2016; Gradisar et al., 2011). Certainly, more studies are needed to determine whether CBT can or cannot enhance light therapy, as well as to investigate the benefits of incorporating exogenous melatonin and/or blue light filtering glasses with CBT for the treatment of DSWPD. Additionally, studies are needed to evaluate the benefit of CBT in combination with chronotherapeutics for the treatment of ASWPD. Finally, it would be worthwhile to test these treatment packages among individuals with DSWPD without a circadian delay per DLMO, as well as among individuals with insomnia with a phase component.

CBT-I/BBT-I for other CRSWDs

The other CRSWDs may benefit from treatment components of CBT-I, though these individuals may be less likely to be identified as having insomnia. Individuals with non-24-h sleep-wake rhythm disorder are unable to entrain their endogenous circadian rhythm to the 24-h environment, and therefore "free run" (their clock shifts earlier or later each day). Effective treatment for these patients may combine exogenous melatonin, bright light therapy (Malkani, Abbott, Reid, & Zee, 2018), and the CBT-I recommendation to wake up at the same time every day. Individuals with irregular sleep-wake rhythm disorder are lacking clearly defined sleep-wake rhythms and may be treated with light therapy, regularity in exercise and social rhythms, and the CBT-I recommendations of reducing time in bed, a 1-h wind-down routine, and waking up at the same time daily (Zee & Vitiello, 2009). Shift work disorder is characterized by a report of insomnia and/or excessive sleepiness associated with a recurring work schedule that occurs during the biological night (American Academy of Sleep Medicine, 2014), and though insomnia occurs entirely during the course of shift work, CBT-I can be used effectively among this group (Järnefelt et al., 2012). Jet lag disorder occurs as a consequence of traveling across time zones and can be prevented with careful pretrip shifts to the clock with light, exogenous melatonin, and adherence to a sleep-wake schedule that changes slowly in the desired direction (Arendt, 2009). In summary, the principles of CBT-I/BBT-I with adjuvant melatonin and bright light may be applied effectively for the treatment of the other CRSWDs.

Treatment course for Jeff

During Jeff's first session of BBT-I, the patient agreed to limit his time in bed to 6.5 h, adhere to a consistent rise time of 9:15 am (even on weekends), avoid retiring unless sleepy (but not earlier than 2:45 am), and avoid staying in bed unless he can sleep. We discussed distracting, relaxing, and low-light activities outside of the bedroom to implement during a 1-h wind-down time before bed, as well as when he cannot fall asleep. We also recommended melatonin (0.5–1 mg) to be taken 4–6 h before bed (~10 pm) to provide a corrective phase advance to his circadian clock.

Jeff reported being happy with his treatment progress at our second session because with his later bedtime he was able to fall asleep and stay asleep more easily. Jeff reports that he was never awake for more than 30 min in bed. His sleep diary suggested that he was maintaining a relatively consistent sleep window of 2:45–9:15 am. However, Jeff reported still feeling sleepy for the first 1–2h after waking up and could not do more than browse the internet. We explained that his continued sleepiness was likely due to a combination of insufficient sleep with the current sleep window, and his tendency toward a delayed circadian rhythm. We recommended that he continue to take melatonin at ~10 pm and that he begin to use blue light filtering glasses for ~2h before bedtime. We also introduced light therapy in the morning for 30–60min; the patient chose to borrow a pair of bright light glasses from the clinic. We did not make any adjustments to his sleep window.

At Jeff's third session, he reported that he continued to experience improvements in falling and staying asleep and that he has experienced an immediate improvement in alertness with the use of the bright light glasses in the morning. Jeff estimated that he wore them 4–5 days per week, sometimes forgetting when he already felt alert upon rising. He stated that he had not tried evening melatonin or blue light filtering glasses because the light therapy was working so well. Jeff noted that he was frustrated on nights when he felt sleepy going to bed, but once in bed, his mind wandered. To address his worry and physiological arousal at bedtime, we introduced the basics of diaphragmatic breathing (including an in-session practice), progressive muscle relaxation, and guided imagery.

During Jeff's fourth and final session (2 months after initiating the treatment plan), he reported that he has been falling asleep and staying asleep during the night and that he has been finding it easier to wake up at the target 9:15 am, including feeling immediately alert upon waking with the continued use of the bright light glasses. Jeff reported that listening to a guided progressive muscle relaxation video he found online helped to quiet his mind and reduce arousal at bedtime; he is now able to guide himself through the relaxation. Jeff maintained a consistent sleep-wake schedule of 2:45–9:15 am for several weeks now, occasionally deviating in his bedtime on nights of drinking. We reviewed with him the principles for modifying his sleep schedule, and what to do if his insomnia symptoms return. Jeff planned to purchase his own pair of bright light glasses to use daily to maintain his sleep-wake schedule.

Conclusion

Patients with a phase disorder or circadian misalignment experience significant clinical impairments and are at risk for negative mental and physical health outcomes. Diagnosis of phase disorders requires careful consideration of ICSD-3 criteria, while being mindful of the dimensionality of these diagnoses, and differentiating from developmentally normative changes in sleep-wake timing as well as primary insomnia. Questionnaires, actigraphy, and DLMO may be informative to clinicians, but cannot be used alone (i.e. without a clinical interview) for diagnosis. For patients who do meet diagnostic criteria for a phase disorder or have insomnia with circadian misalignment, treatment options may include chronotherapeutics (light therapy, exogenous melatonin administration, blue light filtering glasses), and slight modifications to CBT-I/BBT-I. Of note, the research evidence supporting the use of these treatments alone or in combination is limited, as there is a small number of studies overall and large heterogeneity across studies (in dosing and timing). Consequently, much of our advice is informed by clinical experience rather than research studies. In the meantime, while we wait for the research to advance, we hope that this chapter will be useful as an aid for clinicians with patients with phase disorders or insomnia with circadian misalignment to make informed decisions about the optimal treatment options for the individual.

References

Abe, T., Inoue, Y., Komada, Y., Nakamura, M., Asaoka, S., Kanno, M., et al. (2011). Relation between morningness-eveningness score and depressive symptoms among patients with delayed sleep phase syndrome. *Sleep Medicine, 12*(7), 680–684. https://doi.org/10.1016/j.sleep.2010.12.017.

Al-Karawi, D., & Jubair, L. (2016). Bright light therapy for nonseasonal depression: Meta-analysis of clinical trials. *Journal of Affective Disorders, 198*, 64–71. https://doi.org/10.1016/j.jad.2016.03.016.

American Academy of Sleep Medicine. (2014). *International classification of sleep disorders—Third edition (ICSD-3) online version*. Westchester, IL: American Academy of Sleep Medicine.

Amstrup, A. K., Sikjaer, T., Mosekilde, L., & Rejnmark, L. (2015). The effect of melatonin treatment on postural stability, muscle strength, and quality of life and sleep in postmenopausal women: A randomized controlled trial. *Nutrition Journal, 14*(1), 102.

Arendt, J. (2006). Melatonin and human rhythms. *Chronobiology International, 23*(1-2), 21–37.

Arendt, J. (2009). Managing jet lag: Some of the problems and possible new solutions. *Sleep Medicine Reviews, 13*(4), 249–256. https://doi.org/10.1016/j.smrv.2008.07.011.

Auger, R. R., Burgess, H. J., Emens, J. S., Deriy, L. V., Thomas, S. M., & Sharkey, K. M. (2015). Clinical practice guideline for the treatment of intrinsic circadian rhythm sleep-wake disorders: Advanced Sleep-Wake Phase Disorder (ASWPD), Delayed Sleep-Wake Phase Disorder (DSWPD), Non-24-Hour Sleep-Wake Rhythm Disorder (N24SWD), and Irregular Sleep-Wake Rhythm Disorder (ISWRD). An update for 2015. *Journal of Clinical Sleep Medicine, 11*(10), 1199–1236. https://doi.org/10.5664/jcsm.5100.

Auld, F., Maschauer, E. L., Morrison, I., Skene, D. J., & Riha, R. L. (2017). Evidence for the efficacy of melatonin in the treatment of primary adult sleep disorders. *Sleep Medicine Reviews, 34*, 10–22.

Baglioni, C., Battagliese, G., Feige, B., Spiegelhalder, K., Nissen, C., Voderholzer, U., et al. (2011). Insomnia as a predictor of depression: A meta-analytic evaluation of longitudinal epidemiological studies. *Journal of Affective Disorders, 135*(1-3), 10–19.

Barion, A., & Zee, P. C. (2007). A clinical approach to circadian rhythm sleep disorders. *Sleep Medicine, 8*(6), 566–577.

Baron, K. G., Abbott, S., Jao, N., Manalo, N., & Mullen, R. (2017). Orthosomnia: Are some patients taking the quantified self too far? *Journal of Clinical Sleep Medicine, 13*(2), 351–354.

Benedetti, F. (2018). Rate of switch from bipolar depression into mania after morning light therapy: A historical review. *Psychiatry Research, 261*, 351–356.

Bonnar, D., Gradisar, M., Moseley, L., Coughlin, A. M., Cain, N., & Short, M. A. (2015). Evaluation of novel school-based interventions for adolescent sleep problems: Does parental involvement and bright light improve outcomes? *Sleep Health, 1*(1), 66–74.

Borbély, A. A. (1982). A two process model of sleep regulation. *Human Neurobiology, 1*(3), 195–204.

Braun, R., Kath, W. L., Iwanaszko, M., Kula-Eversole, E., Abbott, S. M., Reid, K. J., et al. (2018). Universal method for robust detection of circadian state from gene expression. *PNAS, 115*(39), E9247–E9256. https://doi.org/10.1073/pnas.1800314115.

Burgess, H. J., Crowley, S. J., Gazda, C. J., Fogg, L. F., & Eastman, C. I. (2003). Preflight adjustment to eastward travel: 3 days of advancing sleep with and without morning bright light. *Journal of Biological Rhythms, 18*(4), 318–328.

Burgess, H. J., & Eastman, C. I. (2005). The dim light melatonin onset following fixed and free sleep schedules. *Journal of Sleep Research, 14*(3), 229–237. https://doi.org/10.1111/j.1365-2869.2005.00470.x.

Burgess, H. J., & Fogg, L. F. (2008). Individual differences in the amount and timing of salivary melatonin secretion. *PLoS One, 3*(8), e3055.

Burgess, H. J., Park, M., Wyatt, J. K., & Fogg, L. F. (2016). Home dim light melatonin onsets with measures of compliance in delayed sleep phase disorder. *Journal of Sleep Research, 25*(3), 314–317. https://doi.org/10.1111/jsr.12384.

Burgess, H. J., Park, M., Wyatt, J. K., Rizvydeen, M., & Fogg, L. F. (2017). Sleep and circadian variability in people with delayed sleep–wake phase disorder versus healthy controls. *Sleep Medicine, 34*, 33–39. https://doi.org/10.1016/j.sleep.2017.02.019.

Burgess, H. J., Revell, V. L., Molina, T. A., & Eastman, C. I. (2010). Human phase response curves to three days of daily melatonin: 0.5 mg Versus 3.0 mg. *Journal of Clinical Endocrinology and Metabolism, 95*(7), 3325–3331. https://doi.org/10.1210/jc.2009-2590.

Burgess, H. J., Savic, N., Sletten, T., Roach, G., Gilbert, S. S., & Dawson, D. (2003). The relationship between the dim light melatonin onset and sleep on a regular schedule in young healthy adults. *Behavioral Sleep Medicine, 1*(2), 102–114. https://doi.org/10.1207/S15402010BSM0102_3.

Burke, T. M., Markwald, R. R., Chinoy, E. D., Snider, J. A., Bessman, S. C., Jung, C. M., et al. (2013). Combination of light and melatonin time cues for phase advancing the human circadian clock. *Sleep, 36*(11), 1617–1624.

Burke, T. M., Markwald, R. R., McHill, A. W., Chinoy, E. D., Snider, J. A., Bessman, S. C., et al. (2015). Effects of caffeine on the human circadian clock in vivo and in vitro. *Science Translational Medicine, 7*(305), 305ra146.

Buxton, O. M., L'Hermite-Balériaux, M., Turek, F. W., & Van Cauter, E. (2000). Daytime naps in darkness phase shift the human circadian rhythms of melatonin and thyrotropin secretion. *American Journal of Physiology. Regulatory, Integrative and Comparative Physiology, 278*(2), R373–R382.

Carney, C. E., & Waters, W. F. (2006). Effects of a structured problem-solving procedure on pre-sleep cognitive arousal in college students with insomnia. *Behavioral Sleep Medicine, 4*(1), 13–28.

Carr, R., Wasdell, M. B., Hamilton, D., Weiss, M. D., Freeman, R. D., Tai, J., et al. (2007). Long-term effectiveness outcome of melatonin therapy in children with treatment-resistant circadian rhythm sleep disorders. *Journal of Pineal Research, 43*(4), 351–359.

Carrier, J., Paquet, J., Morettini, J., & Touchette, É. (2002). Phase advance of sleep and temperature circadian rhythms in the middle years of life in humans. *Neuroscience Letters, 320*(1–2), 1–4. https://doi.org/10.1016/S0304-3940(02)00038-1.

Carskadon, M. A., Vieira, C., & Acebo, C. (1993). Association between puberty and delayed phase preference. *Sleep, 16*(3), 258–262. https://doi.org/10.1093/sleep/16.3.258.

Chen, Y. F., Huang, X. Y., Chien, C. H., & Cheng, J. F. (2017). The effectiveness of diaphragmatic breathing relaxation training for reducing anxiety. *Perspectives in Psychiatric Care, 53*(4), 329–336.

Cheng, P., Walch, O. J., Huang, Y., Mayer, C., Sagong, C., Cuamatzi Castelan, A., et al. (2021). Predicting circadian misalignment with wearable technology: Validation of wrist-worn actigraphy and photometry in night shift workers. *Sleep, 44*.

Chinoy, E. D., Cuellar, J. A., Huwa, K. E., Jameson, J. T., Watson, C. H., Bessman, S. C., et al. (2021). Performance of seven consumer sleep-tracking devices compared with polysomnography. *Sleep*, zsaa291.

Colrain, I. M., Nicholas, C. L., & Baker, F. C. (2014). Alcohol and the sleeping brain. In *Vol. 125. Handbook of clinical neurology* (pp. 415–431). Elsevier.

Crowley, S. J., Acebo, C., Fallone, G., & Carskadon, M. A. (2006). Estimating dim light melatonin onset (DLMO) phase in adolescents using summer or school-year sleep/wake schedules. *Sleep, 29*(12), 1632–1641.

Crowley, S. J., & Eastman, C. I. (2015). Phase advancing human circadian rhythms with morning bright light, afternoon melatonin, and gradually shifted sleep: Can we reduce morning bright-light duration? *Sleep Medicine, 16*(2), 288–297.

Czeisler, C. A., & Gooley, J. J. (2007). Sleep and circadian rhythms in humans. In *Vol. 72. Cold Spring Harbor symposia on quantitative biology* (pp. 579–597). Cold Spring Harbor Laboratory Press.

Danielsson, K., Jansson-Fröjmark, M., Broman, J. E., & Markström, A. (2016). Cognitive behavioral therapy as an adjunct treatment to light therapy for delayed sleep phase disorder in young adults: A randomized controlled feasibility study. *Behavioral Sleep Medicine, 14*(2), 212–232. https://doi.org/10.1080/15402002.2014.981817.

Danielsson, K., Jansson-Fröjmark, M., Broman, J. E., & Markström, A. (2018). Light therapy with scheduled rise times in young adults with delayed sleep phase disorder: Therapeutic outcomes and possible predictors. *Behavioral Sleep Medicine, 16*(4), 325–336.

Dijk, D. J., & Duffy, J. F. (1999). Circadian regulation of human sleep and age-related changes in its timing, consolidation and EEG characteristics. *Annals of Medicine, 31*(2), 130–140. https://doi.org/10.3109/07853899908998789.

Dijk, D. J., & Duffy, J. F. (2020). Novel approaches for assessing circadian rhythmicity in humans: A review. *Journal of Biological Rhythms*. 0748730420940483.

Dodson, E. R., & Zee, P. C. (2010). Therapeutics for circadian rhythm sleep disorders. *Sleep Medicine Clinics, 5*(4), 701–715.

Duffy, J. F., Abbott, S. M., Burgess, H., Crowley, S. J., Emens, J. S., Epstein, L. J., et al. (2021). *Workshop report: Circadian rhythm sleep wake disorders: Gaps and opportunities*.

Emens, J. S., & Burgess, H. J. (2015). Effect of light and melatonin and other melatonin receptor agonists on human circadian physiology. *Sleep Medicine Clinics, 10*(4), 435–453. https://doi.org/10.1016/j.jsmc.2015.08.001.

Erland, L. A., & Saxena, P. K. (2017). Melatonin natural health products and supplements: Presence of serotonin and significant variability of melatonin content. *Journal of Clinical Sleep Medicine, 13*(2), 275–281.

Evans, M. A., Buysse, D. J., Marsland, A. L., Wright, A. G., Foust, J., Carroll, L. W., et al. (2021). Meta-analysis of age and actigraphy-assessed sleep characteristics across the lifespan. *Sleep*. https://doi.org/10.1093/sleep/zsab088.

Ferracioli-Oda, E., Qawasmi, A., & Bloch, M. H. (2013). Meta-analysis: Melatonin for the treatment of primary sleep disorders. *PLoS One, 8*(5), e63773.

Folkard, S., & Tucker, P. (2003). Shift work, safety and productivity. *Occupational Medicine, 53*(2), 95–101. https://doi.org/10.1093/occmed/kqg047.

Gaultney, J. F. (2010). The prevalence of sleep disorders in college students: Impact on academic performance. *Journal of American College Health, 59*(2), 91–97. https://doi.org/10.1080/07448481.2010.483708.

Gebara, M. A., Siripong, N., DiNapoli, E. A., Maree, R. D., Germain, A., Reynolds, C. F., et al. (2018). Effect of insomnia treatments on depression: A systematic review and meta-analysis. *Depression and Anxiety, 35*(8), 717–731.

Gradisar, M., Dohnt, H., Gardner, G., Paine, S., Starkey, K., Menne, A., et al. (2011). A randomized controlled trial of cognitive-behavior therapy plus bright light therapy for adolescent delayed sleep phase disorder. *Sleep, 34*(12), 1671–1680. https://doi.org/10.5665/sleep.1432.

Gradisar, M., Smits, M. G., & Bjorvatn, B. (2014). Assessment and treatment of delayed sleep phase disorder in adolescents: Recent innovations and cautions. *Sleep Medicine Clinics, 9*(2), 199–210.

Hamill, K., Jumabhoy, R., Kahawage, P., de Zambotti, M., Walters, E. M., & Drummond, S. P. (2020). Validity, potential clinical utility and comparison of a consumer activity tracker and a research-grade activity tracker in insomnia disorder II: Outside the laboratory. *Journal of Sleep Research, 29*(1), e12944.

Harvey, A. G. (2005). A cognitive theory and therapy for chronic insomnia. *Journal of Cognitive Psychotherapy, 19*(1), 41–59.

Harvey, A. G., & Buysse, D. J. (2017). *Treating sleep problems: A transdiagnostic approach*. Guilford Publications.

Haslam, N., Holland, E., & Kuppens, P. (2012). Categories versus dimensions in personality and psychopathology: A quantitative review of taxometric research. *Psychological Medicine, 42*(5), 903–920. https://doi.org/10.1017/S0033291711001966.

Hasler, B. P., Bruce, S., Scharf, D., Ngari, W., & Clark, D. B. (2019). Circadian misalignment and weekend alcohol use in late adolescent drinkers: Preliminary evidence. *Chronobiology International, 36*(6), 796–810.

Hasler, B. P., Buysse, D. J., & Germain, A. (2016). Shifts toward morningness during behavioral sleep interventions are associated with improvements in depression, positive affect, and sleep quality. *Behavioral Sleep Medicine, 14*(6), 624–635.

Hasler, B., Buysse, D., Ngari, W., & Franzen, P. (2019). 0821 Successful sleep extension and phase advance in adolescents in response to a pilot sleep/circadian manipulation. *Sleep, 42*(Suppl. 1), A329–A330.

Hasler, B. P., Franzen, P. L., de Zambotti, M., Prouty, D., Brown, S. A., Tapert, S. F., et al. (2017). Eveningness and later sleep timing are associated with greater risk for alcohol and marijuana use in adolescence: Initial findings from the national consortium on alcohol and neurodevelopment in adolescence study. *Alcoholism: Clinical and Experimental Research, 41*(6), 1154–1165. https://doi.org/10.1111/acer.13401.

Hoebert, M., Van Der Heijden, K. B., Van Geijlswijk, I. M., & Smits, M. G. (2009). Long-term follow-up of melatonin treatment in children with ADHD and chronic sleep onset insomnia. *Journal of Pineal Research, 47*(1), 1–7.

Horne, J. A., & Östberg, O. (1976). A self-assessment questionnaire to determine morningness-eveningness in human circadian rhythms. *International Journal of Chronobiology, 4*(2), 97–110.

Jansson-Fröjmark, M., Lind, M., & Sunnhed, R. (2012). Don't worry, be constructive: A randomized controlled feasibility study comparing behaviour therapy singly and combined with constructive worry for insomnia. *British Journal of Clinical Psychology, 51*(2), 142–157.

Järnefelt, H., Lagerstedt, R., Kajaste, S., Sallinen, M., Savolainen, A., & Hublin, C. (2012). Cognitive behavioral therapy for shift workers with chronic insomnia. *Sleep Medicine, 13*(10), 1238–1246. https://doi.org/10.1016/j.sleep.2012.10.003.

Kantermann, T., Sung, H., & Burgess, H. J. (2015). Comparing the morningness-eveningness questionnaire and munich chronotype questionnaire to the dim light melatonin onset. *Journal of Biological Rhythms, 30*(5), 449–453. https://doi.org/10.1177/0748730415597520.

Kennaway, D. J. (2015). Potential safety issues in the use of the hormone melatonin in paediatrics. *Journal of Paediatrics and Child Health, 51*(6), 584–589.

Kim, M. J., Lee, J. H., & Duffy, J. F. (2013). Circadian rhythm sleep disorders. *Journal of Clinical Outcomes Management, 20*(11), 513–528. https://doi.org/10.1038/jid.2014.371.

Knutson, K. L., & von Schantz, M. (2018). Associations between chronotype, morbidity and mortality in the UK Biobank cohort. *Chronobiology International, 35*(8), 1045–1053. https://doi.org/10.1080/07420528.2018.1454458.

Kubala, A. G., Barone Gibbs, B., Buysse, D. J., Patel, S. R., Hall, M. H., & Kline, C. E. (2020). Field-based measurement of sleep: Agreement between six commercial activity monitors and a validated accelerometer. *Behavioral Sleep Medicine, 18*(5), 637–652.

Lack, L. C., Lovato, N., & Micic, G. (2017). Circadian rhythms and insomnia. *Sleep and Biological Rhythms, 15*(1), 3–10.

Lack, L. C., & Wright, H. R. (2007). Treating chronobiological components of chronic insomnia. *Sleep Medicine, 8*(6), 637–644. https://doi.org/10.1016/j.sleep.2006.10.003.

Laing, E. E., Möller-Levet, C. S., Poh, N., Santhi, N., Archer, S. N., & Dijk, D. J. (2017). Blood transcriptome based biomarkers for human circadian phase. *eLife, 6*, 1–26. https://doi.org/10.7554/eLife.20214.

Lau, T., Lovato, N., & Lack, L. (2018). Evaluation of a portable light device for phase advancing the circadian rhythm in the home environment. *Sleep and Biological Rhythms, 16*(4), 405–411.

Lewy, A. J., Emens, J., Jackman, A., & Yuhas, K. (2006). Circadian uses of melatonin in humans. *Chronobiology International, 23*(1-2), 403–412.

Lovato, N., Gradisar, M., Short, M., Dohnt, H., & Micic, G. (2013). Delayed sleep phase disorder in an Australian school-based sample of adolescents. *Journal of Clinical Sleep Medicine, 9*(9), 939–944.

Lovato, N., & Lack, L. (2016). Circadian phase delay using the newly developed re-timer portable light device. *Sleep and Biological Rhythms, 14*(2), 157–164.

Magee, M., Marbas, E. M., Wright, K. P., Rajaratnam, S. M. W., & Broussard, J. L. (2016). Diagnosis, cause, and treatment approaches for delayed sleep-wake phase disorder. *Sleep Medicine Clinics, 11*(3), 389–401. https://doi.org/10.1016/j.jsmc.2016.05.004.

Malkani, R. G., Abbott, S. M., Reid, K. J., & Zee, P. C. (2018). Diagnostic and treatment challenges of sighted non-24-hour sleep-wake disorder. *Journal of Clinical Sleep Medicine, 14*(4), 603–613. https://doi.org/10.5664/jcsm.7054.

Malow, B. A., Findling, R. L., Schroder, C. M., Maras, A., Breddy, J., Nir, T., et al. (2020). Sleep, growth, and puberty after two years of prolonged-release melatonin in children with autism spectrum disorder. *Journal of the American Academy of Child and Adolescent Psychiatry*. https://doi.org/10.1016/j.jaac.2019.12.007.

Manzoni, G. M., Pagnini, F., Castelnuovo, G., & Molinari, E. (2008). Relaxation training for anxiety: A ten-years systematic review with meta-analysis. *BMC Psychiatry, 8*(1), 41.

Matthews, E. E., Arnedt, J. T., McCarthy, M. S., Cuddihy, L. J., & Aloia, M. S. (2013). Adherence to cognitive behavioral therapy for insomnia: A systematic review. *Sleep Medicine Reviews, 17*(6), 453–464.

Micic, G., Lovato, N., Ferguson, S. A., Burgess, H. J., & Lack, L. (2020). Circadian tau differences and rhythm associations in delayed sleep-wake phase disorder and sighted non-24-hour sleep-wake rhythm disorder. *Sleep, 44*.

Murray, J. M., Sletten, T. L., Magee, M., Gordon, C., Lovato, N., Bartlett, D. J., et al. (2017). Prevalence of circadian misalignment and its association with depressive symptoms in delayed sleep phase disorder. *Sleep, 40*(1). https://doi.org/10.1093/sleep/zsw002.

Paine, S. J., Fink, J., Gander, P. H., & Warman, G. R. (2014). Identifying advanced and delayed sleep phase disorders in the general population: A national survey of New Zealand adults. *Chronobiology International, 31*(5), 627–636.

Paul, M. A., Gray, G. W., Lieberman, H. R., Love, R. J., Miller, J. C., Trouborst, M., et al. (2011). Phase advance with separate and combined melatonin and light treatment. *Psychopharmacology, 214*(2), 515–523.

Pullman, R. E., Roepke, S. E., & Duffy, J. F. (2012). Laboratory validation of an in-home method for assessing circadian phase using dim light melatonin onset (DLMO). *Sleep Medicine, 13*(6), 703–706.

Qaseem, A., Kansagara, D., Forciea, M. A., Cooke, M., Denberg, T. D., Barry, M. J., et al. (2016). Management of chronic insomnia disorder in adults: A clinical practice guideline from the American college of physicians. *Annals of Internal Medicine, 165*(2), 125–133. https://doi.org/10.7326/M15-2175.

Rahman, S. A., Kayumov, L., Tchmoutina, E. A., & Shapiro, C. M. (2009). Clinical efficacy of dim light melatonin onset testing in diagnosing delayed sleep phase syndrome. *Sleep Medicine, 10*(5), 549–555. https://doi.org/10.1016/j.sleep.2008.03.020.

Richardson, C., Cain, N., Bartel, K., Micic, G., Maddock, B., & Gradisar, M. (2018). A randomised controlled trial of bright light therapy and morning activity for adolescents and young adults with delayed sleep-wake phase disorder. *Sleep Medicine, 45*, 114–123.

Riedel, B. W., & Lichstein, K. L. (2000). Insomnia and daytime functioning. *Sleep Medicine Reviews, 4*(3), 277–298.

Roehrs, T., & Roth, T. (2018). Insomnia as a path to alcoholism: Tolerance development and dose escalation. *Sleep, 41*(8), 1–5. https://doi.org/10.1093/sleep/zsy091.

Roenneberg, T. (2015). *Munich ChronoType Questionnaire (MCTQ) for children and adolescents.* Retrieved from: thewep.org/documentations/mctq.

Roenneberg, T., Kuehnle, T., Juda, M., Kantermann, T., Allebrandt, K., Gordijn, M., et al. (2007). Epidemiology of the human circadian clock. *Sleep Medicine Reviews, 11*(6), 429–438. https://doi.org/10.1016/j.smrv.2007.07.005.

Roenneberg, T., Wirz-Justice, A., & Merrow, M. (2003). Life between clocks: Daily temporal patterns of human chronotypes. *Journal of Biological Rhythms, 18*(1), 80–90. https://doi.org/10.1177/0748730402239679.

Sack, R. L., Hughes, R. J., Edgar, D. M., & Lewy, A. J. (1997). Sleep-promoting effects of melatonin: At what dose, in whom, under what conditions, and by what mechanisms? *Sleep, 20*(10), 908–915.

Shechter, A., Quispe, K. A., Mizhquiri Barbecho, J. S., Slater, C., & Falzon, L. (2020). Interventions to reduce short-wavelength ("blue") light exposure at night and their effects on sleep: A systematic review and meta-analysis. *Sleep Advances, 1*.

Sit, D. K., Terman, M., & Wisner, K. L. (2018). Light therapy and risk of hypomania, mania, or mixed state emergence: Response to Benedetti et al. *American Journal of Psychiatry, 175*(9), 906.

Smith, M. T., McCrae, C. S., Cheung, J., Martin, J. L., Harrod, C. G., Heald, J. L., et al. (2018). Use of actigraphy for the evaluation of sleep disorders and circadian rhythm sleep-wake disorders: An American Academy of Sleep Medicine clinical practice guideline. *Journal of Clinical Sleep Medicine, 14*(07), 1231–1237.

Smith, C. S., Reilly, C., & Midkiff, K. (1989). Evaluation of three circadian rhythm questionnaires with suggestions for an improved measure of morningness. *Journal of Applied Psychology, 74*(5), 728.

Stone, J. E., Aubert, X. L., Maass, H., Phillips, A. J., Magee, M., Howard, M. E., et al. (2019). Application of a limit-cycle oscillator model for prediction of circadian phase in rotating night shift workers. *Scientific Reports, 9*(1), 1–12.

Swanson, L. M., Burgess, H. J., Zollars, J., & Arnedt, J. T. (2018). An open-label pilot study of a home wearable light therapy device for postpartum depression. *Archives of Women's Mental Health, 21*(5), 583–586.

Takahashi, M. (2003). The role of prescribed napping in sleep medicine. *Sleep Medicine Reviews, 7*(3), 227–235.

Taylor, B. J., & Hasler, B. P. (2018). Chronotype and mental health: Recent advances. *Current Psychiatry Reports, 20*(8), 59.

Trotti, L. M. (2017). Waking up is the hardest thing I do all day: Sleep inertia and sleep drunkenness. *Sleep Medicine Reviews, 35*, 76–84.

Troxel, W. M., Germain, A., & Buysse, D. J. (2012). Clinical management of insomnia with brief behavioral treatment (BBTI). *Behavioral Sleep Medicine, 10*(4), 266–279.

Van Geijlswijk, I. M., Korzilius, H. P. L. M., & Smits, M. G. (2010). The use of exogenous melatonin in delayed sleep phase disorder: A meta-analysis. *Sleep, 33*(12), 1605–1614.

van Maanen, A., Meijer, A. M., van der Heijden, K. B., & Oort, F. J. (2016). The effects of light therapy on sleep problems: A systematic review and meta-analysis. *Sleep Medicine Reviews, 29*, 52–62. https://doi.org/10.1016/j.smrv.2015.08.009.

Vyas, M. V., Garg, A. X., Iansavichus, A. V., Costella, J., Donner, A., Laugsand, L. E., et al. (2012). Shift work and vascular events: Systematic review and meta-analysis. *BMJ (Online), 345*(7871), 1–11. https://doi.org/10.1136/bmj.e4800.

Wade, A. G., Ford, I., Crawford, G., McConnachie, A., Nir, T., Laudon, M., et al. (2010). Nightly treatment of primary insomnia with prolonged release melatonin for 6 months: A randomized placebo controlled trial on age and endogenous melatonin as predictors of efficacy and safety. *BMC Medicine, 8*(1), 51.

Wahl, S., Engelhardt, M., Schaupp, P., Lappe, C., & Ivanov, I. V. (2019). The inner clock—Blue light sets the human rhythm. *Journal of Biophotonics, 12*(12), e201900102.

Wasdell, M. B., Jan, J. E., Bomben, M. M., Freeman, R. D., Rietveld, W. J., Tai, J., et al. (2008). A randomized, placebo-controlled trial of controlled release melatonin treatment of delayed sleep phase syndrome and impaired sleep maintenance in children with neurodevelopmental disabilities. *Journal of Pineal Research, 44*(1), 57–64.

Werner, H., Lebourgeois, M. K., Geiger, A., & Jenni, O. G. (2009). Assessment of chronotype in four- to eleven-year-old children: Reliability and validity of the Children's Chronotype Questionnaire (CCTQ). *Chronobiology International, 26*(5), 992–1014. https://doi.org/10.1080/07420520903044505.ASSESSMENT.

Williams, W. P., III, McLin, D. E., III, Dressman, M. A., & Neubauer, D. N. (2016). Comparative review of approved melatonin agonists for the treatment of circadian rhythm sleep-wake disorders. *Pharmacotherapy: The Journal of Human Pharmacology and Drug Therapy, 36*(9), 1028–1041.

Wirz-Justice, A., Benedetti, F., & Terman, M. (2009). *Chronotherapeutics for affective disorders: A clinician's manual for light and wake therapy*. Karger.

Wittenbrink, N., Kunz, D., & Kramer, A. (2018). High-accuracy determination of internal circadian time from a single blood sample. *The Journal of Clinical Investigation, 128*(9), 3826. https://doi.org/10.1172/JCI120874.

Woelders, T., Beersma, D. G., Gordijn, M. C., Hut, R. A., & Wams, E. J. (2017). Daily light exposure patterns reveal phase and period of the human circadian clock. *Journal of Biological Rhythms, 32*(3), 274–286.

Wu, J. Q., Appleman, E. R., Salazar, R. D., & Ong, J. C. (2015). Cognitive behavioral therapy for insomnia comorbid with psychiatric and medical conditions: A meta-analysis. *JAMA Internal Medicine, 175*(9), 1461–1472.

Yan, L. (2009). Expression of clock genes in the suprachiasmatic nucleus: Effect of environmental lighting conditions. *Reviews in Endocrine & Metabolic Disorders, 10*(4), 301–310. https://doi.org/10.1007/s11154-009-9121-9.

Zalta, A. K., Bravo, K., Valdespino-Hayden, Z., Pollack, M. H., & Burgess, H. J. (2019). A placebo-controlled pilot study of a wearable morning bright light treatment for probable PTSD. *Depression and Anxiety, 36*(7), 617–624.

Zee, P. C., & Vitiello, M. V. (2009). Circadian rhythm sleep disorder: Irregular sleep wake rhythm. *Sleep Medicine Clinics, 4*(2), 213–218. https://doi.org/10.1016/j.jsmc.2009.01.009.

CHAPTER

4

CBT-I for patients with shift work disorder

Philip Cheng

Department of Internal Medicine, Thomas Roth Sleep Disorders and Research Center, Henry Ford Health System, Detroit, MI, United States

Introduction

Shift work disorder (SWD), also known as shift work sleep disorder, afflicts a vast number of Americans who work at night or irregular hours. Nightshift work is critical to a 24/7 economy that ensures around-the-clock availability of essential services. The nightshift workforce comprises essential workers, including doctors, nurses, and hospital staff; security, including police officers and security guards; emergency services, including firefighters and paramedics; factories; public transports; energy production; and other sectors that maintain critical safety, healthcare, and economic infrastructures.

SWD impacts between 10% and 38% of shift workers depending on a myriad of factors (e.g., occupation, shift frequency, and duration), and is characterized by complaints of insomnia and excessive sleepiness occurring as a result of work hours during the biological night that also displace nocturnal sleep (American Academy of Sleep Medicine, 2014). Because industries that rely on nightshift workers are often safety-sensitive, SWD can lead to devastating consequences. There are many historical examples of catastrophic accidents on the nightshift, including the infamous Three Mile Island nuclear reactor meltdown, the American Airlines Flight 1420 crash, and the Exxon Valdez oil spill. Additionally, chronic SWD severely compromises the health and functioning of nightshift workers leading to poor metabolic health, cardiovascular difficulties, poor psychiatric health, and even cancer. For example, the International

Adapting Cognitive Behavioral Therapy for Insomnia
https://doi.org/10.1016/B978-0-12-822872-2.00019-0

Agency for Research on Cancer recently classified nightshift work with circadian disruption as a probable carcinogen, with evidence for elevated risk of breast, prostate, and colorectal cancer (Straif, Baan, Grosse, et al., 2007; Ward, Germolec, Kogevinas, et al., 2019; Zhang & Papantoniou, 2019). Other health risks include metabolic dysfunction (e.g., obesity, elevated cholesterol, and raised triglyceride levels) (Karlsson, Knutsson, & Lindahl, 2001; McHill, Melanson, Higgins, et al., 2014), cardiovascular difficulties (Bøggild & Knutsson, 1999; Puttonen, Härmä, & Hublin, 2010), and poor psychiatric health (Kalmbach, Pillai, Cheng, Arnedt, & Drake, 2015; Scott, Monk, & Brink, 1997). Notwithstanding the health risks, the direct and indirect cost of SWD is estimated at over $120 billion annually (Culpepper, 2010). To summarize, SWD is a serious and costly burden on public health and safety, and is an urgent problem needing solutions.

Current landscape of treatments for SWD

Despite being a serious and longstanding problem, the landscape of treatment for SWD continues to face unmet needs. In particular, there is a lack of evidence-based treatments that target the underlying mechanisms of SWD. This is in part because the challenges of SWD suffer from a lack of visibility. Indeed, the difficulties of nightshift work play out at night when most decision makers and stakeholders are asleep. This lack of visibility is a barrier to developing a nuanced understanding of the challenges nightshift workers face, which often leads to oversimplified solutions to SWD. For example, one simple solution recommended for SWD is terminating shiftwork altogether (Sachdeva & Goldstein, 2020). First, as many as one-third of nightshift workers experience excessive sleepiness and insomnia, which is a significant portion of the nightshift workforce (Drake, Roehrs, Richardson, Walsh, & Roth, 2004). If a majority of symptomatic nightshift workers stopped working, these essential services would not be sustainable. Moreover, termination of nightshift work is unrealistic for a significant subset of the workforce. For example, in many industries that require shiftwork (e.g., nursing), many entry positions into the profession are nightshifts, and opportunities to transition out of the nightshift are provided based on seniority. Furthermore, nightshifts often serve as means for socioeconomic mobility or stability in disenfranchised populations. Nightshifts are typically more accessible to those without advanced degrees and commonly pay higher wages than the dayshift. People often turn to nightshifts to provide financial support while they complete educational degrees to advance their careers. Additionally, many individuals (e.g., single mothers) rely on the night shift schedule to minimize childcare costs to maintain financial stability. In sum, avoiding shift work is neither a practical nor a viable solution, and it is imperative that nightshift workers have access to effective treatments that safeguard their health, safety, and productivity.

Advantages of a behavioral treatment for SWD

Current practices in the treatment of SWD largely uses palliative approaches focused on symptom management—namely, the use of stimulants to maintain alertness and hypnotic medications for sleep (Czeisler, Walsh, Roth, et al., 2005; Czeisler, Walsh, Wesnes, Roth, & Arora, 2009; Walsh, Muehlbach, & Schweitzer, 1995). While this approach can improve symptoms, the risk of adverse events and abuse potential is high, particularly with near daily use of medications in this population of workers in safety-sensitive operations. There are some efficacious nonpharmacotherapy strategies that temporarily counteracts fatigue, such as the use of caffeine and naps (American National Standards Institute & American Petroleum Institute, 2010; Schweitzer, Randazzo, Stone, Erman, & Walsh, 2006); however, few strategies have been validated for insomnia symptoms in SWD. Though symptom management is important, it leaves the underlying mechanism unabated which can continue to cause a sequela of acute and long-term problems and morbidities. For example, circadian misalignment has been posited as the mechanism for the increased risk of cardiometabolic dysfunction and cancer in SWD (Barger, Lockley, Rajaratnam, & Landrigan, 2009; Kamdar, Tergas, Mateen, Bhayani, & Oh, 2013; Puttonen et al., 2010). Without treatments that target the underlying mechanisms, shift workers will continue to risk their health while providing essential services.

One potentially promising approach of addressing insomnia symptoms in SWD is to adapt Cognitive Behavioral Therapy for Insomnia (CBT-I) for SWD. CBT-I is brief, highly effective, and is the recommended first line treatment for chronic insomnia (Qaseem, Kansagara, Forciea, Cooke, & Denberg, 2016; Riemann, Baglioni, Bassetti, et al., 2017). However, studies testing adaptations of CBT-I for SWD are still emerging; thus, there is a lack of strong evidence base for what adaptations are efficacious for SWD. As is common with emergent areas of research, no standards have been established for what and how adaptations should be made for SWD. As such, there is significant heterogeneity in approaching adapting CBT-I for SWD. Extant approaches include no adaptations (i.e., testing CBT-I as is), excluding components that may not apply to SWD, adding components that uniquely tailored for SWD, or tweaking CBT-I practices for SWD.

What adaptations have been tried?

Unsurprisingly, studies that have tested the efficacy of CBT-I as is (without any adaptations) find that the effects on CBT-I are more robust in those on the dayshift compared to those on nonday shift schedules (Schiller, Söderström, Lekander, Rajaleid, & Kecklund, 2018); however, results in shift workers have also been inconsistent. For example, one study in nurses on the nightshift utilized an intervention that began with 4 weeks of bibliotherapy using the "Plain Language About Shiftwork" developed by the National Institute for Occupational Safety and Health (NIOSH), which served as the control condition. The bibliotherapy was followed by another 4 weeks of another CBT-I workbook augmented with presleep sound relaxation training delivered via MP3 files. Results showed a moderate improvement in self-reported sleep quality but no changes in objective measures of sleep.

Another study pared full CBT-I down into a brief CBT-I approach comprised of 90 min of didactic training on sleep and reviewing sleep hygiene practices ($n = 156$). A waitlist control condition was included as a comparator ($n = 155$). The adaptations for SWD included recommendations of (1) sleeping as soon as possible following the night shift, (2) minimizing "long periods" of sleep the following morning (assuming it is an off-day), and (3) avoiding daytime naps that are longer than needed. Stimulus control was also included in the sleep hygiene curriculum. The Pittsburgh Sleep Quality Index (PSQI) was measure before and two-months after the intervention. The study reported a significant time × condition interaction suggesting that the reduction in PSQI was larger in the CBT-I condition than in the waitlist control. The postintervention difference in PSQI scores between the conditions was 0.93, corresponding to a small effect size (Cohen's $d = 0.31$).

Another study added light therapy to standard CBT-I (appended to the sleep hygiene session), though details of the parameters of light therapy (e.g., timing, intensity, and duration) were not provided. The study ($n = 12$) found an average decrease of 2.5 points from a pretreatment PSQI score of 11.5, and no significant improvement in sleepiness. However, the lack of a control group precluded inference regarding the specific effect of adding light therapy.

Finally, two other studies incorporated multifaceted in approach in modifications. The modifications included tailoring psychoeducation to shift work, including strategic use of naps for fatigue risk management. Additional strategies were also provided for scheduling sleep and light exposure in accordance with "circadian principles," including the use of anchor sleep. Details regarding implementation of these strategies were not provided. Finally, another modification specifically to sleep restriction was an allowance to extend time in bed by 1 h for up to three sleep periods during the treatment if they experienced "marked shift work-related sleep debt." Results indicated no differences in change in insomnia symptoms compared with a sleep-hygiene only control, though all groups showed a reduction in insomnia symptoms.

Adapting CBT-I for SWD

Pathophysiology of SWD

In considering adapting CBT-I for SWD is important to understand the differences between insomnia disorder and SWD. First, a diagnosis of SWD can arise from two symptoms: insomnia and/or excessive sleepiness. As such, there can be three phenotypes: SWD with insomnia only, SWD with excessive sleepiness only, and SWD with both insomnia and sleepiness. As the principles of CBT-I are designed to target insomnia symptoms, this chapter focuses primarily on the adaptation of CBT-I for insomnia symptoms in SWD.

Although many shift workers experience insomnia symptoms to varying degrees at different points during shift work, not everyone develops SWD with insomnia. The prevailing theory is that insomnia in SWD is driven by circadian misalignment, wherein the individual's internal circadian rhythms are mismatched to their work and sleep schedules. Specifically, the human sleep/wake system is partially governed by an endogenous biological clock that regulates a myriad of functions including sleep and alertness that fluctuate across the 24-h day [i.e., process C in the two-process model of sleep regulation (Borbély, 1982)]. In nonshift workers, this internal clock is aligned with the day-night cycle via natural sunlight (or other sources of bright light). This includes the secretion of melatonin that begins in evening, on average 2-h prior to habitual bedtime (e.g., melatonin secretion begins at 9 pm followed by an 11 pm bedtime). Melatonin secretion peaks in the middle of the night and ends in the morning, after which alerting signals are upregulated to promote wakefulness and performance. In contrast, many nontraditional shifts (especially night shifts) displace the main sleep period into the daytime, causing circadian misalignment between the planned sleep period and the underlying physiology. As a result, the planned sleep during this period occurs against an increasing alerting signal that interrupts or curtails sleep. Though circadian misalignment is sometimes relevant in insomnia disorder, this is likely a much stronger mechanism driving insomnia symptoms in SWD compared with insomnia disorder. As such, the adaptation of CBT-I for SWD should account for circadian misalignment (Fig. 1).

Although there is strong consensus that circadian misalignment is an important mechanism in SWD, emerging evidence suggests that it is

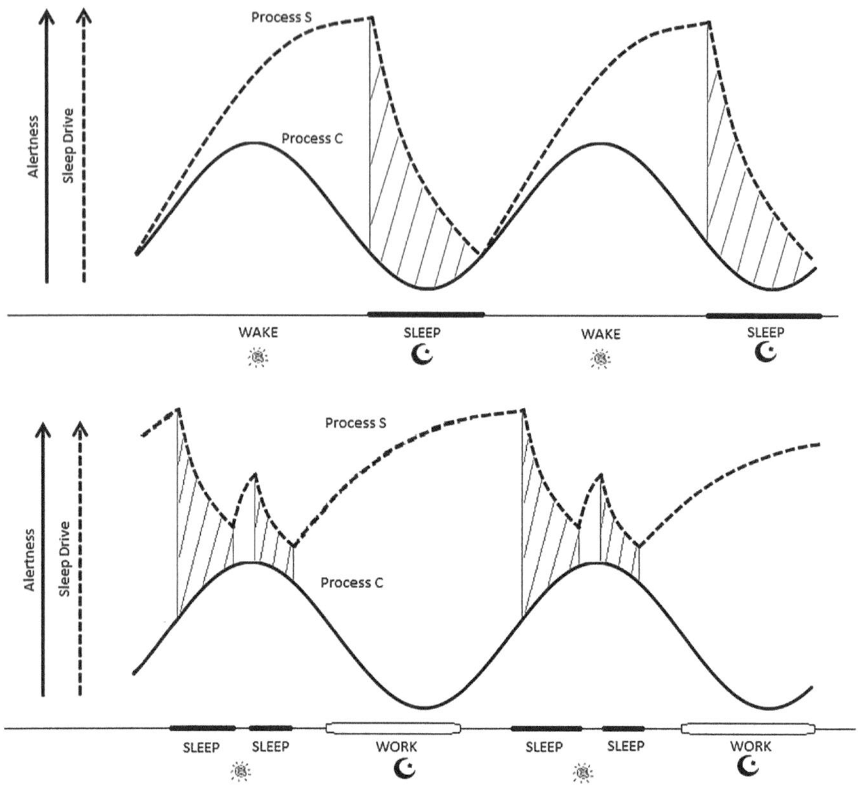

FIG. 1 *Top panel*: Sleep and wake occurring when both the sleep drive (process S) and circadian rhythm (process C) are in harmony. Sleep occurs at night when the circadian signal for alertness is downregulated and sleep drive is high. *Bottom panel*: Typical sleep and wake rhythms in SWD in a nightshift worker. The planned sleep period after the night shift occurs against an increasing circadian signal for alertness, which disrupts and fragments sleep. During work hours, the shift worker is experiencing both a reduction of a circadian alerting signal along with an increase sleep drive.

not the only cause of insomnia symptoms in shift workers. Emerging studies also implicate sleep reactivity as a causal mechanism for insomnia symptoms in SWD (Kalmbach et al., 2015). Sleep reactivity is defined as a sleep system that is particularly vulnerable to perturbations. Sleep reactivity has been determined as a phenotypic trait that shows stability over time (Jarrin, Chen, Ivers, Drake, & Morin, 2016) and is 30%–40% heritable, suggesting a substantial genetic component (Drake, Friedman, Wright, & Roth, 2011). The vulnerability to disturbed sleep associated with high sleep reactivity has been demonstrated across a range of stressors. For example, sleep reactivity has been associated with a worse "first night effect" (Chen et al., 2015; Kalmbach, Anderson, & Drake, 2018), wherein sleep is disturbed due to a new sleep environment (e.g., first night in a hotel room). Individuals with high sleep reactivity also show notably more sleep disturbance in response to caffeine intake close to bedtime. While individuals with low sleep reactivity show a 7-min increase in time to sleep onset following caffeine administration, individuals with high sleep reactivity show a 46 min increase in sleep onset—a response 6.6 times larger in magnitude (Drake, Jefferson, Roehrs, & Roth, 2006). More recently, we have also shown that sleep reactivity prospectively predicts insomnia in response to the COVID-19 pandemic (Cheng, Casement, Kalmbach, Castelan, & Drake, 2021). Specifically, we found that sleep reactivity recorded in 2016–17 was significantly predictive of disturbed sleep in April of 2020 during the first peak of COVID-19 ($B = 0.39 \pm 0.09$ SE, $P < .001$). These studies illustrate that sleep reactivity is a robust predictor of disturbed sleep in response to a wide range of environmental challenges/stressors.

In SWD, the transition to the shift work can trigger insomnia symptoms in those with high sleep reactivity to stress. Shift workers are commonly exposed to occupational and environmental stressors. For example, night-shift workers frequently have less access to workplace resources, including reduced access to important stakeholders (e.g., staff meetings commonly occur during the day), inadequate staff support at night, higher workload associated with inadequate staff, and reduced access to professional development opportunities. Additionally, shift workers who sleep during the day are also more prone to environmental noise as a stressor. Finally, shift workers sometimes note increased social isolation as they often need to choose sleep over attending social or familial functions. As such, the various stressors associated with shift work combined with a predisposition of high sleep reactivity may coalesce, leading to insomnia. Indeed, a prospective study of normal sleeping workers transitioning to shiftwork demonstrated that high sleep reactivity before the onset of shiftwork robustly increased the risk of incident SWD ($OR = 5.6$) 1 year later (Kalmbach et al., 2015). Although sleep reactivity is not a unique mechanism to SWD, the stressors that trigger SWD is often unique to shift work and thus warrant attention when adapting CBT-I for SWD.

Considerations when adapting CBT-I for SWD: Toward a mechanistic approach

Assessment

Adapting CBT-I for SWD begins with an accurate understanding of the relevant mechanisms driving the symptoms of insomnia in SWD. Evaluation of insomnia in shift workers should include an assessment of work history (e.g., occupation, work schedule, years of shift work), and current shift schedule (e.g., morning, afternoon, evenings shifts; fixed vs rotating schedule; if rotating, note direction and speed of rotation), particularly because the goals of treatment may differ based on the shift type. Additionally, a detailed sleep history is also important, making sure to assess daytime and nighttime sleep difficulties separately. Assessing level of sleepiness using standardized measures (e.g., Epworth Sleepiness Scale, Karolinska Sleepiness Scale), accidental dozing (particularly during shift work or while driving), and any performance impairment during work shifts is important to characterize the level of risk that should be accommodated in the treatment. As is standard in CBT-I, patients should also be asked about sleep hygiene and use of medications or substances that may impact sleep.

As is recommended in an ICSD-3 diagnosis of SWD, the assessment should include two-weeks of sleep diaries and actigraphy to capture sleep-wake disturbances on both work-days and off-work days. The combination of sleep diaries and actigraphy is more reliable than retrospective self-report, especially as the day-to-day variation is typically much more erratic than that of nonshift workers. A full two-week period is important to distinguish sleep-wake rhythms on work-days, off-work days, transition to work-days, and transition to off-work days. If actigraphy is not available, the 24-h sleep diary (Fig. 2) is often more informative because of the increased the ease of visual detection of patterns related to circadian rhythms. Conversely, the consensus sleep diary may be preferred for the evaluation of insomnia if it is clear that circadian rhythms are not a primary issue. Some patients may also use a mobile application to log sleep diaries.

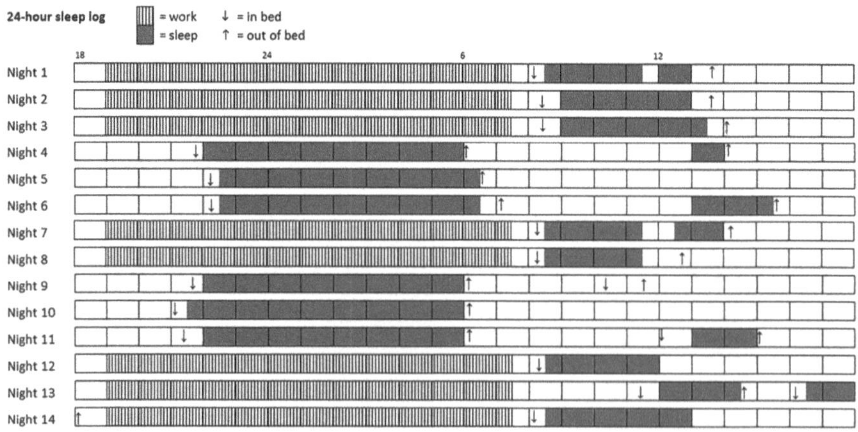

FIG. 2 An example of a 24-h sleep diary. The difference between sleep during work-days and off-work days are easily discerned.

Assessing circadian misalignment

The gold standard method of assessment circadian misalignment are to determine the dim light melatonin onset (DLMO). However, collecting DLMO in shift workers is resource intensive as it requires 24h of saliva samples collected in a laboratory environment under dim light. Other methods include assessment of core body temperature or the use of urinary assays of 6-sulfatoxymelatonin, both of which still require samples over 24h.

Given the infeasibility of using gold standard measurements of circadian phase or DLMO, there has been significant interest in the development of alternatives to DLMO (Braun, Kath, Iwanaszko, et al., 2018; Laing et al., 2017; Sinues, Tarokh, Li, et al., 2014). Many of the alternatives under development extract biomarkers of circadian phase from biological specimens, such as repeated blood samples and tissue biopsies. Another approach under development is the use of light and activity data from wearable technologies processed through a model of the human circadian system to infer the underlying circadian phase. Indeed, this approach has been tested in a sample of nightshift workers, and should be replicated in larger samples (Cheng, Walch, Huang, et al., 2021). A prototype of an internet-based tool has been developed using this method (www.predictDLMO.com) which allows providers to upload light and activity data from actigraphs into a calculator that will generate estimates of DLMO.

Factors to consider when implementing CBT-I for SWD

Circadian rhythms

Circadian misalignment is arguably the most important factor to consider in adapting CBT-I for SWD. When CBT-I is implemented to treat insomnia patients who follow a diurnal schedule, circadian phase is anchored with a stable wake-time in the morning, often combined with recommendations of seeking light exposure on awakening. This approach needs to be adapted for SWD for two reasons. First, the spread of circadian phase in those with SWD is much wider than in those following a diurnal schedule. This means that assessing for circadian phase in SWD can inform treatment recommendations.

Second, if we can access the circadian phase, we can also shift their phase to a more desirable time. There are competing perspectives regarding what an ideal circadian phase is for shift workers, which is often complicated by the specific shift work schedule. In fixed-night shift workers, some have argued that a 12-h shift in DLMO (e.g., form 9pm to 9am) would maximally support sleep following a night shift and alertness during the nocturnal work, especially if the individual works the night shift regularly (9 pm to 5 am, five times a week). However, evidence suggests that most night shift workers do not maintain a nocturnal schedule on their off-work days, especially if they work fewer than five shifts a week (e.g., nurses often work three 12-h shifts a week). Indeed, night shift workers commonly revert to diurnal schedule on off-work days to spend time with their family and friends, or to access services that are only available during the day (e.g., medical appointments and errands). In rotating shifts, the speed and direction of rotations are important considerations. For example, a slow forward rotation (e.g., rotating through day, afternoon, and night shifts every month) may allow adequate time for workers to benefit from circadian adjustment to each of the shift, whereas fast rotating schedules (e.g., rotating through each shift type after 1 day) will likely not accommodate any circadian adjustments. In fact, fast backwards rotating shifts (e.g., rotating counterclockwise through night, afternoon, and day shifts) are designed to have minimal impact on circadian phase. In sum, the shift schedule is an important consideration in the ideal timing of DLMO.

In night shift workers, there is evidence that a *compromised phase position* may be desirable. A compromised phase position places DLMO in the early morning period such that the circadian nadir falls within the daytime sleep window. The circadian nadir corresponds to the period of lowest alertness and typically occurs 7 h following DLMO. For example, a DLMO of 4 am would result in a circadian nadir at 11 am, which means that the period of peak sleepiness is not only outside of the night shift, but is occurring during the daytime sleep period, and thus promoting daytime sleep. On off-work days, individuals would follow a later sleep-wake schedule (e.g., time in bed from 4 am to noon), which would still allow individuals to partake in familial and social activities in the afternoon.

Sleep scheduling

An additional component that works in tandem with circadian rhythms is the timing of sleep on both work days and off-work days. Whenever possible the target should maximize alignment between the planned sleep period and the circadian window of sleep maintenance. For example, in a compromised phase position where the window of sleep maintenance is between 4 am and 4 pm, daytime sleep following a night shift should be placed shortly after returning home following a wind-down period (e.g., 9 am to 4 pm). If sleeping at night on off-days, nighttime sleep should be planned to start as close to the beginning of the sleep maintenance zone as possible (e.g., 4 am to noon).

Sleep restriction

In addition to the unique role of circadian rhythms in SWD, there are also important considerations in translating CBT-I for SWD. Sleep restriction is a core component of CBT-I that requires reconsideration when translated for SWD. First, sleep restriction in insomnia disorder assumes that the sleep period is occurring in the window of sleep maintenance (i.e., period of melatonin secretion) and that the sleep disruptions arise from maladaptive behaviors such as napping and staying in bed when not sleeping. Second, shift workers who are sleeping during the day following a night shift are often already operating under a high homeostatic sleep drive. As such, restricting time in bed may further sleep deprive the patient, leading to worsened sleepiness that increases risk for occupational hazards such as accidents and injuries. Indeed, even in insomnia disorder, the goal of sleep restriction is not sleep deprivation, as evidenced by the fact that most sleep restriction protocols have a minimum time in bed (usually 5–6h). Though some shift workers may be staying in bed for significantly longer than they are sleeping, sleep restriction alone would not account for the fact that their sleep (particularly during the daytime) is likely disturbed due to sleeping against an alerting circadian signal. As such, implementation of sleep restriction should be conducted only after accounting for circadian misalignment.

An adaptation to consider that targets sleep homeostasis is to shift the focus from consolidating sleep to minimizing high sleep drive. For example, to minimize sleep drive during the night shift, you could implement a sleep period closer to the shift start time. This may be implemented in the form of a prolonged nap (e.g., 2–3h) before leaving for work, with a note to leave adequate time for dissipation of sleep inertia before driving. For example, for a work start time of 11pm, one may place a nap from 8pm to 10pm. Some individuals may need to curtail daytime sleep to support this nap. Furthermore, in the 24–48h leading up to a night shift, the patient should engage in sleep banking by prioritizing and maximizing sleep duration and/or supplementing with naps.

Stimulus control

Though stimulus control can and should be implemented in SWD when appropriate, it needs to be balanced with total sleep time for safety. Similar to sleep restriction, stimulus control should be considered in the context of circadian phase and circadian misalignment. In insomnia disorder, patients who are implementing stimulus control are asked to get out of bed and only return when they become sleepy again; however, if stimulus control were to be implemented during the daytime or during window of wake maintenance, the patient may not become sleepy again until after their work shift has started. That said, if there are clear signs of conditioned arousal, stimulus control may be an effective therapeutic approach.

There are a few ways in which stimulus control can be adapted in SWD. One simpler approach may be to only implement stimulus control when sleeping on off-work days, especially if the hazards of sleepiness are lower. When between or transitioning to work days, the goal should still be to achieve a minimum target of total sleep time to support safety. Another approach is to only implement stimulus control during sleep periods that fall within the window of sleep maintenance, and not in supplemental sleep bouts (e.g., prework naps).

Sleep hygiene

Sleep hygiene may be especially important to discuss in the context of SWD, particularly regarding maintaining a dark, cool, and quiet environment during daytime sleep periods as the risk of ambient disruption is much higher during the day. Blackout shades are recommended whenever possible to minimize the intrusion of daylight into the bedroom. Management of noise during daytime sleep can be challenging, and often requires negotiating boundaries and planning for contingencies with family members and friends. Because there is more ambient noise during the day, the use of white noise in the bedroom may provide an acoustic buffer. Caffeine intake should also be monitored as it is often used as a method of countering excessive sleepiness during the night shift. See Table 1 for some recommended adaptations of sleep hygiene for SWD.

Cognitive therapy

The components that fall under cognitive therapy are easily implemented in SWD; however, in addition to the typical dysfunctional beliefs about sleep, there may be other cognitions that may need to be explored and addressed. For many shift workers, the cognitive therapy component may need to address prioritization of sleep and setting/negotiating boundaries around their sleep schedules. Adding a solutions-focused component can be particularly helpful for shift workers whose sleep schedules need to accommodate childcare or other social/familial obligations (e.g., school pick-up times can sometimes curtail sleep window).

Summary

Insomnia in SWD is a common and serious medical problem with few validated treatments that target the underlying mechanisms. Adapting CBT-I for insomnia symptoms in SWD may be a promising approach, though substantial modifications and additions should be added to account for the differences in pathophysiology between insomnia disorder and

TABLE 1 Sleep hygiene recommendations adapted for SWD.

Create a sleep-friendly bedroom environment.
Make sure that the bedroom is *dark*, quiet, and cool (around 65°F). Blackout shades may be particularly important to block out sunlight during daytime sleep. Creating constant background noise in the sleep environment (e.g., a fan, humidifier) can reduce the impact of other ambient sound sounds (e.g., lawn mowers, postal workers).
When possible, maximize regularity in activity and sleep schedule.
Regularity in the timing of sleep, food intake, and social activities help stabilize the biological clock. Minimizing discrepancies in sleep timing between on-shift and off-shift periods may promote adaptation to a fixed-shift schedule, and may also help adaptation to each shift type in a rotating-shift schedule (depending on rotation speed and direction).
Make the last hour before bed a "wind-down" time.
Engage in relaxing and pleasant activities, dim and/or block light in the room, and have a light snack.
Limit exposure to bright light before daytime sleep.
Exposure to bright light (e.g., sunlight during the morning commute home following a night shift) can be alerting and may also set your biological clock to a time that interferes with daytime sleep.
Do not use alcohol to help you sleep or consume alcohol too close to bedtime.
Although alcohol may help you to fall asleep more easily, it can cause frequent awakenings during the sleep bout. One drink of alcohol should not be consumed within 3 h of bedtime.
Smoking and other drugs will disrupt your sleep.
Avoiding smoking too close to bedtime or when awake during the intended sleep period. Most drugs of abuse can disrupt sleep.
Avoid caffeinated products within 6 h of bedtime.
In addition to coffee, these may include tea, chocolate, and various sodas.
Exercise regularly, but avoid activities that raise body temperature close to bedtime.
Regular exercise can improve sleep quality, but exercising or having a warm bath too close to bedtime can disrupt sleep onset. Warm baths should be avoided within 1.5 h of bedtime.
Avoid consuming more than 8–10 oz of liquids close to bedtime.
A full or semi full bladder can contribute to awakenings. Restrict liquids close to bedtime and void right before bed.

insomnia symptoms in SWD (see Table 2). Although emerging studies have tested different modifications, such studies have produced inconsistent results in part because of the lack of assessments that describe the relevant mechanisms to target in SWD. Important considerations for adapting CBT-I for SWD were discussed in this chapter; however, additional research is needed to establish an evidence-based approach for adapting CBT-I for SWD.

TABLE 2 Adaptation of cognitive behavioral therapy for insomnia (CBT-I) for shift work disorder (SWD).

CBT-I components	Standard practice	CBT-I adaptations for SWD
Sleep education	3-P model, 2-process model of sleep regulation, sleep stages	Expand discussion of Process-C, including more in-depth education around endogenous melatonin and circadian misalignment
Sleep restriction	Improve sleep efficiency by limiting time in bed to amount of time sleeping then expanding slowly as long as sleep efficiency is preserved	Implementation of sleep restriction should be conducted only after accounting for circadian misalignment
Stimulus control	Associate bed/bedroom solely as a cue for sleep by eliminating nonsleep activities from the bedroom. Instruction to get out of bed at night if awake >15 minutes	If there are clear signs of conditioned arousal, stimulus control may be an effective therapeutic approach. Stimulus control should be considered in the context of circadian phase and circadian misalignment
Napping/ daytime sleep	Discontinue or restrict daytime napping to 30 min	Naps should be use strategically to increase safety on shift balanced with minimal interruption with the main sleep bout
Sleep hygiene education	Address daytime habits and sleep environment interfering with sleep	See Table 1
Cognitive therapy	Challenge patient's dysfunctional beliefs interfering with sleep and misconceptions about sleep. Replace/restructure to more helpful and realistic thoughts about sleep	Assess for dysfunctional beliefs about sleep in the context of shift work. Patient may require motivational enhancement and solution-focused support for prioritizing daytime sleep among competing demands during the day
Relaxation and meditation techniques	Relaxation can help reduce racing thoughts/tension that accompany lying in bed awake, and may include: deep breathing, progressive muscle relaxation, guided imagery, biofeedback, hypnosis, autogenic training, and meditation practices	Relaxation can be implemented in a similar manner with standard practice

TABLE 2 Adaptation of cognitive behavioral therapy for insomnia (CBT-I) for shift work disorder (SWD)—cont'd

CBT-I components	Standard practice	CBT-I adaptations for SWD
Relapse prevention	Discuss practicing less rigid sleep plan over time and what do to prevent sleep disturbance from turning into another episode of insomnia in the future	Discussing maintain sleep schedules and light exposure when on off-work days. Normalize and plan for how to handle transition periods from vacations
Sleep diaries	Establish baseline sleep patterns, track progress, reinforce appropriate behavior change, problem solve obstacles to adherence	Use a 24-h sleep diary to better detect circadian patterns

References

American Academy of Sleep Medicine. (2014). *The international classification of sleep disorders* (3rd). Darien, IL: American Academy of Sleep Medicine.

American National Standards Institute, & American Petroleum Institute. (2010). *Fatigue risk management systems for personnel in the refining and petrochemical industries*. American Petroleum Institute.

Barger, L. K., Lockley, S. W., Rajaratnam, S. M., & Landrigan, C. P. (2009). Neurobehavioral, health, and safety consequences associated with shift work in safety-sensitive professions. *Current Neurology and Neuroscience Reports, 9*(2), 155–164.

Bøggild, H., & Knutsson, A. (1999). Shift work, risk factors and cardiovascular disease. *Scandinavian Journal of Work, Environment & Health, 25*(2), 85–99. https://doi.org/10.5271/sjweh.410. Published online.

Borbély, A. (1982). A two process model of sleep regulation. *Human Neurobiology, 1*(3), 195–204.

Braun, R., Kath, W. L., Iwanaszko, M., et al. (2018). Universal method for robust detection of circadian state from gene expression. *Proceedings of the National Academy of Sciences, 115*(39), E9247–E9256.

Chen, I. Y., Jarrin, D. C., Rochefort, A., Lamy, M., Ivers, H., & Morin, C. M. (2015). Validation of the French version of the Ford insomnia response to stress test and the association between sleep reactivity and hyperarousal. *Sleep Medicine, 16*, S238. https://doi.org/10.1016/j.sleep.2015.02.1510.

Cheng, P., Casement, M. D., Kalmbach, D. A., Castelan, A. C., & Drake, C. L. (2021). Digital cognitive behavioral therapy for insomnia promotes later health resilience during the coronavirus disease 19 (COVID-19) pandemic. *Sleep, 44*(4), zsaa258.

Cheng, P., Walch, O., Huang, Y., et al. (2021). Predicting circadian misalignment with wearable technology: Validation of wrist-worn actigraphy and photometry in night shift workers. *Sleep, 44*(2), zsaa180.

Culpepper, L. (2010). The social and economic burden of shift-work disorder. *The Journal of Family Practice, 59*(1 Suppl), S3–S11.

Czeisler, C. A., Walsh, J. K., Roth, T., et al. (2005). Modafinil for excessive sleepiness associated with shift-work sleep disorder. *The New England Journal of Medicine, 353*(5), 476–486.

Czeisler, C. A., Walsh, J. K., Wesnes, K. A., Roth, T., & Arora, S. (2009). Armodafinil for treatment of excessive sleepiness associated with shift work disorder: A randomized controlled study. *Mayo Clinic Proceedings, 84*(11), 958–972. https://doi.org/10.1016/S0025-6196(11)60666-6.

Drake, C. L., Friedman, N. P., Wright, K. P., & Roth, T. (2011). Sleep reactivity and insomnia: Genetic and environmental influences. *Sleep*. https://doi.org/10.5665/sleep.1234. Published online September 1.

Drake, C. L., Jefferson, C., Roehrs, T., & Roth, T. (2006). Stress-related sleep disturbance and polysomnographic response to caffeine. *Sleep Medicine, 7*(7), 567–572. https://doi.org/10.1016/j.sleep.2006.03.019.

Drake, C. L., Roehrs, T., Richardson, G., Walsh, J. K., & Roth, T. (2004). Shift work sleep disorder: Prevalence and consequences beyond that of symptomatic day workers. *Sleep, 27*(8), 1453–1462.

Jarrin, D. C., Chen, I. Y., Ivers, H., Drake, C. L., & Morin, C. M. (2016). Temporal stability of the ford insomnia response to stress test (FIRST). *Journal of Clinical Sleep Medicine, 12*(10), 1373–1378. Published online August 22.

Kalmbach, D. A., Anderson, J. R., & Drake, C. L. (2018). The impact of stress on sleep: Pathogenic sleep reactivity as a vulnerability to insomnia and circadian disorders. *Journal of Sleep Research, 27*(6), e12710.

Kalmbach, D. A., Pillai, V., Cheng, P., Arnedt, J. T., & Drake, C. L. (2015). Shift work disorder, depression, and anxiety in the transition to rotating shifts: The role of sleep reactivity. *Sleep Medicine, 16*(12), 1532–1538.

Kamdar, B. B., Tergas, A. I., Mateen, F. J., Bhayani, N. H., & Oh, J. (2013). Night-shift work and risk of breast cancer: A systematic review and meta-analysis. *Breast Cancer Research and Treatment, 138*(1), 291–301. https://doi.org/10.1007/s10549-013-2433-1.

Karlsson, B., Knutsson, A., & Lindahl, B. (2001). Is there an association between shift work and having a metabolic syndrome? Results from a population based study of 27 485 people. *Occupational and Environmental Medicine, 58*(11), 747–752. https://doi.org/10.1136/oem.58.11.747.

Laing, E. E., Möller-Levet, C. S., Poh, N., Santhi, N., Archer, S. N., & Dijk, D.-J. (2017). Blood transcriptome based biomarkers for human circadian phase. *eLife, 6*, e20214.

McHill, A. W., Melanson, E. L., Higgins, J., et al. (2014). Impact of circadian misalignment on energy metabolism during simulated nightshift work. *Proceedings of the National Academy of Sciences, 111*(48), 17302–17307.

Puttonen, S., Härmä, M., & Hublin, C. (2010). Shift work and cardiovascular disease—Pathways from circadian stress to morbidity. *Scandinavian Journal of Work, Environment & Health, 36*, 96–108.

Qaseem, A., Kansagara, D., Forciea, M. A., Cooke, M., & Denberg, T. D. (2016). Management of chronic insomnia disorder in adults: A clinical practice guideline from the American College of Physicians. *Annals of Internal Medicine, 165*(2), 125–133.

Riemann, D., Baglioni, C., Bassetti, C., et al. (2017). European guideline for the diagnosis and treatment of insomnia. *Journal of Sleep Research, 26*(6), 675–700. https://doi.org/10.1111/jsr.12594.

Sachdeva, A., & Goldstein, C. (2020). Shift work sleep disorder. In R. R. Auger (Ed.), *Circadian rhythm sleep-wake disorders: An evidence-based guide for clinicians and investigators* (pp. 149–182). Springer International Publishing. https://doi.org/10.1007/978-3-030-43803-6_11.

Schiller, H., Söderström, M., Lekander, M., Rajaleid, K., & Kecklund, G. (2018). A randomized controlled intervention of workplace-based group cognitive behavioral therapy for insomnia. *International Archives of Occupational and Environmental Health, 91*(4), 413–424.

Schweitzer, P. K., Randazzo, A. C., Stone, K., Erman, M., & Walsh, J. K. (2006). Laboratory and field studies of naps and caffeine as practical countermeasures for sleep-wake problems associated with night work. *Sleep, 29*(1), 39–50.

Scott, A., Monk, T., & Brink, L. (1997). Shiftwork as a risk factor for depression: A pilot study. *International Journal of Occupational and Environmental Health, 3*(Suppl. 2), S2–S9.

Sinues, P. M.-L., Tarokh, L., Li, X., et al. (2014). Circadian variation of the human metabolome captured by real-time breath analysis. *PLoS One, 9*(12), e114422. https://doi.org/10.1371/journal.pone.0114422.

Straif, K., Baan, R., Grosse, Y., et al. (2007). Carcinogenicity of shift-work, painting, and fire-fighting. *The Lancet Oncology*, *8*(12), 1065–1066.

Walsh, J. K., Muehlbach, M. J., & Schweitzer, P. K. (1995). Hypnotics and caffeine as countermeasures for shiftwork-related sleepiness and sleep disturbance. *Journal of Sleep Research*, *4*, 80–83.

Ward, E. M., Germolec, D., Kogevinas, M., et al. (2019). Carcinogenicity of night shift work. *The Lancet Oncology*, *20*(8), 1058–1059.

Zhang, Y., & Papantoniou, K. (2019). Night shift work and its carcinogenicity. *The Lancet Oncology*, *20*(10), e550. https://doi.org/10.1016/S1470-2045(19)30578-9.

CHAPTER

5

CBT-I for patients with hypersomnia disorders

Jason C. Ong and Matthew D. Schuiling

Department of Neurology, Center for Circadian and Sleep Medicine, Northwestern University Feinberg School of Medicine, Chicago, IL, United States

Introduction

Normal levels of alertness are necessary for humans to engage in physical, mental, and social activities. Difficulty maintaining alertness or wakefulness due to excessive daytime sleepiness (EDS) is experienced by 27.8% of the general population (Ohayon, Dauvilliers, & Reynolds, 2012). In most cases, EDS is a symptom due to insufficient sleep quantity, sleep quality, or circadian dysregulation. When EDS is persistent and occurs despite adequate sleep and circadian timing, it is considered a central disorder of hypersomnolence (CDH) (American Academy of Sleep Medicine, 2014). Among CDH, the two most common conditions are narcolepsy and idiopathic hypersomnia (IH). Since these two conditions share the cardinal feature of persistent EDS with similar effects on daytime functioning, they will be referred to as chronic hypersomnia (CH) here. Other CDH conditions such as Kleine-Levin syndrome have different features, such as intermittent episodes of EDS, or have a different etiology (e.g., due to other medical or psychiatric condition). Therefore, the focus of this chapter will be on CH and cognitive-behavioral approaches to managing these conditions. The first section provides an overview of CH, including diagnosis, pathophysiology, epidemiology, with an emphasis on the psychosocial aspects of CH. Next, treatments are discussed, including current pharmacological treatments and the cognitive and behavioral strategies that can be used to help manage CH symptoms and improve

Adapting Cognitive Behavioral Therapy for Insomnia
https://doi.org/10.1016/B978-0-12-822872-2.00018-9

health-related quality of life. Finally, we provide suggestions for future directions in managing CH with cognitive-behavior therapy.

A primer of chronic hypersomnia

Diagnosis

Narcolepsy is the most well-known CH and is characterized by EDS that occurs on a frequent (≥3 times per week) and persistent (≥3 months) basis despite adequate total sleep time (American Psychiatric Association, 2013). Other symptoms include nocturnal sleep fragmentation, hypnogogic hallucinations, sleep paralysis, and vivid dreams, which appear to involve an intrusion of the REM state into wakefulness (Scammell, 2015). Narcolepsy can be further distinguished into subtypes based on clinical evidence of cataplexy, which is the sudden loss of muscle tone often in response to strong emotion, such as laughter, surprise, excitement, anger, or happiness (Krahn, Lymp, Moore, Slocumb, & Silber, 2005). This loss of muscle tone can occur in the jaw, hands, or knees, and result in slurred speech, or in some cases, complete paralysis (Won et al., 2014). Those who show signs of cataplexy are classified as Narcolepsy Type 1 (NT1) while those without cataplexy are categorized as Narcolepsy Type 2 (NT2).

In addition to clinical symptoms, diagnosis of narcolepsy requires laboratory testing through overnight polysomnography (PSG) followed by a next-day multiple sleep latency test (MSLT). A sleep-onset rapid eye movement period (SOREMP) of less than 15 min on the overnight PSG and/or a mean sleep latency of less than 8 min on the MSLT is needed to meet diagnostic criteria for narcolepsy. If available, a hypocretin assay derived from the Cerebrospinal Fluid (CSF) can be used to determine hypocretin levels, where low hypocretin-1 is consistent with a diagnosis of narcolepsy. A value of 110 pg/mL or less than one-third of the normative values on a standardized assay qualifies as a hypocretin deficiency, warranting the diagnosis for Narcolepsy Type 1 (American Academy of Sleep Medicine, 2014).

Similar to narcolepsy, IH shares the core feature of EDS that is present for at least 3 months and is not due to other causes. In addition, people with IH often report sleep inertia, sometimes referred to as "sleep drunkenness," which is characterized by significant difficulty rousing or feeling alert upon awakening. Unlike NT1, people with IH do not report cataplexy and there is an absence of REM-related symptoms, such as hypnogogic hallucinations and sleep paralysis. Furthermore, there is an absence of SOREM on the PSG and MSLT (Bassetti & Aldrich, 1997).

About 30% of individuals with IH also report long nocturnal sleep time (≥10h) and many people with IH also take long unrefreshing naps (≥60min), which are atypical of people with narcolepsy (American Academy of Sleep Medicine, 2014). Moreover, people with IH can exhibit a wide range of symptoms such as irresistible daytime napping, difficulty waking in the morning, or nonrestorative sleep after 9h (Trotti, 2020), making it difficult to determine differential diagnosis from other hypersomnolence disorders such as NT2 and insufficient sleep syndrome (Trotti, 2017).

Recently, there has been a proposal to re-classify CH (Fronczek et al., 2020). Based upon updated findings that IH with long sleep time have distinct features, Fronczek et al. (2020) propose that IH with long sleep time be considered a separate condition. They also propose "lumping" NT2 and IH without long sleep time into a new diagnosis called "narcolepsy spectrum disorder" due to similarities in phenotype and the poor reliability of the MSLT in differentiating NT2 from IH. Finally, they propose to retain NT1 as a diagnostic category given the diagnostic reliability and validity of identifying NT1 and the well-characterized pathophysiology of NT1.

Pathophysiology

Relative to other forms of CH, NT1 has the most established pathophysiological model with a deficiency in hypocretin, a neuropeptide produced in the lateral hypothalamus that contributes to wakefulness and arousal (Ebrahim, Howard, Kopelman, Sharief, & Williams, 2002). Specifically, several studies have demonstrated the destruction of hypocretin (orexin) producing cells in the hypothalamus leading to a deficiency in the hypocretin (Nishino, Ripley, Overeem, Lammers, & Mignot, 2000). This has led some to consider narcolepsy a "hypocretin deficiency syndrome." In addition, there is evidence of a genetic predisposition with the HLA-DR and HLA-DQ alleles. In NT2, hypocretin levels are generally normal. Although there are some cases of hypocretin deficiency in NT2, the findings are not as consistent compared to NT1 and might indicate a different progression in the disease course. About 20% of people who are initially diagnosed with NT2 ultimately develop hypocretin deficiency leading to a diagnosis change to NT1 (Han et al., 2014). Unfortunately, very little is known about the etiology of IH. A survey study showed that 34% of patients with IH reported a family history of excessive daytime sleepiness suggesting a possible genetic influence, though it has not been identified (Anderson, Pilsworth, Sharples, Smith, & Shneerson, 2007).

Epidemiology

Both narcolepsy and IH are considered rare diseases with prevalence estimates of around 25 to 50 people per 100,000, or about 0.025% to 0.05% of the general population (Longstreth Jr., Koepsell, Ton, Hendrickson, & van Belle, 2007). One study that examined the US health care claims database for the years 2008 through 2010 reported that 0.08% of enrolled patients were diagnosed with narcolepsy, including 0.014% with NT1 and 0.065% with NT2 (Scheer et al., 2019). Unfortunately, the prevalence of IH remains unknown with a lack of comprehensive studies investigating the prevalence of IH in the general population (Billiard & Dauvilliers, 2001). However, a study investigating medical/prescription claims to assess the prevalence of IH found that 7.7 per 100,000 people in 2013 were diagnosed with IH and 10.3 per 100,000 people in 2016, suggesting an increasing number of people receiving treatment (Hess et al., 2018).

One challenge with estimating the prevalence of CH is that many people with CH remain undiagnosed, are misdiagnosed, and many have a protracted time between the onset of symptoms and the confirmation of a CH diagnosis. One study found that the median time from the onset of narcolepsy symptoms to diagnosis was 22 months with 18% of the sample reporting at least 5 years between the onset of symptoms and diagnosis (Carter, Acebo, & Kim, 2014). Additionally, 60% of patients in this study had been misdiagnosed with a different disorder, such as depression, insomnia, and sleep apnea, and at least half of the patients required evaluation by multiple providers.

With regards to age, the prevalence of narcolepsy was highest in the 21–30 age group, and incidence was highest in people in their late teens to early twenties (Scheer et al., 2019). Typically, the first symptom to occur is EDS, which emerges between age 15 and 25. With narcolepsy, other symptoms such as cataplexy and other REM-related symptoms typically emerge after the onset of EDS. Therefore, the likely progression is the emergence of symptoms in adolescence to early adulthood, but diagnosis is often not confirmed until the mid to late 20s or early 30s.

Studies have revealed inconsistent findings with regard to gender distribution (Hale, Guan, & Emanuele, 2016). One longitudinal study examining the incidence of narcolepsy between 1960 and 1989 in Minnesota found no significant differences between gender with an incidence rate of 1.72 per 100,000 for men and 1.05 per 100,000 for women (Silber, Krahn, Olson, & Pankratz, 2002). However, a broader study examining the US Health Care Claims database from 2008 to 2010 (Scheer et al., 2019) found a higher prevalence of narcolepsy in females (91.8 per 100,000) compared to males (65.8 per 100,000). These discrepant findings could indicate that females are more likely to access healthcare and seek diagnosis and treatment for narcolepsy symptoms compared to males.

Psychosocial aspects of hypersomnia

The symptoms of CH have a profound impact on daily functioning, leading to a significant impact on health-related quality of life (HRQoL). In studies across different countries around the world (Daniels, King, Smith, & Shneerson, 2001; David, Constantino, dos Santos, & Paiva, 2012; Dodel et al., 2007; Vignatelli et al., 2004; Vignatelli, Plazzi, Peschechera, Delaj, & D'Alessandro, 2011), CH patients consistently reported poor HRQoL, especially in terms of lack of vitality/ energy and problems with carrying out their daily activities or role. A mixed-methods study examining how narcolepsy symptoms impact quality of life found that the constancy of EDS and the unpredictability of other symptoms, such as cataplexy, had the most negative impact on HRQoL (Ong, Fox, Brower, Mazurek, & Moore, 2020). As an example, one participant described significant anxiety when approaching an area on campus where a previous cataplectic attack had occurred and began to avoid that area. When asked how narcolepsy impacted their daily lives, participants reported four major domains (Ong, Fox, et al., 2020). First, patients struggled with self-esteem and self-efficacy. Some described that they were ashamed of having narcolepsy and had low self-worth and others described a loss of productivity and limitations in their ability to participate in activities at a level they were accustomed to in the past. People with narcolepsy also reported the stigma of being diagnosed with narcolepsy, noting that popular media often mock people with narcolepsy through their depiction in movie characters and cartoons and the general public does not recognize it as a serious condition. Second, the cognitive impairment or "brain fog" associated with narcolepsy had detrimental effects on the ability to accomplish tasks and often had difficulty staying organized. Third, the symptoms had a significant impact on social functioning and interpersonal relationships. Patients reported that the limitations caused by their symptoms were detrimental to maintaining social relationships (Ong, Fox, et al., 2020). Many felt that their friends perceived them as unreliable and others reported being unable to travel or not being able to be active in social situations due to fatigue and EDS. Some patients also reported that narcolepsy impacted their decision to have children due to concerns that narcolepsy symptoms might compromise their ability to be a caretaker. Another study found that 72% of patients with narcolepsy reported interpersonal distress (marital and family conflicts) with 20% identifying narcolepsy as the reason for divorce or separation

(Kales et al., 1982). Finally, some people with narcolepsy have changed jobs or abandoned career aspirations due to the impact of narcolepsy symptoms (Ong, Fox, et al., 2020).

These challenges in psychosocial functioning are associated with a greater risk for developing comorbid mood disorders, anxiety disorders, and substance use disorders related to self-medication of stimulants (Ford & Kamerow, 1989; Ohayon, 2013; Ohayon et al., 2012). People with narcolepsy (PWN) report elevated symptoms of depression and anxiety (Dauvilliers et al., 2009; Flores, Villa, Black, Chervin, & Witt, 2016; Neikrug, Crawford, & Ong, 2017) that are two to three times the rate of mood and anxiety disorders and significantly higher work absenteeism compared to matched controls (Flores et al., 2016). Furthermore, PWN uses twice the amount of medications for comorbid medical and psychiatric conditions compared to matched controls (Black et al., 2014) with 37% of PWN taking antidepressant medications (Ohayon, 2013). One study also found that poor HRQoL is present even when treated with pharmacotherapy (Dauvilliers et al., 2009). Collectively, these studies indicate that poor psychosocial functioning is a significant problem that is not adequately addressed with current therapies (see Fig. 1).

Unfortunately, much less attention has been given to investigating the psychosocial aspects of IH specifically. Studies that have included IH with narcolepsy (e.g., (Neikrug et al., 2017; Ozaki et al., 2012) have generally found deficits in HRQoL, which are comparable to those found in narcolepsy. There is a clear need for further research in examining specific aspects of HRQoL associated with IH.

Treatments for chronic hypersomnia

Pharmacological treatments

To date, no cure has been discovered for either narcolepsy or IH. Pharmacotherapy is the standard treatment for CH and is primarily targeted at EDS, with some medications also targeting other symptoms such as cataplexy and consolidation of nighttime sleep (see Table 1). Traditionally, stimulants have been used as the first-line treatment for EDS given their wake-promoting effects. However, these medications are tightly regulated and can produce undesirable side effects such as anxiety or appetite suppression. Stimulants are also contraindicated in patients with hypertension. One study showed that 60% of patients taking stimulants for CH reported side effects, and 30% reporting that these side effects were treatment-limiting (Thakrar et al., 2018). The same study found that combination treatment was associated with fewer side effects when compared with monotherapy. In addition to stimulants, newer medications for CH

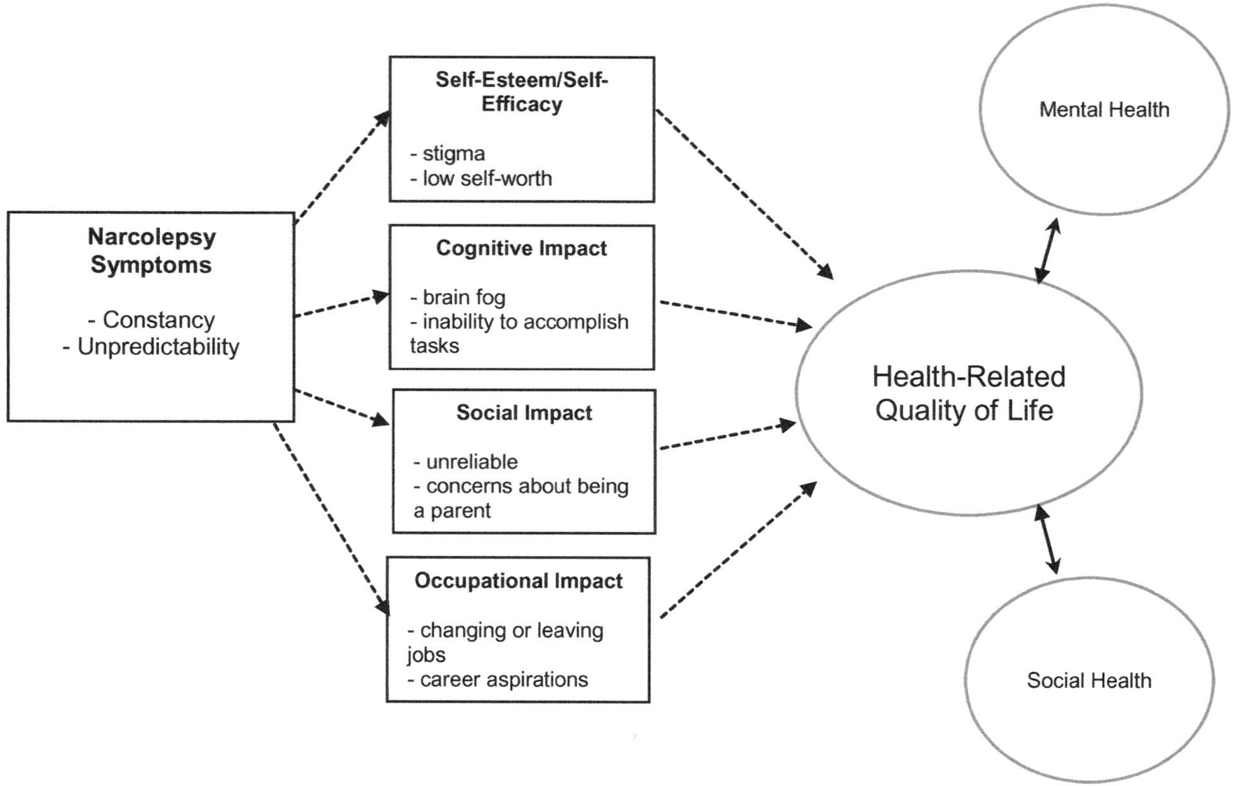

FIG. 1 Psychosocial model for the impact of narcolepsy on health-related quality of life.

TABLE 1 Pharmacotherapy for chronic hypersomnia.

Drug	Class	Indication
Pitolisant	Histamine inverse agonists	EDS & cataplexy
Sodium oxybate	CNS depressant	EDS & cataplexy
Modafinil	Nonamphetamine stimulant	EDS
Armodafinil	Nonamphetamine stimulant	EDS
Dextroamphetamine	Stimulant	EDS
Methylphenidate	Stimulant	EDS
Imipramine	TCA	Cataplexy
Nortriptyline	TCA	Cataplexy
Fluoxetine	SSRI	Cataplexy
Venlafaxine	SNRI	Cataplexy
Selegiline	MAO-B inhibitor	EDS & cataplexy

have included other drug classes. Sodium oxybate is a central nervous depressant that has been shown to reduce cataplexy in addition to reducing EDS. As a result, it has emerged as a standard treatment for narcolepsy, particularly for NT1. Pitolisant is a histamine antagonist/inverse agonist that has demonstrated effectiveness for EDS and cataplexy. In addition, there is low potential for abuse and therefore is currently the only FDA-approved nonscheduled drug for narcolepsy.

Cognitive and behavioral treatments for hypersomnia

Previous studies have found some support for using behavioral strategies to reduce subjectively and objectively measured sleepiness and to improve functional performance (Helmus et al., 1997; Mullington & Broughton, 1993; Rogers, Aldrich, & Lin, 2001). The most common behavioral recommendation for coping with EDS is scheduled daytime naps, whereby the clinician establishes a structure of prescheduled, prophylactic nap periods during the day with the intent of improving alertness and cognitive functioning. One study also examined the impact of adding a consistent nocturnal sleep schedule with or without the scheduled naps (Rogers et al., 2001). In general, these studies found indications that regular scheduled sleep periods can reduce sleepiness and improve some aspects of performance, but the effects were heterogeneous, transient, and often limited to those with more profound EDS despite the use of stimulant medications. Moreover, these studies included small sample sizes and were relatively short in duration (1 to 2 weeks). Finally, none of these studies evaluated mood or HRQoL so it is unclear if behavioral treatments can improve other patient-reported outcomes. Unfortunately, very little research has been conducted to further test these behavioral strategies since the early 2000s.

A cognitive-behavioral program for hypersomnia

With the increased focus on HRQoL in CH, opportunities are emerging for Behavioral Sleep Medicine to provide services to help people with narcolepsy and IH manage symptoms and improve psychosocial functioning. Recent work has been conducted to develop and test cognitive and behavioral strategies that include components of cognitive-behavior therapy for insomnia (CBT-I) to optimize nighttime sleep, daytime components such as scheduled naps and daytime activities to manage sleepiness and energy throughout the day, and novel strategies for emotion regulation and interpersonal functioning to improve self-efficacy with regards to managing the impact of hypersomnia on HRQoL (see Table 2). Given the heterogeneity of symptoms and intensity across narcolepsy and IH, these techniques are intended to be delivered in modules that allow clinicians to select and customize the techniques based on the patient's symptom profile. Finally, these techniques were designed to be delivered as adjunctive therapy to patients who are receiving standard care for CH. The following sections describe these components that collectively form a novel cognitive-behavior therapy for hypersomnia (CBT-H) program.

Education about hypersomnia

Many patients with CH and their family members are very interested in learning about their condition. However, there are many misconceptions about CH, and some might not have a proper understanding of the condition, the nature of the symptoms, and the potential impact it might have on their functioning and HRQOL. In other cases, patients might have received education from a sleep specialist upon diagnosis of their condition, but other questions arise as their condition progresses or they encounter challenges with their symptoms in new situations. Therefore, assessing the patient's knowledge about their condition, their understanding of treatment options, and their expectations of living with hypersomnia can provide an opportunity to provide education as needed. The level of information should be customized to the appropriate patient demographics (e.g., patient's level of education, living situation). In some cases, having a partner or family member present can be important so that

TABLE 2 Adaptation of CBT-I Components for Hypersomnia.

CBT-I Components	Standard practice	Modifications/Adaptions
Sleep education	3-P model, 2-process model of sleep regulation, sleep stages	– Education about the basics of hypersomnia – Education about treatment options for hypersomnia – Provide resources for further educational opportunities (e.g., patient organizations, online materials)
Sleep restriction	Improve sleep efficiency by limiting time in bed to the amount of time sleeping then expanding slowly as long as sleep efficiency is preserved	– Rather than reducing TIB, the focus is on regulating TIB – Set alarms or reminders for bedtime and wake up time
Stimulus control	Associate bed/bedroom solely as a cue for sleep by eliminating non-sleep activities from the bedroom. Instruction to get out of bed at night if awake >15 min	– No modifications – Not typically needed for hypersomnia patients, since prolonged awakenings are uncommon
Napping/daytime sleep	Discontinue or restrict daytime napping to 30 min	– Use scheduled naps and scheduled activities to manage energy and alertness during the day – Split up the day into smaller segments or "windows" for sleep and activities – Schedules should be customized
Sleep hygiene education	Address daytime habits and sleep environment interfering with sleep	– No modifications

Cognitive therapy	Challenge patient's dysfunctional beliefs interfering with sleep and misconceptions about sleep. Replace/restructure to more helpful and realistic thoughts about sleep	– Cognitive strategies aimed at improving self-efficacy for managing hypersomnia symptoms – Cognitive strategies aimed at improving self-esteem and self-image related to the stigma of hypersomnia
Mindfulness and acceptance	N/A	– Self-compassion can be used as a tool work with low self-esteem and/or self-efficacy – Active acceptance can help reduce anxiety or depression related to hypersomnia symptoms – Value-based living can help patients identify modifications to activities while still maintaining their core values
Sleep diaries	Establish baseline sleep patterns, track progress, reinforce appropriate behavior change, problem-solve obstacles to adherence	– Data should be gathered on the timing and duration of daytime naps – Gathering additional data on the timing of daytime activities can be used to develop a structure for daytime naps and activities

members of the patient's household are well-informed about the patient's condition and potential limitations. Specific areas to explore and provide education include: (1) prevalence, etiology, and symptoms of CH; (2) current treatment options; and (3) resources for further educational opportunities.

Ideally, the educational component is delivered early during the course of treatment. Clinicians who are not familiar with CH can review the section above (see Section "A primer of chronic hypersomnia") for reference. As part of the educational component, the clinician can also ask the patient to describe their journey to getting diagnosed with CH, since it takes most patients several years to get diagnosed and they are often referred to several providers before seeing a sleep specialist. This can provide an important first step in understanding the patient's perspective, establish rapport, and correct any misconceptions about their condition. Furthermore, being well-informed about their condition can empower patients to educate others (e.g., friends, co-workers, and acquaintances) about CH, which can improve interpersonal functioning, one of the main complaints of people with CH.

Regulating nighttime sleep

CH is not typically associated with severe symptoms of insomnia but people with narcolepsy can experience frequent awakenings and difficulty staying asleep. In addition, the sleepiness associated with CH can lead to irregular bedtimes and wake-up times, which can potentially exacerbate daytime sleepiness (Manber, Bootzin, Acebo, & Carskadon, 1996). Therefore, regulation of nighttime sleep is an important behavioral strategy that adopts elements from Sleep Restriction Therapy and Sleep Hygiene that are used in CBT-I. Instead of reducing time in bed as is typically done in CBT-I, the focus in hypersomnia is to set aside a regular "sleep window" that is established by having a regular bedtime and rise time. The rationale for not reducing time in bed is to avoid the exacerbation of daytime sleepiness that can occur as part of Sleep Restriction Therapy. Similar to sleep restriction, the sleep window can be set based on the average sleep duration obtained through sleep/wake diaries and collaborative discussion with the patient regarding factors such as chronotype, lifestyle preferences, and other responsibilities (e.g., occupational, child care). It is also important to discuss ways to protect the sleep window by encouraging patients to set reminder alarms for bedtime (e.g., "30-min warning") and alarms for the rise time. Patients should also be reminded that the sleep window should be followed on the weekends or off days in addition to weekdays or workdays.

Although sleep hygiene is typically associated with insomnia, clinical observations suggest that sleep hygiene is often inadequate in people with hypersomnia. Consequently, the removal or minimization of electronic devices and other items that might interfere with sleep during the sleep window should be emphasized. Similarly, an assessment of the sleep environment should be conducted and avoidance of activities such as work or watching TV in bed should be discussed as needed.

Clinicians should be aware that sodium oxybate is taken in two doses—one at bedtime and the second dose 2.5 to 4h later. Since this second dose typically requires patients to wake up in the middle of the night, some patients can have difficulty falling back to sleep. In these situations, discussing stimulus control techniques, such as not attempting to go back to sleep until sleepy, could be useful to minimize the nocturnal sleep disturbance over time.

Regulation of daytime naps and activities

Regulation of daytime naps and activities is an important component for managing energy and alertness during the day. Although most people with CH will report taking naps, it is often ad hoc and used when they are at the point of exhaustion. Instead, developing a consistent schedule for prophylactic naps and activities that require high cognitive or physical resources can be a more efficient and effective way to manage energy throughout the day. Similar to the concept of a sleep window at night, this approach allows clinicians and patients to develop scheduled "nap windows" during the day and other windows for work, school, or leisurely activities.

Rather than approaching the day as one continuous period of wakefulness, patients with hypersomnia are encouraged to break up their waking hours from rising time to bedtime in smaller segments. For example, there can be a morning segment that is designated as a window for work, followed by a brief nap window (e.g., 20–30min). For some patients with IH who might not be able to take short naps, a window of rest or relaxation can be substituted for the nap window. An afternoon window for work or physical activity can also be scheduled, followed by a second nap window (if appropriate) or a window for leisure activities. Finally, a window for evening activities can be scheduled, which could consist of social or leisure activities, leading to the nighttime sleep window. This approach is based on a time management strategy designed to split up larger intervals of time into smaller, more manageable components. This technique is used to improve focus and attention, and frequent breaks can improve cognitive functioning.

Unfortunately, the current evidence base has not revealed consistent evidence to provide guidelines on the optimal length or timing of naps. In addition, people with IH might have difficulty limiting naps to short periods. Therefore, clinicians should customize the daytime schedule to each CH patient based upon their symptoms, daytime responsibilities, and other schedule requirements. Having patients keep "daytime diaries" for activities and naps can be very helpful in developing the schedule and monitoring progress with adherence to the sleep schedule. Also, setting alarms or reminders can help to facilitate the transition from one window to the next. Some patients will be resistant to the idea of a daytime schedule, perceiving it to be constraining. In these cases, clinicians can explain that the purpose is not to be rigid, where one adheres regardless of circumstances, but to be consistent, which allows for some flexibility when needed with a return to the regular schedule when circumstances permit. In contrast to insomnia, people with hypersomnia generally do not have difficulty falling asleep during naps. However, in case this happens, clinicians should be prepared to adjust the nap timing by working with the patient to identify other times when they might be more sleepy and therefore more likely to nap.

Self-efficacy and self-esteem

In addition to the behavioral components, cognitive strategies directed at improving psychosocial functioning are essential, given the high rates of depression and anxiety in people with CH. For people with narcolepsy, there are issues related to self-image, self-esteem, and self-efficacy, which results from the stigma of narcolepsy, the constancy of low energy and sleepiness that adversely affects functioning, and the unpredictability of symptoms such as cataplexy (Ong, Dawson, Mundt, & Moore, 2020; Ong, Fox, et al., 2020). Although research is still in the nascent stages, preliminary work and clinical anecdotes have revealed a few promising techniques.

First, clinicians can assess the patient's understanding of their diagnosis and, if appropriate, help patients process their self-image as a person with CH. Those who have been recently diagnosed might not have accepted their diagnosis or processed their self-perception or how others see them. For example, some patients still have expectations to function at their premorbid condition. The clinician can discuss what it means to the patient to be diagnosed with hypersomnia and whether or not this has changed their career or family goals. This could lead to cognitive restructuring of the patient's expectations to more realistic levels that are commensurate with their symptoms and current level of functioning. If appropriate, clinicians can review the patient's stated values and help patients establish new goals. This can improve both self-esteem and self-efficacy as patients are no longer judging their performance based on unrealistic expectations.

Addressing interpersonal issues can be very beneficial for patients who are encountering negative interpersonal interactions due to CH. In our pilot study (Ong, Dawson, et al., 2020), therapists engaged in discussions about the patient's experience in disclosing their CH diagnosis and any stigma that was associated with their experience. Clinicians can provide guidance about assertive communication, a style of communication that expresses both positive and negative feelings in an open, honest, and direct way, versus aggressive communication, a demanding or authoritarian style of communication that involves personal attacks and threats. In addition, it can be helpful to discuss social support. Clinicians should assess the support structure in the patient's current home or work environment and discuss ways to increase support. If there are issues related to managing hypersomnia symptoms at work or school, a discussion about disability accommodations and how to approach employers or teachers could be appropriate. Given that CH is a rare condition, many patients might not have met another person with CH. Providing resources for patients to connect with organizations that support people with narcolepsy (Wake up Narcolepsy, Narcolepsy Network) and Idiopathic Hypersomnia (Hypersomnia Foundation) can enhance psychosocial support.

Mindfulness and acceptance

Mindfulness and acceptance-based techniques can also be used for managing the emotional burden associated with CH symptoms. Patients may not be able to fully engage in social settings at times due to feelings of sleepiness or may choose not to socialize altogether. Discussion of the principles of self-compassion can be very helpful since patients often feel guilty or disappointed about their level of functioning.

Since there is currently no cure for narcolepsy or IH, the concept of active acceptance can be useful to manage frustrations and disappointments related to the constant feeling of sleepiness and fatigue or the unpredictability of certain symptoms such as cataplexy. In active acceptance, the individual makes an *active* decision to accept or embrace the situation even if the outcome cannot be changed. In the case of CH, it is to acknowledge or embrace the fact that one has a diagnosis of CH and that it cannot be changed, yet still choose to make decisions that are value-congruent. By practicing active acceptance, one is not denying that hypersomnia has limitations but rather working within those limitations to still engage in meaningful activities. For example, a person with CH might have had career ambitions of being a surgeon, but due to CH symptoms did not have the stamina to complete surgical training. Instead, they *choose* to re-direct their interest in medicine by becoming involved in teaching medical students and residents and doing administrative roles in a medical clinic. This is in contrast to passive acceptance, which involves giving up, or the resignation that one has no control over the problem. By practicing active acceptance, it provides a way to work with the unpredictability of hypersomnia symptoms without always trying to control them, which can sometimes exacerbate feelings of depression and anxiety.

Helping patients identify personal values can help to establish priorities and maintain goals consistent with their personal values. The challenges of managing CH symptoms can results in significant functional limitations, making it difficult to maintain career or family ambitions. Clinicians can help patients identify core values by developing a values inventory, or list of values using the following questions:

- What is important to you?
- What gives your life meaning?
- At the end of the day, what really matters to you?
- What are the priorities and principles that guide your life?

Patients are then encouraged to set a goal or each of the values in their inventory. The focus should be on how they can achieve their specific goals in their current life or situation. Although some modifications might be needed, the key point is to help patients establish the possibility of living a life with activities that are consistent with their core values.

Conclusions and future directions

Behavioral Sleep Medicine is expanding in areas beyond insomnia and cognitive-behavioral strategies can play an important role in improving the HRQoL in people with CH. Building upon previous work using scheduled naps and regulating nighttime sleep, additional behavioral components of scheduled daytime activities can be used to reinforce structure for managing EDS. In addition, cognitive strategies designed to improve self-esteem and self-efficacy related to the unique psychosocial aspects of hypersomnia can provide important tools for CH patients to accept their diagnosis, cope with their symptoms, and address interpersonal issues related to living with hypersomnia.

The approach described in this chapter should be considered a starting point and future directions should be aimed at testing these approaches and other cognitive and behavioral strategies. Although preliminary findings support the feasibility of delivering these strategies into a CBT-H program (Ong, Dawson, et al., 2020) further research is needed to evaluate the efficacy of the program, individual components, or optimal combination of components through randomized controlled trials. Research is also needed to examine the appropriate method of delivery for these strategies. A pilot study revealed that this CBT program can be delivered individually or in groups, although the group approach had somewhat more favorable outcomes (Ong, Dawson, et al., 2020) and has the benefit of peer support. Given that narcolepsy and IH are considered rare conditions, scalable delivery methods such as telehealth or digital programs (i.e., apps) can be particularly important to enhance the accessibility of these treatments for patients with CH due to their location or if their symptoms preclude traveling long distances. Additionally, components such as adherence to CH medications or family support groups could be considered or developed as separate intervention programs. Management of diet can be very important given the connections between orexin and diet regulation and could be examined as a possible module in CBT-H. Finally, research is needed to determine if this program is appropriate for patients with narcolepsy and IH or if separate programs with different approaches are needed. Moving forward, there is a clear need for more nonpharmacological interventions for hypersomnia to accompany the pharmacological treatments so that patients with hypersomnia can manage their symptoms effectively and achieve a high HRQoL.

References

American Academy of Sleep Medicine. (2014). *International classification of sleep disorders* (3rd ed.). Darien, IL: American Academy of Sleep Medicine.

American Psychiatric Association. (2013). *Diagnostic and statistical manual of mental disorders* (5th ed.).

Anderson, K. N., Pilsworth, S., Sharples, L. D., Smith, I. E., & Shneerson, J. M. (2007). Idiopathic hypersomnia: A study of 77 cases. *Sleep*, *30*(10), 1274–1281. https://doi.org/10.1093/sleep/30.10.1274.

Bassetti, C., & Aldrich, M. S. (1997). Idiopathic hypersomnia. A series of 42 patients. *Brain*, *120*(8), 1423–1435. https://doi.org/10.1093/brain/120.8.1423.

Billiard, M., & Dauvilliers, Y. (2001). Idiopathic hypersomnia. *Sleep Medicine Reviews*, *5*(5), 349–358. https://doi.org/10.1053/smrv.2001.0168.

Black, J., Reaven, N. L., Funk, S. E., McGaughey, K., Ohayon, M., Guilleminault, C., et al. (2014). The burden of narcolepsy disease (BOND) study: Health-care utilization and cost findings. *Sleep Medicine*, *15*(5), 522–529.

Carter, L. P., Acebo, C., & Kim, A. (2014). Patients' journeys to a narcolepsy diagnosis: A physician survey and retrospective chart review. *Postgraduate Medicine*, *126*(3), 216–224. https://doi.org/10.3810/pgm.2014.05.2769.

Daniels, E., King, M. A., Smith, I. E., & Shneerson, J. M. (2001). Health-related quality of life in narcolepsy. *Journal of Sleep Research*, *10*(1), 75–81. Retrieved from https://www.ncbi.nlm.nih.gov/pubmed/11285058.

Dauvilliers, Y., Paquereau, J., Bastuji, H., Drouot, X., Weil, J. S., & Viot-Blanc, V. (2009). Psychological health in central hypersomnias: The French harmony study. *Journal of Neurology, Neurosurgery, and Psychiatry*, *80*(6), 636–641. https://doi.org/10.1136/jnnp.2008.161588.

David, A., Constantino, F., dos Santos, J. M., & Paiva, T. (2012). Health-related quality of life in Portuguese patients with narcolepsy. *Sleep Medicine, 13*(3), 273–277. https://doi.org/10.1016/j.sleep.2011.06.021.

Dodel, R., Peter, H., Spottke, A., Noelker, C., Althaus, A., Siebert, U., et al. (2007). Health-related quality of life in patients with narcolepsy. *Sleep Medicine, 8*(7–8), 733–741. https://doi.org/10.1016/j.sleep.2006.10.010.

Ebrahim, I. O., Howard, R. S., Kopelman, M. D., Sharief, M. K., & Williams, A. J. (2002). The hypocretin/orexin system. *Journal of the Royal Society of Medicine, 95*(5), 227–230. https://doi.org/10.1258/jrsm.95.5.227.

Flores, N. M., Villa, K. F., Black, J., Chervin, R. D., & Witt, E. A. (2016). The humanistic and economic burden of narcolepsy. *Journal of Clinical Sleep Medicine: JCSM: Official Publication of the American Academy of Sleep Medicine, 12*(3), 401–407. https://doi.org/10.5664/jcsm.5594.

Ford, D. E., & Kamerow, D. B. (1989). Epidemiologic study of sleep disturbances and psychiatric disorders. An opportunity for prevention? *JAMA, 262*(11), 1479–1484. Retrieved from: https://www.ncbi.nlm.nih.gov/pubmed/2769898.

Fronczek, R., Arnulf, I., Baumann, C. R., Maski, K., Pizza, F., & Trotti, L. M. (2020). To split or to lump? Classifying the central disorders of hypersomnolence. *Sleep, 43*(8). https://doi.org/10.1093/sleep/zsaa044, zsaa044.

Hale, L., Guan, S., & Emanuele, E. (2016). Epidemiology of narcolepsy. In M. Goswami, M. J. Thorpy, & S. R. Pandi-Perumal (Eds.), *Narcolepsy: A clinical guide* (pp. 37–43). Cham: Springer International Publishing.

Han, F., Lin, L., Schormair, B., Pizza, F., Plazzi, G., Ollila, H. M., et al. (2014). HLA DQB1*06:02 negative narcolepsy with Hypocretin/orexin deficiency. *Sleep, 37*(10), 1601–1608. https://doi.org/10.5665/sleep.4066.

Helmus, T., Rosenthal, L., Bishop, C., Roehrs, T., Syron, M. L., & Roth, T. (1997). The alerting effects of short and long naps in narcoleptic, sleep deprived, and alert individuals. *Sleep, 20*(4), 251–257. https://doi.org/10.1093/sleep/20.4.251.

Hess, G., Mehra, R., Carls, G., Profant, J., Altenburger, J., Pasenchenko, O., et al. (2018). 0625 US prevalence of narcolepsy and other sleep disorders from 2013–2016: A retrospective, epidemiological study utilizing Nationwide claims. *Sleep, 41*(suppl_1), A232. https://doi.org/10.1093/sleep/zsy061.624.

Kales, A., Soldatos, C. R., Bixler, E. O., Caldwell, A., Cadieux, R. J., Verrechio, J. M., et al. (1982). Narcolepsy-cataplexy. II. Psychosocial consequences and associated psychopathology. *Archives of Neurology, 39*(3), 169–171. Retrieved from https://www.ncbi.nlm.nih.gov/pubmed/7065935.

Krahn, L. E., Lymp, J. F., Moore, W. R., Slocumb, N., & Silber, M. H. (2005). Characterizing the emotions that trigger cataplexy. *The Journal of Neuropsychiatry and Clinical Neurosciences, 17*(1), 45–50. https://doi.org/10.1176/jnp.17.1.45.

Longstreth, W. T., Jr., Koepsell, T. D., Ton, T. G., Hendrickson, A. F., & van Belle, G. (2007). The epidemiology of narcolepsy. *Sleep, 30*(1), 13–26. https://doi.org/10.1093/sleep/30.1.13.

Manber, R., Bootzin, R. R., Acebo, C., & Carskadon, M. A. (1996). The effects of regularizing sleep-wake schedules on daytime sleepiness. *Sleep, 19*(5), 432–441. https://doi.org/10.1093/sleep/19.5.432.

Mullington, J., & Broughton, R. (1993). Scheduled naps in the management of daytime sleepiness in narcolepsy-cataplexy. *Sleep, 16*(5), 444–456. https://doi.org/10.1093/sleep/16.5.444.

Neikrug, A. B., Crawford, M. R., & Ong, J. C. (2017). Behavioral sleep medicine Services for Hypersomnia Disorders: A survey study. *Behavioral Sleep Medicine, 15*(2), 158–171. https://doi.org/10.1080/15402002.2015.1120201.

Nishino, S., Ripley, B., Overeem, S., Lammers, G. J., & Mignot, E. (2000). Hypocretin (orexin) deficiency in human narcolepsy. *The Lancet, 355*(9197), 39–40. https://doi.org/10.1016/S0140-6736(99)05582-8.

Ohayon, M. M. (2013). Narcolepsy is complicated by high medical and psychiatric comorbidities: A comparison with the general population. *Sleep Medicine, 14*(6), 488–492. https://doi.org/10.1016/j.sleep.2013.03.002.

Ohayon, M. M., Dauvilliers, Y., & Reynolds, C. F. (2012). Operational definitions and algorithms for excessive sleepiness in the general population: Implications for DSM-5 nosology. *Archives of General Psychiatry, 69*(1), 71–79.

Ong, J. C., Dawson, C. S., Mundt, M. J., & Moore, C. (2020). Developing a cognitive behavioral therapy for hypersomnia using telehealth: A feasibility study. *Journal of Clinical Sleep Medicine, 16*(12), 2047–2062.

Ong, J. C., Fox, R. S., Brower, R. F., Mazurek, S., & Moore, C. (2020). How does narcolepsy impact health-related quality of life? A mixed-methods study. *Behavioral Sleep Medicine*, 1–14. https://doi.org/10.1080/15402002.2020.1715411.

Ozaki, A, Inoue, Y, Hayashida, K, Nakajima, T, Honda, M, Usui, A, et al. (2012). Quality of life in patients with narcolepsy with cataplexy, narcolepsy without cataplexy, and idiopathic hypersomnia without long sleep time: Comparison between patients on psychostimulants, drug-naive patients and the general Japanese population. *Sleep Medicine, 13*(2), 200–206.

Rogers, A. E., Aldrich, M. S., & Lin, X. (2001). A comparison of three different sleep schedules for reducing daytime sleepiness in narcolepsy. *Sleep, 24*(4), 385–391. https://doi.org/10.1093/sleep/24.4.385.

Scammell, T. E. (2015). Narcolepsy. *New England Journal of Medicine, 373*(27), 2654–2662. https://doi.org/10.1056/NEJMra1500587.

Scheer, D., Schwartz, S. W., Parr, M., Zgibor, J., Sanchez-Anguiano, A., & Rajaram, L. (2019). Prevalence and incidence of narcolepsy in a US health care claims database, 2008–2010. *Sleep, 42*(7). https://doi.org/10.1093/sleep/zsz091.

Silber, M. H., Krahn, L. E., Olson, E. J., & Pankratz, V. S. (2002). The epidemiology of narcolepsy in Olmsted County, Minnesota: A population-based study. *Sleep, 25*(2), 197–202. https://doi.org/10.1093/sleep/25.2.197.

Thakrar, C., Patel, K., D'ancona, G., Kent, B. D., Nesbitt, A., Selsick, H., et al. (2018). Effectiveness and side-effect profile of stimulant therapy as monotherapy and in combination in the central hypersomnias in clinical practice. *Journal of Sleep Research, 27*(4). https://doi.org/10.1111/jsr.12627, e12627.

Trotti, L. M. (2017). Idiopathic hypersomnia. *Sleep Medicine Clinics, 12*(3), 331–344. https://doi.org/10.1016/j.jsmc.2017.03.009.

Trotti, L. M. (2020). Central disorders of Hypersomnolence. *Continuum: Lifelong Learning in Neurology, 26*(4), 890–907. https://doi.org/10.1212/con.0000000000000883.

Vignatelli, L., D'Alessandro, R., Mosconi, P., Ferini-Strambi, L., Guidolin, L., De Vincentiis, A., et al. (2004). Health-related quality of life in Italian patients with narcolepsy: The SF-36 health survey. *Sleep Medicine, 5*(5), 467–475. https://doi.org/10.1016/j.sleep.2004.04.003.

Vignatelli, L., Plazzi, G., Peschechera, F., Delaj, L., & D'Alessandro, R. (2011). A 5-year prospective cohort study on health-related quality of life in patients with narcolepsy. *Sleep Medicine, 12*(1), 19–23. https://doi.org/10.1016/j.sleep.2010.07.008.

Won, C., Mahmoudi, M., Qin, L., Purvis, T., Mathur, A., & Mohsenin, V. (2014). The impact of gender on timeliness of narcolepsy diagnosis. *Journal of Clinical Sleep Medicine, 10*(01), 89–95. https://doi.org/10.5664/jcsm.3370.

CHAPTER

6

CBT-I for patients with orthosomnia

Kelly Glazer Baron

Department of Family and Preventive Medicine, University of Utah, Salt Lake City, UT, United States

The growing interest in sleep tracking

The market for consumer sleep technology is rapidly increasing. It is estimated that nearly 57 million adults in the US own a fitness tracker, and the market is continuing to expand among all age groups.(eMarketer, 2018) Sleep tracking apps are consistently in the top-selling fitness apps. (Analytics V. Verto Index, 2019) Although wrist-worn wearables have been the most common devices, there are numerous other devices on the market designed to measure sleep and provide feedback, including apps, rings, bedside monitors, mattresses, and even pillows. Some monitors, called nearables, are contactless sensors that are even able to track sleep and respiration, by being placed on the bedside table. This popularity has provided some interesting opportunities and challenges for the field of behavioral sleep medicine, as patients are bringing in their data to discuss and also suggesting in some cases that they abandon the "tried and true" paper and pencil sleep diaries in favor of their sleep tracker. The focus of this chapter is adaptations of CBT-I among patients who have orthosomnia (Baron, Abbott, Jao, Manalo, & Mullen, 2017) or preoccupation with correct or right sleep. This chapter will also provide some recommendations on how to use sleep trackers in those without orthosomnia, who are interested in using a sleep tracker in CBT-I.

Orthosomnia

Around 2016, when I was faculty at Northwestern University, my practicum students and I began to notice an increasing number of patients who came to our CBT-I clinic and wanted to discuss their sleep tracker data.

Adapting Cognitive Behavioral Therapy for Insomnia
https://doi.org/10.1016/B978-0-12-822872-2.00002-5

The majority of patients had general questions about how to interpret the data "My son/daughter bought me this device to track my sleep, does this tell you anything? I'm not sure to make of this." In those discussions, we generally reviewed the data from the app and discussed what we thought we could learn from it. However, a selection of patients presented their sleep tracker data with significant anxiety or concern about their data. They often were worried about having too many periods of "restless sleep" or not enough "deep sleep" or reporting that they could not function unless their sleep tracker reported 7h of sleep at night. The most interesting thing is that at that time, the sleep trackers on the market were movement-based, and thus less precise than current trackers that use heart rate to estimate REM versus non-REM sleep. For example, studies have demonstrated that "light" and "deep sleep" did not decipher sleep stages (de Zambotti, Goldstone, Claudatos, Colrain, & Baker, 2018; Fonseca et al., 2017). The sleep log below was completed by one patient who printed out their sleep tracker data and pasted it on the sleep log provided by the sleep clinic. This patient felt that the sleep log did not accurately represent their periods of light sleep (Fig. 1).

As we began to discuss this growing phenomenon, we collected and published a case series of 3 patients. Overall, we found that the patients felt that the sleep tracker data was accurate, and they were fairly inflexible about examining their beliefs about the tracker data. There is not a diagnostic test or questionnaire to diagnose orthosomnia, but rather it is

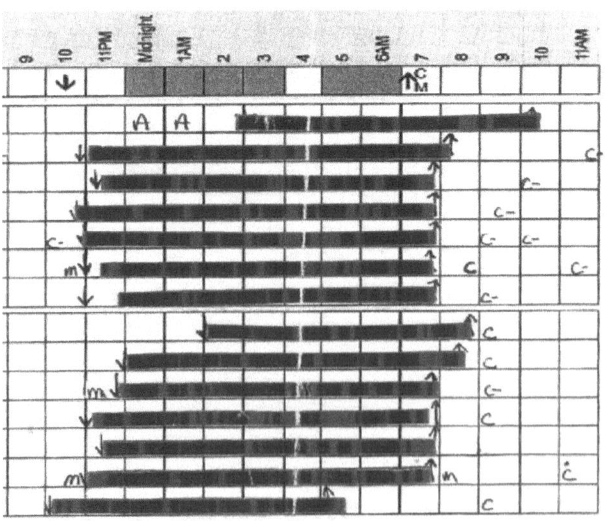

FIG. 1 This patient was concerned about "light sleep" and to demonstrate this, printed out then cut out their sleep tracker data and pasted it in our clinic sleep log.

reflected in how patients are overly reliant on their sleep tracker data. For example, one patient reported that his sleep apnea was diagnosed by his sleep tracker. What actually happened is that he purchased a sleep tracker because he was concerned about his sleep. He showed the data to his primary care physician, who ordered a sleep study. Had this 65-year-old patient merely brought up his sleep concerns of snoring and daytime fatigue with his physician, a sleep study would have been ordered, even without the tracker data. However, somehow this patient conflated that his data was the reason the study was ordered. On the positive side, the data did encourage the patient to discuss sleep with the physician.

How valid are sleep tracking devices?

I should add a caveat to the story above, these devices are improving over time. In the mid-2010s, the devices were only movement-based. Now, with the inclusion of heart rate through photoplethysmography, they are increasingly moving toward more clinically useful measures. The generation devices with heart rate sensors are slightly better than actigraphy at detecting sleep and improved in the detection of sleep stages (Haghayegh, Khoshnevis, Smolensky, Diller, & Castriotta, 2020). In addition, Fitbit has released an oxygen desaturation index. This has not been validated or approved by the FDA, but there is a potential that these devices could play a role in clinical care at some point. Had the patient above brought in data that said "I'm noticing that my oxygen levels are variable overnight," it would have been much more believable that the device "diagnosed" his condition. However, with the patient above, this predates any of these features. This was a movement-only tracker. There has been a tremendous amount of research aimed at validating sleep trackers. We published a scoping review in 2018 and reported that over half of all published sleep wearables studies (23 of 43 studies) were focused on validation. The limitations to these validation studies are that (1) Most were conducted in small samples, (2) validation studies will show more concordance between wearables and the criterion (either polysomnography or actigraphy) among healthy sleepers, (3) most are conducted in a laboratory rather than a home environment (Baron et al., 2018). Another issue in the validation of any particular device is that the company can change the algorithm without any notice and that there are always new devices being released, so it is really impossible to keep up on which is the most "accurate." There are some efforts in the field to publish standards or keep up on the evidence for validation of devices. For example, the American Academy of Sleep Medicine has a section of their website devoted to reviewing consumer technology and providing supporting citations. The Journal of Clinical Sleep Medicine also has a focus on publishing articles with consumer technology.

With all of those limitations, here is what is known about the most popularly worn current sleep technology, which uses movement and heart rated (Fitbit). A study by de Zambotti and colleagues (2018) conducted a single night recording to compare epoc-by-epoc scoring of PSG with the Fitbit Charge 2 (de Zambotti et al., 2018). Results indicated that the TST estimate of this device was quite close to the PSG estimate (overestimated by 9 min), and the device was accurate at identifying REM and WASO. However, the device overestimated light sleep (N1 and N2, overestimated by 34 min) and underestimated N3 (34 min). This suggests that participants may perceive they are not achieving deep sleep when this is a function of the algorithm not picking it up. A study published by Lee and colleagues demonstrated that both the Fitbit Alta HR and Actiwatch 2 similarly underestimated TST and overestimated WASO in adolescents by approximately 40 min (Lee et al., 2019). These studies represent only two devices from one company, and therefore should not be applied to other devices or algorithms. However, these studies do suggest that consumer sleep technology as an estimate of objective sleep data is improving over time and the newest technology is likely as good as actigraphy.

Why do patients track their sleep?

When deciding how to engage with a patient who is using a sleep tracker, it is important to consider the reason why patients are tracking their sleep. Consumer survey data show that sleep is one of the most desirable features of fitness tracking devices, but the motivation for purchasing devices is variable. Some may purchase sleep trackers for only the desire to understand their sleep, self-discovery about what is happening overnight. Others may be interested in identifying whether they have a sleep problem. Furthermore, the information provided by sleep trackers may be confusing or even at times misleading. These devices are not regulated by the FDA and are classified as entertainment devices. As pointed out by a review by Russo and colleagues, claims made by these devices (e.g., "start improving your sleep on the first night") may lead consumers to believe the devices can change their sleep (Russo, Goparaju, & Bianchi, 2015). Although some devices do provide advice or suggestions, there are no current studies demonstrating the efficacy of these programs. Patients with sleep problems are probably at the greatest risk of purchasing a device with the hope that it will improve their sleep. A survey completed by my laboratory among individuals with short sleep duration (6 h or less) found that sleep trackers were highly desirable to this group (preferred by >80% of those surveyed) (Adkins, DeYonker, Duffecy, Hooker, & Baron,

2019). The only predictor of interest was sleep quality (higher interest with worse sleep quality). This highlights the mismatch between what individuals with short sleep duration desire from trackers versus what they deliver.

Challenges in CBT-I for patients with orthosomnia

Overall, we have found that patients with orthosomnia are challenging to engage in CBT-I. The most noticeable aspect is the rigidity of their sleep beliefs. We have found that a core feature of orthosomnia is that they believe the tracker data above all. Therefore, the clinician is perceived as trying to talk them out of their belief or perhaps even not knowledgeable compared to the research they have done online. In the adaptation section, I provide some suggestions for challenging unhelpful beliefs about their sleep tracker using cognitive behavioral techniques. Another challenge is that the preoccupation with tracking can interfere with sleep and undermine adherence to CBT-I. For example, patients are "rewarded" by spending excessive time in bed to reach their sleep duration goal, and that engaging in the recommended sleep schedule will result in lowering that number. They may be more likely to compensate for a lower sleep duration number on the tracker by taking a nap. They tend to worry about their sleep duration, which increases their effort to sleep. These behaviors are similar to other patients in CBT-I except, in this case, the patient is following the "score" on their sleep tracker device.

Adaptation of CBT-I for orthosomnia (Table 1)

Below, I have listed some considerations and recommendations for patients with orthosomnia who are attending sessions of CBT-I. The decision to continue using vs. discontinue the tracker is an important discussion. Some patients may be reluctant to discontinue using their device because they are using it for other types of tracking, but perhaps they could remove it at night only, or try skipping some nights. The advice below may help patients and clinicians come to that decision.

Education: The first recommendation is to add education about sleep tracking to the sleep education session. Clinicians may find it helpful to make this an interactive discussion versus "telling" participants about the limitations of their device. For example, using techniques to elicit patients' thoughts and beliefs, then providing information, then eliciting their reactions. For example, patients may be interested to learn about how sleep is measuring in the laboratory and the pros and cons of sleep tracker

TABLE 1 CBT-I adaptations.

CBT-I Components	Standard practice	Modifications/Adaptions
Sleep education	3-P model, 2-process model of sleep regulation, sleep stages	– Include education about the limitations of sleep trackers, particularly for sleep stages – Emphasize the variability in "normal" sleep stages
Sleep restriction	Improve sleep efficiency by limiting time in bed to the amount of time sleeping then expanding slowly as long as sleep efficiency is preserved	– Discuss anxieties about sleep restriction – Consider taking a break from tracking
Stimulus control	Associate bed/bedroom solely as a cue for sleep by eliminating nonsleep activities from the bedroom. Instruction to get out of bed at night if awake >15 min	– Discuss anxieties about sleep restriction – Consider taking a break from tracking
Napping/ daytime sleep	Discontinue or restrict daytime napping to 30 min	– Patients may require more discussion about not compensating by napping to catch up on sleep
Sleep hygiene education	Address daytime habits and sleep environment interfering with sleep	– Consider stopping tracking
Cognitive therapy	Challenge patient's dysfunctional beliefs interfering with sleep and misconceptions about sleep. Replace/restructure to more helpful and realistic thoughts about sleep	– Focus on beliefs about tracking that interfere with compliance to CBT-I – Address beliefs about how sleep "should" be – Impact of sleep numbers on daytime function
Relapse Prevention	Discuss practicing less rigid sleep plan over time and what do to prevent sleep disturbance from turning into another episode of insomnia in the future	– No change
Sleep diaries	Establish baseline sleep patterns, track progress, reinforce appropriate behavior change, problem-solve obstacles to adherence	– Work on anxiety about tracking – Consider simplifying diary if needed

data. In addition, I spend time discussing the meaning of the sleep stage data, that it is not as accurate as polysomnography yet, and even in polysomnography, there is a wide range of normal values. I even show the participants my data, which often says I get very little deep sleep, even though I'm a healthy person who exercises regularly and does not have insomnia. For patients who are complaining about "not enough REM sleep," I explain that there is not a diagnosis or treatment based on sleep stages but our treatment is focused on improving the quality of their sleep and how they feel during the day. Overall, this is an interactive discussion, and patients are invited to learn about how we measure sleep, what the measurements mean and the goals of treatment.

Sleep restriction: The second consideration is during sleep restriction. Seeing the sleep duration decrease may be anxiety-provoking and lead the patient to disengage with treatment. Consider discontinuing tracking or the number of days tracked, prepare the patient for seeing the change (gets worse before it gets better). For example, one patient in our case series became anxious when tapering off his hypnotic when the numbers decreased. However, with some encouragement, he continued the taper and eventually tapered off. When he saw the numbers begin to rise again, he felt encouraged to see this progress. Therefore, the tracker was at first a barrier to treatment but then it gave him encouraging feedback that helped him feel more confident to continue with treatment.

Cognitive therapy: One of the most challenging areas in orthosomnia is working with strongly held beliefs about sleep and sleep tracking. As in typical CBT-I, clinicians should identify maladaptive beliefs and work with patients to alter the beliefs that are causing distress and interfering with treatment. The maladaptive sleep beliefs in orthosomnia are similar to those typically seen in CBT-I, but they are more focused on the tracker data. For example, "I can't function if I don't sleep 7 hours." The patient should discuss with the clinician if the data from the tracker is making those thoughts better or worse. If the tracker is contributing to anxiety, the clinician may want to develop behavioral experiments (tracking for 1 week vs. not tracking for 1 week). The clinician could ask the patient to track a log of their tracker data and ratings of alertness, mood, or other daytime function to see the correlation between sleep and functioning throughout the day.

Sleep logs: A consideration for orthosomnia is to discuss with the patient how will trackers be used; will a tracker continue to be worn or will the patient use sleep logs. If the patient is feeling more anxious due to the device, it may be advisable to discontinue. Otherwise, it may be helpful for the patient to fill out the sleep log as well as bring in their tracker data. I would not advise clinicians to use only sleep tracker data. I find that the sleep tracker is missing other key information that is collected on the paper log, such as alcohol, caffeine, and exercise timing, or other notes in the margins. I also find the automatic data collection versus the act of writing a log seems to leave out an important part of keeping a log; the intentional writing down of sleep promotes adherence to CBT-I. If patients do want to wear a sleep tracker and use it to help complete their log, I recommend giving the instruction "write down only the awakenings that you remember," as not to reinforce writing down unimportant arousals in the night.

Enhancing adherence to CBT-I in orthosomnia

I also encourage clinicians to maintain a collaborative relationship when working with patients who have orthosomnia. It will not be helpful to tell them, "tracking is not accurate" because the patient is telling us that they feel that the experience of their sleep is captured well by the device. Dismissing their data will potentially undermine treatment and also jeopardize the working relationship with the patient. As with any CBT patient, it is important to work together to align together on shared goals ("I'm not sure we could make it that you would have 7 hours of sleep each night but we could work to decrease the amount of time you are awake each night and how you feel during the day" does that sound ok). Then in the process of working together, the clinician can evaluate and dispel some of the beliefs of orthosomnia.

Can you use wearable devices among patients who do not have orthosomnia?

Given all of the discussion about the negative aspects of tracking, a clinician may wonder why anyone at all would want to track sleep during CBT-I. Behavioral sleep medicine has used actigraphy to enhance treatment for patients with insomnia, particularly among patients who have limited ability to complete logs (e.g., adolescents, children, disabled adults) (Ancoli-Israel et al., 2015). Although consumer devices are not as widely used as validated clinical actigraphy programs, there may be a place for their use in some patients, when clinical actigraphy is not practical. For example, I had a young adult patient (age 20) with severe learning disabilities. He could hardly read or write. After completing 4 weeks of actigraphy in the assessment of his circadian rhythm disorder, we continued using a commercial sleep tracker during the course of treatment, as an adjunct to his sleep diaries. This approach was not only lowered cost than an actigraphy device, it provided him with immediate feedback, rather than needing to come into the clinic.

Sample questions/language

Here is some language that may be useful in discussing whether to use or not use a consumer sleep technology.

1. What is the reason the patient is interested in this technology?
   a. Are they interested in self-discovery? Assistance in completing sleep logs?
   b. How do they anticipate the data will make them feel? Will it increase or decrease anxiety?
2. How do they want to review/share data?
   a. Will you create a shared password so you can review it between sessions? This should prompt a discussion about confidentiality, as the consumer tech platforms are not part of their healthcare record but it is personal healthcare information.
   b. Do they just want to show it to you in follow-up sessions? Will they send screenshots if you are on telehealth? Otherwise, it would be difficult to view the screen.
3. What do they hope the information will accomplish?
   a. Are they looking for information about their sleep pattern?
   b. If they are looking for treatment, they should be advised that wearing the device alone is unlikely to improve their sleep. However, if they are wearing it in the CBT-I program, they may observe some changes as their sleep improves.
4. How to discuss validation and sleep staging.
   a. Here is some language about validation: "These devices provide an estimate of your sleep. They are not a substitute for a sleep study, but they can estimate your sleep based on whether you are still vs. moving and your heart rate. Overall, they tend to overestimate a little (may say that you are sleeping when you are awake") but they are within the ballpark.
   b. Adjusting the sleep log in the app: One reason these devices can give inaccurate numbers is if the log does not capture the whole time you are trying to sleep. You can improve the accuracy of the device if you make sure that the device catches the whole time you are trying to sleep.
   c. Small awakenings: You may notice that the device picks up a lot of small awakenings. You shouldn't worry about these too much. Everyone has awakenings at night between changing sleep stages or moving around at night. This is normal and if you don't remember them, they are not important to track.
   d. Beware of sleep staging data: Lastly, you should be aware that the devices out now are better at estimating how long you sleep than

they are at estimating the sleep stages, such as how much light vs. deep sleep that you get. Also, even if they were accurate, people vary a lot in how much of each stage of sleep they have. It's more important to focus on the pattern of your sleep, amount of sleep, and how solid vs. broken your sleep is at night.

Future directions in sleep wearables in CBT-I

It is my observation, orthosomnia is less prevalent in 2020 than it was in 2015. Although I do still see patients who are anxious about their sleep tracker data, over the past 2years or so, the number of patients who are anxious about their data has seemed to decrease. Perhaps the public is getting more accustomed to seeing their data? On the other hand, am seeing more patients bring their devices into the clinic in the course of treatment. Existing research really cannot determine if using a device in CBT-I is helpful, although there is no evidence that using a device harms treatment. One study conducted a CBT-I intervention (app-based with telephone sessions) and a selection of participants randomized to wear a sleep tracker. Results of the intervention were comparable between the two groups (Kang et al., 2017). Another interesting study used a sleep tracker in a just-in-time intervention, which could adapt treatment based on sleep data (Pulantara, Parmanto, & Germain, 2018). This is an innovative use of the device, but the intervention is still in the preliminary phases.

Summary

In summary, orthosomnia, or the preoccupation with sleep tracking, can interfere with CBT-I due to rigidly held beliefs that interfere with treatment adherence. We recommend that clinicians focus on education about sleep trackers, challenge maladaptive beliefs with cognitive therapy techniques, and plan with the patient how they will use the sleep tracker in treatment (e.g., still use paper logs). We caution clinicians that "telling" patients their data is not accurate will not be helpful because it undermines the patient experience. Furthermore, the use of sleep trackers among patients without orthosomnia could be considered for those who find it to be helpful/reassuring if the tracker is used along with traditional sleep logs.

References

Adkins, E. C., DeYonker, O., Duffecy, J., Hooker, S. A., & Baron, K. G. (2019). Predictors of intervention interest among individuals with short sleep duration. *Journal of Clinical Sleep Medicine, 15*(8), 1143–1148.

Analytics V. Verto Index. (2019). *Health and fitness.* Charles Koch Institute. www.emarketer.com.

Ancoli-Israel, S., Martin, J. L., Blackwell, T., Buenaver, L., Liu, L., Meltzer, L. J., et al. (2015). The SBSM guide to actigraphy monitoring: Clinical and research applications. *Behavioral Sleep Medicine, 13*(Suppl 1), S4–S38.

Baron, K. G., Abbott, S., Jao, N., Manalo, N., & Mullen, R. (2017). Orthosomnia: Are some patients taking the quantified self too far? *Journal of Clinical Sleep Medicine, 13*(02), 351–354.

Baron, K. G., Duffecy, J., Berendsen, M. A., Cheung Mason, I., Lattie, E. G., & Manalo, N. C. (2018). Feeling validated yet? A scoping review of the use of consumer-targeted wearable and mobile technology to measure and improve sleep. *Sleep Medicine Reviews, 40*, 151–159.

de Zambotti, M., Goldstone, A., Claudatos, S., Colrain, I. M., & Baker, F. C. (2018). A validation study of Fitbit charge 2™ compared with polysomnography in adults. *Chronobiology International, 35*(4), 465–476.

eMarketer. (2018). *US adult wearable users and penetration 2018-2022.*

Fonseca, P., Weysen, T., Goelema, M. S., Møst, E. I., Radha, M., Lunsingh Scheurleer, C., et al. (2017). Validation of photoplethysmography-based sleep staging compared with polysomnography in healthy middle-aged adults. *Sleep, 40*(7), zsx097.

Haghayegh, S., Khoshnevis, S., Smolensky, M. H., Diller, K. R., & Castriotta, R. J. (2020). Performance assessment of new-generation Fitbit technology in deriving sleep parameters and stages. *Chronobiology International, 37*(1), 47–59.

Kang, S.-G., Kang, J. M., Cho, S.-J., Ko, K.-P., Lee, Y. J., Lee, H.-J., et al. (2017). Cognitive behavioral therapy using a mobile application synchronizable with wearable devices for insomnia treatment: A pilot study. *Journal of Clinical Sleep Medicine, 13*(4), 633–640.

Lee, X. K., Chee, N. I., Ong, J. L., Teo, T. B., van Rijn, E., Lo, J. C., et al. (2019). Validation of a consumer sleep wearable device with actigraphy and polysomnography in adolescents across sleep opportunity manipulations. *Journal of Clinical Sleep Medicine, 15*(9), 1337–1346.

Pulantara, I. W., Parmanto, B., & Germain, A. (2018). Development of a just-in-time adaptive mHealth intervention for insomnia: Usability study. *JMIR Human Factors, 5*(2), e21.

Russo, K., Goparaju, B., & Bianchi, M. T. (2015). Consumer sleep monitors: Is there a baby in the bathwater? *Nature and Science of Sleep, 7*, 147–157.

PART 3

CBT-I in psychiatric disorders

CHAPTER

7

CBT-I for patients with depression

Jennifer Goldschmied[a] *and Philip Gehrman*[a,b]

[a]Department of Psychiatry, Perelman School of Medicine of the University of Pennsylvania, Philadelphia, PA, United States, [b]Department of Behavioral Health, Corporal Michael J. Crescenz VA Medical Center, Philadelphia, PA, United States

Major depressive disorder (MDD) is often referred to as the "common cold" of mental illness because of its high prevalence. Roughly one in five (20.6%) US adults will meet the criteria for MDD in their lifetime, and half of those (10.4%) will meet criteria over the past year (Hasin et al., 2018). The symptoms of MDD include depressed mood, anhedonia (loss of interest or pleasure in activities), low energy and motivation, hopelessness, and suicidality, among others (American Psychiatric Association, 2013). Symptoms must last for a minimum of 2 weeks, although they can last for months or even years in chronic cases. Individuals with MDD often report the symptom of sleep disturbance, which includes both insomnia and hypersomnia, although insomnia is more common by far, affecting 67%–84% of adults with the disorder (Ford & Kamerow, 1989) compared to 47% who report hypersomnia (Geoffroy et al., 2018). It is noteworthy that some individuals report both insomnia and hypersomnia simultaneously. In terms of patterns of insomnia across the night, there is a long-standing dictum that depression is associated with early morning awakenings, whereas anxiety causes sleep onset insomnia, although there has not yet been empirical support for these generalizations.

There is a long history of polysomnographic (PSG) studies comparing individuals with MDD to healthy controls. In terms of the overall patterns of sleep across the night, a representative comparison of MDD patients ($n = 178$) and good sleeper subjects ($n = 108$) found a number of significant differences between groups (Riemann, Hohagen, Bahro, & Berger, 1994).

Adapting Cognitive Behavioral Therapy for Insomnia
https://doi.org/10.1016/B978-0-12-822872-2.00006-2

Sleep latency was increased by ~5 min, wakefulness after sleep onset (WASO) was increased by ~20 min, the frequency of awakenings was increased by ~6 episodes per night, early morning awakening was advanced by ~15 min, total sleep time (TST) was reduced by ~35 min, and sleep efficiency was reduced by ~8%. In terms of sleep architecture, most research has focused on REM sleep abnormalities in MDD. A number of studies have found a decreased latency to the first episode of REM sleep (i.e., reduced REM latency), a prolonged first REM period, increased percent of the night spent in REM, and increased REM density (i.e., number of eye movements per minute of REM sleep) (Pillai, Kalmbach, & Ciesla, 2011; Srinivasan et al., 2009). A classic meta-analysis found that, of all the PSG abnormalities found in MDD, only the shortened REM latency was unique to depression, with all other findings being shared with other psychiatric disorders (Benca, Obermeyer, Thisted, & Gillin, 1992). A more recent meta-analysis found that REM latency and density were altered only in depressed men, with results only approaching marginal significance in women (Baglioni et al., 2016), but these sex differences remain poorly understood.

It was long thought that insomnia was *just* one of the symptoms of depression and that it played a no more important role than other symptoms. Over the past several decades, this view has changed as evidence has accumulated that insomnia plays a significant role in the course of the disorder. *First, insomnia often precedes the development of a first depressive episode and increases the risk of developing depression.* A meta-analysis of 34 prospective cohort studies of over 170,000 subjects with an average follow-up period of over 60 months found that individuals with insomnia had more than twice the risk of developing depression (Li, Wu, Gan, Qu, & Lu, 2016). Individuals who report insomnia, but not depression, at one timepoint have an approximately 3.5-fold increased risk of reporting depression at a later time point compared to those with no insomnia. Further, the development of insomnia can be an early indicator of an impending major depressive episode. In a prospective, 42-week study of patients in remission from MDD, weekly monitoring of depression symptoms found that those who relapsed into depression exhibited a progressive worsening of their insomnia during the 5 weeks before the onset of the recurrent episode (Perlis, Giles, Buysse, Tu, & Kupfer, 1997). This evidence demonstrates that insomnia increases vulnerability to MDD but the mechanisms underlying these effects are unknown.

Second, the severity of insomnia is independently associated with the severity of depressive symptoms, degree of functional impairment, and response to treatment over and above the severity of other symptoms (Soehner, Kaplan, & Harvey, 2014; Taylor, Lichstein, Durrence, Reidel, & Bush, 2005). In one cohort study that assessed patients with depression at baseline and 6 months later, those with persistent insomnia were 1.8 to 3.5 times more like to remain depressed and achieve less than 50% improvement in depressive symptoms compared with patients with no insomnia (Pigeon et al., 2008). In a separate multisite study of acute and continuation-phase cognitive therapy for depression, individuals with less overall sleep disturbance and greater reduction in sleep disturbance throughout treatment achieved remission and recovery sooner (Boland, Vittengl, Clark, Thase, & Jarrett, 2020). In recent years there has been considerable interest in the relationship between insomnia and suicidality, with a number of studies finding that greater insomnia severity is associated with increased suicidal thoughts and attempts, over and above the overall severity of depression (Lopez-Castroman & Jaussent, 2020).

Third, insomnia frequently persists even after resolution of depression, indicating that it was more than just a component of the mood disturbance. Rates of residual insomnia have been found to be as high as 71% following treatment with antidepressant medications (Nierenberg et al., 2010) and 92% following cognitive-behavioral treatment (Carney, Harris, Friedman, & Segal, 2011) despite clinical improvements in overall depression. Further, those with residual insomnia symptoms were less likely to return to healthy social and occupational functioning (Romera et al., 2013).

These lines of research clearly demonstrate that insomnia is more than just a symptom of depression. It is critical that providers, when treating depression, take insomnia into account in treatment planning. Conversely, it is important for insomnia treatment providers to consider the presence of depression in their patients, beginning with a comprehensive assessment of depressive symptoms.

Assessment of depression

Diagnosis of depression has historically been based on the Diagnostic and Statistical Manual of Mental Disorders, now in its 5th edition (DSM-V). The diagnostic structure of the DSM-V is categorical in nature, yielding a yes/no determination based on nine primary symptoms. More recently, there has been some movement in the field toward a more dimensional approach, which would forego the idea of categorical diagnosis, and transition to the identification of certain symptom clusters. The National Institutes of Mental Health Research Domain Criteria (RDOC), for example, is an initiative aimed at understanding depression based on varying degrees of dysfunction along six domains including negative and positive valence, cognitive, arousal, and sensorimotor systems, and systems for social processes. However, at present, most research and clinical operations continue to use diagnostic criteria to determine if an individual is experiencing an episode of major depression.

According to the DSM-V, to meet the criteria for a major depressive episode (MDE), one must either exhibit depressed mood most of the day, nearly every day, and/or loss of interest in all or almost all activities for at least 2 weeks. In addition to these "gateway" symptoms, the individual must also exhibit at least five total symptoms of the remaining seven that can include weight loss or gain, insomnia or hypersomnia, psychomotor agitation or retardation, fatigue or loss of energy, feelings of worthlessness or excessive guilt, decreased concentration, and thoughts of suicide. These symptoms must also cause significant distress or functional impairment and must not be better explained by substance use or other psychiatric conditions like mania or psychosis.

In addition to the diagnosis of MDE, the DSM-V also provides guidelines for the diagnosis of mood specifiers for MDE. These include mixed, melancholic, and atypical features, in addition to anxious distress. These features represent depression phenotypes that could potentially respond differently to treatment interventions. For example, melancholic features include the absence of mood reactivity, defined as the lack of effect brightening following positive experiences, anhedonia, defined as the inability to experience pleasure, excessive guilt, the significant diurnal variation in mood, specifically with symptoms of depression worse in the morning than in the evening. This last symptom is in contrast to typical circadian patterns of increasing positive affect across the day for healthy individuals (Murray, Allen, & Trinder, 2002). Finally, there may also be the presence of early morning awakenings. This is an important consideration as early morning awakenings are, in itself, an independent presentation of insomnia. Thus, when considering the possibility of comorbid depression and insomnia, the presence of the early morning phenotype of insomnia may actually reflect depression with melancholic features rather than insomnia.

The severity of the diagnosis is then determined according to the intensity of symptoms and their perceived impact on functioning. Mild severity is indicated when only those symptoms required to meet diagnostic criteria are present and functional impairment is minor. Severe symptomatology is indicated where the symptoms present are in excess of those required for diagnosis and functional impairment is marked. Moderate severity is indicated for those between mild and severe. The determination of illness severity is beneficial as it may inform treatment decisions. For example, according to the American Psychiatric Association practice guidelines (Gelenberg et al., 2010), published in 2010, treatment for individuals with moderate to severe depression or those with specifiers should include a combination of medication and psychotherapy, while treatment for individuals with mild to moderate depression should include either psychotherapy or medications.

It is important to distinguish major depressive disorder from other mood disorders as treatment interventions vary according to the symptoms characteristic of the specific disorder present. For example, one of the most important distinctions is between that of unipolar and bipolar depression as both disorders can include a major depressive episode, but modifications to CBT-I for bipolar disorder are significantly different than for unipolar depression. Criteria for bipolar disorder include the presence of at least one manic episode, as defined as a period of at least 4 days where the individual experiences abnormally and persistently elevated or irritable mood, in addition to at least three additional symptoms including an increase in goal-directed activity, feelings of grandiosity, decreased need for sleep, pressured speech, racing thoughts, distractibility, and engagement in risky behaviors that are not otherwise accounted for by substance use or other medical conditions. Although it is not necessary to have experienced a major depressive episode to meet diagnostic criteria for bipolar disorder, research has shown that most individuals who have experienced an episode of mania will go on to experience episodes of depression more frequently than episodes of mania (Weinstock, Strong, Uebelacker, & Miller, 2009).

Another important differential diagnosis is that of persistent depressive disorder (PDD), formerly dysthymic disorder. PDD is defined as chronic low mood, lasting at least two years that is associated with at least two other depressive symptoms. The important distinction from MDE is that of chronicity and severity, with symptoms of PDD being present for a longer period of time but with a more mild presentation. It is possible for an individual to experience an MDE during the course of PDD, and therapists and researchers have termed this "double depression." Although PDD is, by definition, a more mild manifestation of depressive symptoms than MDE, individuals who experience PDD can respond less favorably to treatment interventions. This may be due to the nature of the longstanding illness and the belief in these individuals that their mental health will not improve. Additionally, research has also shown that individuals with PDD and MDE respond more poorly to pharmacotherapy than those with MDE (Hung, Liu, & Yang, 2019). These authors reason that the poorer outcomes in PDD may result from alterations in neurobiology, or effects on socioeconomics including finances and occupational functioning that are associated with long-lasting psychiatric illness.

To appropriately assess depressive symptoms and determine the most accurate diagnosis, several tools are available. As previously mentioned, most clinicians currently rely on the DSM-V for diagnostic guidelines. As such, the *Structured Clinical Interview for the DSM (SCID)* (First, 2014) was developed as a guide for using the DSM criteria for diagnostic purposes. The SCID is a standardized, semistructured interview administered by clinicians or trained professionals that assesses the presence of each symptom using a categorical (yes/no) response that yields a categorical determination (yes/no) of the presence of the disorder. The SCID is organized into diagnostic modules, with the mood disorders module including the assessment of current MDE (in the past month) including specifiers, past MDE, current mania, past mania, current PDD, and past PDD. The SCID also includes guidelines for conducting a thorough differential diagnosis for mood disorders. The SCID has been shown to have adequate reliability and validity for most diagnoses and is currently the most widely used diagnostic instrument for psychiatric assessment.

Several instruments are also available to assess depression severity. These include both clinician-administered scales including the *Hamilton Rating Scale for Depression (HRSD)* and the *Montgomery-Asberg Depression Rating Scale (MADRS)* and self-report scales including the *Beck Depression Inventory II (BDI-II)*.

The HRSD (Hamilton, 1960) is a 17-item, semistructured interview that assesses depression severity in the past week. Items include questions about depressed mood, suicidal ideation, interest and motivation, difficulties with sleep, irritability, and libido. Items are scored from 0 to 4, with not all items utilizing the entire score range. Total scores can range from 0 to 52, with higher scores indicating greater severity of depressive symptomatology. The HRSD has been shown to have adequate reliability and validity (Bagby, Ryder, Schuller, & Marshall, 2004).

The MADRS (Montgomery & Åsberg, 1979) is a 10-item scale used to assess depression severity in the past week. To improve reliability and provide a structured format when administering the assessment, the Structured Interview Guide for the MADRS (SIGMA) can be used. Items on the MADRS include statements regarding apparent and reported sadness, difficulties with concentration, reduced interest, suicidal ideation, and difficulties with sleep. Items are scored from 0 to 6, with qualitative anchors are provided for even-numbered scores. Odd scores are available for symptoms severities that fall between even-numbered anchors. Total scores can range from 0 to 60, with higher scores indicating greater severity of depressive symptomatology. The MADRS has been shown to have adequate reliability and validity (Mulder, Joyce, & Frampton, 2003).

The *BDI-II* (Beck, Steer, & Brown, 1996) is a 21-item scale with a focus on symptoms experienced in the past 2 weeks. Items include statements regarding sadness, anhedonia, suicidal ideation, feelings of worthlessness, sleep changes, and difficulties concentrating. Each item has four response options ranging from 0 to 3. Total scores can range from 0 to 63, with higher scores indicating greater severity of depressive symptomatology. The BDI-II has been shown to have adequate reliability and validity (Dozois, Dobson, & Ahnberg, 1998).

Does CBT-I work in people with depression?

There have been a number of clinical trials published examining the efficacy of CBT-I in patients with both insomnia and MDD. A recent meta-analysis found 17 randomized trials encompassing 1756 participants and conducted a meta-analysis on the effects on insomnia severity in this population (Feng, Han, Li, Geng, & Miao, 2020). In studies that used a no-treatment comparator, CBT-I was more effective on the Insomnia Severity Index (ISI) (mean difference = −4.88 points) in a patient with insomnia and depression. In some trials, subjects could have comorbidities in addition to depression, and in this group the mean difference was −4.47 points, suggesting that effects were comparable in more complicated cases. In two trials that compared CBT-I to hypnotic medication, CBT-I led to greater improvements (mean difference = −2.82 points). The largest study to date is the Treatment of Insomnia and Depression (TRIAD) study that examined the effect of combining CBT-I or a control therapy to antidepressant medication in 150 participants with insomnia and MDD (Manber et al., 2016). CBT-I led to a greater reduction in insomnia severity on the ISI compared to the control condition and greater rates of remission from insomnia (54% vs. 29%). These results are noteworthy given the more stringent control therapy used rather than a no-treatment control. Overall, these results indicate that CBT-I is effective in reducing insomnia severity in patients with MDD.

A related question is whether CBT-I is associated with secondary improvements in the severity of depressive symptoms. Given the extent to which insomnia and depressive symptoms are interrelated, it seems reasonable that improving sleep could lead to improvements in mood. In the Feng et al. meta-analysis reported in the preceding paragraph this question was investigated (Feng et al., 2020). They found that CBT-I produced larger improvements than no treatment in depression severity assessed with the CES-D and QIDS but not with the BDI, although the number of trials for each measure was very small. A separate meta-analysis focused on the effects of self-help CBT-I on depressive symptoms, including 30 randomized trials with 5945 participants (Ho, Chan, Lo, & Leung, 2020). Note that subjects in these studies did not have to meet the criteria for MDD so the focus is on depressive symptoms more broadly and control conditions included waitlists, no treatment, and psychoeducation. Across studies the improvement in depressive symptoms was larger in CBT-I compared to control with a standardized mean difference of −0.35, indicating a modest effect size. In the TRIAD study, CBT-I did not lead to greater improvements in depression symptoms than the control condition, although improvements in insomnia-mediated improvements in depression. It appears that CBT-I can produce improvements in depressive symptoms, but results are variable across studies. Future research is needed to understand the factors contributing to this heterogeneity and to understand the mechanisms through which improving insomnia benefits depression.

Adaptations to CBT-I for depression

Because CBT-I has been shown to improve some symptoms of depression, it follows that these improvements could be enhanced with protocol adaptations that are made specifically for individuals with depression. In the following section, we review several adaptations that can be easily incorporated into existing CBT-I protocols that may address depression symptomatology (Table 1). It is important to note that these adaptations are based on clinical experience and there have not been studies explicitly comparing them to standard CBT-I.

As discussed previously, one of the two gateway symptoms for MDE is loss of interest and motivation to participate in activities. Because many individuals with an MDE will report difficulty with motivation, adhering to treatment recommendations for both sleep restriction and stimulus control, the two most effective components of CBT-I, can be challenging. Although the rationale for sleep restriction is fairly easy to understand, the practice of getting out of bed in the morning or avoiding napping while experiencing daytime sleepiness can be quite difficult to follow, especially when intrinsic levels of motivation are low. This is especially true for those individuals who do not engage in many activities throughout the day, and instead, spend more time in bed or dozing on the couch. Additionally, many individuals with MDE report early morning awakening, and due to low motivation to wake up, they may end up staying in bed even longer to try and extend total sleep time.

Cognitive-behavioral approaches to address issues of low motivation in depression can be integrated into CBT-I. For example, behavioral activation, or the practice of activity scheduling as a means to increase engagement, can be incorporated into the individual's daily homework to increase motivation for getting out of bed. Studies have shown that behavioral activation, as a stand-alone intervention, is efficacious in improving symptoms of depression and can increase motivation (Sturmey, 2009). Tip sheets and worksheets for identifying pleasurable activities for the morning can be particularly helpful. In addition to identifying these pleasurable activities, the scheduling of specific times to engage in these activities is essential. For example, scheduling breakfast at a local café at 7:30 am. Additionally, it can be beneficial to encourage clients to set alarms or share plans with friends to increase accountability.

Behavioral activation can also be a very effective approach for individuals with depression that experience significant diurnal variation in mood

TABLE 1 Adaptation of cognitive behavioral therapy for insomnia (CBT-I) for depression.

CBT-I Components	Standard practice	CBT-I Adaptations for depression
Sleep education	3-P model, 2-process model of sleep regulation, sleep stages	– Provide sufficient information around treatment goals and anticipated timeline to elicit appropriate expectations and reduce hopelessness during the initial stages of treatment – Provide additional education around the effects of antidepressants on sleep – Provide additional education around the presence of low motivation, sleepiness, and early morning awakenings as symptoms of MDD
Sleep restriction	Improve sleep efficiency by limiting time in bed to the amount of time sleeping then expanding slowly as long as sleep efficiency is preserved	– Encourage the patient to identify pleasurable activities for times not spent sleeping
Stimulus control	Associate bed/bedroom solely as a cue for sleep by eliminating nonsleep activities from the bedroom. Instruction to get out of bed at night if awake >15 min	– Provide sufficient information about the rationale for stimulus control including the association between bed/sleep and reducing excessive time in bed – Incorporate behavioral activation approaches to encourage individuals not to spend time in bed when not sleeping. This includes identifying approaches to enhance accountability including engaging with friends or setting alarms
Napping/daytime sleep	Discontinue or restrict daytime napping to 30 min	– Provide additional education about sleep homeostasis/sleep pressure to ensure adherence to non-napping
Sleep hygiene education	Address daytime habits and sleep environment interfering with sleep	– Discuss the potential use of light therapy if morning/evening sleepiness is problematic

Continued

TABLE 1 Adaptation of cognitive behavioral therapy for insomnia (CBT-I) for depression.—cont'd

CBT-I Components	Standard practice	CBT-I Adaptations for depression
Cognitive therapy	Challenge patient's dysfunctional beliefs interfering with sleep and misconceptions about sleep. Replace/ restructure to more helpful and realistic thoughts about sleep	– Address automatic thoughts and core beliefs about the self that may be associated with spending excessive time in bed – Discuss how behavioral avoidance maintains depression and worsens sleep due to inactivity – Challenge feelings and thoughts around hopelessness
Relaxation and meditation techniques	Relaxation can help reduce racing thoughts/tension that accompanies lying in bed awake, and may include: deep breathing, progressive muscle relaxation, guided imagery, biofeedback, hypnosis, autogenic training, and meditation practices	
Relapse prevention	Discuss practicing less rigid sleep plan over time and what do to prevent sleep disturbance from turning into another episode of insomnia in the future	
Sleep diaries	Establish baseline sleep patterns, track progress, reinforce appropriate behavior change, problem solve obstacles to adherence	

such that they feel worse in the evening. Scheduling pleasurable activities for the evening may allow individuals practicing sleep restriction to adhere more closely to their recommended bedtime. In this way, individuals are encouraged to engage in those activities rather than focus on increasing sleepiness or the desire to go to sleep.

The use of light therapy in those experiencing diurnal mood variation has also been suggested as a potential treatment (Wirz-Justice, 2008). For those individuals who experience difficulties with mood or with waking in the morning, the use of a lightbox for 30 min in the morning is recommended. This morning bright light can help suppress endogenous melatonin production, thereby increasing alertness, and making it easier to wake up. For those individuals who exhibit worse mood or excessive sleepiness in the evening, the use of a lightbox for 30 min in the evening can likewise suppress early melatonin onset that may be due to low ambient light at night. This increase in evening alertness can improve the ability to engage in pleasurable activities and adhere to treatment recommendations.

For some patients with MDD, the bed and bedroom are a place to escape from the difficulties of waking life so they may spend excessive time in bed for reasons unrelated to sleep. This can lead to poor stimulus control and the association between the bed and arousal. It also can make it particularly difficult for these patients to adhere to stimulus control guidelines. If a patient is reporting or demonstrating this pattern, it will be especially important to make sure they understand the rationale for stimulus control and the impact that excessive time in bed during the day can have on the ability to sleep at night. It may also be helpful to use cognitive therapy approaches to identify the negative automatic thoughts that patients are having that are leading them to spend in bed, which may include the use of thought records. These negative thoughts, such as negative core beliefs about themselves or their sleep, can then be addressed with cognitive restructuring or other approaches. Behavioral experiments may be useful and can be implemented by having the patient spend certain days in bed and other days out of the bedroom with ratings at the end of the day about how they feel. It is likely that they will report feeling better when they left the bedroom. If there is a particular time of day when the tendency to escape in bed is especially strong, it may also be helpful to add light therapy at this time to promote alertness.

Other depressogenic beliefs and attitudes can also interfere with the implementation of CBT-I. The hopelessness that patients with MDD experience is likely to lead to the belief that there is no point in engaging in CBT-I since their insomnia, like their depression, is unlikely to ever improve. They may believe that CBT-I is not going to have any benefit since nothing they have tried in the past to improve their sleep has ever worked. Indeed, insomnia patients without MDD often express these beliefs. The result is often poor adherence to CBT-I guidelines and homework. It is important to make sure patients understand the process of CBT-I and have accurate expectations of how long it will take to experience improvements in sleep. Otherwise, they may follow the guidelines for a few days and then give up because they aren't feeling better and, in fact, may be feeling worse if they have been prescribed sleep restriction therapy. This is another situation in which cognitive therapy techniques will be essential to address the automatic thoughts and core beliefs driving the hopelessness.

As discussed, it is critically important to adequately assess individuals with symptoms of depression before initiating CBT-I. Research has indicated that sleep deprivation can trigger mania in those with bipolar disorder (Wehr, Sack, & Rosenthal, 1987). Thus, in contrast to individuals with unipolar depression who have been shown to respond positively to behavioral components of CBT-I, sleep restriction may be contraindicated in individuals with bipolar disorder. A study published in 2013 (Kaplan & Harvey, 2013) has suggested that behavioral treatments for insomnia in those with bipolar disorder focus on utilizing sleep schedules to regularize bedtimes and wake times. Indeed, the authors demonstrated that regularizing the sleep/wake schedule improved middle-of-the-night awakenings in most patients without the introduction of sleep restriction or stimulus control. Their data, however, also show preliminary evidence that sleep restriction and stimulus control may be used safely in this population. Their summary recommendations for practicing brief behavioral treatment for insomnia include regularizing sleep/wake schedules with the use of daily sleep diaries and implementing sleep restriction and stimulus control only if sleep efficiency does not improve following this regularization. They also suggest regular monitoring of symptoms of mania and depression throughout the course of treatment, in addition to the monitoring of sleepiness and education regarding drowsy driving. Furthermore, the authors encourage providers to use positive reinforcement approaches, encourage accountability, and focus some attention on relapse prevention to maintain gains following treatment termination.

Finally, it is imperative that CBT-I providers be aware of any antidepressant medications patients with MDD are taking because many of them have significant effects on sleep (for a review see Steiger & Pawlowski, 2019). Some antidepressant medications, such as tricyclics, trazodone, and mirtazapine, tend to be very sedating and may be selected for patients with MDD and insomnia. Of note, trazodone is commonly used for the treatment of insomnia irrespective of the presence of MDD. If patients are taking sedating medications during the day, they may be more likely to nap or doze. Other antidepressants can be activating, such as bupropion. If these medications are taken at night they can cause insomnia. The selective serotonin reuptake inhibitors often produce insomnia as a side effect and can complicate CBT-I. It is important to ascertain whether insomnia is occurring purely due to the precipitating effects of antidepressant medications, since in these cases CBT-I may not even be warranted. Of note, tricyclic antidepressants and monoamine oxidase inhibitors have both been shown to be potent REM sleep suppressants but it is not known whether REM suppression would affect the process of CBT-I. If it is suspected that antidepressant medications are negatively impacting sleep or the process of CBT-I it is important to work with the patient's prescriber to see if medications can be adjusted. Sometimes just taking the antidepressant at a different time of day can make a significant difference.

Conclusions

Major depression is one of the most common psychiatric disorders and has been intimately linked to sleep disturbance. Although historically, insomnia has been viewed as one of the hallmark symptoms of depression, it is now evident that insomnia and depression can coexist simultaneously and interact to impact treatment trajectory. Thus, it is critical to effectively evaluate depressive symptoms before initiating CBT-I. The diagnosis of depression typically requires the administration of a clinical interview by a trained clinician, in addition to the use of both clinician-administered and self-report instruments to assess the severity of symptoms. It is critical to conduct a thorough differential diagnosis to adequately distinguish major depression from bipolar disorder and persistent depressive disorder, in addition to determining if any diagnostic specifiers are present as these may guide treatment recommendations. To date, CBT-I has been shown to be effective for individuals with comorbid insomnia and depression. However, adaptations to CBT-I to specifically target depressive symptomatology may not only improve its effectiveness on sleep but may also improve mood. These adaptations include the use of behavioral activation, cognitive restructuring with a focus on negative automatic thoughts and core beliefs around sleep, and the use of light therapy.

References

American Psychiatric Association. (2013). *Diagnostic and statistical manual of mental disorders* (5th ed.). APA. https://doi.org/10.1176/appi.books.9780890425596.

Bagby, R. M., Ryder, A. G., Schuller, D. R., & Marshall, M. B. (2004). The Hamilton depression rating scale: Has the gold standard become a lead weight? *The American Journal of Psychiatry, 161*(12), 2163–2177.

Baglioni, C., Nanovska, S., Regen, W., Spiegelhalder, K., Feige, B., Nissen, C., et al. (2016). Sleep and mental disorders: A meta-analysis of polysomnographic research. *Psychological Bulletin, 142*(9), 969.

Beck, A. T., Steer, R. A., & Brown, G. (1996). Beck depression inventory–II. *Psychological Assessment.*

Benca, R. M., Obermeyer, W. H., Thisted, R. A., & Gillin, J. C. (1992). Sleep and psychiatric disorders: A meta-analysis. *Archives of General Psychiatry, 49*(8), 651–668.

Boland, E. M., Vittengl, J. R., Clark, L. A., Thase, M. E., & Jarrett, R. B. (2020). Is sleep disturbance linked to short-and long-term outcomes following treatments for recurrent depression? *Journal of Affective Disorders, 262*, 323–332.

Carney, C. E., Harris, A. L., Friedman, J., & Segal, Z. V. (2011). Residual sleep beliefs and sleep disturbance following cognitive behavioral therapy for major depression. *Depression and Anxiety, 28*(6), 464–470.

Dozois, D. J., Dobson, K. S., & Ahnberg, J. L. (1998). A psychometric evaluation of the Beck depression inventory–II. *Psychological Assessment, 10*(2), 83.

Feng, G., Han, M., Li, X., Geng, L., & Miao, Y. (2020). The clinical effectiveness of cognitive behavioral therapy for patients with insomnia and depression: A systematic review and meta-analysis. *Evidence-based Complementary and Alternative Medicine, 2020.*

First, M. B. (2014). Structured clinical interview for the DSM (SCID). *The Encyclopedia of Clinical Psychology*, 1–6.

Ford, D. E., & Kamerow, D. B. (1989). Epidemiologic study of sleep disturbances and psychiatric disorders: An opportunity for prevention? *JAMA, 262*(11), 1479–1484.

Gelenberg, A. J., Freeman, M. P., Markowitz, J. C., Rosenbaum, J. F., Thase, M. E., Trivedi, M. H., et al. (2010). American Psychiatric Association practice guidelines for the treatment of patients with major depressive disorder. *The American Journal of Psychiatry, 167*(Suppl. 10), 9–118.

Geoffroy, P. A., Hoertel, N., Etain, B., Bellivier, F., Delorme, R., Limosin, F., et al. (2018). Insomnia and hypersomnia in major depressive episode: Prevalence, sociodemographic characteristics and psychiatric comorbidity in a population-based study. *Journal of Affective Disorders, 226*, 132–141.

Hamilton, M. (1960). A rating scale for depression. *Journal of Neurology, Neurosurgery, and Psychiatry, 23*(1), 56.

Hasin, D. S., Sarvet, A. L., Meyers, J. L., Saha, T. D., Ruan, W. J., Stohl, M., et al. (2018). Epidemiology of adult DSM-5 major depressive disorder and its specifiers in the United States. *JAMA Psychiatry, 75*(4), 336–346.

Ho, F. Y., Chan, C. S., Lo, W., & Leung, J. C. (2020). The effect of self-help cognitive behavioral therapy for insomnia on depressive symptoms: An updated meta-analysis of randomized controlled trials. *Journal of Affective Disorders, 265*, 287–304.

Hung, C., Liu, C., & Yang, C. (2019). Persistent depressive disorder has long-term negative impacts on depression, anxiety, and somatic symptoms at 10-year follow-up among patients with major depressive disorder. *Journal of Affective Disorders, 243*, 255–261.

Kaplan, K. A., & Harvey, A. G. (2013). Behavioral treatment of insomnia in bipolar disorder. *The American Journal of Psychiatry, 170*(7), 716–720.

Li, L., Wu, C., Gan, Y., Qu, X., & Lu, Z. (2016). Insomnia and the risk of depression: A meta-analysis of prospective cohort studies. *BMC Psychiatry, 16*(1), 1–16.

Lopez-Castroman, J., & Jaussent, I. (2020). *Sleep disturbances and suicidal behavior*. Springer.

Manber, R., Buysse, D. J., Edinger, J., Krystal, A., Luther, J. F., Wisniewski, S. R., et al. (2016). Efficacy of cognitive-behavioral therapy for insomnia combined with antidepressant

pharmacotherapy in patients with comorbid depression and insomnia: A randomized controlled trial. *The Journal of Clinical Psychiatry, 77*(10), 1316–1323.
Montgomery, S. A., & Åsberg, M. (1979). A new depression scale designed to be sensitive to change. *The British Journal of Psychiatry, 134*(4), 382–389.
Mulder, R. T., Joyce, P. R., & Frampton, C. (2003). Relationships among measures of treatment outcome in depressed patients. *Journal of Affective Disorders, 76*(1–3), 127–135.
Murray, G., Allen, N. B., & Trinder, J. (2002). Mood and the circadian system: Investigation of a circadian component in positive affect. *Chronobiology International, 19*(6), 1151–1169.
Nierenberg, A. A., Husain, M. M., Trivedi, M. H., Fava, M., Warden, D., Wisniewski, S. R., et al. (2010). Residual symptoms after remission of major depressive disorder with citalopram and risk of relapse: A STAR* D report. *Psychological Medicine, 40*(1), 41.
Perlis, M. L., Giles, D. E., Buysse, D. J., Tu, X., & Kupfer, D. J. (1997). Self-reported sleep disturbance as a prodromal symptom in recurrent depression. *Journal of Affective Disorders, 42.*
Pigeon, W. R., Hegel, M., Unützer, J., Fan, M., Sateia, M. J., Lyness, J. M., et al. (2008). Is insomnia a perpetuating factor for late-life depression in the IMPACT cohort? *Sleep, 31*(4), 481–488.
Pillai, V., Kalmbach, D. A., & Ciesla, J. A. (2011). A meta-analysis of electroencephalographic sleep in depression: Evidence for genetic biomarkers. *Biological Psychiatry, 70*(10), 912–919.
Riemann, D., Hohagen, F., Bahro, M., & Berger, M. (1994). Sleep in depression: The influence of age, gender and diagnostic subtype on baseline sleep and the cholinergic REM induction test with RS 86. *European Archives of Psychiatry and Clinical Neuroscience, 243*(5), 279–290.
Romera, I., Pérez, V., Caballero, L., Roca, M., Polavieja, P., & Gilaberte, I. (2013). Residual symptoms and functioning in depression, does the type of residual symptom matter? A post-hoc analysis. *BMC Psychiatry, 13*(1), 1–7.
Soehner, A. M., Kaplan, K. A., & Harvey, A. G. (2014). Prevalence and clinical correlates of co-occurring insomnia and hypersomnia symptoms in depression. *Journal of Affective Disorders, 167*, 93–97.
Srinivasan, V., Pandi-Perumal, S. R., Trakht, I., Spence, D. W., Hardeland, R., Poeggeler, B., et al. (2009). Pathophysiology of depression: Role of sleep and the melatonergic system. *Psychiatry Research, 165*(3), 201–214.
Steiger, A., & Pawlowski, M. (2019). Depression and sleep. *International Journal of Molecular Sciences, 20*(3), 607.
Sturmey, P. (2009). Behavioral activation is an evidence-based treatment for depression. *Behavior Modification, 33*(6), 818–829.
Taylor, D. J., Lichstein, K. L., Durrence, H. H., Reidel, B. W., & Bush, A. J. (2005). Epidemiology of insomnia, depression, and anxiety. *Sleep, 28*(11), 1457–1464.
Wehr, T. A., Sack, D. A., & Rosenthal, N. E. (1987). Sleep reduction as a final common pathway in the genesis of mania. *The American Journal of Psychiatry, 144.*
Weinstock, L. M., Strong, D., Uebelacker, L. A., & Miller, I. W. (2009). Differential item functioning of DSM-IV depressive symptoms in individuals with a history of mania versus those without: An item response theory analysis. *Bipolar Disorders, 11*(3), 289–297.
Wirz-Justice, A. (2008). Diurnal variation of depressive symptoms. *Dialogues in Clinical Neuroscience, 10*(3), 337.

CHAPTER

8

CBT-I for patients with schizophrenia and other psychotic disorders

Andrew Scott Tubbs[a] *and Michael A. Grandner*[b,c,d]

[a]Sleep and Health Research Program, Department of Psychiatry, The University of Arizona College of Medicine – Tucson, Tucson, AZ, United States, [b]Sleep and Health Research Program, University of Arizona, Tucson, AZ, United States, [c]Behavioral Sleep Medicine Clinic, Banner—University Medical Center Tucson, Tucson, AZ, United States, [d]Department of Psychiatry and Medicine, UA College of Medicine, Tucson, AZ, United States

Introduction

Although cognitive-behavioral therapy for insomnia (CBT-I) is the first-line treatment for insomnia, there are not enough providers to meet demand in the general population. Consequently, insomnia can go for months or years without being diagnosed or adequately treated which then contributes to deteriorating physical and mental health. Unfortunately, issues around access to care are magnified in psychotic disorders. The patients are medically and psychologically complex and many providers lack the competence and/or confidence to treat these individuals. Thus, even if a patient can access a CBT-I provider, the provider may not feel comfortable or capable of providing treatment. The goal of this chapter is to give providers the knowledge, skills, and confidence to work with patients with psychotic disorders. This chapter will review the current literature on sleep in psychotic illness, provide a basic overview of the patient with psychosis, and then explore the current use and adaptation of CBT-I in this population.

https://doi.org/10.1016/B978-0-12-822872-2.00015-3

The problem

Psychotic disorders are devastating mental illnesses characterized by hallucinations, delusions, and disorganized thinking (American Psychiatric Association and American Psychiatric Association. DSM-5 Task Force, 2013). Despite a population prevalence of less than 1% (Moreno-Kustner, Martin, & Pastor, 2018; Saha, Chant, Welham, & McGrath, 2005), schizophrenia and other psychotic disorders account for 13 million disability-adjusted life years globally (Charlson et al., 2018) and may cost as much as $100 billion annually in the US due to medical expenses, lost productivity, and premature mortality (Chong et al., 2016). Schizophrenia reduces an individual's lifespan by approximately 20 years due to poor lifestyle, cardiometabolic disease (e.g., diabetes, obesity, hypertension), minimal social support, adverse medication events, and a 40% suicide attempt rate (Fuller-Thomson & Hollister, 2016; Laursen, 2019; Olfson, Gerhard, Huang, Crystal, & Stroup, 2015; Seeman, 2019).

Disrupted sleep features prominently in psychotic disorders. Half of the individuals with schizophrenia report insomnia symptoms, 48% have a nightmare disorder, another 30% have hypersomnia, and 15% have obstructive sleep apnea (Stubbs et al., 2016; Waite, Sheaves, Isham, Reeve, & Freeman, 2020). Circadian rhythm disturbances are also common and may affect as many as 50% of patients (Afonso, Figueira, & Paiva, 2014; Wulff, Dijk, Middleton, Foster, & Joyce, 2012). Moreover, these disorders are often comorbid; one study reported an average of three disorders per patient (Reeve, Sheaves, & Freeman, 2019). Addressing these sleep disturbances is critical because the cost of poor sleep in psychosis is nontrivial. Insomnia triggers hallucinations and delusions, reduces the quality of life, and increases the risk of suicide (Li et al., 2016; Miller, Parker, Rapaport, Buckley, & McCall, 2019; Mulligan, Haddock, Emsley, Neil, & Kyle, 2016; Reeve, Sheaves, & Freeman, 2019; Waite et al., 2020). Additionally, disrupted sleep in psychosis likely contributes to or exacerbates cardiometabolic disease as has been demonstrated in other populations (St-Onge et al., 2016).

Behavioral sleep medicine can significantly improve these sleep disturbances. A pilot trial of CBT-I in the United Kingdom substantially improved insomnia in patients with psychotic illness (Freeman et al., 2015), and similar results were shown in a nonrandomized trial in South Korea (Hwang, Nam, & Lee, 2019). Furthermore, treating insomnia may reduce psychotic symptoms (Bradley et al., 2018), although larger studies are needed to confirm this finding. For inpatient settings, traditional CBT-I can be modified to a brief, intensive format with reasonable results (Sheaves et al., 2018). Additionally, the Transdiagnostic Sleep and Circadian Intervention (Trans-C) (Allison G. Harvey & Buysse, 2018), which addresses the broader issues of sleep/wake dysregulation in psychiatric illness, represents an exciting new opportunity to improve sleep in psychotic disorders.

While patients (Faulkner & Bee, 2017; Waite et al., 2016; Waite et al., 2018; Waters, Chiu, Janca, Atkinson, & Ree, 2015) and providers (Rehman et al., 2017) acknowledge insomnia as a significant problem, sleep is often assessed informally and treated using sleep hygiene interventions, sedative medications, or not at all (Hou et al., 2017; Rehman et al., 2017). This is troubling because (1) medications are not an effective long-term solution for insomnia (Sateia, Buysse, Krystal, Neubauer, & Heald, 2017), and (2) patients often express a preference for behavioral/psychological treatment of insomnia (Faulkner & Bee, 2017; Waite et al., 2018; Waters et al., 2015). Consequently, access to CBT-I in this population remains poor.

The patient

It is not necessary to be a psychosis expert to do CBT-I in psychotic disorders. However, having some general information can be helpful in treatment, so this section will address some common issues therapists may face, namely, psychotic symptoms, poor insight and demotivation, and cognitive/memory impairment.

Being stable enough for CBT-I does not mean being symptom-free. While patients with more severe psychosis are less likely to respond to treatment (Waters, Chiu, Dragovic, & Ree, 2020), many individuals with chronic low-level hallucinations or delusional thinking can benefit from therapy. As an example, one of my patients struggled with unintelligible auditory hallucinations which he believed were from extradimensional entities. However, these symptoms never interfered with his ability to follow my instructions, and I never addressed them directly; we just monitored their intensity severity over the course of treatment to ensure they were not getting worse. Thus, even though he was not symptom-free, his hallucinations were not a barrier to treatment.

Do not be afraid to ask about auditory or visual hallucinations. You can explain that you do not need to know specifics (e.g., what the voices say, what the visions look like), but you need to know if these symptoms are interfering with their sleep and that you would like to monitor these symptoms during therapy to help keep them safe. Ultimately, all that may be needed is a daily or weekly 1 to 10 severity rating to ensure things are not getting worse. Additionally, if they see a psychiatrist or physician outside of your organization, have the patient sign a release of information so that you can communicate with their providers. Not only does this open the door for useful collateral information, but it gives you someone to contact if the patient's symptoms are getting worse. A release of information with the patient's caregiver (if one exists) is similarly useful.

Beyond hallucinations and delusions, psychotic illness is characterized by poor insight and a lack of motivation (Subotnik et al., 2020). A patient may believe they sleep soundly despite the claims of family or friends that they are up at all hours of the night. Alternatively, a patient may understand that spending 10h in bed to only get 3 to 4h of sleep may be a problem, but if her only goal is to get a job then she is unlikely to change this behavior. Even if sleep is perceived as an issue, patients may find the burden of treatment more troublesome than its worth.

Overcoming these issues often requires rapport and time. An additional week or two of baseline data collection (preferably with actigraphy) can help patients to see problems they did not realize were there. Behavioral experiments help patients explore their beliefs about sleep and allow for shared decision-making and greater patient autonomy. Motivational interviewing can help you frame interventions as steps toward a patient's goals. While these techniques can be time-consuming, they help patients retain information, improve motivation, and increase self-efficacy in addressing their sleep.

Cognitive and memory deficits are also a significant barrier to care, as these make delivery and retention of psychoeducational content more difficult. While this is not true for everyone, some patients often have trouble remembering what was discussed at previous visits or generalizing specific solutions to new problems. To overcome these issues, patients may need more reminders, handouts, and other visual aids, and simpler explanations to help concepts stick. Introducing fewer concepts at each session, actively reviewing concepts from previous sessions, and asking patients to apply concepts to issues in their own life are all good ways to improve retention and treatment adherence.

The plan

While it is tempting to focus on insomnia as the primary sleep disorder, insomnia likely occurs in the context of broader sleep/wake dysregulation. Patients who cannot sleep at night are sedentary/lethargic during the day, are prone to napping, have inconsistent sleep schedules, and may use the bed as a coping strategy for psychotic symptoms and other emotional stressors. Treating insomnia requires addressing all of this, which may seem time-consuming and complicated. Fortunately, there is a unified approach.

The Transdiagnostic Sleep and Circadian Intervention (Trans-C) (Harvey & Buysse, 2018) is a comprehensive, modular behavioral sleep medicine intervention that addresses multifactorial sleep disturbances. As a transdiagnostic intervention, Trans-C frames individual sleep disorders in the broader context of sleep/wake rhythms and then develops an individualized treatment plan to address each factor contributing to poor sleep. *Trans*-C might employ traditional CBT-I tools such as sleep restriction and stimulus control but may add elements of Interpersonal and

Social Rhythm Therapy such as regularizing sleep schedules and increasing daytime activity, as well as Imagery Rehearsal Therapy for nightmares. While Trans-C has only been tested in adolescents (Dong, Dolsen, Martinez, Notsu, & Harvey, 2020), a randomized controlled trial of Trans-C in serious mental illness recently concluded (Harvey et al., 2016), which may show efficacy in psychotic disorders.

This section presents a general treatment plan for addressing insomnia in patients with psychotic disorders. The approach described is heavily influenced by Trans-C, and the reader is strongly encouraged to read the Trans-C treatment manual, "Treating Sleep Problems: A Transdiagnostic Approach" (Harvey & Buysse, 2018) by Allison Harvey and Daniel Buysse to learn more. A summary of this plan as a series of adaptations/modifications to CBT-I is presented in Table 1.

Assessment

Screening tools

Questionnaires and other screening tools are an efficient way to collect information about your patient's sleep. Because of cognitive impairments and lack of insight, however, these measures are not necessarily valid in individuals with psychosis (Faulkner & Sidey-Gibbons, 2019). Consequently, data collected by screening tools should be reviewed directly with the patient to ensure accuracy.

Because of the comorbidity issue in psychotic illness, patients should be thoroughly assessed for other sleep disorders, including nightmares, parasomnias, circadian rhythm disorders, and restless legs syndrome. Sleep apnea is of particular importance, as antipsychotic medications are known to cause weight gain and metabolic disturbances that increase the risk for sleep apnea. The Sleep Disorders Symptoms Check List-25 (Klingman, Jungquist, & Perlis, 2017) is a simple, initial screening tool that assesses the common symptoms of a number of sleep disorders. Individuals who screen positive on the SDS-CL-25 can then be screened using more specific measures (e.g., STOP-Bang) and referred to a sleep physician as necessary. Screening should also address daytime activity (or lack thereof), and measures such as the Fatigue Severity Scale and the Epworth Sleepiness Scale are helpful in this regard.

The clinical interview

When interviewing a patient with psychotic illness, there are a few things to keep in mind. As mentioned above, try to assess the patient's psychotic symptoms, including how they manage these symptoms and whether these symptoms are interfering with sleep. It is also important to know what medications the patient is taking and when they are taking them; for example, taking high dose olanzapine in the morning may result in significant daytime somnolence that could be avoided by taking the medication at night. Finally, a thorough assessment of substance use is important; many patients use cigarettes or other tobacco products to manage anxiety (even at night), and cannabis use is common in this population.

Sleep diary

As usual, the sleep diary is the most powerful tool in the sleep clinician's arsenal for understanding their patient's sleep. Unfortunately, it is often difficult to deploy among individuals with psychotic illnesses. Patients will forget to fill it out, not remember what happened during the night, forget to bring it to the session, or simply report inaccurate information. While there are solutions to this (e.g., repeated coaching on how to fill out the sleep diary, use of an electronic format which patients can complete on their phone or computer), actigraphy is a useful complementary approach. Using an actigraph increases the chances of accurate data, reduces patients' barriers to participating in therapy, and provides data in a visual format (often a graph or chart) that can be more easily explained. While all patients should be asked to complete a sleep diary, the addition of actigraphy in this population can be particularly helpful.

Core treatment approaches

When treating insomnia in psychotic disorders, there are three major issues that typically need to be addressed: sleep scheduling, stimulus control, and daytime activity.

Sleep scheduling

Circadian rhythm disturbances such as advanced or delayed sleep phase are common in patients with psychosis (Afonso et al., 2014; Wulff et al., 2012). While this may be due to the direct effects of psychotic illness on the brain, it is also likely influenced by disrupted social and environmental rhythms. Patients are often unemployed and have no reason to adhere to regular sleeping hours. They may use a computer, phone, or TV late into the night to avoid psychotic symptoms or simply alleviate boredom, resulting in delayed sleep times. Alternatively, they may take their antipsychotic medications with dinner at 6pm, become sedated, and go to bed early because they have no activities or social interactions to engage them in the evening. Additionally, patients often lack wind down or wake up routines that help them to transition to and from sleep, resulting in significant sleep onset insomnia and delayed morning awakenings.

The first step is to help the patient identify a consistent 7- to 8-h sleep schedule that they believe will work best for them. This will likely involve some negotiation: patients may want to go to bed late (e.g., 4 am) to avoid troublesome family members or to stay up playing video games, while others may want to go to bed early (e.g., 7 pm) because that is when they are tired. As a collaborator, try to avoid making direct suggestions and instead work with the patient to identify the benefits and drawbacks of these times. An early bedtime may alleviate sleep pressure, but may also result in taking a long time to fall asleep and waking up too early, while a late bedtime may result in sleeping through the morning, thus missing appointments or making it difficult to work a morning job shift. While it is tempting to suggest or advocate for a more typical sleep schedule (e.g., 11 pm to 7 am), the primary goal here is to find a schedule that the patient can adhere to consistently. You can always adjust the schedule in a later session.

Once you have identified a schedule, the next step is the wind-down routine. The goal here is to reduce light exposure (particularly blue light) and to engage in calming/soothing activities that facilitate sleep. Help the patient identify specific quiet activities they can engage in for 30 to 60 min before their preferred bedtime. In developing this routine, you may need to consider whether a "quiet" activity is still too stimulating; reading a comic book may seem appropriate, but a patient may become engrossed and miss their bedtime. Additionally, patients may suggest activities using their phone or computer, so psychoeducation on blue light exposure and melatonin may be warranted. I frequently recommend an "electronic curfew" of at least 1 h before bedtime to facilitate falling asleep. If patients are resistant or unconvinced about the curfew, suggest testing it in a behavioral experiment for a week to see if it helps or hurts their ability to fall asleep.

Getting up in the morning can be a difficult problem for most patients for two reasons: sleep inertia and lack of daytime structure. While everyone experiences some degree of sleep inertia when they wake up, sleep inertia in psychosis may last for an hour or more, either due to the disorder or medication hangover. Many patients interpret this sleep inertia as insufficient or poor sleep and will stay in bed to get more sleep, particularly if they are unemployed and/or out of school and have no reason to get up. Consequently, psychoeducation about sleep inertia can help normalize expectations about morning energy, and a wake-up routine gives patients specific activities they can do to increase their energy and wakefulness. While many activities can be planned, this routine should at least involve increased exposure to sunlight (e.g., opening curtains/blinds, going outside) and having breakfast, as light exposure and food intake are known to have potent effects on circadian functioning.

Ideally, all of this can be accomplished in a single 1-h session, although it can be spread across sessions depending on the patient. Additionally, it is important to remind your client that even a single week of strong adherence may not lead to profound changes; sleep/wake rhythms take time to adapt, and it will take many days of consistency for the brain to learn and practice the new routines.

Stimulus control

Stimulus control is a core component of traditional CBT-I and its implementation in psychotic illness is not substantially different than usual: use the bed for sleep (and sex) only. What makes this difficult is that patients often use the bed as a coping strategy for depression, anxiety, or psychotic symptoms. Beds are generally comfortable and safe so patients will retreat there when their mental health symptoms are at their worst. Unfortunately, this is rarely effective and can lead to an opposite effect whereby psychotic symptoms become exacerbated when patients get into bed, either through unintentional conditioning or because there is nothing to distract patients.

Replacing the bed as a coping strategy is a key to stimulus control in psychotic illness. If patients use the bed to avoid hallucinations during the day, then you can help them find and test alternative activities to reduce these experiences: going outside for a walk, talking to a friend or relative, or watching a television program. Have them rate their symptoms during each of these activities so they can see whether they are more, or less, effective than lying in bed.

Dealing with hallucinations at bedtime or during the night can be more challenging, since immediately leaving the bed to reduce symptoms may reinforce nighttime wakefulness. Since stress is a major trigger for hallucinations, using stress reduction strategies ahead of time can help; a scheduled worry time earlier in the day coupled with a calming wind-down routine can alleviate stress and reduce the likelihood of hallucinations. Once patients are in bed (or if they wake up in the night), it is important that patients spend 15 to 20 min trying to fall asleep before they get up to avoid negatively reinforcing the hallucinations. During this time, patients can engage in grounding techniques (e.g., focusing on the physical sensations of being in the bed), relaxation exercises (e.g., progressive muscle relaxation), or reality testing to directly challenge the hallucinations (e.g., the bed is real, the voices are not real). Patients still have to get up after 15 to 20 min to limit excess time in bed, so building an alternative coping location, such as a comfortable armchair or a "cozy corner" with blankets and pillows, provides patients a place to go where they can stay awake until they are ready to try sleeping again. Regardless of how the night went, patients should be reminded to adhere to the sleep schedule established in the prior session—no sleeping in to compensate.

Daytime activity

Insomnia is a 24-h problem that requires a 24-h solution (Waite et al., 2016). This is especially true in psychotic illness, where poor sleep coupled with avolition and sedative medications can produce daytime lethargy, inactivity, and napping that exacerbates nighttime sleep disturbances. However, it is possible to break this cycle. Increasing daytime activity can improve nighttime sleep, which then decreases daytime dysfunction and enables further daytime activity. Thus, effective treatment of insomnia requires interventions to improve daytime activity and functioning.

Building a daily schedule can improve activity levels. Start by writing down their wake-up and wind-down routines, which they developed in previous sessions. As a reminder, these routines should include increased light exposure in the morning and decreased exposure at night. Next, plan out mealtimes. Food intake is an important zeitgeber, or circadian cue, and irregular eating can weaken circadian rhythms and increase daytime drowsiness/fatigue. Thus, building a consistent breakfast, lunch, and dinner schedule can help increase daytime energy levels while containing unhealthy snacking. From here, you can add additional scheduled activities depending on the patient's needs. For example, if patients find they get drowsy or sleepy at a certain time of day, perhaps scheduling exercise, a social activity, or a phone call to a friend is an appropriate response. If patients have high levels of anxiety or worry at bedtime, then a scheduled worry time may be appropriate earlier in the day. Generally, it is better to start with just a few activities and only add to the schedule as needed in subsequent sessions; if the schedule becomes too complex, then patients may feel overwhelmed and unable to follow any of them. Start small and monitor progress to see if the schedule needs to be amended.

Motivation is a major hurdle when trying to increase daytime activities. Patients (with or without psychotic illness) often believe that their daytime fatigue, lack of motivation, and poor energy are the direct result of poor sleep and that only sleep can help increase their energy. Consequently, patients may spend time during the day napping to try to increase energy or may feel unmotivated to try other activities because they do not believe they will help. In both cases, behavioral experiments are critical to helping patients challenge these beliefs. Patients can try napping one day and then not napping the next day and see if that affects their sense of fatigue. Alternatively, patients can compare their energy levels when sitting on the couch or lying in bed to when they are on a walk or engaging in moderate exercise. Regardless of the particulars, make sure to add a relevant row to the sleep diary for the data collection on that experiment; patients are unlikely to record how an experiment went unless they have a specific prompt to do so.

Additional treatment approaches

Sleep restriction/compression

While sleep restriction is typically a core component of CBT-I, there are compelling reasons to not use sleep restriction in psychotic disorders. The most obvious reason is the belief that it may provoke psychotic symptoms in the same way that sleep restriction can trigger manic episodes in bipolar disorders. While there is no direct evidence on this point (i.e., no studies have tested whether sleep restriction in CBT-I leads to increased hallucinations), reduced sleep duration has been associated with worse psychotic experiences (Reeve et al., 2019), and so, there is some merit to this concern.

In practice, however, sleep restriction may prove too difficult or ineffective. Patients may already have low motivation to participate in sleep therapy and the unpleasant increases in daytime fatigue and sleepiness may drive patients out of your office. Additionally, sleep restriction depends on the core components described above (e.g., regularizing sleep schedules and eliminating excess time in bed), and addressing these factors is often all that is needed anyway.

Ultimately, the choice of whether to use sleep restriction rests with the clinician: if you believe the patient could benefit from a restricted sleep schedule, then don't be afraid to try it. Just make sure to talk with your patient about monitoring for worsening symptoms.

Nightmares

Nightmares are extremely common in psychotic disorders and contribute to significant distress. As in PTSD, some patients may actively avoid the bed due to their fear of nightmares, resulting in reduced sleep duration and/or delayed bedtimes. In many cases, patients may cite nightmares as a higher treatment priority than insomnia.

Imagery rehearsal therapy (IRT) is the primary behavioral treatment for nightmares (Aurora et al., 2010), and studies in other populations show significant reductions in nightmares after 2 to 3 sessions. While there are no studies of IRT in psychotic patients, there is no reason this approach cannot be used, and anecdotally patients report it is both tolerable and effective in reducing nightmares. While readers interested in IRT are encouraged to read more in-depth treatment manuals (Krakow & Zadra, 2010), a brief overview of the approach is described here.

First, patients choose a nightmare to rescript. If patients have multiple nightmares, they should not choose the most severe nightmare for rescripting as this decreases the likelihood of success. Once they have successfully rescripted one or two other nightmares, it is more reasonable to tackle the most severe dream.

Having chosen a nightmare, patients should write it down in as much detail as they feel comfortable using. While it is possible that using more detail can act as a sort of exposure therapy, this is not necessary for IRT to be effective. Once they have written the original dream, patients should then rewrite the dream, starting in a similar manner to the original dream but quickly changing into a different story. The only requirement is that the new dream be something the patient *wants* to experience. In the new script, patients should be as specific as possible with details, particularly around the positive emotions the dream conveys. While patients should be encouraged to be creative in their rescripting, make sure the new dream does not play into any delusions or hallucinations that the patient experiences. For example, if a patient struggles with delusions thinking around being a messiah, rescripting of nightmares should not involve the patient using magical messianic powers.

TABLE 1 Recommended modifications and adaptations of CBT-I for patients with psychotic disorders.

CBT-I Components	Standard practice	Modifications/Adaptions
Sleep education	3-P model, 2-process model of sleep regulation, sleep stages	Add education as needed about: sleep inertia, medication effects on sleep and daytime energy, melatonin and blue light exposure, circadian rhythms and zeitgebers, nightmares. Handouts and other visual materials are very helpful
Sleep restriction	Improve sleep efficiency by limiting time in bed to the amount of time sleeping then expanding slowly as long as sleep efficiency is preserved	Not generally needed or recommended in this population. If necessary, make sure to monitor for psychotic symptoms (e.g., increased hallucinations) resulting from reduced sleep duration. Sleep compression may be preferable
Stimulus control	Associate bed/bedroom solely as a cue for sleep by eliminating nonsleep activities from the bedroom. Instruction to get out of bed at night if awake >15 min	Because the bed is often used to cope with mood/psychotic symptoms, patients may need alternative coping strategies/ locations for dealing with symptoms to reduce time in bed
Napping/ daytime sleep	Discontinue or restrict daytime napping to 30 min	May require adjusting timing of medications to reduce daytime sleepiness
Sleep hygiene education	Address daytime habits and sleep environment interfering with sleep	Build wind down and wake up routines and implement an evening electronics curfew

Continued

TABLE 1 Recommended modifications and adaptations of CBT-I for patients with psychotic disorders—cont'd

CBT-I Components	Standard practice	Modifications/Adaptions
Cognitive therapy	Challenge patient's dysfunctional beliefs interfering with sleep and misconceptions about sleep. Replace/restructure to more helpful and realistic thoughts about sleep	Behavioral experiments are generally most effective for challenging dysfunctional beliefs, increasing insight, and motivating behavior change
Relapse Prevention	Discuss practicing less rigid sleep plan over time and what do to prevent sleep disturbance from turning into another episode of insomnia in the future	Decatastrophize future poor sleep and reinforce not compensating for a bad night of sleep
Sleep diaries	Establish baseline sleep patterns, track progress, reinforce appropriate behavior change, problem-solve obstacles to adherence	If possible, add objective measures (i.e., actigraphy) due to unreliable reporting. Add questions to the diary to monitor particular symptoms/behaviors as part of behavioral experiments and/or behavior change

Once the patient has developed a replacement dream, they need to practice visualizing the new dream at least 2 to 3 times per day whenever the patient wants. While response times vary, patients should generally stick to the same script for 3 to 7 days before trying to rescript a new nightmare.

CPAP compliance

As mentioned before, obstructive sleep apnea is prevalent and often undertreated in psychotic disorders. Moreover, even if patients have access to sleep medicine and are diagnosed by polysomnography, they frequently have difficulty using positive airway pressure (PAP) machines, which coupled with low motivation, results in high rates of PAP noncompliance. While PAP adherence therapy is not typically part of CBT-I, untreated sleep apnea is likely to maintain and exacerbate a patient's insomnia. Thus, it is often beneficial to help patients increase their use of the PAP. This may involve psychoeducation around what sleep apnea is and how PAP treats it, problem-solving challenges to PAP use (such as remembering to clean it and/or remembering to put it on), and helping patients adjust straps and settings to make it more comfortable. Additionally, patients who report claustrophobia from wearing the mask will benefit from graded exposure to help reduce anxiety and increase comfort.

Conclusion

Patients with psychotic disorders have difficulties engaging in treatment and often have more complex sleep disturbances than other patient populations. Consequently, treatment often takes longer and requires more planning/investment. However, the benefits are significant: better sleep can significantly improve patients' quality of life, reduce psychotic symptoms, and increase daytime activities and social interactions. Suicide is common in psychotic disorders and poor sleep only increases that risk, so treating insomnia can protect patients from suicidal thoughts and behaviors. Moreover, regularizing sleep and reducing insomnia can allow patients to discontinue adjunct sedative medications they are receiving from prescribers (e.g., trazodone, Z-drugs), which is particularly important in a patient population already struggling with polypharmacy. Hopefully, the information provided in this chapter has bolstered your competence and confidence in working with people with psychosis.

References

Afonso, P., Figueira, M. L., & Paiva, T. (2014). Sleep-wake patterns in schizophrenia patients compared to healthy controls. *The World Journal of Biological Psychiatry, 15*(7), 517–524. https://doi.org/10.3109/15622975.2012.756987.

American Psychiatric Association, & American Psychiatric Association. DSM-5 Task Force. (2013). *Diagnostic and statistical manual of mental disorders: DSM-5* (5th ed.). Washington, D.C.: American Psychiatric Association.

Aurora, R. N., Zak, R. S., Auerbach, S. H., Casey, K. R., Chowdhuri, S., Karippot, A., et al. (2010). Best practice guide for the treatment of nightmare disorder in adults. *Journal of Clinical Sleep Medicine, 6*(4), 389–401.

Bradley, J., Freeman, D., Chadwick, E., Harvey, A. G., Mullins, B., Johns, L., et al. (2018). Treating sleep problems in young people at ultra-high risk of psychosis: A feasibility case series. *Behavioural and Cognitive Psychotherapy, 46*(3), 276–291. https://doi.org/10.1017/S1352465817000601.

Charlson, F. J., Ferrari, A. J., Santomauro, D. F., Diminic, S., Stockings, E., Scott, J. G., et al. (2018). Global epidemiology and burden of schizophrenia: Findings from the global burden of disease study 2016. *Schizophrenia Bulletin*. https://doi.org/10.1093/schbul/sby058.

Chong, H. Y., Teoh, S. L., Wu, D. B., Kotirum, S., Chiou, C. F., & Chaiyakunapruk, N. (2016). Global economic burden of schizophrenia: A systematic review. *Neuropsychiatric Disease and Treatment, 12*, 357–373. https://doi.org/10.2147/NDT.S96649.

Dong, L., Dolsen, M. R., Martinez, A. J., Notsu, H., & Harvey, A. G. (2020). A transdiagnostic sleep and circadian intervention for adolescents: Six-month follow-up of a randomized controlled trial. *Journal of Child Psychology and Psychiatry, 61*(6), 653–661. https://doi.org/10.1111/jcpp.13154.

Faulkner, S., & Bee, P. (2017). Experiences, perspectives and priorities of people with schizophrenia spectrum disorders regarding sleep disturbance and its treatment: A qualitative study. *BMC Psychiatry, 17*(1), 158. https://doi.org/10.1186/s12888-017-1329-8.

Faulkner, S., & Sidey-Gibbons, C. (2019). Use of the Pittsburgh sleep quality index in people with schizophrenia spectrum disorders: A mixed methods study. *Frontiers in Psychiatry, 10*, 284. https://doi.org/10.3389/fpsyt.2019.00284.

Freeman, D., Waite, F., Startup, H., Myers, E., Lister, R., McInerney, J., et al. (2015). Efficacy of cognitive behavioural therapy for sleep improvement in patients with persistent delusions and hallucinations (BEST): A prospective, assessor-blind, randomised controlled pilot trial. *Lancet Psychiatry, 2*(11), 975–983. https://doi.org/10.1016/S2215-0366(15)00314-4.

Fuller-Thomson, E., & Hollister, B. (2016). Schizophrenia and suicide attempts: Findings from a representative community-based Canadian sample. *Schizophrenia Research and Treatment, 2016*, 3165243. https://doi.org/10.1155/2016/3165243.

Harvey, A. G., & Buysse, D. J. (2018). *Treating sleep problems: A transdiagnostic approach*. New York: The Guilford Press.

Harvey, A. G., Hein, K., Dong, L., Smith, F. L., Lisman, M., Yu, S., et al. (2016). A transdiagnostic sleep and circadian treatment to improve severe mental illness outcomes in a community setting: Study protocol for a randomized controlled trial. *Trials, 17*(1), 606. https://doi.org/10.1186/s13063-016-1690-9.

Hou, C. L., Li, Y., Cai, M. Y., Ma, X. R., Zang, Y., Jia, F. J., et al. (2017). Prevalence of insomnia and clinical and quality of life correlates in Chinese patients with schizophrenia treated in primary care. *Perspectives in Psychiatric Care, 53*(2), 80–86. https://doi.org/10.1111/ppc.12139.

Hwang, D. K., Nam, M., & Lee, Y. G. (2019). The effect of cognitive behavioral therapy for insomnia in schizophrenia patients with sleep disturbance: A non-randomized, assessor-blind trial. *Psychiatry Research, 274*, 182–188. https://doi.org/10.1016/j.psychres.2019.02.002.

Klingman, K. J., Jungquist, C. R., & Perlis, M. L. (2017). Questionnaires that screen for multiple sleep disorders. *Sleep Medicine Reviews, 32*, 37–44. https://doi.org/10.1016/j.smrv.2016.02.004.

Krakow, B., & Zadra, A. (2010). Imagery rehearsal therapy: Principles and practice. *Sleep Medicine Clinics, 5*(2), 289–298. https://psycnet.apa.org/doi/10.1016/j.jsmc.2010.01.004.

Laursen, T. M. (2019). Causes of premature mortality in schizophrenia: A review of literature published in 2018. *Current Opinion in Psychiatry, 32*(5), 388–393. https://doi.org/10.1097/YCO.0000000000000530.

Li, S. X., Lam, S. P., Zhang, J., Yu, M. W., Chan, J. W., Chan, C. S., et al. (2016). Sleep disturbances and suicide risk in an 8-year longitudinal study of schizophrenia-spectrum disorders. *Sleep, 39*(6), 1275–1282. https://doi.org/10.5665/sleep.5852.

Miller, B. J., Parker, C. B., Rapaport, M. H., Buckley, P. F., & McCall, W. V. (2019). Insomnia and suicidal ideation in nonaffective psychosis. *Sleep, 42*(2). https://doi.org/10.1093/sleep/zsy215.

Moreno-Kustner, B., Martin, C., & Pastor, L. (2018). Prevalence of psychotic disorders and its association with methodological issues. A systematic review and meta-analyses. *PLoS One, 13*(4), e0195687. https://doi.org/10.1371/journal.pone.0195687.

Mulligan, L. D., Haddock, G., Emsley, R., Neil, S. T., & Kyle, S. D. (2016). High resolution examination of the role of sleep disturbance in predicting functioning and psychotic symptoms in schizophrenia: A novel experience sampling study. *Journal of Abnormal Psychology, 125*(6), 788–797. https://doi.org/10.1037/abn0000180.

Olfson, M., Gerhard, T., Huang, C., Crystal, S., & Stroup, T. S. (2015). Premature mortality among adults with schizophrenia in the United States. *JAMA Psychiatry, 72*(12), 1172–1181. https://doi.org/10.1001/jamapsychiatry.2015.1737.

Reeve, S., Nickless, A., Sheaves, B., Hodgekins, J., Stewart, S. L. K., Gumley, A., et al. (2019). Sleep duration and psychotic experiences in patients at risk of psychosis: A secondary analysis of the EDIE-2 trial. *Schizophrenia Research, 204*, 326–333. https://doi.org/10.1016/j.schres.2018.08.006.

Reeve, S., Sheaves, B., & Freeman, D. (2019). Sleep disorders in early psychosis: Incidence, severity, and association with clinical symptoms. *Schizophrenia Bulletin, 45*(2), 287–295. https://doi.org/10.1093/schbul/sby129.

Rehman, A., Waite, F., Sheaves, B., Biello, S., Freeman, D., & Gumley, A. (2017). Clinician perceptions of sleep problems, and their treatment, in patients with non-affective psychosis. *Psychosis, 9*(2), 129–139. https://doi.org/10.1080/17522439.2016.1206955.

Saha, S., Chant, D., Welham, J., & McGrath, J. (2005). A systematic review of the prevalence of schizophrenia. *PLoS Medicine, 2*(5). https://doi.org/10.1371/journal.pmed.0020141, e141.

Sateia, M. J., Buysse, D. J., Krystal, A. D., Neubauer, D. N., & Heald, J. L. (2017). Clinical practice guideline for the pharmacologic treatment of chronic insomnia in adults: An American Academy of sleep medicine clinical practice guideline. *Journal of Clinical Sleep Medicine, 13*(2), 307–349. https://doi.org/10.5664/jcsm.6470.

Seeman, M. V. (2019). Schizophrenia mortality: Barriers to progress. *The Psychiatric Quarterly, 90*(3), 553–563. https://doi.org/10.1007/s11126-019-09645-0.

Sheaves, B., Freeman, D., Isham, L., McInerney, J., Nickless, A., Yu, L. M., et al. (2018). Stabilising sleep for patients admitted at acute crisis to a psychiatric hospital (OWLS): An assessor-blind pilot randomised controlled trial. *Psychological Medicine, 48*(10), 1694–1704. https://doi.org/10.1017/S0033291717003191.

St-Onge, M. P., Grandner, M. A., Brown, D., Conroy, M. B., Jean-Louis, G., Coons, M., et al. (2016). Sleep duration and quality: Impact on lifestyle behaviors and cardiometabolic health: A scientific statement from the American Heart Association. *Circulation, 134*(18), e367–e386. https://doi.org/10.1161/CIR.0000000000000444.

Stubbs, B., Vancampfort, D., Veronese, N., Solmi, M., Gaughran, F., Manu, P., et al. (2016). The prevalence and predictors of obstructive sleep apnea in major depressive disorder, bipolar disorder and schizophrenia: A systematic review and meta-analysis. *Journal of Affective Disorders, 197*, 259–267. https://doi.org/10.1016/j.jad.2016.02.060.

Subotnik, K. L., Ventura, J., Hellemann, G. S., Zito, M. F., Agee, E. R., & Nuechterlein, K. H. (2020). Relationship of poor insight to neurocognition, social cognition, and psychiatric symptoms in schizophrenia: A meta-analysis. *Schizophrenia Research, 220*, 164–171. https://doi.org/10.1016/j.schres.2020.03.038.

Waite, F., Bradley, J., Chadwick, E., Reeve, S., Bird, J. C., & Freeman, D. (2018). The experience of sleep problems and their treatment in young people at ultra-high risk of psychosis: A thematic analysis. *Frontiers in Psychiatry, 9*, 375. https://doi.org/10.3389/fpsyt.2018.00375.

Waite, F., Evans, N., Myers, E., Startup, H., Lister, R., Harvey, A. G., et al. (2016). The patient experience of sleep problems and their treatment in the context of current delusions and hallucinations. *Psychology and Psychotherapy, 89*(2), 181–193. https://doi.org/10.1111/papt.12073.

Waite, F., Myers, E., Harvey, A. G., Espie, C. A., Startup, H., Sheaves, B., et al. (2016). Treating sleep problems in patients with schizophrenia. *Behavioural and Cognitive Psychotherapy, 44*(3), 273–287. https://doi.org/10.1017/S1352465815000430.

Waite, F., Sheaves, B., Isham, L., Reeve, S., & Freeman, D. (2020). Sleep and schizophrenia: From epiphenomenon to treatable causal target. *Schizophrenia Research, 221*, 44–56. https://doi.org/10.1016/j.schres.2019.11.014.

Waters, F., Chiu, V. W., Dragovic, M., & Ree, M. (2020). Different patterns of treatment response to cognitive-behavioural therapy for insomnia (CBT-I) in psychosis. *Schizophrenia Research, 221*, 57–62. https://doi.org/10.1016/j.schres.2020.03.054.

Waters, F., Chiu, V. W., Janca, A., Atkinson, A., & Ree, M. (2015). Preferences for different insomnia treatment options in people with schizophrenia and related psychoses: A qualitative study. *Frontiers in Psychology, 6*, 990. https://doi.org/10.3389/fpsyg.2015.00990.

Wulff, K., Dijk, D. J., Middleton, B., Foster, R. G., & Joyce, E. M. (2012). Sleep and circadian rhythm disruption in schizophrenia. *The British Journal of Psychiatry, 200*(4), 308–316. https://doi.org/10.1192/bjp.bp.111.096321.

CHAPTER

9

CBT-I for people diagnosed with bipolar disorder: Moving from a disorder-focused to a transdiagnostic conceptualization

Allison G. Harvey and Caitlin E. Gasperetti

Department of Psychology, University of California, Berkeley, CA, United States

Empirical basis for treatment adaptations

In a recent systematic review of evidence-based psychosocial treatments (EBPTs), we found that clinical intuition was a common basis for conducting treatment adaptations (Harvey, Lammers, et al., 2021). On one hand, we can use clinical intuition as a source of new hypotheses to be tested empirically (Clark, 1999; Salkovskis, 2002). In other words, clinical intuition can be effective when combined with an empirical approach (Witteman, Spaanjaars, & Aarts, 2012). On the other hand, clinical intuition is prone to cognitive biases (Lilienfeld, Ritschel, Lynn, Cautin, & Latzman, 2013), and feedback as to the veracity of intuition is unlikely to be available (Witteman et al., 2012).

Following the treatment development traditions described by Clark (1999, 2004), Salkovskis (2002), and Onken, Carroll, Shoham, Cuthbert, and Riddle (2014), the use of an empirical process involving scientific data should be the cornerstone of all treatment development and adaptation efforts. The sources of data that can be used are wide-ranging and include epidemiologic studies, questionnaires and surveys, stakeholder interviews, focus groups, or experiments that identify if there is a need for

https://doi.org/10.1016/B978-0-12-822872-2.00007-4

the adaptation, as well as experiments that test the proposed adapted treatment element(s). These perspectives have been a major influence on the adaptation process reported here.

In the early 2000s, we were working on improving treatment for chronic insomnia when Professor Guy Goodwin, from Oxford University, encouraged us to apply our findings to people diagnosed with bipolar disorder (BP). He alerted us to the great need for sleep treatment among this group of people. This started a steep learning curve for our team, and we were grateful to have the opportunity to collaborate with Dr. Daniel Buysse at every step. The goal of this chapter is to describe our process of working out how to treat sleep problems among people diagnosed with bipolar disorder as well as the outcome from the process.

Bipolar disorder and sleep disturbance

Bipolar Disorder is common, severe, and chronic. The spectrum of bipolar disorders—Bipolar I disorder (BP1), Bipolar II disorder, Bipolar Not Otherwise Specified (BP-NOS)—is increasingly being recognized as a valid and clinically important dimension. Even the "softer" end of the spectrum (BP-NOS) was known to be associated with moderate to severe clinical and role impairment (Judd & Akiskala, 2003; Merikangas et al., 2007). For this reason, unless otherwise specified, we will use "BP" across this chapter to refer to the entire bipolar spectrum. The lifetime prevalence of BP is 2.6%–6.5% (Angst, 1998; Dunner, 2003; Merikangas et al., 2011). The impact of episodes of mania, hypomania, and depression is enormous. Those who have been hospitalized spend 20% of their life in episodes (Angst & Sellaro, 2000) and 50% of their time unwell (Judd, Akiskal, & Schettler, 2002). In fact, BP is one of the leading causes of medical disability according to the World Health Organization (UN World Health Organization (Producer), 2011). While there have been important advances in pharmacological (Keck, 2000) and nonpharmacological (Miklowitz & Johnson, 2006) treatments for BP, even with continued adherence and adjunctive interventions, many patients are seriously symptomatic in the interepisode period (Judd et al., 2003; MacQueen et al., 2003; Robb, Cooke, Devins, Young, & Joffe, 1997) and the risk of another mood episode is high (Gitlin, Swendsen, Heller, & Hammen, 1995). Clearly, new treatment strategies are urgently needed.

Sleep disturbance is among the most prominent correlates of mood episodes and inadequate recovery. Reduced need for sleep is a classic symptom of mania (American Psychiatric Association, 2013). During episodes of depression, insomnia or hypersomnia are common. Even in the interepisode period, sleep is disturbed; up to 70% of people diagnosed with BP report insomnia (Harvey, Schmidt, Scarna, Semler, & Goodwin, 2005), which is associated with risk for relapse and previous suicide attempts (Sylvia et al., 2011). Sleep is a common prodrome—or early warning signal—for mood episodes (Jackson, Cavanagh, & Scott, 2003).

Sleep disturbances such as insomnia contribute to mood symptoms in BP. Short sleepers exhibit more symptoms of mania, depression, anxiety, and irritability, and lower scores on functioning and life satisfaction compared to people diagnosed with BP with longer sleep times (Gruber et al., 2009). Moreover, shorter total sleep time is associated with increased mania and depression severity over 12 months (Gruber et al., 2011). In a 7-day diary study, total wake time was associated with next day morning negative mood in BP while evening negative mood was associated with subsequent total wake time in both BP and insomnia (Talbot et al., 2012). Sleep disturbance is a common prodrome of relapse (Jackson et al., 2003). Experimentally induced sleep deprivation is associated with the onset of hypomania or mania (e.g., Wehr, Sack, & Rosenthal, 1987). Together, these data raised the possibility that treating insomnia in patients who meet diagnostic criteria for BP could improve mood and functioning. These findings also generate the more general hypothesis that insomnia is an important, but understudied pathway contributing to the provocation and/or maintenance of symptoms and impairment in BP.

Development of an insomnia treatment for bipolar disorder

Despite the clear importance of sleep disturbance in BP, at the time we were starting to work in this field, there were very little empirical data that specifically addressed the treatment of sleep problems experienced by people with BP. We found a chart review, a handful of case reports, and an open trial of sleep medications, but we could not find any test of a psychosocial insomnia treatment, nor any controlled clinical trials for insomnia in BP. Existing nonpharmacologic interventions for BP included psychoeducation, prodrome monitoring, interpersonal and social rhythms therapy (IPSRT), family-focused therapy, and cognitive behavior therapy (CBT), as well as combination approaches. These treatments reduce relapse in adults with BP (Craighead, Miklowitz, Frank, & Vajk, 2002) and several included sleep components. However, to the best of our knowledge, none included sleep outcome measures. As such, we did not know if these approaches were effective for sleep.

We elected to focus on developing a nonpharmacologic insomnia treatment because there are fewer side effects and interactions with concurrent treatments. Hypnotics are efficacious and clinically indicated in some situations, but concerns remain about residual effects, dependence, tolerance, and rebound insomnia (Harvey & Li, 2009) and some insomnia medications pose a risk of abuse, a concern given the prevalence of comorbid substance use in BP (Levin & Hennessy, 2004).

Our first approach was to recruit individuals who met diagnostic criteria for bipolar disorder who also had insomnia and treat them with cognitive behavior therapy for insomnia (CBT-I). We expected that CBT-I would be an excellent match. To our surprise, as we started to treat patients, examine the literature, and collect our data, it quickly became apparent that in addition to insomnia, a range of other sleep and circadian problems was often present, either at the full syndromal or subsyndromal levels, including reduced sleep need (Kanady, Soehnera, & Harvey, 2015), hypersomnia or too much time in bed (Kaplan et al., 2015; Kaplan, Gruber, Eidelman, Talbot, & Harvey, 2011; Kaplan & Harvey, 2009), delayed sleep phase (Giglio et al., 2010) and irregular sleep-wake schedules (Gruber et al., 2009) were all common among people diagnosed with BP. Also, we became concerned about the risk of mania with sleep restriction (Colombo, Benedetti, Barbini, Campori, & Smeraldi, 1999; Leibenluft, Albert, Rosenthal, & Wehr, 1996; Wehr et al., 1987), as the sleep restriction aspect of CBT-I involves mild short-term sleep deprivation. Due to the tendency toward goal/reward pursuit (Johnson, 2005) during prolonged awakenings, we had some reservations about the CBT-I recommendation to get out of the bed/bedroom if unable to fall asleep in case it prompted engagement in nonsleep promoting activities. Also, it was clear that there was a need to address the highly variable sleep-wake schedules, a tendency toward delayed bedtimes, sensitivity to light (Barbini et al., 2005; Benedetti, Colombo, Barbini, Campori, & Smeraldi, 2001; Sit, Wisner, Hanusa, Stull, & Terman, 2007), sleep inertia, and daytime sleepiness.

Taken together, we concluded that there was a need to modify traditional CBT-I to address this broader range of sleep and circadian dysfunctions. We again scoured the scientific literature to seek guidance on *how* to target these complicated features of sleep and circadian functioning in BP. We decided that we would focus the modifications on improving safety and targeting the unique features of sleep experienced by people diagnosed with BP by integrating elements from Interpersonal and Social Rhythms Therapy (IPSRT) (Frank et al., 1999; Frank, Swartz, & Kupfer, 2000) and chronotherapy (Wirz-Justice, Benedetti, & Terman, 2009). We also included a strong emphasis on motivational interviewing (Miller & Rollnick, 2002) and habit formation (Harvey, Callaway, Zieve, Gumport, & Armstrong, 2020). CBT-I was selected as the basis for the adaptation, which we started to refer to as CBT-I-BP, because (a) the evidence base is impressive (Morin et al., 2006; Qaseem, Kansagara, Forciea, Cooke, & Denberg, 2016; Riemann et al., 2017), including for insomnia comorbid with depression and schizophrenia (Ball et al., 1997; Manber et al., 2008; Manber et al., 2016; Myers, Startup, & Freeman, 2011), (b) previous treatments for BP have not been informed by the principles underlying CBT-I (Harvey, 2008), and (c) CBT-I improves sleep efficiency, reduces night-to-night variability, and improves the time taken to get to sleep, all of which are characteristic of the sleep of patients diagnosed with BP (Eidelman, Talbot, Gruber, & Harvey, 2010; Gruber et al., 2009).

Other influences on *how* to conduct the adaptation process included the strong "circadian" theme that had developed in the literature on BP well before our work began, including the work of Wehr (e.g., Wehr, 1989; Wehr et al., 1985), Frank (e.g., Frank et al., 1997), Kupfer (e.g., Kupfer, 2000; Kupfer, Wyatt, Greenspan, Scott, & Snyder, 1970), and other colleagues. More recently, Murray and colleagues have clearly demonstrated the circadian contributions to BP (Morton & Murray, 2020; Murray, 2019).

Description of CBT-I for bipolar disorder

In this section, we offer a summary of the elements of CBT-I for BP, including the specific adaptations made to CBT-I (see also Table 1). Further details and handouts are available in other publications (Harvey & Buysse, 2017). Of note, we deliver this approach regardless of whether or not patients have been prescribed sleep medications. Although future studies are needed to determine the "dose" of treatment that is necessary, we have typically delivered CBT-I-BP in 8 weekly, 50-min sessions.

Sleep diary, functional analysis/case formulation, and goal setting

The daily sleep diary is an essential element of CBT-I-BP, as it is in standard CBT-I-I. Via the sleep diary we can assess where to focus treatment and we can evaluate if the treatment is effective. In our experience, the most common pattern observed within the sleep diary of people diagnosed with BP is irregular bed and wake times, which often vary by 3+ hours across 1 week (Gruber et al., 2009). The functional analysis/case formulation continues by assessing the interplay between sleep-related behaviors, thoughts, emotions, and consequences before bed (e.g., bedtime routine), during the night (e.g., cell phone left on), on waking (e.g., sleepiness, lethargy), and during the day (e.g., caffeine use). This is a highly collaborative process. Including the period of first waking in the morning and the daytime is particularly important in BP given that sleep inertia can be experienced for several hours into the day and some people diagnosed with BP exhibit hypersomnia or too much time in bed. The information from the functional analysis/case formation process is the basis for generating hypotheses about modifiable maintaining processes, which become the basis of the treatment. Taking all of this information together, the patient and therapists work together to set specific and realistic goals for treatment.

TABLE 1 Summary of the adaptations to CBT-I components for bipolar disorder.

CBT-I components	Standard practice	Modifications/adaptions
Sleep education	3-P model, 2-process model of sleep regulation, sleep stages	Standard practice is included plus: – Education about light exposure and other environmental influences on sleep – Education about circadian rhythms to provide additional rationale for reducing variability in bed and wake times – Education about creating an evening wind-down routine and morning rise-up routine to support regular bed and wake-times – Education about regularizing social rhythms (e.g. mealtimes, exercise, socializing) to promote daytime energy – Education about sleep inertia can be highly impairing for people with BP
Sleep restriction	Improve sleep efficiency by limiting time in bed to the amount of time sleeping then expanding slowly as long as sleep efficiency is preserved	– Given the risk of mania or hypomania associated with sleep restriction, start by regularizing bed and wake times, emphasizing dim light exposure before bedtime and bright light exposure on waking. This step alone may improve sleep efficiency. If not then, standard practice is included with the following modifications: – Consult first with treating psychiatrist – Consider utilizing a sleep compression approach to restrict time in bed gradually by 15–30 min per week – Never allow time in bed to go below 6.5 h – Knowing that sleep deprivation can trigger hypomania/mania, create a safety plan to ensure safe implementation

Stimulus control	Associate bed/bedroom solely as a cue for sleep by eliminating nonsleep activities from the bedroom. Instruction to get out of bed at night if awake >15 min	Standard practice is included plus: – If there are concerns about engagement in goal/reward-seeking, modify by asking the patient to go to bed (and into darkness) at bedtime that has been derived based on circadian principles, even if they are not yet sleepy (often darkness is needed to promote sleepiness) – Decide on specific relaxing activities to complete when leaving the bed during the night to avoid engaging in goal/reward-seeking behaviors. In some cases, consider if it preferable for the patient to stay in bed during waking
Napping/ daytime sleep	Discontinue or restrict daytime napping to 30 min	Standard practice is included plus: – Behavioral experiments are used to test the energy-generating effects of activity – Develop a list of energy generating and energy-sapping activities – Focus on regularizing daytime rhythms like mealtimes, exercise, and social activities to encourage a more consistent routine
Sleep hygiene education	Address daytime habits and sleep environment interfering with sleep	Standard practice is included plus: – Increase social contact and activities during the day to avoid getting back into bed (behavioral activation) – Avoid caffeine in the afternoon – Address possible stimulating or distracting elements of the bedroom environment, including adding blinds or drapes

Continued

TABLE 1 Summary of the adaptations to CBT-I components for bipolar disorder.—cont'd

CBT-I components	Standard practice	Modifications/adaptions
		to darken the room, using a bedside lamp instead of overhead lights, adding a sound machine or fan to block out external noise, and removing the television and other electronics from the bedroom – Create a relaxing evening routine of 30–60 min that includes relaxing activities and dim light conditions – Create a stimulating morning routine that includes no snoozing, increasing light exposure and activity, and engaging in activities to increase energy and reduce sleep inertia
Cognitive therapy	Challenge patient's dysfunctional beliefs interfering with sleep and misconceptions about sleep. Replace/restructure to more helpful and realistic thoughts about sleep	Standard practice is included plus: – Provide strategies to reduce bedtime worry, rumination, and vigilance including cognitive therapy (e.g., negative automatic thought forms, positive data logs), scheduled worry, relaxation, diary writing, imagery, gratitude practice and savoring. Practice each in a treatment session. Develop behavioral experiments to test which strategies are helpful – Behavioral experiments are devised to test unhelpful beliefs about sleep and to develop new beliefs about sleep – Note that certain beliefs that are unhelpful for insomnia patients to hold, may be *helpful* for people diagnosed with bipolar disorder (e.g., I am worried that if I go for 1 or 2 nights without sleep, I may have a nervous breakdown)

Relapse Prevention	Discuss practicing less rigid sleep plan over time and what do to prevent sleep disturbance from turning into another episode of insomnia in the future	Standard practice is included plus: – Generate a long-term sleep plan that addresses the variety of sleep problems that can emerge during episodes of depression (e.g., hypersomnia) or mania (e.g., reduced sleep need), as well as interepisode periods and describe the steps to help get sleep back on track
Sleep diaries	Establish baseline sleep patterns, track progress, reinforce appropriate behavior change, problem-solve obstacles to adherence	Standard practice is included plus – Track relevant daytime and/or nighttime behavior including daytime energy, medications, caffeine, evening activities completed during the wind-down period, technology use, and/or morning activities completed during the first hour after waking

Sleep restriction/sleep compression

Restricting time in bed (Spielman, Saskin, & Thorpy, 1987) is derived from the observations that excessive time in bed perpetuates insomnia and increases homeostatic drive improves sleep. Several adaptations of this element of CBT-I were warranted, given the risk of relapse into a mood episode from sleep deprivation that can be associated with sleep restriction. In particular, there was an emphasis on regularizing bed and wake times, which was often sufficient to improve sleep efficiency (Kaplan & Harvey, 2013). This approach is described below. If regularizing bed and wake times was not sufficient, a sleep compression approach was considered. The exact method used to compress sleep varied enormously across patients. Often reducing time in bed to around 8 h was sufficient to improve sleep efficiency. If sleep restriction was used, time in bed was restricted to no less than 6.5 h. The treating psychiatrist was consulted and a carefully devised safety plan ensured safe implementation. Interestingly, there is a sizable subgroup of people diagnosed with BP who start treatment with limited time in bed and thus inadequate opportunity to sleep. In these cases, there was a need to gradually increase time in bed back to an optimal sleep time.

Stimulus control

Stimulus control (Bootzin, 1972) is one of the most effective treatment components of CBT-I (Morin et al., 2006). It focuses on regularizing the sleep-wake cycle and strengthening associations between the bed and sleep (Bootzin, 1972). Based on the functional analysis/case formation, as well as the results of behavioral experiments, basic stimulus control instructions sometimes needed to be altered for BP. For example, the recommendation to only go to bed when sleepy and get up if unable to sleep, often needed to be modified to reduce the risk of engagement in goal-seeking and/or rewarding behaviors (Johnson, 2005) that could further reduce sleep opportunity (e.g., shopping on the internet). Also, lying in bed in darkness was a necessary step to getting more sleep for many people with BP disorder. This perhaps reflects the light sensitivity discussed below. The latter, of course, is an adaptation of the standard recommendations of CBT-I.

Circadian approaches

Relative to CBT-I, a heavier emphasis was placed on circadian rhythm education to provide the rationale and the motivation for regularizing 24-h rhythms and for the behavioral adjustments required to reduce variability in bed and wake times. Sleep and circadian education include environmental influences (particularly light), circadian rhythmicity, social jetlag, the importance of aligning the many biological clocks within the body, and the tendency toward delayed sleep phase. Sleep inertia is defined and normalized (Tassi & Muzet, 2000). We also address the role of sleep disturbance in mood regulation and as a prodrome of relapse (Cartwright, Luten, Young, Mercer, & Bears, 1998; Perlis & Nielsen, 1993). The latter is often particularly helpful for increasing patient's motivation to regularize their bed and wake times.

Intertwined with education, specific behavioral adjustments are collaboratively derived, using the sleep diary as a guide. Examples of these adjustments will now be described.

Regularizing sleep-wake times. Regularizing sleep and wake times and avoiding naps promote consistent sleepiness in the evening and scaffold patients who have a tendency to very late bedtimes to progressively move their bedtime forward by 20–30 min per week (small enough to promote mastery and motivation). A personalized wind-down and wake-up support the process of establishing regular bed and wake times.

Wind-down. To support regular bedtimes, patients often need assistance to devise a "wind-down" of 30–60 min in which relaxing, sleep-enhancing activities are introduced, *in dim light conditions*. This helps the circadian phase advance among patients who are evening-types and maintains entrainment (Wyatt, Stepanski, & Kirkby, 2006). A central issue is restricting the use of interactive electronic media (internet, cell phones, MP3 players). Motivational interviewing and behavioral experiments are used to facilitate voluntarily *choosing* an electronic vacation. This is particularly important in bipolar disorder as patients are more sensitive to light (Barbini et al., 2005; Benedetti et al., 2001; Lewy, Wehr, Goodwin, Newsome, & Rosenthal, 1981; Nathan, Burrows, & Norman, 1999; Sit et al., 2007). Although not included within our work to date, the use of blue-blocking technologies and formal light and dark therapy should be explored in future research.

Wake-up. To support regular wake-ups, the "brisk wake-up" was developed to assist patients with the extended sleep inertia (2–3+ hours) that is commonly experienced (Kanady & Harvey, 2015; Kaplan, Talavera, & Harvey, 2018). CBT-I-BP also includes behavioral activation, activity scheduling, and goal setting to reinforce getting out of bed. Wake-up plans are individualized and often include not hitting snooze, opening the curtains to let sunlight in, and making the bed so the incentive to get back in is reduced. This intervention, along with activity scheduling, was particularly important for BP patients who exhibited hypersomnia or spending too much time in bed.

Darkness and Light. We consider and teach the potential value of a therapeutic sleep extension (or "dark therapy") procedure (Barbini et al., 2005) if a participant develops manic symptoms, particularly reduced sleep need. There is also an emphasis on exposure to natural sources of light if a participant develops symptoms of depression (Wirz-Justice et al., 2009).

Interpersonal and social rhythms therapy

Continuing the emphasis on rhythmicity and regularizing sleep and wake times, principles from IPSRT (Frank, 2005) were added to CBT-I-BD. These assist with regularizing daily social rhythms, which build upon the regular bed and wake-up times. In particular, through activity scheduling, there was an emphasis on developing regular mealtimes, exercise times, and social activities and avoiding naps.

Cognitive approaches

People diagnosed with BP are often anxious about their sleep, in part, because they are aware that sleep loss can herald relapse (Harvey et al., 2005). As anxiety is antithetical to sleep (Espie, 2002), we included treatment elements to work with unhelpful beliefs which often fuel anxiety as well bedtime worry, rumination, and anxiety. Examples of the cognitive approaches used within CBT-I-BP will now be described.

In CBT-I we know that working with *unhelpful beliefs about sleep* is important (Edinger, Wohlgemuth, Radtke, Marsh, & Quillian, 2001). We also know that unhelpful beliefs about sleep are common in BP (Harvey et al., 2005). They include "the TV helps me fall asleep" and "medication is the only factor that contributes to my feeling drowsy." Guided discovery and individualized experiments test the validity and utility of the beliefs (Harvey, Sharpley, Ree, Stinson, & Clark, 2007; Ree & Harvey, 2004). For example, a commonly held belief is that the only way one can feel less tired in the day is to sleep more. Hence, a behavioral experiment is devised to allow the patient to *experience* the energy-generating effects of activity (Ree & Harvey, 2004) and develop a list of "energy generating" and "energy sapping" activities to better manage daytime tiredness. For further details and examples of behavioral experiments, see our prior publications (Harvey et al., 2007; Ree & Harvey, 2004). Importantly, the CBT-I approach to unhelpful beliefs about sleep was adapted to the clinical realities of BP. For instance, sleep deprivation in BP (unlike insomnia) *can* be dangerous because it can trigger a manic episode.

We also used individualized strategies to *reduce bedtime worry, rumination, and vigilance* including cognitive therapy (e.g., teaching negative automatic thought forms), diary writing, a scheduled "worry period," relaxation, imagery, gratitude practice, and savoring. Each skill is practiced and honed in the treatment session, and between sessions, experiments are planned to determine 1–3 of this "menu of options" is preferred by the patient. These skills then become "rolling interventions" that are checked on each week to promote habitual use of the skill.

Behavior change and habit formation

Behavior change is difficult for all of us, particularly because many sleep-incompatible behaviors are rewarding. Accordingly, we found it was very important to include approaches to promote uptake of treatment elements. For example, we interweaved Motivational interviewing (Miller & Rollnick, 2002) into all treatment sessions. This is a method that emphasizes accepting the patient as an individual, avoiding argumentation, giving lectures or ultimatums, and focuses on the process of eliciting and shaping language in favor of change (i.e., change talk). Motivational interviewing also includes regular straightforward reviews of perceived pros and cons of change, recognizing that many sleep-incompatible/interfering behaviors are rewarding. In addition, we incorporated habit formation approaches (Harvey et al., 2020) in an attempt to ensure that the skills and strategies learned during CBT-I-BP will endure, even with changes in mood state and across the course of a lifetime. For example, all skills and strategies become "rolling interventions" that are checked on each week, as repetition is an essential element of habit formation.

Relapse prevention and generalization of skills

A standard part of CBT, the purpose of relapse prevention is to consolidate gains and prepare for setbacks using an individualized summary of learning across the course of treatment. Goals for continuing progress over the months ahead are also developed. Unique to CBT-I-BP, the therapist and patient also develop a decision tree and menu of options for managing the range of sleep problems that may be experienced during the course of BP mood episodes (e.g., hypomania, depression, reduced sleep need, delayed phase). An individualized decision tree provides guidance and adaptations of the skills learned during treatment for each kind of sleep problem. For example, "dark therapy" is appropriate for mania but not depression.

Efficacy of CBT-I-BP

To evaluate the efficacy of CBT-I-BP, adults meeting diagnostic criteria for insomnia and BP1 disorder who were also interepisode were recruited. The comparison condition was psychoeducation (PE). PE was an active condition in which education on the reciprocal relationships between sleep, stress, diet, mood, health, and exercise was provided. It controlled for therapeutic attention and expectation of improvement. The hypothesis tested was that CBT-I-BP, relative to PE, would be more efficacious for improving sleep and mood symptoms and reducing functional impairment. Of note, we referred to this treatment as "transdiagnostic" because we aimed to treat insomnia along with the broader group of sleep and circadian problems commonly experienced by people with BP. In past studies on the treatment of insomnia, individuals with conditions comorbid to insomnia such as hypersomnia or delayed sleep phase tended to be excluded. We decided to include individuals who exhibit these comorbidities to (a) ensure the findings generalize to the sleep and circadian problems experienced by "real life" patients and (b) recruiting pure "insomnia" was very difficult.

All participants were receiving standard psychiatric care. Half of the participants were randomly allocated to the new treatment (CBT-I-BP; $n = 30$), and the other half received Psychoeducation (PE; $n = 28$). Outcomes were assessed at baseline, at the end of 8 sessions of treatment, and 6 months later. The results were encouraging. During the 6-month follow-up, the CBT-I-BP group had fewer days in a bipolar episode relative to PE (3.3 days vs. 25.5 days). The CBT-I-BP group also experienced a significantly lower hypomania/mania relapse rate (4.6% vs. 31.6%) and a marginally lower overall mood episode relapse rate (13.6% vs. 42.1%) compared to the PE group. Relative to PE, CBT-I-BP reduced insomnia severity. Both CBT-I-BP and PE showed statistically significant improvement on selected sleep and functional impairment measures. The effects of treatment were well sustained through follow-up for most outcomes (Harvey et al., 2015). Furthermore, it appeared that CBT-I-BP was safe for individuals with BP (Kaplan & Harvey, 2013). This outcome was encouraging as it seemed that a broader approach to sleep and circadian problems was feasible and helpful to participants. Based on these findings, CBT-I-BP was recommended by an expert task force as a maintenance treatment for people with BP and insomnia (Gottlieb et al., 2019).

Moving from a disorder-focused approach to a transdiagnostic approach

As our experiences working with BD, schizophrenia (Waite et al., 2016), and depression (Clarke et al., 2015), it started to become clear that real sleep and circadian problems are not so neatly categorized in many mental illnesses. Meanwhile, the majority of prior treatment studies on sleep and circadian dysfunction in severe mental illness, like BP, have been disorder-focused. That is, most studies aim to treat a specific sleep problem (e.g., insomnia) in a specific diagnostic group (e.g., MDD, PTSD). Indeed, insomnia can overlap with hypersomnia (Kaplan et al., 2011; Kaplan & Harvey, 2009; Liu et al., 2007), delayed sleep phase (Giglio et al., 2010), and irregular sleep-wake schedules (Gruber et al., 2009). Also, various types of sleep and circadian dysfunction coexist with mental illness. For example, insomnia, hypersomnia, delayed sleep phase, and irregular sleep-wake schedules are commonly comorbid with mental illness (Benca, Obermeyer, Thisted, & Gillin, 1992; Kaplan & Harvey, 2009; NIH, 2005; Roth et al., 2006; Smith, Huang, & Manber, 2005). Also, sleep dysfunction predicts and predates the onset and worsening of severe mental illness symptoms (Breslau, Roth, Rosenthal, & Andreski, 1996; Bryant, Creamer, O'Donnell, Silove, & McFarlane, 2010; Chang, Ford, Mead, Cooper-Patrick, & Klag, 1997; Ford & Kamerow, 1989; Jansson-Fromark & Lindblom, 2008; Johnson, Roth, & Breslau, 2006; McLay, Klam, & Volkert, 2010; Perlis et al., 2006; Perlis, Giles, Buysse, Tu, & Kupfer, 1997; Sivertsen, Harvey, Lundervold, & Hysing, 2013). Moreover, sleep and circadian problems often persist even with "best practice" treatment for the mental illness (Gruber et al., 2009; Gruber et al., 2011; Nierenberg et al., 1999; Nierenberg et al., 2010; Sachs et al., 2003).

Furthermore, it is clear that sleep and circadian dysfunction contributes to vicious cycles in mental illness including: *emotional dysfunction* (Cartwright et al., 1998; Perlis & Nielsen, 1993), involving the loss of top-down regulatory control usually exerted by the medial-prefrontal cortex on the amygdala (Yoo, Gujar, Hu, Jolesz, & Walker, 2007); *cognitive dysfunction* (Goel, Rao, Durmer, & Dinges, 2009; Van Dongen, Maislin, Mullington, & Dinges, 2003), coincident with altered activation patterns in prefrontal cortex, including lateral regions associated with cognitive control (Drummond et al., 2000; Killgore, 2010); *behavioral problems* (Adan, Natale, Caci, & Prat, 2010; Medeiros, Carvalho, Silva, Prado, & Prado, 2005) via reward seeking and impulsivity centered on ventral striatum (Chuah, Huettel, & Chee, 2007) and *poor health* (Buysse, Grunstein, Horne, & Lavie, 2010; Roth et al., 2011), via immune system dysregulation including increased proinflammatory marker activity (Motivala, 2011; Motivala & Irwin, 2007). In other words, across mental illnesses—not just BP—sleep and circadian dysfunction is likely to be important contributors in the multifactorial causation of mental illness.

Given the high prevalence of sleep problems, alongside the paucity of treatment providers, there is a pressing need for continued innovation to improve the transportability and usefulness of current treatments to front-line providers. Indeed, further disorder-focused variants of CBT-I (like CBT-I-BP) add to the burden on providers who often do not have the resources or time to learn multiple disorder-focused treatments (Weisz, Ng, & Bearman, 2014). Taken together, we began considering if it is possible to develop a sleep-focused treatment that applies to a *variety of sleep and circadian problems* comorbid with a *variety of mental disorders*, and that can be used confidently by a *variety of mental health professionals*. If it were possible, it would assist with scalability nationally and internationally relative to multiple disorder-focused treatments (e.g., CBT-I-BP). Also, a key advantage of one treatment that tackles multiple problems is the substantial cost advantage to training providers (McHugh & Barlow, 2010). These observations motivated the development of Transdiagnostic Sleep and Circadian Intervention (TranS-C) (Harvey & Buysse, 2017).

Transdiagnostic sleep and circadian intervention (TranS-C)

Inspired by the research of Dr. Chorpita and Dr. Weisz (e.g., Weisz et al., 2012), TranS-C takes a modular approach. It is comprised of cross-cutting core and optional modules, which allows the treatment sessions to be more time-efficient and "personalized" to the specific sleep problem(s) experienced by each patient. The process for deriving TranS-C from the sleep and circadian literature and its grounding in the sleep health framework (Buysse, 2014) is described elsewhere (Harvey & Buysse, 2017). In brief, TranS-C includes four cross-cutting interventions in every session, four core modules that apply to most participants, and seven optional modules applied based on patient presentation. Two initial tests of TranS-C—one with 178 teenage night-owls (Harvey et al., 2018) and one with 121 adults with mixed mental illness diagnoses (Harvey, Dong, et al., 2021)—yielded encouraging findings.

Concluding comments

In sum, this chapter has described one process for adapting CBT-I to bipolar disorder (CBT-I-BP). The sources for the adaptation included published scientific findings on the sleep and circadian functioning of people with bipolar disorder, studies conducted within our team as well as clinical experience. Adaptations were made to address the broader range of sleep and circadian problems that are common to BP and to improve safety. A small randomized controlled trial indicates the adapted approach (CBT-I-BP) is promising. However, larger studies are needed to determine replicability. We have also described how the development of CBT-I-BP prompted a full transdiagnostic approach (TranS-C) that aims to provide one approach that applies to a variety of sleep and circadian problems experienced by people with a range of mental health problems. It is also hoped that this approach will be useful to a variety of mental health professionals and be useful in a variety of clinical settings. If this so, there may be considerable advantages for scaling TranS-C, relative to disorder-focused treatments (e.g., CBT-I-BP).

Acknowledgment

This research program has been supported by the National Institutes of Mental Health (R01MH079188, R34 MH080958, R34MH082034, R01MH120147, and R01MH105513). The authors are grateful to Dr. Daniel Buysse for his important contributions to this research.

References

Adan, A., Natale, V., Caci, H., & Prat, G. (2010). Relationship between circadian typology and functional and dysfunctional impulsivity. *Chronobiology International, 27*, 606–619.

American Psychiatric Association. (2013). *Diagnostic and statistical manual of mental disorders (DSM-5®)*. American Psychiatric Association.

Angst, J. (1998). The emerging epidemiology of hypomania and bipolar II disorder. *Journal of Affective Disorders, 50*, 143–151.

Angst, J., & Sellaro, R. (2000). Historical perspectives and natural history of bipolar disorder. *Biological Psychiatry, 48*, 445–457.

Ball, D., Hill, L., Freeman, B., Eley, T. C., Strelau, J., Riemann, R., et al. (1997). The serotonin transporter gene and peer-rated neuroticism. *Neuroreport, 8*(5), 1301–1304.

Barbini, B., Benedetti, F., Colombo, C., Dotoli, D., Bernasconi, A., Cigala-Fulgosi, M., et al. (2005). Dark therapy for mania: A pilot study. *Bipolar Disorders, 7*, 98–101.

Benca, R. M., Obermeyer, W. H., Thisted, R. A., & Gillin, J. C. (1992). Sleep and psychiatric disorders. A meta-analysis. *Archives of General Psychiatry, 49*, 651–668 (discussion 669-670).

Benedetti, F., Colombo, C., Barbini, B., Campori, E., & Smeraldi, E. (2001). Morning sunlight reduces length of hospitalization in bipolar depression. *Journal of Affective Disorders, 62*(3), 221–223.

Bootzin, R. R. (1972). Stimulus control treatment for insomnia. *Proceedings of the American Psychological Association, 7*, 395–396.

Breslau, N., Roth, T., Rosenthal, L., & Andreski, P. (1996). Sleep disturbance and psychiatric disorders: A longitudinal epidemiological study of young adults. *Biological Psychiatry, 39*, 411–418.

Bryant, R. A., Creamer, M., O'Donnell, M., Silove, D., & McFarlane, A. C. (2010). Sleep disturbance immediately prior to trauma predicts subsequent psychiatric disorder. *Sleep, 33*(1), 69.

Buysse, D. J. (2014). Sleep health: Can we define it? Does it matter. *Sleep, 37*(1), 9–17.

Buysse, D., Grunstein, R., Horne, J., & Lavie, P. (2010). Can an improvement in sleep positively impact on health? *Sleep Medicine Reviews, 14*, 405–410.

Cartwright, R., Luten, A., Young, M., Mercer, P., & Bears, M. (1998). Role of REM sleep and dream affect in overnight mood regulation: A study of normal volunteers. *Psychiatry Research, 81*, 1–8.

Chang, P. P., Ford, D. E., Mead, L. A., Cooper-Patrick, L., & Klag, M. J. (1997). Insomnia in young men and subsequent depression. The Johns Hopkins Precursors Study. *American Journal of Epidemiology, 146*, 105–114.

Clark, D. M. (1999). Anxiety disorders: Why they persist and how to treat them. *Behaviour Research and Therapy, 37*(Suppl. 1), S5–27.

Clark, D. M. (2004). Developing new treatments: On the interplay between theories, experimental science and clinical innovation. *Behaviour Research and Therapy, 42*(9), 1089–1104.

Clarke, G., McGlinchey, E. L., Hein, K., Gullion, C. M., Dickerson, J. F., Leo, M. C., et al. (2015). Cognitive-behavioral treatment of insomnia and depression in adolescents: A pilot randomized trial. *Behaviour Research and Therapy, 69*, 111–118.
Colombo, C., Benedetti, F., Barbini, B., Campori, E., & Smeraldi, E. (1999). Rate of switch from depression into mania after therapeutic sleep deprivation in bipolar depression. *Psychiatry Research, 86*, 267–270.
Craighead, W. E., Miklowitz, D. J., Frank, E., & Vajk, F. C. (2002). Psychosocial treatments for bipolar disorder. In P. E. Nathan, & J. M. Gorman (Eds.), *A guide to treatments that work* (2nd ed., pp. 263–275). London: Oxford University Press.
Drummond, S. P., Brown, G. G., Gillen, J. C., Stricker, J. L., Wong, E. C., & Buston, R. B. (2000). Altered brain response to verbal learning following sleep deprivation. *Nature, 403*, 655–657.
Dunner, D. L. (2003). Clinical consequences of under-recognized bipolar spectrum disorder. *Bipolar Disorders, 5*, 456–463.
Edinger, J. D., Wohlgemuth, W. K., Radtke, R. A., Marsh, G. R., & Quillian, R. E. (2001). Does cognitive-behavioral insomnia therapy alter dysfunctional beliefs about sleep? *Sleep, 24*, 591–599.
Eidelman, P., Talbot, L. S., Gruber, J., & Harvey, A. G. (2010). Sleep, illness course, and concurrent symptoms in inter-episode bipolar disorder. *Journal of Behavior Therapy and Experimental Psychiatry, 41*, 145–149.
Espie, C. A. (2002). Insomnia: Conceptual issues in the development, persistence, and treatment of sleep disorder in adults. *Annual Review of Psychology, 53*, 215–243.
Ford, D. E., & Kamerow, D. B. (1989). Epidemiologic study of sleep disturbances and psychiatric disorders. An opportunity for prevention? *Journal of the American Medical Association, 262*, 1479–1484.
Frank, E. (2005). *Treating bipolar disorder: A clinician's guide to interpersonal and social rhythm therapy*. NY: Guilford Press.
Frank, E., Hlastala, S., Ritenour, A., Houck, P., Tu, X. M., Monk, T. H., et al. (1997). Inducing lifestyle regularity in recovering bipolar disorder patients: Results from the maintenance therapies in bipolar disorder protocol. *Biological Psychiatry, 41*, 1165–1173.
Frank, E., Swartz, H. A., & Kupfer, D. J. (2000). Interpersonal and social rhythm therapy: Managing the chaos of bipolar disorder. *Biological Psychiatry, 48*, 593–604.
Frank, E., Swartz, H. A., Mallinger, A. G., Thase, M. E., Weaver, E. V., & Kupfer, D. J. (1999). Adjunctive psychotherapy for bipolar disorder: Effects of changing treatment modality. *Journal of Abnormal Psychology, 108*, 579–587.
Giglio, L. M., Magalhães, P., Andersen, M. L., Walz, J. C., Jakobson, L., & Kapczinski, F. (2010). Circadian preference in bipolar disorder. *Sleep & Breathing, 14*, 153–155.
Gitlin, M. J., Swendsen, J., Heller, T. L., & Hammen, C. (1995). Relapse and impairment in bipolar disorder. *American Journal of Psychiatry, 152*, 1635–1640.
Goel, N., Rao, H., Durmer, J. S., & Dinges, D. F. (2009). Neurocognitive consequences of sleep deprivation. *Seminal Neurology, 29*, 320–329.
Gottlieb, J. F., Benedetti, F., Geoffroy, P. A., Henriksen, T. E., Lam, R. W., Murray, G., et al. (2019). The chronotherapeutic treatment of bipolar disorders: A systematic review and practice recommendations from the ISBD task force on chronotherapy and chronobiology. *Bipolar Disorders, 21*(8), 741–773.
Gruber, J., Harvey, A. G., Wang, P. W., Brooks, J. O., III, Thase, M. E., Sachs, G. S., et al. (2009). Sleep functioning in relation to mood, function, and quality of life at entry to the systematic treatment enhancement program for bipolar disorder (STEP-BD). *Journal of Affective Disorders, 114*(1–3), 41–49.
Gruber, J., Miklowitz, D. J., Harvey, A. G., Frank, E., Kupfer, D., Thase, M. E., et al. (2011). Sleep matters: Sleep functioning and course of illness in bipolar disorder. *Journal of Affective Disorders, 134*.

Harvey, A. G. (2008). Sleep and circadian rhythms in bipolar disorder: Seeking synchrony, harmony, and regulation. *American Journal of Psychiatry, 165*, 820–829.

Harvey, A. G., & Buysse, D. J. (2017). *Treating sleep problems: A transdiagnostic approach*. New York: Guilford.

Harvey, A. G., Callaway, C. A., Zieve, G. G., Gumport, N. B., & Armstrong, C. C. (2020). Applying the science of habit formation to evidence-based psychological treatment: Improving outcomes for mental illness. *Perspectives in Psychological Science*. In press.

Harvey, A. G., Dong, L., Hein, K., Yu, S., Martinez, A., Gumport, N., et al. (2021). A randomized controlled trial of the transdiagnostic intervention for sleep and circadian dysfunction (TranS-C) to improve serious mental illness outcomes in a community setting. *Journal of Consulting and Clinical Psychology*. In press.

Harvey, A. G., Hein, K., Dolsen, M. R., Dong, L., Rabe-Hesketh, S., Gumport, N. B., et al. (2018). Modifying the impact of eveningness chronotype ("night-owls") in youth: A randomized controlled trial. *Journal of the American Academy of Child & Adolescent Psychiatry, 57*(10), 742–754.

Harvey, A. G., Lammers, H. S., Dolsen, M. R., Mullin, A. C., Hilmoe, H. E., Tran, M., … Lee, C. (2021). Systematic review to examine the methods used to adapt evidence-based psychological treatments for adults diagnosed with a mental illness. *Evidence-Based Mental. Health, 24*(1), 33–40.

Harvey, A. G., & Li, D. (2009). Managing sleep disturbance in bipolar disorder. *Current Psychiatry Reviews, 5*, 194–201.

Harvey, A. G., Schmidt, D. A., Scarna, A., Semler, C. N., & Goodwin, G. M. (2005). Sleep-related functioning in euthymic patients with bipolar disorder, patients with insomnia, and subjects without sleep problems. *American Journal of Psychiatry, 162*, 50–57.

Harvey, A. G., Sharpley, A. L., Ree, M. J., Stinson, K., & Clark, D. M. (2007). An open trial of cognitive therapy for chronic insomnia. *Behaviour Research and Therapy, 45*, 2491–2501.

Harvey, A. G., Soehner, A. M., Kaplan, K. A., Hein, K., Lee, J., Kanady, J., et al. (2015). Treating insomnia improves sleep, mood and functioning in bipolar disorder: A pilot randomized controlled trial. *Journal of Consulting and Clinical Psychology, 83*(3), 564–577.

Jackson, A., Cavanagh, J., & Scott, J. (2003). A systematic review of manic and depressive prodromes. *Journal of Affective Disorders, 74*, 209–217.

Jansson-Fromark, M., & Lindblom, K. (2008). A bidirectional relationship between anxiety and depression, and insomnia? A prospective study in the general population. *Journal of Psychosomatic Research, 64*(4), 443–449.

Johnson, S. L. (2005). Mania and dysregulation in goal pursuit: A review. *Clinical Psychology Review, 25*, 241–262.

Johnson, E. O., Roth, T., & Breslau, N. (2006). The association of insomnia with anxiety disorders and depression: Exploration of the direction of risk. *Journal of Psychiatric Research, 40*(8), 700–708.

Judd, L. L., Akiskal, H. S., & Schettler, P. J. (2002). The long-term natural history of a weekly symptomatic status of bipolar 1 disorder. *Archives of General Psychiatry, 39*, 530–537.

Judd, L. L., Akiskal, H. S., Schettler, P. J., Coryell, W., Endicott, J., Maser, J. D., et al. (2003). A prospective investigation of the natural history of the long-term weekly symptomatic status of bipolar II disorder. *Archives of General Psychiatry, 60*, 261–269.

Judd, L. L., & Akiskala, H. S. (2003). The prevalence and disability of bipolar spectrum disorders in the US population: Re-analysis of the ECA database taking into account subthreshold cases. *Journal of Affective Disorders, 73*, 123–131.

Kanady, J. C., & Harvey, A. G. (2015). Development and validation of the sleep inertia questionnaire (SIQ) and assessment of sleep inertia in analogue and clinical depression. *Cognitive Therapy and Research, 39*(5), 601–612.

Kanady, J. C., Soehnera, A. M., & Harvey, A. G. (2015). A retrospective examination of sleep disturbance across the course of bipolar disorder. *Journal of Sleep Disorders & Therapy, 4*(2).

Kaplan, K. A., Gruber, J., Eidelman, P., Talbot, L. S., & Harvey, A. G. (2011). Hypersomnia in inter-episode bipolar disorder: Does it have prognostic significance? *Journal of Affective Disorders, 132*(3), 438–444.

Kaplan, K. A., & Harvey, A. G. (2009). Hypersomnia across mood disorders: A review and synthesis. *Sleep Medicine Reviews, 13*(4), 275–285.

Kaplan, K. A., & Harvey, A. G. (2013). Behavioral treatment of insomnia in bipolar disorder. *American Journal of Psychiatry, 170*(7), 716–720.

Kaplan, K. A., McGlinchey, E. L., Soehner, A., Gershon, A., Talbot, L. S., Eidelman, P., et al. (2015). Hypersomnia subtypes, sleep and relapse in bipolar disorder. *Psychological Medicine, 45*(8), 1751–1763.

Kaplan, K. A., Talavera, D. C., & Harvey, A. G. (2018). Rise and shine: A treatment experiment testing a morning routine to decrease subjective sleep inertia in insomnia and bipolar disorder. *Behaviour Research and Therapy, 111*, 106–112.

Keck, J. P. (2000). Treatment advances in bipolar disorder–making up for lost time. *Biological Psychiatry, 48*, 430–432.

Killgore, W. D. S. (2010). Effects of sleep deprivation on cognition. *Progress in Brain Research, 185*, 105–129.

Kupfer, D. J. (2000). Models of bipolar disease and their clinical implications. *Biological Psychiatry, 48*, 428–429.

Kupfer, D. J., Wyatt, R. J., Greenspan, K., Scott, J., & Snyder, F. (1970). Lithium carbonate and sleep in affective illness. *Archives of General Psychiatry, 23*, 35–40.

Leibenluft, E., Albert, P. S., Rosenthal, N. E., & Wehr, T. A. (1996). Relationship between sleep and mood in patients with rapid-cycling bipolar disorder. *Psychiatry Research, 63*, 161–168.

Levin, F. R., & Hennessy, G. (2004). Bipolar disorder and substance abuse. *Biological Psychiatry, 56*, 738–748.

Lewy, A., Wehr, T., Goodwin, F., Newsome, D., & Rosenthal, N. (1981). Manic-depressive patients may be supersensitive to light. *The Lancet, 317*(8216), 383–384.

Lilienfeld, S. O., Ritschel, L. A., Lynn, S. J., Cautin, R. L., & Latzman, R. D. (2013). Why many clinical psychologists are resistant to evidence-based practice: Root causes and constructive remedies. *Clinical Psychology Review, 33*(7), 883–900.

Liu, X., Buysse, D. J., Gentzler, A. L., Kiss, E., Mayer, L., Kapornai, K., et al. (2007). Insomnia and hypersomnia associated with depressive phenomenology and comorbidity in childhood depression. *Sleep, 30*, 83–90.

MacQueen, G. M., Marriott, M., Begin, H., Robb, J., Joffe, R. T., & Young, L. T. (2003). Subsyndromal symptoms assessed in longitudinal, prospective follow-up of a cohort of patients with bipolar disorder. *Bipolar Disorders, 5*, 349–355.

Manber, R., Buysse, D. J., Edinger, J., Krystal, A., Luther, J. F., Wisniewski, S. R., et al. (2016). Efficacy of cognitive-behavioral therapy for insomnia combined with antidepressant pharmacotherapy in patients with comorbid depression and insomnia: A randomized controlled trial. *The Journal of Clinical Psychiatry, 77*(10), e1316–e1323.

Manber, R., Edinger, J. D., Gress, J. L., San Pedro-Salcedo, M. G., Kuo, T. F., & Kalista, T. (2008). Cognitive behavioral therapy for insomnia enhances depression outcome in patients with comorbid major depressive disorder and insomnia. *Sleep, 31*, 489–495.

McHugh, R. K., & Barlow, D. H. (2010). The dissemination and implementation of evidence-based psychological treatments: A review of current efforts. *American Psychologist, 65*(2), 73.

McLay, R. N., Klam, W. P., & Volkert, S. L. (2010). Insomnia is the most commonly reported symptom and predicts other symptoms of post-traumatic stress disorder in US service members returning from military deployments. *Military Medicine, 175*(10), 759–762.

Medeiros, M., Carvalho, L. B., Silva, T. A., Prado, L. B., & Prado, G. F. (2005). Sleep disorders are associated with impulsivity in school children aged 8 to 10 years. *Arquivos de Neuro-Psiquiatria, 63*(3B), 761–765.

Merikangas, K. R., Akiskal, H. S., Angst, J., Greenberg, P. E., Hirschfeld, R. M., Petukhova, M., et al. (2007). Lifetime and 12-month prevalence of bipolar spectrum disorder in the National Comorbidity Survey replication. *Archives of General Psychiatry*, *64*(5), 543–552.

Merikangas, K. R., Jin, R., He, J.-P., Kessler, R. C., Lee, S., Sampson, N. A., et al. (2011). Prevalence and correlates of bipolar spectrum disorder in the world mental health survey initiative. *Archives of General Psychiatry*, *68*, 241–251.

Miklowitz, D. J., & Johnson, S. L. (2006). The psychopathology and treatment of bipolar disorder. *Annual Review of Clinical Psychology*, 199–235.

Miller, W. R., & Rollnick, S. (2002). *Motivational interviewing: Preparing people for change*. New York: Guilford Press.

Morin, C. M., Bootzin, R. R., Buysse, D. J., Edinger, J. D., Espie, C. A., & Lichstein, K. L. (2006). Psychological and behavioral treatment of insomnia: An update of recent evidence (1998-2004). *Sleep*, *29*, 1396–1406.

Morton, E., & Murray, G. (2020). Assessment and treatment of sleep problems in bipolar disorder—A guide for psychologists and clinically focused review. *Clinical Psychology & Psychotherapy*.

Motivala, S. J. (2011). Sleep and inflammation: Psychoneuroimmunology in the context of cardiovascular disease. *Annals of Behavioral Medicine*.

Motivala, S. J., & Irwin, M. R. (2007). Sleep and immunity: Cytokine pathways linking sleep and health outcomes. *Current Directions in Psychological Science*, *16*, 21–25.

Murray, G. (2019). *Circadian science and psychiatry: Of planets, proteins and persons*. London, England: SAGE Publications Sage UK.

Myers, E., Startup, H., & Freeman, D. (2011). Cognitive behavioural treatment of insomnia in individuals with persistent persecutory delusions: A pilot trial. *Journal of Behavior Therapy and Experimental Psychiatry*, *42*, 330–336.

Nathan, P. J., Burrows, G. D., & Norman, T. R. (1999). Melatonin sensitivity to dim white light in affective disorders. *Neuropsychopharmacology*, *21*(3), 408–413.

Nierenberg, A., Husain, M., Trivedi, M., Fava, M., Warden, D., Wisniewski, S., et al. (2010). Residual symptoms after remission of major depressive disorder with citalopram and risk of relapse: A STAR* D report. *Psychological Medicine*, *40*(01), 41–50.

Nierenberg, A. A., Keefe, B. R., Leslie, V. C., Alpert, J. E., Pava, J. A., Worthington, J. J., III, et al. (1999). Residual symptoms in depressed patients who respond acutely to fluoxetine. *Journal of Clinical Psychiatry*, *60*, 221–225.

NIH. (2005). National Institutes of Health state of the science conference statement: Manifestations and management of chronic insomnia in adults. June 13-15, 2005. *Sleep*, *28*, 1049–1057.

Onken, L. S., Carroll, K. M., Shoham, V., Cuthbert, B. N., & Riddle, M. (2014). Re-envisioning clinical science: Unifying the discipline to improve the public health. *Clinical Psychological Science*, *2*(1), 22–34.

Perlis, M. L., Giles, D. E., Buysse, D. J., Tu, X., & Kupfer, D. J. (1997). Self-reported sleep disturbance as a prodromal symptom in recurrent depression. *Journal of Affective Disorders*, *42*, 209–212.

Perlis, M. L., & Nielsen, T. A. (1993). Mood regulation, dreaming and nightmares: Evaluation of a desensitization function for REM sleep. *Dreaming*, *3*, 243–257.

Perlis, M. L., Smith, L. J., Lyness, J. M., Matteson, S. R., Pigeon, W. R., Jungquist, C., et al. (2006). Insomnia as a risk factor for onset of depression in the elderly. *Behavioral Sleep Medicine*, *4*, 104–113.

Qaseem, A., Kansagara, D., Forciea, M. A., Cooke, M., & Denberg, T. D. (2016). Management of chronic insomnia disorder in adults: A clinical practice guideline from the American College of Physicians. *Annals of Internal Medicine*, *165*(2), 125–133.

Ree, M., & Harvey, A. G. (2004). Insomnia. In J. Bennett-Levy, G. Butler, M. Fennell, A. Hackman, M. Mueller, & D. Westbrook (Eds.), *Oxford guide to behavioural experiments in cognitive therapy* (pp. 287–305). Oxford: Oxford University Press.

Riemann, D., Baglioni, C., Bassetti, C., Bjorvatn, B., Dolenc Groselj, L., Ellis, J. G., et al. (2017). European guideline for the diagnosis and treatment of insomnia. *Journal of Sleep Research, 26*(6), 675–700.

Robb, J. C., Cooke, R. G., Devins, G. M., Young, L. T., & Joffe, R. T. (1997). Quality of life and lifestyle disruption in bipolar disorder—Euthymic phase. *Journal of Psychiatric Research, 31*, 509–517.

Roth, T., Coulouvrat, C., Hajak, G., Lakoma, M. D., Sampson, N. A., Shahly, V., et al. (2011). Prevalence and perceived health associated with insomnia based on DSM-IV-TR; international statistical classification of diseases and related health problems, tenth revision; and research diagnostic criteria/international classification of sleep disorders, second edition criteria: Results from the America insomnia survey. *Biological Psychiatry, 69*, 592–600.

Roth, T., Jaeger, S., Jin, R., Kalsekar, A., Stang, P. E., & Kessler, R. C. (2006). Sleep problems, comorbid mental disorders, and role functioning in the national comorbidity survey replication. *Biological Psychiatry, 60*(12), 1364–1371.

Sachs, G. S., Thase, M. E., Otto, M. W., Bauer, M., Miklowitz, D., Wisniewski, S. R., et al. (2003). Rationale, design, and methods of the systematic treatment enhancement program for bipolar disorder (STEP-BD). *Biological Psychiatry, 53*(11), 1028–1042.

Salkovskis, P. M. (2002). Empirically grounded clinical interventions: Cognitive-behavioural therapy progresses through a multi-dimensional approach to clinical science. *Behavioural and Cognitive Psychotherapy, 30*, 3–9.

Sit, D., Wisner, K. L., Hanusa, B. H., Stull, S., & Terman, M. (2007). Light therapy for bipolar disorder: A case series in women. *Bipolar Disorders, 9*, 918–927.

Sivertsen, B., Harvey, A. G., Lundervold, A. J., & Hysing, M. (2013). Sleep problems and depression in adolescence: Results from a large population-based study of Norwegian adolescents aged 16–18 years. *European Child and Adolescent Psychiatry*, 1–9.

Smith, M. T., Huang, M. I., & Manber, R. (2005). Cognitive behavior therapy for chronic insomnia occurring within the context of medical and psychiatric disorders. *Clinical Psychology Review, 25*, 559–592.

Spielman, A. J., Saskin, P., & Thorpy, M. J. (1987). Treatment of chronic insomnia by restriction of time in bed. *Sleep, 10*, 45–56.

Sylvia, L. G., Dupuy, J. M., Ostacher, M. J., Cowperthwait, C. M., Hay, A. C., Sachs, G. S., et al. (2011). Sleep disturbance in euthymic bipolar patients. *Journal of Psychopharmacology, 26*.

Talbot, L. S., Stone, S., Gruber, J., Hairston, I. S., Eidelman, P., & Harvey, A. G. (2012). A test of the bidirectional association between sleep and mood in bipolar disorder and insomnia. *Journal of Abnormal Psychology, 121*(1), 39–50.

Tassi, P., & Muzet, A. (2000). Sleep inertia. *Sleep Medicine Reviews, 4*, 341–353.

UN World Health Organization (Producer). (2011). *World report on disability: Summary.* WHO/NMH/VIP/11.01. 3 September 2020.

Van Dongen, H. P., Maislin, G., Mullington, J. M., & Dinges, D. F. (2003). The cumulative cost of additional wakefulness: Dose-response effects on neurobehavioral functions and sleep physiology from chronic sleep restriction and total sleep deprivation. *Sleep, 26*, 117–126.

Venkatraman, V., Chuah, Y. L., Huettel, S. A., & Chee, M. W. (2007). Sleep deprivation elevates expectation of gains and attenuates response to losses following risky decisions. *Sleep-New York Then Westchester, 30*(5), 603.

Waite, F., Myers, E., Harvey, A. G., Espie, C. A., Startup, H., Sheaves, B., et al. (2016). Treating sleep problems in patients with schizophrenia. *Behavioural and Cognitive Psychotherapy, 44*(3), 273–287.

Wehr, T. A. (1989). Sleep loss: A preventable cause of mania and other excited states. *The Journal of Clinical Psychiatry, 50*(Suppl), 8–16 (discussion 45-17).

Wehr, T. A., Sack, D. A., Duncan, W. C., Mendelson, W. B., Rosenthal, N. E., Gillin, J. C., et al. (1985). Sleep and circadian rhythms in affective patients isolated from external time cues. *Psychiatry Research, 15*(4), 327–339.

Wehr, T. A., Sack, D. A., & Rosenthal, N. E. (1987). Sleep reduction as a final common pathway in the genesis of mania. *American Journal of Psychiatry, 144*, 201–204.

Weisz, J. R., Chorpita, B. F., Palinkas, L. A., Schoenwald, S. K., Miranda, J., Bearman, S. K., et al. (2012). Testing standard and modular designs for psychotherapy treating depression, anxiety, and conduct problems in youth: A randomized effectiveness trial. *Archives of General Psychiatry, 69*(3), 274–282.

Weisz, J. R., Ng, M. Y., & Bearman, S. K. (2014). Odd couple? Reenvisioning the relation between science and practice in the dissemination-implementation era. *Clinical Psychological Science, 2*(1), 58–74.

Wirz-Justice, A., Benedetti, F., & Terman, M. (2009). *Chronotherapeutics for affective disorders: A clinician's manual for light & wake therapy* (1st ed.). Basel: Karger.

Witteman, C. L., Spaanjaars, N. L., & Aarts, A. A. (2012). Clinical intuition in mental health care: A discussion and focus groups. *Counselling Psychology Quarterly, 25*(1), 19–29.

Wyatt, J. K., Stepanski, E. J., & Kirkby, J. (2006). Circadian phase in delayed sleep phase syndrome: Predictors and temporal stability across multiple assessments. *Sleep, 29*, 1075–1080.

Yoo, S., Gujar, N., Hu, P., Jolesz, F., & Walker, M. (2007). The human emotional brain without sleep: A prefrontal-amygdala disconnect? *Current Biology, 17*, R877–R878.

CHAPTER

10

CBT-I in patients with alcohol use and cannabis use disorders

Gabrielle E. Bowyer, Trevor M. Brooks, and Deirdre A. Conroy

Sleep and Circadian Research Laboratory, Department of Psychiatry, University of Michigan, Ann Arbor, MI, United States

Introduction

All substances of abuse can negatively affect sleep quality and continuity. This chapter will discuss the use of Cognitive Behavioral Therapy for Insomnia (CBT-I) in patients with insomnia who also use alcohol and/or cannabis. As with any comprehensive sleep assessment, the clinician is urged to first conduct a comprehensive evaluation of sleep disorders in the SUD patient such as sleep-disordered breathing, parasomnias, and movement disorders (Chakravorty, Chaudhary, & Brower, 2016). The diagnosis and treatment of these other underlying sleep disorders can play a key part in the management of the patient's sleep disturbance.

Alcohol and insomnia

Assessment of the insomnia patient using alcohol

About three-quarters of patients who are actively using alcohol also have sleep disturbance (Hartwell, Bujarski, Glasner-Edwards, & Ray, 2015). When discussing treatment options with active suspected substance abuse or dependence, the clinician is encouraged to first discuss motivation to enter addiction treatment focused on use reduction or sobriety. Insomnia symptoms may improve during the detoxification process. However, even after drinking has stopped, insomnia can persist even into

Adapting Cognitive Behavioral Therapy for Insomnia
https://doi.org/10.1016/B978-0-12-822872-2.00016-5

the recovery period (defined as >3months after stopping drinking) (Brower, 2003). For the patient who has stopped drinking and has persistent insomnia, the clinician may inquire about the patient's history of alcohol use and how it related to bouts of insomnia in the past. This can provide rich insight into their presenting complaint and inform the treatment process. Assessing and treating insomnia is important because the persistence of insomnia during recovery from AUD can increase the risk of relapse (Brower & Perron, 2010).

Spielman's three P model of insomnia is still a helpful model to formulate the case conceptualization, e.g., identifying predisposing, precipitating, and perpetuating factors (Spielman & Glovinsky, 1991). When assessing insomnia in a patient with a history of alcohol use disorder (AUD), the clinician should keep in mind that insomnia can be perpetuated by multiple factors including but not limited to biological factors (e.g., circadian rhythm disturbances) and psychological factors (e.g., dysfunctional beliefs) (Chakravorty et al., 2016). Many patients with a history of AUD report having used alcohol to decrease the time to fall asleep. When the act of drinking alcohol before bed stops during early recovery, the patient may not know what new behaviors or habits should replace the old ones (e.g., drinking alcohol to fall asleep). Educating the patient that it may be normal for it to take about 30min to fall asleep might reduce the pressure to fall asleep immediately, which may have been their only experience while drinking alcohol to "pass out." Moreover, providing specific activities of what to do during the time before bed such as winding down may be helpful. The app developed through the Veteran's Administration CBT-I coach application (Kuhn et al., 2016) includes many of these suggestions, such as "sort out junk mail and bills (but don't pay bills), make a grocery shopping list for the week, etc. These recommendations are not unique to the AUD population but can be especially helpful as substitutes for the old behaviors of drinking alcohol during the night to fall or stay asleep.

Effects of alcohol on sleep

It has been well established that alcohol assists in falling asleep but can contribute to middle-of-the-night awakenings or early terminal awakenings (Ebrahim, Shapiro, Williams, & Fenwick, 2013; Feige et al., 2006). When consumed before normal bedtime, alcohol results in shortened sleep onset latency and delayed onset of rapid eye movement (REM) sleep (Chakravorty et al., 2016; Colrain, Nicholas, & Baker, 2014). Alcohol has been shown to increase total sleep time, sleep efficiency, and amount of slow-wave sleep (SWS) in the first half of the night, consistent with observations that it increases levels of adenosine in the basal forebrain, a neuromodulator involved in sleep homeostasis and generation of SWS

(Alam & McGinty, 2017). During the second half of the night, alcohol use is associated with decreased total sleep time, decreased sleep efficiency, and increased nighttime awakenings (Thakkar, Sharma, & Sahota, 2015).

Sleep psychologists will often cite this data as a way to explain how insomnia manifests itself during a time of heavy drinking. This vicious cycle is eloquently described in Dr. Kirk Brower's model of insomnia, alcohol use, and relapse (Brower, 2003). Over time, the frequent and heavy use of alcohol may change the brain chemistry such that the user requires more alcohol to achieve the same sleep-promoting effects (Chaudhary, Wong, Kolla, Kampman, & Chakravorty, 2020).

Other physiological changes occur in the circadian system with some studies suggest that levels of melatonin in the brain are lower (Kuhlwein, Hauger, & Irwin, 2003) and onset delayed (Conroy et al., 2012) in AUD patients compared to non-AUD patients. Consideration of judicious use of OTC melatonin or ramelteon (Brower, Conroy, Kurth, & Stein, 2011) may help in combination with a CBT-I plan. Ramelteon is also preferred as it is not targeting the GABA receptors with a lower risk of abuse or dependence.

CBT-I in individuals with AUD

Nonpharmacological options are often preferred to pharmacotherapy for insomnia due to the addiction potential in many of the commonly prescribed hypnotics. Three randomized controlled pilot trials of CBT for insomnia have been conducted to date in adults with AUD, all of which found improvements in sleep and daytime symptoms at post-treatment and follow-up. There is evidence that CBT-I in AUD is effective in improving insomnia (Chakravorty et al., 2019) (Currie, Clark, Hodgins, & El-Guebaly, 2004) and insomnia plus daytime functioning (Arnedt, Conroy, Armitage, & Brower, 2011). However, it is still unclear whether the intervention changes drinking behavior after the intervention as differences in relapse rates have not yet been found. This may be related, in part, to methodological differences in the few studies conducted to date. Many sleep and addiction specialists would agree that targeting sleep disturbance seems like a promising target to reduce drinking and such protocols are in progress.

In addition to sleep disturbance, depression is one of the most common symptoms in patients with AUD in early recovery (Chaudhary et al., 2020). Therefore, CBT-I in AUD should include components that might also be helpful when working with patients with depression, such as avoiding using the bed for escape and targeting the low level of activity or napping during the daytime. Other modifications to consider in this patient population are listed in Table 1.

TABLE 1 Adaptation of cognitive behavioral therapy for insomnia (CBT-I) for alcohol and cannabis users.

CBT-I components	Standard practice	CBT-I adaptations for alcohol and cannabis users
Sleep education	3-P model, 2-process model of sleep regulation, sleep stages	– Educate patient about how the specific substance of use affects sleep – Highlight subjective versus objective effects of the substance (i.e., subjective improvement of sleep but objective worsening of sleep) – Educate patient about worsening insomnia with substance withdrawal – Educate about the co-occurrence of sleep disorders in substance users (e.g., sleep apnea)
Sleep restriction	Improve sleep efficiency by limiting time in bed to the amount of time sleeping then expanding slowly as long as sleep efficiency is preserved	– Explore reasons for an excessive time in bed – Plan ahead for the next day increased sleepiness/tiredness (avoid substance use to cope) – Avoid using substances in the additional time spent awake
Stimulus control	Associate bed/bedroom solely as a cue for sleep by eliminating nonsleep activities from the bedroom. Instruction to get out of bed at night if awake >15 min	– Avoid using substance while out of bed to return to sleep
Napping/ daytime sleep	Discontinue or restrict daytime napping to 30 min	– Educate patient on next day effects (e.g., hangover) on daytime functioning
Sleep hygiene education	Address daytime habits and sleep environment interfering with sleep	– Avoid late-night snacking – Highlight avoiding substances before bedtime
Cognitive therapy	Challenge patient's dysfunctional beliefs interfering with sleep and misconceptions about sleep. Replace/restructure to more helpful and realistic thoughts about sleep	– Discuss patient's expectations about sleep latency and wakefulness at night versus normal sleep onset and time awake at night – Emphasize nonsubstance related behaviors and cognitive tools as an alternative to substance use for sleep

TABLE 1 Adaptation of cognitive behavioral therapy for insomnia (CBT-I) for alcohol and cannabis users—cont'd

CBT-I components	Standard practice	CBT-I adaptations for alcohol and cannabis users
Relaxation and meditation techniques	Relaxation can help reduce racing thoughts/tension that accompanies lying in bed awake, and may include: deep breathing, progressive muscle relaxation, guided imagery, biofeedback, hypnosis, autogenic training, and meditation practices	- Engage in nonsubstance related activities for coping and stress relief
Relapse prevention	Discuss practicing less rigid sleep plan over time and what do to prevent sleep disturbance from turning into another episode of insomnia in the future	- Consider using language common in substance use treatment, e.g., lapse versus relapse to discuss the possibility of future sleep disturbance in the future
Sleep diaries	Establish baseline sleep patterns, track progress, reinforce appropriate behavior change, problem-solve obstacles to adherence	- Use the daytime section or comment section of the sleep diary to document the amount and frequency of substance use each night

Clinical pearls

A strong focus on sleep expectations may be of benefit. For example, normalizing that even a "normal" sleeper may take about 30 min to fall asleep and awaken during the night. However, AUD patients may be using other substances such as nicotine, cannabis, or other substances that impact sleep and these must be addressed according to their sleep disruption profiles. For example, nicotine is a stimulant and when used before bedtime or during the night this might disrupt sleep.

There is also a number of co-occurring psychiatric disorders with AUD that must be monitored. For example, patients may continue to experience co-occurring depression. Depression carries its sleep characteristics such as early morning awakenings, hypersomnia, or using the bed as a place to escape. Identifying and targeting these symptoms with behavioral activation, stimulus control, and cognitive therapy may also be of benefit.

Areas for future consideration

As mentioned above, laboratory-based studies using polysomnography indicate increased sleep latency, decreased total sleep time and sleep efficiency, and altered sleep architecture (e.g., reduced slow-wave sleep (SWS) and increased rapid eye movement [REM] sleep) among abstinent adults with AUD. This can persist long-term despite continued abstinence (Drummond, Gillin, Smith, & DeModena, 1998). Future trials might include using CBT-I to target the specific mechanisms (e.g., reduced SWS), which might underlie the association between insomnia and relapse (TRLS-D-20-01479).

Cannabis and insomnia

Assessment of the insomnia patient using cannabis

The frequency, dose, timing, and subjective experience of using cannabis are important factors in case conceptualization and treatment planning. Patients may present with myriad reasons for cannabis use. Assessment should attempt to gain a thorough understanding of primary and secondary reasons for use as well as contributing comorbid conditions. It is important to gain an understanding of the patient's attitudes toward cannabis and how they believe it affects their sleep. To provide further context, a patient can be asked when they started using cannabis for sleep, what their sleep resembled prior, and what they notice when they do not use cannabis on any particular night.

Assessing the patient's frequency of past cannabis use and current use throughout a day, a typical week, and how it is used in relation to their nighttime routine will provide important information about the salience of their use. Since there may be differential effects of dose or THC concentration on sleep parameters (Schierenbeck, Riemann, Berger, & Hornyak, 2008), it is important to assess dose (if known) and route of administration. Combined with the frequency of use, this will likely give further information regarding physical dependence, tolerance, and the likelihood of withdrawal symptoms.

In addition to assessing their current sleep pattern and insomnia symptoms, it is important to know if periods of wakefulness throughout the night are also accompanied by cannabis use or the side effects of cannabis use. For example, dry mouth and increased appetite, common side effects of cannabis use may have a direct impact on nighttime routines and behaviors. Cannabis may also explain early morning "grogginess" that would not necessarily be related to the poorer quality of sleep related to insomnia. A thorough assessment will include capturing the nuances of cannabis use and its effects.

Effects of substance use on sleep

Recent research demonstrates that cannabis can no longer be considered a monolithic substance of use or abuse. Dissecting the plant into its constituent compounds and exploring the effects of those specific cannabinoids has obligated researchers to regard cannabis as existing on a spectrum of varying chemical compositions, causing varied effects in its users. The human body produces its endogenous cannabinoids. In contrast, cannabis is a phytocannabinoid—an exogenous cannabinoid derived from a plant. The two most extensively researched phytocannabinoids within cannabis are delta-9 tetrahydrocannabinol (THC) and cannabidiol (CBD) (Babson, Sottile, & Morabito, 2017).

THC is the primary cannabinoid responsible for the psychotropic effects associated with cannabis use (Grotenhermen & Russo, 2002). As a mood-altering substance used by increasingly larger numbers, its impact on sleep quality and quantity is of import. Studies have generally shown that acute THC administration affects sleep by decreasing sleep onset latency and altering the percentages of time a user spends in REM and Stage 3 Non-REM sleep (decrease in the former, increase in the latter) (Chakravorty, Vandrey, He, & Stein, 2018).

The effects of THC on sleep seem to change over time, however. There is evidence that users develop a tolerance to the sedating, hypnotic effects as a result of alterations in the endocannabinoid system (ECS) that can lead to even greater sleep disturbances when contrasted with those who use less often (Chakravorty et al., 2018). Nonetheless, these studies remain rather preliminary, and the sequelae of whole-plant cannabis use must be investigated further due to its aforementioned varying chemical make-up.

Additionally, cannabis can be ingested through varying routes of administration, which is yet to be understood in terms of impact on sleep. Subjectively, cannabis is often reported to aid sleep. For example, survey data from 800 people seeking medical cannabis for chronic pain suggest 80% also used it to improve sleep, and over three-quarters believed strongly that it helped in that regard (Cranford et al., 2017). From the same survey data, 65% reported disturbed sleep when attempting to cease use. Indeed, sleep disturbance appears to be among the most severe cannabis withdrawal symptoms and it remains to be determined whether disordered sleep stems primarily from cannabis use in this population or if it simply exacerbates a preexisting condition.

CBT-I in individuals using cannabis

Research on CBT-I for cannabis users specifically is scant and still in its infancy. Despite robust demonstration across numerous randomized clinical trials of the efficacy and reliability of CBT for primary insomnia, research on its potential for the amelioration of insomnia symptoms in those who use cannabis for sleep is curiously sparse. Of the extant research, participants have not received the full course of CBT-I, which is generally considered 6–8 weekly sessions delivered by a trained therapist.

One such study, aimed to assess the feasibility and preliminary outcome measures, delivered CBT-I via mobile phone application for 2 weeks to four participants with a DSM-5 cannabis use disorder diagnosis (Babson, Ramo, Baldini, Vandrey, & Bonn-Miller, 2015). While improvements in sleep were found, this study serves more to highlight and pressure the research community to focus on this area of inquiry rather than veritably demonstrating the efficacy of CBT-I in this population. Fortunately, there has been a re-emergence of interest in the therapeutic boons and detrimental effects of cannabis in the last decade, in part, due to a more nuanced understanding of the plant and its complex chemical composition.

Most of this interest, however, is geared toward noninsomnia areas of psychopathology, such as anxiety, pain, and affective disorders. Further, while strain-type and route of administration have emerged as important factors for future consideration, the diverse array of products available render controlling for these variables difficult (Walsh et al., 2017). Methodologically, many studies have simply contrasted outcomes among groups who tested positive for cannabis with groups who have not. Controlling for such nuance is rare to date.

Clinical pearls

Conversations about cannabis use and sleep can require some clinical finesse. Medical marijuana users who found relief in only marijuana use for their insomnia may be less swayed to reduce marijuana use based on research findings described above. Moreover, if cannabis is used for other salient conditions or symptoms, changes to use may involve a more comprehensive discussion that weighs pros and cons. For example, the client with concurrent PTSD may have a strong motivation to continue using cannabis specifically due to its ability to suppress REM sleep; they notice that they no longer have recurring nightmares or dream as frequently when using cannabis before bed and therefore report less worry and hyperarousal at bedtime. In this instance, among many other potentially complex interactions, client goals and concurrent symptoms will help guide treatment planning, potential referrals, and recommendations as it relates to treating insomnia.

Given what is known about withdrawal symptoms and sleep (Bolla et al., 2008), it is important to normalize a potential worsening of symptoms when discontinuing cannabis. Clients may present with sleep-related anxiety, especially if they hold the belief that only cannabis is effective or have learned through experience that sleep is worse when they do not use cannabis. Reassurance that sleep disruptions are normal and temporary during this period, along with providing other strategies, is likely a necessary step for enhancing buy-in and reducing anxiety.

CBT-I has promising clinical implications even for those who continue the use of cannabis, however. Abstinence from cannabis is not a requirement for the therapy; many use it for comorbid medical or mental health conditions and still reap the benefits of better quality sleep and less daytime functional impairment. It is important to note that CBT-I is a treatment to enhance sleep quality, not necessarily to decrease cannabis use, although that may occur naturally following CBT-I and research is underway to better understand this. CBT-I focuses on changing maladaptive thoughts and behaviors that maintain and exacerbate sleep difficulty. Cannabis use may constitute one of those behaviors, but there are often others that patients may be more willing to challenge or alter first. Motivational interviewing can be used within the context of CBT-I to ascertain readiness for such change. Additional modifications to CBT-I in cannabis-using individuals can be found in Table 1.

Areas for future consideration

The paucity of research at the intersection of cannabis use and CBT-I presents plentiful intriguing research opportunities. First, the efficacy and reliability of CBT-I in this population is yet to be established. Second, the therapeutic benefits and detriments of cannabis in an insomnia context remains obscure as research is not just nascent but has also yielded mixed findings and has been investigated in studies with small samples that lack control populations or long-term follow-up (Babson et al., 2017).

Differences among cannabinoids, in particular, seem fertile ground for useful findings. As mentioned previously, more nuanced knowledge of the constitution of the cannabis flower suggests that different cannabinoids may impact sleep differentially. Further, the concentration of THC and CBD varies widely across different strains of cannabis (Walsh et al., 2017). While initial research findings suggest a fairly uniform effect of THC on short- and long-term sleep, the effect of CBD appears to depend upon its dose, with low doses acting as stimulants and higher doses acting as sedatives.

Motives for cannabis use as well as the subjective versus the objective experience of use confers interesting research possibilities as well. Users of cannabis often report feeling that cannabis aids their sleep across several parameters that do not always coincide with what objective measures indicate. It is possible that the psychoactive effects of cannabis simply lessen the negative effect during bouts of insomnia that would otherwise incite anxiety, dread, or anger.

Of course, psychiatric and medical comorbidities complicate the clinical picture, and more research is needed on these fronts as well. For example, research indicates that those with relatively higher post-traumatic stress are more likely to use cannabis to cope with heightened hyperarousal, a predominant cause of sleep disturbance (Bonn-Miller, Babson, & Vandrey, 2014). Those with night-related trauma may experience fear of sleep itself. Other worthwhile comorbid conditions for investigation include depression, general anxiety, chronic pain, cancer, and more severe psychopathology such as bipolar disorder and schizophrenia.

Summary

Alcohol and cannabis are substances that in the short term can reduce sleep latency and time awake during the night, particularly in the first half of the night. However, chronic use and withdrawal may lead to increased sleep disruption. During this time, insomnia may be perpetuating by maladaptive sleep behaviors and beliefs. CBT-I in patients with a history of SUD may be a beneficial part of their treatment program.

References

Alam, M., & McGinty, D. (2017). Acute effects of alcohol on sleep are mediated by components of homeostatic sleep regulatory system: An editorial highlight for 'lesions of the basal forebrain cholinergic neurons attenuates sleepiness and adenosine after alcohol consumption' on page 710. *Journal of Neurochemistry*, *142*(5), 620–623.

Arnedt, J., Conroy, D., Armitage, R., & Brower, K. (2011). Cognitive-behavioral therapy for insomnia in alcohol dependent patients: A randomized controlled pilot trial. *Behaviour Research and Therapy*, *49*(4), 227–233.

Babson, K., Ramo, D., Baldini, L., Vandrey, R., & Bonn-Miller, M. (2015). Mobile app-delivered cognitive behavioral therapy for insomnia: Feasibility and initial efficacy among veterans with cannabis use disorders. *JMIR Research Protocols*, *4*(3), e87.

Babson, K., Sottile, J., & Morabito, D. (2017). Cannabis, cannabinoids, and sleep: A review of the literature. *Current Psychiatry Reports*, *19*(4), 23.

Bolla, K., Lesage, S., Gamaldo, C., Neubauer, D., Funderburk, F., Cadet, J., et al. (2008). Sleep disturbance in heavy marijuana users. *Sleep*, *31*(6), 901–908.

Bonn-Miller, M., Babson, K., & Vandrey, R. (2014). Using cannabis to help you sleep: Heightened frequency of medical cannabis use among those with PTSD. *Drug and Alcohol Dependence*, *136*, 162–165.

Brower, K. (2003). Insomnia, alcoholism and relapse. *Sleep Medicine Reviews*, *7*(6), 523–539.

Brower, K., Conroy, D., Kurth, M., & Stein, M. (2011). Ramelteon and improved insomnia in alcohol-dependent patients: A case series. *Journal of Clinical Sleep Medicine*, *7*(3), 274–275.

Brower, K., & Perron, B. (2010). Sleep disturbance as a universal risk factor for relapse in addictions to psychoactive substances. *Medical Hypotheses*, *74*, 928–933.

Chakravorty, S., Chaudhary, N., & Brower, K. (2016). Alcohol dependence and its relationship with insomnia and other sleep disorders. *Alcoholism, Clinical and Experimental Research*, *40*(11), 2271–2282.

Chakravorty, S., Morales, K., Arnedt, J., Perlis, M., Oslin, D., Findley, J., et al. (2019). Cognitive behavioral therapy for insomnia in alcohol-dependent veterans: A randomized, controlled pilot study. *Alcoholism, Clinical and Experimental Research, 43*(6), 1244–1253.

Chakravorty, S., Vandrey, R., He, S., & Stein, M. (2018). Sleep management among patients with substance use disorders. *Medical Clinics, 102*(4), 733–743.

Chaudhary, N., Wong, M., Kolla, B., Kampman, K., & Chakravorty, S. (2020). The relationship between insomnia and the intensity of drinking in treatment-seeking individuals with alcohol dependence. *Drug and Alcohol Dependence, 1*(215), 108189.

Colrain, I., Nicholas, C., & Baker, F. (2014). Alcohol and the sleeping brain. *Handbook of Clinical Neurology, 125*, 415–431.

Conroy, D. A., Hairston, I. S., Arnedt, J. T., Hoffmann, R. F., Armitage, R., & Brower, K. J. (2012). Dim light melatonin onset in alcohol-dependent men and women compared with healthy controls. *Chronobiology International, 29*(1), 35–42. https://doi.org/10.3109/07420528.2011.636852.

Cranford, J., Arnedt, J., Conroy, D., Bohnert, K., Bourque, C., Blow, F., et al. (2017). Prevalence and correlates of sleep-related problems in adults receiving medical cannabis for chronic pain. *Drug and Alcohol Dependence, 180*, 227–233.

Currie, S., Clark, S., Hodgins, D., & El-Guebaly, N. (2004). Randomized controlled trial of brief cognitive-behavioural interventions for insomnia in recovering alcoholics. *Addiction, 99*(9), 1121–1132.

Drummond, S., Gillin, J., Smith, T., & DeModena, A. (1998). The sleep of abstinent pure primary alcoholic patients: Natural course and relationship to relapse. *Alcoholism, Clinical and Experimental Research, 22*, 1796–1802.

Ebrahim, I., Shapiro, C., Williams, A., & Fenwick, P. (2013). Alcohol and sleep: Effects on normal sleep. *Alcoholism, Clinical and Experimental Research, 37*(4), 539–549.

Feige, B., Gann, H., Brueck, R., Hornyak, M., Litsch, S., Hohagen, F., et al. (2006). Effects of alcohol on polysomnographically recorded sleep in healthy subjects. *Alcoholism, Clinical and Experimental Research, 30*(9), 1527–1537.

Grotenhermen, F., & Russo, E. (2002). *Cannabis and cannabinoids: Pharmacology, toxicology, and therapeutic potential*. New York: Haworth Press Inc.

Hartwell, E., Bujarski, S., Glasner-Edwards, S., & Ray, L. (2015). The association of alcohol severity and sleep quality in problem drinkers. *Alcohol and Alcoholism, 50*(536–541).

Kuhlwein, E., Hauger, R., & Irwin, M. (2003). Abnormal nocturnal melatonin secretion and disordered sleep in abstinent alcoholics. *Biological Psychiatry, 54*(12), 1437–1443.

Kuhn, E., Weiss, B., Taylor, K., Hoffman, J., Ramsey, K., Manber, R., et al. (2016). CBT-I coach: A description and clinician perceptions of a Mobile app for cognitive behavioral therapy for insomnia. *Journal of Clinical Sleep Medicine, 12*(4), 597–606.

Schierenbeck, T., Riemann, D., Berger, M., & Hornyak, M. (2008). Effect of illicit recreational recreational drug use upon sleep: Cocaine, ecstasy, and marijuana. *Sleep Medicine Reviews, 12*, 381–389.

Spielman, A., & Glovinsky, P. (1991). The varied nature of insomnia. In P. Hauri (Ed.), *Case studies in insomnia*. New York: Plenum Publishing Corporation.

Thakkar, M., Sharma, R., & Sahota, P. (2015). Alcohol disrupts sleep homeostasis. *Alcohol, 49*(4), 299–310.

Walsh, Z., Gonzalez, R., Crosby, K., Thiessen, M., Carroll, C., & Bonn-Miller, M. (2017). Medical cannabis and mental health: A guided systematic review. *Clinical Psychology Review, 51*, 15–29.

PART 4

CBT-I in medical disorders

CHAPTER

11

CBT-I for patients with chronic pain

Leisha J. Cuddihy[a], *Sara Nowakowski*[b,c,d], *Michael A. Grandner*[e], *Jessica M. Meers*[b,c,d], *and Michael T. Smith*[f]

[a]Pediatric Behavioral Health, Spectrum Health Helen DeVos Children's Hospital, Grand Rapids, MI, United States, [b]Department of Medicine, Baylor College of Medicine, Houston, TX, United States, [c]Department of Medicine—Health Services Research, Center for Innovations in Quality, Effectiveness, and Safety, Michael E. DeBakey VA Medical Center, Houston, TX, United States, [d]South Central Mental Illness Research Education Clinical, Centers of Excellence (MIRECC), Michael E. DeBakey VA Medical Center, Houston, TX, United States, [e]Department of Psychiatry and Medicine, UA College of Medicine, Tucson, AZ, United States, [f]Psychiatry and Behavioral Sciences, Johns Hopkins University, Baltimore, MD, United States

Sleep and pain are strongly connected. Sleep disturbance is reported by 67%–88% (Morin, LeBlanc, Daley, Gregoire, & Mérette, 2006; Smith & Haythornthwaite, 2004) of patients with chronic pain, and 50% of patients with insomnia suffer from chronic pain (Taylor et al., 2007). Patients with chronic pain may have difficulty implementing strategies of traditional CBT-I, such as stimulus control or sleep restriction, due to physical limitations (e.g., unable to get in-and-out of bed easily) or behavioral strategies of pain management (e.g., "sleeping off" headaches). This chapter is a guide to modifications to CBT-I that may help patients with chronic pain adhere to and benefit more from treatment.

https://doi.org/10.1016/B978-0-12-822872-2.00021-9

What is chronic pain?

The most basic definition of chronic pain is pain that lasts for at least 3 months or beyond the expected time of healing after injury. From a neurologic standpoint, one of the key concepts in chronic pain is known as central sensitization, which is the idea that pain is modulated by multiple levels of the neural axis (Melzack, 1999). Ascending circuits send pain signals from the periphery through the spinothalamic tract to the areas of the brain that process pain. Equally important are descending circuits that modulate the flow of pain signals in the spinal cord. These descending circuits are both facilitatory and inhibitory. Central sensitization posits that there is some dysregulation of this system that causes amplification of the pain signal by either facilitating or failing to inhibit it at the level of the spine or higher order brain structures.

Emerging research shows that sleep loss has a substantial impact on the pain inhibitory (Iacovides, George, Kamerman, & Baker, 2017; Smith, Edwards, McCann, & Haythomthwaite, 2007) and facilitatory systems (Smith et al., 2019). Furthermore, longitudinal studies show that poor sleep is a significant risk factor for new onset chronic pain (Bonvanie, Oldehinkel, Rosmalen, & Janssens, 2016; Gupta et al., 2007; Harrison, Wilson, & Munafò, 2014; Mikkelsson, Sourander, Salminen, Kautiainen, & Piha, 1999; Sanders et al., 2016; Smith et al., 2008). Put together, these studies indicate that sleep disruption is an independent risk factor for the emergence chronic pain, and a great deal of research suggests that when poor sleep leads to more negative pain outcomes, greater pain amplification, increased pain, and more pain flare ups (Campbell et al., 2015; Gerhart et al., 2017; Krause, Prather, Wager, Lindquist, & Walker, 2019); however, little work has been done to investigate the mechanisms of this relationship.

One possible mechanism of the relationship between pain and sleep is that sleep loss can lead to central sensitization by impairing the body's natural ability to inhibit pain, thereby amplifying it, aggravating it, and making pain persist longer than it normally would. Research has shown evidence that pain inhibits further pain via the descending inhibitory system. When a pain stimulus is applied (for example, to the right forearm), the pain threshold (level of stimulus at which a person reports feeling pain) increases in the opposite body part (e.g., left forearm) (Ramaswamy & Wodehouse, 2021). This is also known as conditioned pain modulation (CPM). This inhibitory effect may be mediated by the endogenous opioid system—if Naloxone is administered, the increase in pain threshold is not seen (Anderson, Sheth, Bencherif, Frost, & Campbell, 2002; Julien & Marchand, 2006; Willer, Le Bars, & De Broucker, 1990). There is also evidence that this increase in pain threshold is present even in the absence of perceived pain (De Broucker, Cesaro, Willer, & Le Bars, 1990). Studies show that CPM is impaired in patients with chronic pain, including fibromyalgia (Kosek & Hansson, 1997; Lautenbacher & Rollman, 1997; Staud, Robinson, Vierck, & Price, 2003), temporomandibular dental pain (Kashima, Rahman, Sakoda, & Shiba, 1999; Maixner, Fillingim, Booker, & Sigurdsson, 1995), irritable bowel syndrome (Wilder-Smith, Schindler, Lovblad, Redmond, & Nirkko, 2004), low back pain (Peters, Schmidt, Van den Hout, Koopmans, & Sluijter, 1992), and tension headaches (Pielsticker, Haag, Zaudig, & Lautenbacher, 2005). Other studies suggest that patients with impaired CPM at baseline are more likely to develop chronic pain following surgery (Granovsky & Yarnitsky, 2013; Wilder-Smith, Schreyer, Scheffer, & Arendt-Nielsen, 2010). We can infer from this research that the failure of the pain inhibitory system plays a significant role in the development and maintenance of chronic pain.

In 2007, Smith and colleagues measured the impact of experimentally induced sleep loss on CPM in healthy women (Smith et al., 2007). They manipulated sleep loss in two ways. The forced awakening group was given an 8-hour opportunity to sleep but were awoken for 20 minutes out of each hour, the precise timing of this awakening being randomized across the hour. This condition was designed to mimic the severe loss associated with mixed insomnia typically experienced by patients with chronic pain. In the sleep restriction group, sleep opportunity was limited to the total sleep time of a randomly selected participant in the forced awakening condition, allowing for experimental control of total sleep time. Participants completed three nights of the sleep loss condition, one night of total sleep deprivation, and a night of recovery sleep. Participants in the forced awakening group showed reductions in CMP after one night of sleep fragmentation and stayed low even after recovery sleep. Interestingly, participants in the restricted sleep condition did not show significant change in CMP. These findings have since been replicated in two separate studies (Iacovides et al., 2017; Matre, Andersen, Knardahl, & Nilsen, 2016) and have implications for CBT-I, as it highlights the importance of sleep consolidation and suggests that sleep restriction is not necessarily contraindicated in this population although it should be practiced more judiciously and less aggressively.

Assessing sleep in patients with chronic pain

A thorough assessment is essential to effective treatment, and there are several issues that arise when assessing sleep in patients with chronic pain. Chronic insomnia is one of the most common sleep disorders associated with chronic pain with conservatively estimated prevalence rate of ~50% (Morin et al., 2006; Smith & Haythornthwaite, 2004; Taylor et al., 2007). There are also high rates of sleep apnea in patients with chronic pain (39%–75%; Webster, Choi, Desai, Webster, & Grant, 2008). The incidence of circadian rhythm disorders and restless legs syndrome in patients with chronic pain is unknown. It is important to evaluate not only for insomnia, but other sleep disorders, and have a fairly low threshold for referral for sleep studies or medical evaluation.

Patients with chronic pain typically take medication for pain management, many of which can affect sleep. Opioid medications are known to decrease respiratory drive and are associated with central sleep apnea. The incidence of central sleep apnea in patients taking opioid agents is between 11% and 36% (Filiatrault et al., 2016; Javaheri, Germany, & Greer, 2016; Shear et al., 2014). Opioids are also ineffective sedatives. They reduce slow wave sleep and REM sleep and are associated with increased wakefulness after sleep onset (Cutrufello, Ianus, & Rowley, 2020; Wang & Teichtahl, 2007). Patients report that opioid use helps sleep; however, this is more likely due to the impairments in memory associated with the sedation produced by opioids. SSRIs and SNRIs can be helpful for pain but reduce REM sleep and sometimes contribute to insomnia (Ferreira et al., 2021; Wichniak, Wierzbicka, Walęcka, & Jernajczyk, 2017). Anticonvulsants such as gabapentin and pregabalin are often prescribed for neuropathic pain and fibromyalgia. These medications can actually increase slow wave sleep, and there is research to suggest that this is the mechanism by which they improve pain (Lo et al., 2010; Roth, Van Seventer, & Murphy, 2010; Vinik, Emir, Parsons, & Cheung, 2014).

It is also important to consider mental health when assessing sleep in patients with chronic pain. As many as 50% of patients with chronic pain who present to tertiary care settings (such as pain clinics) meet diagnostic criteria for depression (Bair, Robinson, Katon, & Kroenke, 2003). Anxiety disorders, particularly PTSD, are also prominent in this population (Beckham et al., 1997; Fishbain, Goldberg, Robert Meagher, Steele, & Rosomoff, 1986). The negative mood symptoms that are a hallmark of these disorders are consistent predictors of pain outcomes and higher pain severity (Bair et al., 2003; Bair, Outcalt, Ang, Wu, & Yu, 2020). Suicidality is also elevated in patients with chronic pain (Tang & Crane, 2006), and extensive research has shown that insomnia is an independent risk factor for suicide (McCall et al., 2010; Pigeon, Pinquart, & Conner, 2012). It is extremely important to evaluate suicidal ideation in patients with chronic pain, as both depression and insomnia increase the risk of this symptom.

CBT-I in chronic pain

Pain fits into Spielman's (Spielman, Caruso, & Glovinsky, 1987) 3-P model of insomnia. Most obviously, pain can be a precipitating factor contributing to the onset of insomnia. Over time, pain also becomes a perpetuating factor for insomnia and contributed to the conditioned arousal that patients develop with their bed and bedroom. Often patients will go to bed when in pain, either to sleep it off to avoid triggering stimuli (as in headaches) or because they feel that there is no other place that they can be comfortable. Sleep can help alleviate pain (particularly in headache disorder or migraines), and the reclined position may provide some relief, but the tendency to repeatedly retire to bed when in pain sets up the bed as a conditioned stimulus for pain and weakening the association between the bed and sleep. Patients may also take more pain medication (such as opioids or gabapentin) to try to put themselves to sleep, which can negatively impact sleep architecture as described above (Table 1).

A great deal of research indicates that unmodified CBT-I is effective at improving insomnia symptoms in patients with chronic pain, and that the effects are large and maintained in long-term follow-up (Currie, Wilson, Pontefract, & DeLaplante, 2000; Edinger, Wohlgemuth, Krystal, & Rice, 2005; Jungquist et al., 2010; Mccrae et al., 2019; Smitherman et al., 2018). The literature is mixed on whether CBT-I improves pain symptoms, but some research has shown clinically significant reductions in pain following CBT-I (Tang et al., 2015). This research indicates that modifications may be helpful in achieving optimal outcomes.

We know that sleep consolidation is important for patients with chronic pain because of the CMP research described above, suggesting that sleep restriction can consolidate sleep quickly. There is research that indicates that severely restricted sleep can also increase sensitivity to pain (Roehrs, Hyde, Blaisdell, Greenwald, & Roth, 2006), however. Therefore, it is important to balance the goal of sleep consolidation with the need for adequate sleep duration when considering sleep restriction recommendations. A study by Smith et al. (2015) showed that patients with knee osteoarthritis who got at least 6.5 hours of sleep by the midpoint of CBT-I were more likely to have a long-term treatment response than those who got less than 6.5 hours of sleep. Furthermore, when sleep was restricted by more than 90 minutes (compared to habitual sleep opportunity), patients were less likely to be adherent to sleep restriction. This study indicates that limiting sleep restriction in patients with chronic pain may improve both treatment adherence and long-term outcomes. There are several ways to approach this, including restricting sleep to total sleep time plus 30 minutes, avoiding restricting sleep opportunity by more than 90 minutes (as compared to baseline sleep opportunity), or using sleep

TABLE 1 Adaptation of cognitive behavioral therapy for insomnia (CBT-I) for chronic pain.

CBT-I components	Standard practice	CBT-I adaptions for chronic pain
Sleep education	3-P model, 2-process model of sleep regulation, sleep stages	- Education about the reciprocal relationship of pain and sleep - Education about injury, illness, surgery, hospitalization, comorbid conditions, and medication effects on sleep - Education about pain as component of conditioned arousal
Sleep restriction	Improve sleep efficiency by limiting time in bed to amount of time sleeping then expanding slowly as long as sleep efficiency is preserved	- Restrict sleep by no more than 90 min - Goal to get to at least 6.5 h as quickly as possible.
Stimulus control	Associate bed/bedroom solely as a cue for sleep by eliminating nonsleep activities from the bedroom. Instruction to get out of bed at night if awake >15 min.	- If patient using bed to "rest" when pain is severe, identify other places patient can "rest" when not sleeping. - Omit instruction to leave bedroom when awake to reduce risk for falls—can sit in chair in bedroom instead - Use countercontrol—advise patient to sit in bed doing sleep promoting activities until feeling sleepy
Napping/daytime sleep	Discontinue or restrict daytime napping to 30 min	- No change
Sleep hygiene education	Address daytime habits and sleep environment interfering with sleep	- Encourage physical activity consistent with medical rehabilitation/physical therapy advice - Encourage sound machine or white noise to prevent environmental noses from disrupting sleep - Encourage hot baths about 2 h before bed to promote slow wave sleep

Cognitive therapy	Challenge patient's dysfunctional beliefs interfering with sleep and misconceptions about sleep. Replace/restructure to more helpful and realistic thoughts about sleep	- Provide realistic expectation for sleep with comorbid conditions and schedule of needed medications - Utilize cognitive therapy to challenge maladaptive thoughts about pain catastrophizing and kinesiophobia
Relaxation and meditation techniques	Relaxation can help reduce racing thoughts/tension that accompany lying in bed awake, and may include: deep breathing, progressive muscle relaxation, guided imagery, biofeedback, hypnosis, autogenic training, and meditation practices.	- Progressive Muscle Relaxation (PMR) may be difficult because tensing muscles could increase pain. - Instead, introduce/focus on meditation, breathing techniques, or guided imagery.
Relapse prevention	Discuss practicing less rigid sleep plan over time and what do to prevent sleep disturbance from turning into another episode of insomnia in the future	- Discuss how to get sleep back on track after health or life events - Generate long-term sleep plan in writing
Sleep diaries	Establish baseline sleep patterns, track progress, reinforce appropriate behavior change, problem solve obstacles to adherence	- Consider tracking pain severity/intensity, medication, and pain coping strategies (stretching, PT)

compression strategies instead of strict sleep restriction. Another alternative could be to implement standard sleep restriction but expand sleep more rapidly with the goal of achieving 6.5 hours of sleep by the midpoint of treatment. Aggressive sleep expansion could be accomplished by adjusting the benchmark at which sleep is expanded (e.g., expanding if sleep efficiency is 80%–85% instead of 90%). This may be especially helpful for patients with chronic pain and older adults who may have extremely difficulty achieving sleep efficiencies greater than 80%–85%. Alternatively, sleep could be expanded in 30-minute increments instead of 15-minute increments. A third strategy could be to expand sleep every 3–4 days instead of waiting a full week or until the next appointment.

It is also important to consider modifications to stimulus control therapy in patients with chronic pain. An important step in determining how to implement stimulus control is completing a functional analysis of the patients' behavior during a pain flare. As noted above, behaviors such as retiring to bed or taking additional pain medications can contribute to insomnia and are important to address in treatment. Patients with pain having lower extremity issues or older adults with compromise balance are also vulnerable to falls and hip fractures, particularly if they are taking opioids or benzodiazepines, so getting out of bed when awake may not always be a safe option. Additionally, the simple act of getting out of bed and moving around may exacerbate pain and further disrupt sleep. Patients with chronic pain may also have significant mobility limitations, making the implementation of traditional stimulus control difficult. There are a variety of ways that stimulus control can be modified to be safer and accommodate these patients. The goal of stimulus control is to only use the bed for sleeping; however, patients with chronic pain may need a dark environment and may need to lie down to cope with or manage pain successfully. Finding a location that the patient can make comfortable enough for management as an alternative to the bedroom is important for reducing the association between pain and the bed/bedroom. It is also important to develop safe strategies for implementing stimulus control at night. One option is to ask the patient to set up a chair in their bedroom so that they do not have to move far when they get out of bed when awake. Another strategy could be to change location or position in the bed, such as moving to the other side or flipping head/feet to the opposite end of the bed. Countercontrol has also been shown to be an effective strategy for improving sleep-maintenance insomnia and is a good alternative for patients who cannot safely implement stimulus control (Davies, Lacks, Storandt, & Bertelson, 1986). Countercontrol is similar to stimulus control, except patients do not leave the bed. They are instructed to sit up in bed and engage in some noncognitive (boring) activity until drowsy. This activity consisted of things such as reading dull material, watching brief television shows, or listening to the radio with lights off and/or using blue blocking glasses to prevent melatonin suppression.

Cognitive therapy in CBT-I typically focuses on maladaptive thoughts related to sleep, anticipation of sleep, or hyperarousal. Pain-related thoughts and beliefs predict pain and disability in patients with chronic pain (Keefe, Rumble, Scipio, Giordano, & Perri, 2004) and are important to bear in mind when implementing cognitive therapy in this population. There are two types of cognitive processes related to chronic pain that should be considered. "Pain catastrophizing" is a set of negative cognitions, emotions, and attitudes about pain that are activated by pain. These thoughts fall into three main categories: magnification and exaggeration, rumination and hypervigilance, and helplessness and pessimism. Pain catastrophizing predicts the development and exacerbation of chronic pain, the spread of pain from one body part to the entire body, and is one of the major psychological contributors to poor outcomes in chronic pain. Examples of thoughts that might be expressed by chronic pain patients include, "my pain is never going to get better," or "this is the worst pain I can imagine." You could approach these thoughts the same way you would approach a negative sleep-related thought, but it is important to assess for pain-related thoughts, in addition to sleep-related thoughts, in the course of cognitive therapy. Another important cognitive factor in chronic pain is kinesiophobia, which is the fear of movement causing reinjury or intense pain. In most circumstances, this is an exaggerated if not inaccurate belief, and in chronic conditions such as back pain or knee osteoarthritis, movement is important for improving pain. Eliciting this fear and using cognitive techniques (in addition to talking to medical providers) to evaluate whether this fear is realistic can be an important part of cognitive therapy as well.

There are several components of sleep hygiene that can be particularly helpful for patients with chronic pain. As discussed above, sleep in this population is often lighter and more fragmented than healthy sleep. White noise machines may be especially helpful in minimizing the disruption that may be caused by sounds occurring in the sleep environment (Smith, Perlis, Carmody, Smith, & Giles, 2001). Slow wave sleep is reduced in chronic pain (Bjurstrom & Irwin, 2015; Drewes et al., 1995; Nielsen, Drewes, Svendsett, Bjerregard, & Taagholt, 1994), and reduced slow wave sleep can increase pain sensitivity (Lentz, Landis, Rothermel, & Shaver, 1999; Moldofsky & Scarisbrick, 1976). Passive body heating (such as taking a 30-minute hot bath about 2 hours before bedtime) may increase slow wave sleep and potentially help with pain the following day (Bunnell, Agnew, Horvath, Jopson, & Wills, 1988; Liao, 2002). Setting exercise goals is also an important component of sleep hygiene for patients with chronic pain. Exercise (particularly aerobic exercise) has been shown to improve both sleep and pain and enhance CPM (Lima, Abner, & Sluka, 2017; Yang,

Ho, Chen, & Chien, 2012). It is important to address any kinesiophobia before implementing exercise and to pace exercise appropriately to avoid pain flares.

There have been some studies that attempt to combine CBT-I with CBT for pain. At face value, a hybrid therapy makes a lot of sense because many components overlap, such as relaxation training, cognitive restructuring, and behavioral activation. Unfortunately, studies conducted to date have tried to include full CBT-I and full CBT for pain. This combination results in longer and more burdensome treatment protocols. Findings of these studies indicate the combining the two approaches shows similar effect on sleep as CBT-I alone, and so to date, there is no incremental benefit of simply adding CBT for pain to a CBT-I protocol (Pigeon et al., 2012; Tang, Goodchild, & Salkovskis, 2012; Vitiello et al., 2013, 2014). It may be that in these situations, patients were given too much information too quickly and could not learn any of the skills very well. A better approach may be to create a novel hybrid CBT for both pain and insomnia that consolidates the overlapping aspects of both treatments, incorporates the most important independent aspects of each, is tailored to the patients' needs and preferences, and sequences treatment components in a way that optimizes adherence and outcomes. This type of treatment optimization has yet to be explored.

Other areas for future work include investigation of the roles that melatonin and light therapy play in sleep treatments for chronic pain patients. Melatonin is a natural analgesic and may reduce pain in patients with chronic pain (de Zanette et al., 2014; Schwertner et al., 2013). A study by Burgess shows that bright light therapy reduced clinical pain and improves sleep quality in veterans with low back pain (Burgess et al., 2019). While these effects were not large, there is some promise that incorporating melatonin and/or bright light into CBT-I when appropriate may provide some incremental benefit for pain.

Summary

In summary, not only do pain symptoms contribute to insomnia and sleep disruption, but sleep disruption also predicts new onset chronic pain and impairs CPM, creating a complex sleep-pain relationship. Thorough assessment is critical when treating patients with chronic pain. Other sleep disorders (such as sleep apnea), pain medications (such as opioids), suicidal ideation, and other mental health disorders (such as depression and PTSD) are common in this population and have implications for treatment. Standard CBT-I improves sleep in patients with chronic pain, and may reduce pain, but modifications may be needed to improve adherence and outcomes. In particular, sleep restriction therapy should aim to achieve more than 6.5 hours of total sleep time by midtreatment, and sleep opportunity should not be restricted by more than 90 minutes (compared to baseline sleep opportunity). Patients should be encouraged to avoid the bed/bedroom during daytime pain flares, and modifications to stimulus control may be needed if pain limits mobility or creates safety concerns. Further research and development are needed to create hybrid therapies for insomnia and pain. The sequence and number of skills addressed in a hybrid treatment are important to consider, although relaxation therapy and cognitive restructuring (addressing pain catastrophizing and kinesiophobia) appear to have benefits for both pain and insomnia. Further research is also needed to determine the role that melatonin and bright light play in pain management and how this could enhance CBT-I in this population.

References

Anderson, W. S., Sheth, R. N., Bencherif, B., Frost, J. J., & Campbell, J. N. (2002). Naloxone increases pain induced by topical capsaicin in healthy human volunteers. *Pain, 99*(1–2), 207–216. https://doi.org/10.1016/S0304-3959(02)00103-3.

Bair, M. J., Outcalt, S. D., Ang, D., Wu, J., & Yu, Z. (2020). Pain and psychological outcomes among Iraq and Afghanistan veterans with chronic pain and PTSD: ESCAPE trial longitudinal results. *Pain Medicine (United States), 21*(7), 1369–1376. https://doi.org/10.1093/PM/PNAA007.

Bair, M. J., Robinson, R. L., Katon, W., & Kroenke, K. (2003). Depression and pain comorbidity: A literature review. *Archives of Internal Medicine, 163*, 2433–2445. https://doi.org/10.1001/archinte.163.20.2433.

Beckham, J. C., Crawford, A. L., Feldman, M. E., Kirby, A. C., Hertzberg, M. A., Davidson, J. R. T., et al. (1997). Chronic posttraumatic stress disorder and chronic pain in Vietnam combat veterans. *Journal of Psychosomatic Research, 43*(4), 379–389. https://doi.org/10.1016/S0022-3999(97)00129-3.

Bjurstrom, M. F., & Irwin, M. R. (2015). Polysomnographic characteristics in nonmalignant chronic pain populations: A review of controlled studies. *Sleep Medicine Reviews, 26*, 74–86. https://doi.org/10.1016/j.smrv.2015.03.004.

Bonvanie, I. J., Oldehinkel, A. J., Rosmalen, J. G. M., & Janssens, K. A. M. (2016). Sleep problems and pain: A longitudinal cohort study in emerging adults. *Pain, 157*(4), 957–963. https://doi.org/10.1097/j.pain.0000000000000466.

Bunnell, D. E., Agnew, J. A., Horvath, S. M., Jopson, L., & Wills, M. (1988). Passive body heating and sleep: Influence of proximity to sleep. *Sleep, 11*(2), 210–219. https://doi.org/10.1093/sleep/11.2.210.

Burgess, H. J., Rizvydeen, M., Kimura, M., Pollack, M. H., Hobfoll, S. E., Rajan, K. B., et al. (2019). An open trial of morning bright light treatment among US military veterans with chronic low back pain: A pilot study. *Pain Medicine (United States), 20*(4), 770–778. https://doi.org/10.1093/pm/pny174.

Campbell, C. M., Buenaver, L. F., Finan, P., Bounds, S. C., Redding, M., McCauley, L., et al. (2015). Sleep, pain catastrophizing, and central sensitization in knee osteoarthritis patients with and without insomnia. *Arthritis Care and Research, 67*(10), 1387–1396. https://doi.org/10.1002/acr.22609.

Currie, S. R., Wilson, K. G., Pontefract, A. J., & DeLaplante, L. (2000). Cognitive-behavioral treatment of insomnia secondary to chronic pain. *Journal of Consulting and Clinical Psychology, 68*(3), 407–416. https://doi.org/10.1037/0022-006X.68.3.407.

Cutrufello, N. J., Ianus, V. D., & Rowley, J. A. (2020). Opioids and sleep. *Current Opinion in Pulmonary Medicine, 26*, 634–641. https://doi.org/10.1097/MCP.0000000000000733.

Davies, R., Lacks, P., Storandt, M., & Bertelson, A. D. (1986). Countercontrol treatment of sleep-maintenance insomnia in relation to age. *Psychology and Aging, 1*(3), 233–238. https://doi.org/10.1037/0882-7974.1.3.233.

De Broucker, T. H., Cesaro, P., Willer, J. C., & Le Bars, D. (1990). Diffuse noxious inhibitory controls in man: Involvement of the spinoreticular tract. *Brain, 113*(4), 1223–1234. https://doi.org/10.1093/brain/113.4.1223.

de Zanette, S. A., Vercelino, R., Laste, G., Rozisky, J. R., Schwertner, A., Machado, C. B., et al. (2014). Melatonin analgesia is associated with improvement of the descending endogenous pain-modulating system in fibromyalgia: A phase II, randomized, double-dummy, controlled trial. *BMC Pharmacology & Toxicology, 15*, 40. https://doi.org/10.1186/2050-6511-15-40.

Drewes, A. M., Nielsen, K. D., Taagholt, S. J., Bjerregård, K., Svendsen, L., & Gade, J. (1995). Sleep intensity in fibromyalgia: Focus on the microstructure of the sleep process. *Rheumatology, 34*(7), 629–635. https://doi.org/10.1093/rheumatology/34.7.629.

Edinger, J. D., Wohlgemuth, W. K., Krystal, A. D., & Rice, J. R. (2005). Behavioral insomnia therapy for fibromyalgia patients: A randomized clinical trial. *Archives of Internal Medicine, 165*(21), 2527–2535. https://doi.org/10.1001/archinte.165.21.2527.

Ferreira, G. E., McLachlan, A. J., Lin, C. W. C., Zadro, J. R., Abdel-Shaheed, C., O'Keeffe, M., et al. (2021). Efficacy and safety of antidepressants for the treatment of back pain and osteoarthritis: Systematic review and meta-analysis. *The BMJ, 372*. https://doi.org/10.1136/bmj.m4825.

Filiatrault, M. L., Chauny, J. M., Daoust, R., Roy, M. P., Denis, R., & Lavigne, G. (2016). Medium increased risk for central sleep apnea but not obstructive sleep apnea in long-term opioid users: A systematic review and meta-analysis. *Journal of Clinical Sleep Medicine, 12*(4), 617–625. https://doi.org/10.5664/jcsm.5704.

Fishbain, D. A., Goldberg, M., Robert Meagher, B., Steele, R., & Rosomoff, H. (1986). Male and female chronic pain patients categorized by DSM-III psychiatric diagnostic criteria. *Pain, 26*(2), 181–197. https://doi.org/10.1016/0304-3959(86)90074-6.

Gerhart, J. I., Burns, J. W., Post, K. M., Smith, D. A., Porter, L. S., Burgess, H. J., et al. (2017). Relationships between sleep quality and pain-related factors for people with chronic low Back pain: Tests of reciprocal and time of day effects. *Annals of Behavioral Medicine: A Publication of the Society of Behavioral Medicine, 51*(3), 365. https://doi.org/10.1007/S12160-016-9860-2.

Granovsky, Y., & Yarnitsky, D. (2013). Personalized pain medicine: The clinical value of psychophysical assessment of pain modulation profile. *Rambam Maimonides Medical Journal, 4*(4), e0024. https://doi.org/10.5041/RMMJ.10131.

Gupta, A., Silman, A. J., Ray, D., Morriss, R., Dickens, C., MacFarlane, G. J., et al. (2007). The role of psychosocial factors in predicting the onset of chronic widespread pain: Results from a prospective population-based study. *Rheumatology, 46*(4), 666–671. https://doi.org/10.1093/rheumatology/kel363.

Harrison, L., Wilson, S., & Munafò, M. R. (2014). Exploring the associations between sleep problems and chronic musculoskeletal pain in adolescents: A prospective cohort study. *Pain Research and Management, 19*(5), e139–e145. https://doi.org/10.1155/2014/615203.

Iacovides, S., George, K., Kamerman, P., & Baker, F. C. (2017). Sleep fragmentation hypersensitizes healthy young women to deep and superficial experimental pain. *Journal of Pain, 18*(7), 844–854. https://doi.org/10.1016/j.jpain.2017.02.436.

Javaheri, S., Germany, R., & Greer, J. J. (2016). Novel therapies for the treatment of central sleep apnea. *Sleep Medicine Clinics, 11*(2), 227–239. https://doi.org/10.1016/j.jsmc.2016.01.004.

Julien, N., & Marchand, S. (2006). Endogenous pain inhibitory systems activated by spatial summation are opioid-mediated. *Neuroscience Letters, 401*(3), 256–260. https://doi.org/10.1016/j.neulet.2006.03.032.

Jungquist, C. R., O'Brien, C., Matteson-Rusby, S., Smith, M. T., Pigeon, W. R., Xia, Y., et al. (2010). The efficacy of cognitive-behavioral therapy for insomnia in patients with chronic pain. *Sleep Medicine, 11*(3), 302–309. https://doi.org/10.1016/j.sleep.2009.05.018.

Kashima, K., Rahman, O. I. F., Sakoda, S., & Shiba, R. (1999). Increased pain sensitivity of the upper extremities of TMD patients with myalgia to experimentally-evoked noxious stimulation: Possibility of worsened endogenous opioid systems. *Cranio, 17*(4), 241–246. https://doi.org/10.1080/08869634.1999.11746100.

Keefe, F. J., Rumble, M. E., Scipio, C. D., Giordano, L. A., & Perri, L. C. M. (2004). Psychological aspects of persistent pain: Current state of the science. *Journal of Pain, 5*(4), 195–211. https://doi.org/10.1016/j.jpain.2004.02.576.

Kosek, E., & Hansson, P. (1997). Modulatory influence on somatosensory perception from vibration and heterotopic noxious conditioning stimulation (HNCS) in fibromyalgia patients and healthy subjects. *Pain, 70*(1), 41–51. https://doi.org/10.1016/S0304-3959(96)03295-2.

Krause, A. J., Prather, A. A., Wager, T. D., Lindquist, M. A., & Walker, M. P. (2019). The pain of sleep loss: A brain characterization in humans. *Journal of Neuroscience, 39*(12), 2291–2300. https://doi.org/10.1523/JNEUROSCI.2408-18.2018.

Lautenbacher, S., & Rollman, G. B. (1997). Possible deficiencies of pain modulation in fibromyalgia. *Clinical Journal of Pain, 13*(3), 189–196. https://doi.org/10.1097/00002508-199709000-00003.

Lentz, M. J., Landis, C. A., Rothermel, J., & Shaver, J. L. F. (1999). Effects of selective slow wave sleep disruption on musculoskeletal pain and fatigue in middle aged women. *Journal of Rheumatology, 26*(7), 1586–1592.

Liao, W. C. (2002). Effects of passive body heating on body temperature and sleep regulation in the elderly: A systematic review. *International Journal of Nursing Studies, 39*(8), 803–810. https://doi.org/10.1016/S0020-7489(02)00023-8.

Lima, L. V., Abner, T. S. S., & Sluka, K. A. (2017). Does exercise increase or decrease pain? Central mechanisms underlying these two phenomena. *Journal of Physiology, 595*(13), 4141–4150. https://doi.org/10.1113/JP273355.

Lo, H. S., Yang, C. M., Lo, H. G., Lee, C. Y., Ting, H., & Tzang, B. S. (2010). Treatment effects of gabapentin for primary insomnia. *Clinical Neuropharmacology, 33*(2), 84–90. https://doi.org/10.1097/WNF.0b013e3181cda242.

Maixner, W., Fillingim, R., Booker, D., & Sigurdsson, A. (1995). Sensitivity of patients with painful temporomandibular disorders to experimentally evoked pain. *Pain, 63*(3), 341–351. https://doi.org/10.1016/0304-3959(95)00068-2.

Matre, D., Andersen, M. R., Knardahl, S., & Nilsen, K. B. (2016). Conditioned pain modulation is not decreased after partial sleep restriction. *European Journal of Pain (United Kingdom), 20*(3), 408–416. https://doi.org/10.1002/ejp.741.

McCall, W. V., Blocker, J. N., D'Agostino, R., Kimball, J., Boggs, N., Lasater, B., et al. (2010). Insomnia severity is an indicator of suicidal ideation during a depression clinical trial. *Sleep Medicine, 11*(9), 822–827. https://doi.org/10.1016/j.sleep.2010.04.004.

Mccrae, C. S., Williams, J., Roditi, D., Anderson, R., Mundt, J. M., Miller, M. B., et al. (2019). Cognitive behavioral treatments for insomnia and pain in adults with comorbid chronic insomnia and fibromyalgia: Clinical outcomes from the SPIN randomized controlled trial. *Sleep, 42*(3). https://doi.org/10.1093/sleep/zsy234.

Melzack, R. (1999). Pain—An overview. *Acta Anaesthesiologica Scandinavica, 43*(9), 880–884. https://doi.org/10.1034/j.1399-6576.1999.430903.x.

Mikkelsson, M., Sourander, A., Salminen, J. J., Kautiainen, H., & Piha, J. (1999). Widespread pain and neck pain in schoolchildren. A prospective one-year follow-up study. *Acta Paediatrica, International Journal of Paediatrics, 88*(10), 1119–1124. https://doi.org/10.1080/08035259950168199.

Moldofsky, H., & Scarisbrick, P. (1976). Induction of neurasthenic musculoskeletal pain syndrome by selective sleep stage deprivation. *Psychosomatic Medicine, 38*(1), 35–44. https://doi.org/10.1097/00006842-197601000-00006.

Morin, C. M., LeBlanc, M., Daley, M., Gregoire, J. P., & Mérette, C. (2006). Epidemiology of insomnia: Prevalence, self-help treatments, consultations, and determinants of help-seeking behaviors. *Sleep Medicine, 7*(2), 123–130. https://doi.org/10.1016/j.sleep.2005.08.008.

Nielsen, K. D., Drewes, A. M., Svendsett, L., Bjerregard, K., & Taagholt, S. (1994). Ambulatory recording and power spectral analysis by autoregressive modelling of polygraphic sleep signals in patients suffering from chronic pain. *Methods of Information in Medicine, 33*(1), 76–78. https://doi.org/10.1055/s-0038-1634963.

Peters, M. L., Schmidt, A. J. M., Van den Hout, M. A., Koopmans, R., & Sluijter, M. E. (1992). Chronic back pain, acute postoperative pain and the activation of diffuse noxious inhibitory controls (DNIC). *Pain, 50*(2), 177–187. https://doi.org/10.1016/0304-3959(92)90159-9.

Pielsticker, A., Haag, G., Zaudig, M., & Lautenbacher, S. (2005). Impairment of pain inhibition in chronic tension-type headache. *Pain, 118*(1–2), 215–223. https://doi.org/10.1016/j.pain.2005.08.019.

Pigeon, W. R., Moynihan, J., Matteson-Rusby, S., Jungquist, C. R., Xia, Y., Tu, X., et al. (2012). Comparative effectiveness of CBT interventions for co-morbid chronic pain & insomnia: A pilot study. *Behaviour Research and Therapy, 50*(11), 685–689. https://doi.org/10.1016/j.brat.2012.07.005.

Pigeon, W. R., Pinquart, M., & Conner, K. (2012). Meta-analysis of sleep disturbance and suicidal thoughts and behaviors. *Journal of Clinical Psychiatry, 73*(9). https://doi.org/10.4088/JCP.11r07586.

Ramaswamy, S., & Wodehouse, T. (2021). Conditioned pain modulation—A comprehensive review. *Neurophysiologie Clinique, 51*(3), 197–208. https://doi.org/10.1016/J.NEUCLI.2020.11.002.

Roehrs, T., Hyde, M., Blaisdell, B., Greenwald, M., & Roth, T. (2006). Sleep loss and REM sleep loss are hyperalgesic. *Sleep, 29*(2), 145–151. https://doi.org/10.1093/sleep/29.2.145.

Roth, T., Van Seventer, R., & Murphy, T. K. (2010). The effect of pregabalin on pain-related sleep interference in diabetic peripheral neuropathy or postherpetic neuralgia: A review of nine clinical trials. *Current Medical Research and Opinion, 26*(10), 2411–2419. https://doi.org/10.1185/03007995.2010.516142.

Sanders, A. E., Akinkugbe, A. A., Bair, E., Fillingim, R. B., Greenspan, J. D., Ohrbach, R., et al. (2016). Subjective sleep quality deteriorates before development of painful temporomandibular disorder. *Journal of Pain, 17*(6), 669–677. https://doi.org/10.1016/j.jpain.2016.02.004.

Schwertner, A., Conceição Dos Santos, C. C., Costa, G. D., Deitos, A., De Souza, A., De Souza, I. C. C., et al. (2013). Efficacy of melatonin in the treatment of endometriosis: A phase II, randomized, double-blind, placebo-controlled trial. *Pain, 154*(6), 874–881. https://doi.org/10.1016/j.pain.2013.02.025.

Shear, T. C., Balachandran, J. S., Mokhlesi, B., Spampinato, L. M., Knutson, K. L., Meltzer, D. O., et al. (2014). Risk of sleep apnea in hospitalized older patients. *Journal of Clinical Sleep Medicine, 10*(10), 1061–1066. https://doi.org/10.5664/jcsm.4098.

Smith, M. T., Edwards, R. R., McCann, U. D., & Haythomthwaite, J. A. (2007). The effects of sleep deprivation on pain inhibition and spontaneous pain in women. *Sleep, 30*(4), 494–505. https://doi.org/10.1093/sleep/30.4.494.

Smith, M. T., Finan, P. H., Buenaver, L. F., Robinson, M., Haque, U., Quain, A., et al. (2015). Cognitive-behavioral therapy for insomnia in knee osteoarthritis: A randomized, double-blind, active placebo-controlled clinical trial. *Arthritis and Rheumatology, 67*(5), 1221–1233. https://doi.org/10.1002/art.39048.

Smith, M. T., & Haythornthwaite, J. A. (2004). How do sleep disturbance and chronic pain inter-relate? Insights from the longitudinal and cognitive-behavioral clinical trials literature. *Sleep Medicine Reviews, 8*, 119–132. https://doi.org/10.1016/S1087-0792(03)00044-3.

Smith, M. T., Klick, B., Kozachik, S., Edwards, R. E., Holavanahalli, R., Wiechman, S., et al. (2008). Sleep onset insomnia symptoms during hospitalization for major burn injury predict chronic pain. *Pain, 138*(3), 497–506. https://doi.org/10.1016/j.pain.2008.01.028.

Smith, M. T., Perlis, M. L., Carmody, T. P., Smith, M. S., & Giles, D. E. (2001). Presleep cognitions in patients with insomnia secondary to chronic pain. *Journal of Behavioral Medicine, 24*(1), 93–114. https://doi.org/10.1023/A:1005690505632.

Smith, M. T., Remeniuk, B., Finan, P. H., Speed, T. J., Tompkins, D. A., Robinson, M., et al. (2019). Sex differences in measures of central sensitization and pain sensitivity to experimental sleep disruption: Implications for sex differences in chronic pain. *Sleep, 42*(2). https://doi.org/10.1093/sleep/zsy209.

Smitherman, T. A., Kuka, A. J., Calhoun, A. H., Walters, A. B. P., Davis-Martin, R. E., Ambrose, C. E., et al. (2018). Cognitive-behavioral therapy for insomnia to reduce chronic migraine: A sequential Bayesian analysis. *Headache, 58*(7), 1052–1059. https://doi.org/10.1111/head.13313.

Spielman, A. J., Caruso, L. S., & Glovinsky, P. B. (1987). A behavioral perspective on insomnia treatment. *Psychiatric Clinics of North America, 10*(4), 541–553. https://doi.org/10.1016/s0193-953x(18)30532-x.

Staud, R., Robinson, M. E., Vierck, C. J., & Price, D. D. (2003). Diffuse noxious inhibitory controls (DNIC) attenuate temporal summation of second pain in normal males but not in normal females or fibromyalgia patients. *Pain, 101*(1–2), 167–174. https://doi.org/10.1016/S0304-3959(02)00325-1.

Tang, N. K. Y., & Crane, C. (2006). Suicidality in chronic pain: A review of the prevalence, risk factors and psychological links. *Psychological Medicine, 36*(5), 575–586. https://doi.org/10.1017/S0033291705006859.

Tang, N. K. Y., Goodchild, C. E., & Salkovskis, P. M. (2012). Hybrid cognitive-behaviour therapy for individuals with insomnia and chronic pain: A pilot randomised controlled trial. *Behaviour Research and Therapy, 50*(12), 814–821. https://doi.org/10.1016/j.brat.2012.08.006.

Tang, N. K. Y., Lereya, S. T., Boulton, H., Miller, M. A., Wolke, D., & Cappuccio, F. P. (2015). Nonpharmacological treatments of insomnia for long-term painful conditions: A systematic review and meta-analysis of patient-reported outcomes in randomized controlled trials. *Sleep, 38*(11), 1751–1764E. https://doi.org/10.5665/sleep.5158.

Taylor, D. J., Mallory, L. J., Lichstein, K. L., Durrence, H. H., Riedel, B. W., & Bush, A. J. (2007). Comorbidity of chronic insomnia with medical problems. *Sleep, 30*(2), 213–218. https://doi.org/10.1093/sleep/30.2.213.

Vinik, A., Emir, B., Parsons, B., & Cheung, R. (2014). Prediction of pregabalin-mediated pain response by severity of sleep disturbance in patients with painful diabetic neuropathy and post-herpetic neuralgia. *Pain Medicine (United States), 15*(4), 661–670. https://doi.org/10.1111/pme.12310.

Vitiello, M. V., McCurry, S. M., Shortreed, S. M., Baker, L. D., Rybarczyk, B. D., Keefe, F. J., et al. (2014). Short-term improvement in insomnia symptoms predicts long-term improvements in sleep, pain, and fatigue in older adults with comorbid osteoarthritis and insomnia. *Pain, 155*(8), 1547–1554. https://doi.org/10.1016/j.pain.2014.04.032.

Vitiello, M. V., McCurry, S. M., Shortreed, S. M., Balderson, B. H., Baker, L. D., Keefe, F. J., et al. (2013). Cognitive-behavioral treatment for comorbid insomnia and osteoarthritis pain in primary care: The lifestyles randomized controlled trial. *Journal of the American Geriatrics Society, 61*(6), 947–956. https://doi.org/10.1111/jgs.12275.

Wang, D., & Teichtahl, H. (2007). Opioids, sleep architecture and sleep-disordered breathing. *Sleep Medicine Reviews, 11*, 35–46. https://doi.org/10.1016/j.smrv.2006.03.006.

Webster, L. R., Choi, Y., Desai, H., Webster, L., & Grant, B. J. B. (2008). Sleep-disordered breathing and chronic opioid therapy. *Pain Medicine, 9*(4), 425–432. https://doi.org/10.1111/j.1526-4637.2007.00343.x.

Wichniak, A., Wierzbicka, A., Walęcka, M., & Jernajczyk, W. (2017). Effects of antidepressants on sleep. *Current Psychiatry Reports, 19*(9). https://doi.org/10.1007/S11920-017-0816-4.

Wilder-Smith, C. H., Schindler, D., Lovblad, K., Redmond, S. M., & Nirkko, A. (2004). Brain functional magnetic resonance imaging of rectal pain and activation of endogenous inhibitory mechanisms in irritable bowel syndrome patient subgroups and healthy controls. *Gut, 53*(11), 1595–1601. https://doi.org/10.1136/gut.2003.028514.

Wilder-Smith, O. H., Schreyer, T., Scheffer, G. J., & Arendt-Nielsen, L. (2010). Patients with chronic pain after abdominal surgery show less preoperative endogenous pain inhibition and more postoperative hyperalgesia: A pilot study. *Journal of Pain and Palliative Care Pharmacotherapy, 24*(2), 119–128. https://doi.org/10.3109/15360281003706069.

Willer, J. C., Le Bars, D., & De Broucker, T. (1990). Diffuse noxious inhibitory controls in man: Involvement of an opioidergic link. *European Journal of Pharmacology, 182*(2), 347–355. https://doi.org/10.1016/0014-2999(90)90293-F.

Yang, P. Y., Ho, K. H., Chen, H. C., & Chien, M. Y. (2012). Exercise training improves sleep quality in middle-aged and older adults with sleep problems: A systematic review. *Journal of Physiotherapy, 58*(3), 157–163. https://doi.org/10.1016/S1836-9553(12)70106-6.

CHAPTER

12

CBT-I during and after a cancer diagnosis

Sheila N. Garland

Department of Psychology, Faculty of Science, Memorial University of Newfoundland, St. John's, NL, Canada
Discipline of Oncology, Faculty of Medicine, Memorial University of Newfoundland, St. John's, NL, Canada

Importance of identifying and treating insomnia in cancer survivors

Cancer is one of the leading causes of global morbidity and mortality, second only to heart disease (Global Burden of Disease Cancer Collaboration et al., 2017). Early detection and improved treatment methods have increased overall cancer survival rates (Siegel, Naishadham, & Jemal, 2012). As of 2019, it is estimated that there are 16.9 million cancer survivors in the United States (American Cancer Society, 2019). This number is projected to increase to 21.7 million by 2029 and 26.1 million by 2040. Improved survival rates mean that most people will spend more time recovering from the persistent physical and psychological side effects of cancer than being treated for it.

An important, but often overlooked, comorbidity or side effect of a cancer diagnosis and treatment is insomnia (Leysen et al., 2019; Schieber et al., 2019). Individuals will present with insomnia at the time of their cancer diagnosis, during treatment, and long after treatment has ended (Barsevick et al., 2013; Palesh et al., 2012). In one of the best studies to assess the prevalence of insomnia throughout the cancer trajectory, close to 1000 patients were assessed before surgery for cancer and then again at 2, 6, 10, 14, and 18 months later, during which they would have received and completed cancer treatments (Savard, Ivers, Villa, Caplette-Gingras, & Morin, 2011; Savard, Villa, Ivers, Simard, & Morin, 2009). After

Adapting Cognitive Behavioral Therapy for Insomnia
https://doi.org/10.1016/B978-0-12-822872-2.00003-7

diagnosis but before receiving any cancer treatment, 59% of the individuals had symptoms of insomnia and 28% met the criteria for insomnia disorder. Based on a diagnostic criteria duration of 3 months, more than half of all patients would have had insomnia symptoms before their cancer diagnosis. Despite some improvement in the rate of insomnia over time, 36% of the individuals still experienced insomnia symptoms 18 months later, whereas 21% met the criteria for insomnia disorder. Considering that the prevalence of insomnia in the general population is roughly 10% (LeBlanc et al., 2009), cancer survivors are 2–6 times more likely to experience insomnia, depending on the time of assessment, whether the study was assessing insomnia symptoms or a disorder, and the measurement tool used (Hoang, Molassiotis, Chan, Nguyen, & Liep Nguyen, 2019; Maguire, Drummond, Hanly, Gavin, & Sharp, 2019; Palesh et al., 2010; Savard et al., 2005).

Insomnia is one of the longest-lasting symptoms reported by cancer survivors (Lowery-Allison et al., 2018). While many other symptoms resolve, insomnia once established tends to be unrelenting. In the study by Savard, Ivers, et al. (2011), 51% of those patients who had insomnia at one time point continued to experience it at a subsequent assessment, and 35% of patients had insomnia persisting for at least three consecutive time points over the 18 months. Even 5-years after their diagnosis, women with breast cancer experience greater sleep problems despite rating their quality of life to be equal to or better than peers without cancer (Schmidt, Wiskemann, & Steindorf, 2018). Similarly, 83% of patients with head and neck cancer who were assessed 3 or more years after surgery reported poor sleep (Li, Otomaru, & Taniguchi, 2017), and 57% of elderly lung cancer survivors who were assessed more than 5 years after diagnosis had poor sleep as compared to only 30% of controls (Gooneratne et al., 2007). Furthermore, 49% of the participants who did not have sleep difficulties before their lung cancer diagnosis would go on to develop these problems over the average 8-year survival time. Considering the number of people projected to be cancer survivors in the next 20 years, insomnia represents a significant additional burden to the individual and society.

Insomnia has significant implications for overall cancer recovery. Insomnia is associated with impaired neurocognitive function (Dzierzewski, Dautovich, & Ravyts, 2018), as well as an increased risk of developing and worsened recovery from many mental health disorders (Garland, Vargas, Grandner, & Perlis, 2018). Specifically, in cancer survivors, insomnia is associated with worse quality of life (Ancoli-Israel, 2009; Arndt, Merx, Stegmaier, Ziegler, & Brenner, 2005), immune function impairments (Blask et al., 2011; Payne, Piper, Rabinowitz, & Zimmerman, 2006), problems with memory (Caplette-Gingras, Savard, Savard, & Ivers, 2013; Jean-Pierre et al., 2015), and cancer-related fatigue (Balachandran, Faiz, Bashoura, & Manzullo, 2013; Roscoe et al., 2007). Disturbed sleep and insomnia may also have implications for tumor progression (Cash et al., 2015; Filipski et al., 2003; Filipski, Li, & Lévi, 2006), response to cancer treatment (Innominato et al., 2015), and overall survival time (Gottfried et al., 2020; Innominato et al., 2009).

Despite its prevalence and importance, insomnia is often unrecognized and poorly managed (Savard & Morin, 2001). Cancer survivors may be reluctant to discuss their insomnia with their cancer care team, perceiving it to be of less importance than their cancer treatment or a normal reaction to the experience (Reynolds-Cowie & Fleming, 2020). Oncology care providers may also not inquire about the presence of insomnia, or if they do are more likely to prescribe pharmacological interventions as opposed to recommending CBT-I (Zhou, Partridge, Syrjala, Michaud, & Recklitis, 2017). There is still much work to be done to educate cancer survivors and clinicians about the existence and efficacy of CBT-I and integrate insomnia treatment as part of routine cancer care. The first section of this chapter discusses the conceptualization of insomnia in cancer survivors with reference to predisposing, precipitating, and perpetuating factors and the relative impact of cancer and its treatments. The second section discusses a general approach to CBT-I and potential modifications to the delivery of insomnia interventions in cancer with attention paid to those who may be currently undergoing cancer treatment, have comorbid conditions, and the unique health and existential concerns that cancer can bring. All recommendations herein are based on evidence from peer-reviewed research, and, when unavailable, clinical experiences have been used to supplement the evidence base.

Conceptualizing insomnia in cancer survivors

Predisposing factors

In many cases, insomnia in cancer can be understood using the diathesis-stress model, which suggests that the disorder arises from a combination of latent predispositions and vulnerabilities that can be triggered by and interact with environmental stress (Drake, Pillai, & Roth, 2014). Cancer survivors share many of the same predisposing factors for insomnia as the general population. These predisposing factors are female sex and/or gender (Zhang & Wing, 2006), high neuroticism (Harvey, Gehrman, & Espie, 2014), and genetic heritability (Jarrin et al., 2017). Cancer survivors also present with some unique predisposing factors. Older age is seen as a predisposing factor for insomnia in the general population (Morin & Jarrin, 2013), and while this is also the case in cancer survivors, younger age is also often associated with insomnia (Davidson,

MacLean, Brundage, & Schulze, 2002; Desai et al., 2013; Palesh et al., 2012). The prevalence of insomnia appears to vary as a function of cancer sites, being more frequent in patients with breast, ovarian, or gynecologic cancer and lower in those with prostate cancer (Davidson et al., 2002; Portenoy et al., 1994; Zhou, Clark, Recklitis, Obenchain, & Loscalzo, 2018), but higher rates of insomnia are not solely attributable to sex (Savard et al., 2009). Other cancer types with high rates of insomnia include head, neck, and lung cancer where the prevalence by sex tends to be more equal (Harrington, Hansen, Moskowitz, Todd, & Feuerstein, 2010; Otte, Carpenter, Russell, Bigatti, & Champion, 2010; Santoso et al., 2019; Slade, Waters, & Serrano, 2019).

Precipitating factors

The diagnosis and treatment of cancer can bring with it a wide variety of short- and long-term psychological and physical side effects that have the potential to cause or worsen insomnia. Many of these psychological and physical conditions have their chapters in this book, and it would be helpful to be familiar with the adaptation of CBT-I for those conditions as well. Although insomnia might be initially triggered by these other conditions, it may not be sufficient to treat only those factors and expect that insomnia will resolve. While some of the side effects may remit with treatment and/or time, insomnia becomes rapidly self-reinforcing. The ability to consult with other health professionals involved in the care of your patient can be helpful to identify and reduce the contribution of these to the patient's insomnia.

Hospitalizations

For many patients, being in the hospital can lead to severe disruptions in sleep that can persist after discharge. Nocturnal awakenings by hospital staff or nurses, be it to change the garbage or check blood pressure, can be very disruptive. Patients report a median of 5 (range 4–7) interruptions each night, and those who experience more than 3 sleep interruptions are more likely to report poor sleep than those with 3 or fewer interruptions (Mouch, Baskin, Yearling, Miller, & Dossett, 2020). Many hospitals are getting better at prioritizing patients' sleep over routines, but one of the most common causes of sleep disruptions in hospital settings is still elevated noise levels. Telephones, alarms, and staff talking are among the most reported noises that cause the most disruption in sleep (Aydın Sayılan, Kulakaç, & Sayılan, 2020). Sleep promotion in hospitals can include the use of sleep masks, earplugs, white noise machines, and bundling care to avoid unnecessary nocturnal interruptions (Graham et al., 2020; Kamdar et al., 2013). While it is likely that the patient will seek treatment for insomnia well after their hospitalization, this is sometimes identified as the time that sleep-related worries begin to take hold. It may also be possible to prepare patients to preserve their sleep if a future hospitalization is anticipated. Patients may be concerned that their lack of sleep may impact their ability to heal and this initial worry can worsen over time, especially when combined with the effects of cancer treatment described below.

The effects of cancer diagnosis and treatment

Roughly half of cancer survivors have preexisting insomnia that will be worsened by cancer treatment (Garland et al., 2018; Savard, Ivers, et al., 2011; Zhou et al., 2018). For the remaining individuals, their insomnia is thought to be brought on by the impact of the cancer diagnosis and/or treatment. Treatment for cancer can include a combination of surgery, chemotherapy, radiation therapy, targeted therapies, immunotherapy, and/or hormone therapy, all of which have the potential to provoke or intensify insomnia because of their emotional impact, their direct physiologic effects, or their side effects (Hoogland et al., 2019; Miaskowski & Lee, 1999; Savard, Ivers, Savard, & Morin, 2015; Savard & Savard, 2013).

Of all the treatments, chemotherapy is had been demonstrated to be particularly disruptive to sleep (Beck et al., 2010; Enderlin et al., 2010). The link between chemotherapy and insomnia is likely due in part to the use of corticosteroids during chemotherapy regimens. Corticosteroids can be used to treat the cancer itself, reduce inflammation, reduce the body's immune response, reduce sickness when having chemotherapy, and improve appetite. A common side effect of corticosteroid use is insomnia (Ismail, Lavelle, & Cassidy, 2017). Many patients are not prepared for steroid-induced insomnia, which can cause concern and initiate maladaptive behaviors to try and cope with this sleeplessness. Indeed, patients report more subjective sleep disturbance (lower sleep quality and less total sleep time) during the active phases of chemotherapy compared with rest periods (Chen, Yu, & Yang, 2008). These patterns can get worse over time and longitudinal studies have shown gradual increases in sleep impairment over the course of chemotherapy (Van Onselen et al., 2013) as well as the persistence of elevated insomnia rates across chemotherapy cycles (Palesh et al., 2010). In patients with early-stage disease, some research suggests that rest–activity patterns improve once the active phase of cancer treatment is over, but the disturbance remains worse than in matched controls (Ancoli-Israel et al., 2014). The prolonged nature of cancer treatment and survivorship means that an acute episode of insomnia triggered by stress and/or the effects of treatment can easily turn into a chronic condition.

Emotional distress

The emotional stress that can accompany a cancer diagnosis can certainly be sufficient to trigger an episode of insomnia in someone with an existing predisposition. Cancer survivors with high levels of psychological distress are 4.5 times more likely to report sleep difficulties than those with low levels (Sharma et al., 2012). Further, in 213 patients undergoing chemotherapy, insomnia was associated with symptoms of anxiety and depression but not with individual participant characteristics, cancer-related, or treatment-related factors (Hoang et al., 2019). While it is important not to overlook the possibility that insomnia in cancer survivors may be comorbid with a mood or anxiety disorder, there is also a significant proportion of patients who have isolated insomnia (Savard et al., 2005). As such, providers should conduct a thorough assessment of psychological functioning to assess whether adjunctive therapies for emotional distress may also be indicated.

Pain

Pain can be a cause of sleep disruption in patients with cancer (Fleming, Gillespie, & Espie, 2010). Indeed, cancer-related pain has been demonstrated to significantly predict the incidence or exacerbation of sleep difficulties (Palesh et al., 2007; Shi et al., 2013). The risk of reporting insomnia symptoms is close to 3 times higher for cancer survivors who also experience pain (Sharma et al., 2012). While pain may be the initial cause of the sleep problem, psychological distress regarding the pain can prevent the patient from falling back to sleep (Engstrom, Strohl, Rose, Lewandowski, & Stefanek, 1999). Opioid use is another factor influencing the relationship between sleep disturbance and pain. To help control pain, patients diagnosed with cancer are often prescribed opioids (Gress, Charipova, Kaye, Viswanath, & Urits, 2020); however, opioids decrease rapid eye movement and slow-wave sleep and may actually contribute to sleep disturbances experienced by these patients (Dimsdale, Norman, DeJardin, & Wallace, 2007). In any case, a cycle of pain and poor sleep may become a self-perpetuating positive feedback loop.

Hormonal factors

Endocrine therapy is a primary treatment for breast, prostate, and many other hormonally mediated cancers, and this treatment can continue for years or indefinitely. In women, the estrogen deficiency induced by chemotherapy and hormone therapy, the abrupt cessation of hormone replacement therapy at cancer diagnosis, or the removal of female reproductive organs may trigger or exacerbate preexisting hot flashes. The vasomotor symptoms experienced are often being more intense than in women undergoing natural menopause (Kaplan, Mahon, Lubejko, &

Ginex, 2020). Indeed, change in self-reported vasomotor symptoms is significantly associated with parallel changes in insomnia complaints in women with breast cancer (Savard, Savard, et al., 2011). In men with prostate cancer, the association between androgen deprivation therapy and insomnia is partly explained by nocturia and hot flash interference (Gonzalez et al., 2018). In some cases, the sleep interference caused by hot flashes resulting from treatment with aromatase inhibitors can be reduced by having the patient take their medication in the morning as opposed to the evening before bed. Considering that poor sleep and insomnia symptoms are one of the main reasons why people discontinue these life preserving medications (Henry et al., 2012; Moscetti et al., 2015), treatment of insomnia is a clinical priority.

Fatigue

Cancer-related fatigue is another frequent and disturbing concern for cancer survivors (Barsevick et al., 2013; Minton et al., 2013). Cancer-related fatigue is defined as a "persistent, subjective sense of tiredness related to cancer and cancer treatment that interferes with usual functioning and does not resolve with rest" (Bower, 2014). Unlike transient acute fatigue that can be attributed to a clearly identifiable cause (Jason, Evans, Brown, & Porter, 2010), fatigue associated with cancer is persistent throughout the day, not time-limited, impairs functioning, cannot be managed with sleep and/or stimulants (such as caffeine), and cannot be tied to health behaviors. More than 70% of patients during active treatment reporting feeling fatigued, and approximately 30% continue to struggle with fatigue after the treatment phase is finished (Howell et al., 2013).

The association between insomnia and fatigue in cancer survivors is well-established (Banthia, Malcarne, Ko, Varni, & Sadler, 2009; Jim et al., 2013; Roscoe et al., 2007; Stepanski et al., 2009), but less is known about the temporal relationships. Prospective research showed that fatigue significantly predicted a subsequent increase in insomnia symptoms during the cancer care trajectory, whereas insomnia was not found to predict subsequent fatigue (Trudel-Fitzgerald, Savard, & Ivers, 2013). The potential behavioral mechanisms for fatigue to affect the development of insomnia are described in the perpetuating factors section below. Certainly, once insomnia develops alongside fatigue, the combination has the potential to exacerbate both conditions.

Fatigue can be challenging to treat directly. Physical activity is the intervention with the strongest evidence of efficacy to reduce and even prevent cancer-related fatigue (Fuller, Hartland, Maloney, & Davison, 2018), but adherence to these recommendations can be difficult for some patients and populations (Burse, Bhuiyan, Mama, & Schmitz, 2020). Other adjunctive therapies with some evidence of efficacy include bright light therapy (Johnson et al., 2018), cognitive behavioral therapy (Poort et al., 2020), and mindfulness-based interventions (Cillessen, Johannsen, Speckens, & Zachariae, 2019). Stimulant medications like methylphenidate and modafinil have been evaluated as potential treatments for cancer-related fatigue, but the effects of these medications are underwhelming and have the potential for unwanted side effects (Qu et al., 2016).

Cognitive impairment

One of the most salient barriers to resuming normal functioning among cancer survivors is perceived cognitive impairment, sometimes referred to as "chemobrain" despite the fact that it is reported by people who receive other treatments as well. Approximately 75% of cancer patients report a decline across a variety of cognitive domains during treatment, and up to 35% continue to experience cognitive difficulties for months or years following treatment (Janelsins, Kesler, Ahles, & Morrow, 2014). Cognitive impairment can negatively impact return to work, impair performance, and result in prolonged leaves of absence or early retirement, which have significant negative impacts on quality of life and earning potential (Henderson, Cross, & Baraniak, 2019). Inadequate sleep has negative consequences for cognition in the general population (Banks & Dinges, 2007), and poor sleep and insomnia are significantly associated with subjective and objective cognitive complaints in cancer populations (Caplette-Gingras et al., 2013; Hartman, Marinac, Natarajan, & Patterson, 2015; Von Ah & Tallman, 2015). Recent evidence challenges the conventional idea that the cancer treatment itself is responsible for the changes in cognition and places sleep in the spotlight as a potent contributor (Xu et al., 2018).

Perpetuating factors

Similar to the general population, cancer survivors engage in several behaviors that are known to maintain insomnia, including taking naps during the day, using backlit electronics before bed, canceling daytime activities because of poor sleep, going to bed earlier, trying harder to sleep, and sleeping-in to make up for the effects of a poor night's sleep. It is important to understand that many of these behaviors are influenced by their experience of cancer and their intended purpose is to cope with the frustration and distress caused by insomnia. In cancer survivors who are not currently working because of treatment and recovery, they may continue to go to bed at the same time as before their diagnosis but spend more time in bed in the morning because they do not have to be at work for a specific time. Most people are unaware that this behavior can negatively influence their ability to fall asleep and how consolidated their sleep will be (Goldman et al., 2008; Owens et al., 2010).

Many cancer survivors have difficulty distinguishing between being tired (aka, fatigued) and being sleepy. This lack of attributional clarity may prompt the individual to think, "I am tired [aka, fatigued]. I must, therefore, need more sleep." An understandable behavioral response is for the individual to attempt to get more sleep. Many survivors are aware of the negative impact of napping but feel that they do not have better options to manage their levels of daytime fatigue. This may be particularly the case during cancer treatments when patients suffer from higher levels of fatigue and are very likely encouraged to rest to recuperate. In the case of cancer-related fatigue, the fatigue may not be related to sleep loss, and thus, no amount of increased sleep will diminish the experience of fatigue. This can lead to a host of maladaptive behaviors that, while intended to cope with the fatigue, can actually make it more likely that sleep problems will continue.

The use of prescribed and over-the-counter sleeping medications is very common in cancer survivors both on and off treatment (Moore, Berger, & Dizona, 2011) and is frequently encouraged and normalized by their doctors. In a survey of close to 2000 people who had received treatment for breast, prostate, lung, or colorectal cancer, 41% were given a prescription for medication to help with sleep (Casault, Savard, Ivers, Savard, & Simard, 2012). Further, the majority of cancer survivors (78%) who use sleeping medications do so three or more nights per week (Casault et al., 2012). In a qualitative study of 63 cancer survivors enrolled in an insomnia treatment study, participants reported having tried several medications or having to switch or alternate between different medications to maintain an effect (Garland, Barg, et al., 2018). Female gender, older age, and concomitant use of painkillers have been with the use of sleeping medication (Paltiel et al., 2004). Unfortunately, the use of sleeping medication is associated with the poorer overall quality of life, reducing the reliance on sleeping medications an important treatment target in cancer survivors.

Empirical support for CBT-I in cancer

Delivering CBT-I in the context of cancer is particularly challenging because of the overlap and chronicity of cancer-related side effects that may influence the development, severity, and persistence of insomnia symptoms. The treatment of cancer-related sleep disturbances should employ a combined approach that targets any contributing factors (e.g., hot flashes, pain, fatigue) and the factors that are believed to maintain the sleep difficulties over time (i.e., maladaptive sleep behaviors, dysfunctional beliefs about sleep) (Howell et al., 2013). CBT-I providers may benefit from consulting the other chapters in this book for guidance on how to manage insomnia that occurs in cancer in the context of other comorbidities.

Guidelines for the treatment of cancer-related sleep disturbances and insomnia recommend CBT-I as the treatment of choice (Howell, Keller-Olaman, et al., 2013; Howell et al., 2014; Matthews, Carter, Page, Dean, & Berger, 2018); however, patients may require short-term use of pharmacological interventions until cognitive behavioral therapy takes effect or is available. Meta-analytic findings compiled from 8 studies of cancer survivors ($n = 752$) were consistent in demonstrating that CBT-I (combining stimulus control, sleep restriction, cognitive restructuring, sleep hygiene, and sometimes relaxation) was associated with clinically significant and durable improvements in multiple insomnia outcomes including sleep efficiency, sleep onset latency, wake after sleep onset, and insomnia symptom severity (Johnson et al., 2016). A number of other randomized controlled trials have been published, which further support the efficacy of CBT-I in cancer since the time of the meta-analysis (Garland et al., 2016; Roscoe et al., 2015). In addition to improving insomnia, CBT-I reduces depression (Peoples et al., 2019) and cancer-related fatigue (Espie et al., 2008; Fleming, Randell, Harvey, & Espie, 2014; Heckler et al., 2016; Savard, Ivers, Savard, & Morin, 2014), and increases the overall quality of life in cancer survivors (Peoples et al., 2017). Preliminary research suggests that CBT-I may also improve perceived cognitive impairment (Quesnel, Savard, Simard, Ivers, & Morin, 2003), making it a potent intervention for many co-occurring symptoms.

Most of the trials completed to date have recruited post-treatment cancer survivors, which means we know less about how to adapt CBT-I for people currently undergoing cancer treatment. Recent studies have tested briefer versions of CBT-I for use during chemotherapy, which focus on education, sleep compression, stimulus control, limiting napping, and circadian entrainment (Palesh et al., 2019, 2018, 2020). These preliminary studies demonstrate that it is possible to intervene during chemotherapy using the abbreviated and tailored approaches described below.

Important considerations in the delivery of CBT-I in cancer populations

In cancer survivors, CBT-I is typically delivered to individuals over the course of 6–8 weeks; however, CBT-I can also be delivered successfully to groups and in less intensive doses. The briefer interventions delivered during cancer treatments have employed a combination of two 60-min in-person sessions and four 15-min telephone sessions (Palesh et al., 2020). Lack of access to CBT-I in cancer centers has limited its dissemination (Morin, 2017); therefore, CBT-I has also been delivered to cancer survivors using online (Zachariae et al., 2018) and self-led formats (Casault, Savard, Ivers, & Savard, 2015; Mercier, Ivers, & Savard, 2018; Savard et al., 2014; Savard, Ivers, Savard, & Morin, 2016). However, these appear to be less effective than therapist-delivered CBT-I.

Overall treatment approach

CBT-I is more than a set of instructions (see Table 1). Encouraging patient buy-in and adherence to treatment begin with the first session, and there are a number of nonspecific techniques that can help promote

TABLE 1 Adaptation of CBT-I for cancer survivors.

CBT-I components	Standard practice	Adaptations for cancer survivors
Sleep education	3-P model, 2-process model of sleep regulation, sleep stages	– Education about the role of physical and cognitive hyperarousal in maintaining insomnia – Education about how cancer and treatments, comorbid conditions, and cancer medications affect sleep – Education on distinguishing sleepiness from fatigue – Education about how other lifestyle factors can influence cancer recovery
Sleep restriction	Improve sleep efficiency by limiting time in bed to the amount of time sleeping then expanding slowly as long as sleep efficiency is preserved	– Use a sleep efficiency cutoff of 85% instead of 90% to increase the sleep window – If a person has high anxiety, multiple comorbidities, or is in active treatment, utilize sleep compression to restrict time in bed gradually by 15–30 min each week until sleep efficiency ≥85% is reached – Use light therapy in the morning to reduce cancer-related fatigue and promote circadian entrainment
Stimulus control	Associate bed/bedroom solely as a cue for sleep by eliminating non-sleep activities from the bedroom. Instruction to get out of bed at night if awake >15 min	– If a person is hospitalized, in active treatment, or if unsafe to get out of bed at night, use counter conditioning instead of stimulus control

Continued

TABLE 1 Adaptation of CBT-I for cancer survivors—cont'd

CBT-I components	Standard practice	Adaptations for cancer survivors
		– Change bedroom environment to make it less like the place they spent time when ill – Make other places more comfortable to rest so that bed is reserved for sleep
Napping/daytime sleep	Discontinue or restrict daytime napping to 30 min	– Naps may be needed during times of treatment – Limit naps to early in the day – Naps should be taken in the bed as opposed to the couch or other areas
Relaxation strategies		– Implement a 60–90 min "buffer zone" before bed in which to perform sedentary activities in dim light which are pleasant and relaxing. The use of backlit devices before bed or in the middle of the night is prohibited – If significant hyperarousal is present, according to patient preference, provide instruction on progressive muscle relaxation, imagery, meditation, etc.
Sleep hygiene education	Address daytime habits and sleep environment interfering with sleep	– Use of sleep-promoting eye masks, earplugs, and efforts to reduce noise interference – Work with other professionals to address cancer-specific factors that may influence comfort at night (e.g., dry mouth, hot flashes, pain, nocturnal enuresis, etc.)
Cognitive therapy	Challenge patient's dysfunctional beliefs interfering with sleep and misconceptions about sleep. Replace/restructure to more helpful and realistic thoughts about sleep	– Use throughout to promote adherence and address barriers – Address fears of the impact of insomnia on overall health and risk of cancer recurrence – Challenge perceived benefits of rest versus sleep – Implement a "worry time" or a "clear your head" time in which to address concerns during the day – Use behavioral activation/energy generation techniques to manage daytime fatigue

TABLE 1 Adaptation of CBT-I for cancer survivors—cont'd

CBT-I components	Standard practice	Adaptations for cancer survivors
Relapse prevention	Discuss practicing less rigid sleep plan over time and what do to prevent sleep disturbance from turning into another episode of insomnia in the future	– Anticipate short-term sleep disruption in advance of cancer-related tests and develop a plan to manage these
Sleep diaries	Establish baseline sleep patterns, track progress, reinforce appropriate behavior change, problem-solve obstacles to adherence	– Track additional concerns and medications to explore possible contributions of these to sleep problems

the development of patient adherence. First, the therapeutic relationship is critical to the success of treatment, and the patient should leave their first interaction with the clinician trusting that the provider can help them and feeling a sense of hope, no matter how small. The therapist's confidence in the techniques of CBT-I will help develop this relationship and present the process as collaborative, taking time to make each patient feel understood and unique. It is important to anticipate and address potential obstacles to adherence to sleep restriction and stimulus control in advance and develop plans to overcome these. The ability of the therapist to anticipate barriers enhances the appearance of experience and fosters the development of trust and hope.

This general overall approach often requires that cognitive techniques be employed throughout CBT-I to modify beliefs that may impact the patient's willingness to engage with the other aspects of therapy, in addition to a session dedicated to cognitive restructuring. It is recommended to acknowledge the patient's skepticism and the development of an attitude of exploration. Many patients finally find their way to CBT-I after many years of struggling with insomnia and failed attempts to address their problems. They may have even tried some CBT-I techniques, albeit in an unstructured or haphazard way. Acknowledging the patient's doubt and rolling with resistance can minimize the patient's defenses and help them feel safe to try new ways of behaving or thinking. It is also important to emphasize that plans are re-evaluated on a weekly basis so that the patient feels better able to cope with the discomfort if they know it is short-term.

Reminding the patient of their ability to manage the effects of poor sleep can sometimes help to build their self-efficacy if they are concerned about the impact of sleep restriction and stimulus control. This can be a simple as saying "You have been managing to function with insomnia for the past 5 years, so you already have the skills to make it through this next week." It is also helpful to normalize any discomfort and prevent them from withdrawing from treatment prematurely. For example, the therapist might tell them that it is normal to feel worse, more tired, and/or irritable than they did before they started CBT-I. It may also be helpful to encourage them to contact the therapist, rather than abandoning the plan, during the first and/or second weeks of sleep restriction and stimulus control if they are unable or unwilling to continue with the individualized program developed. This helps retain the patient in therapy and allows the therapist to modify any aspect of treatment that might not have been practical or feasible (e.g., placement of sleep window).

Clinical interview and assessment

Treatment should begin with a semistructured clinical interview and at least 1 week of prospective sleep monitoring with a sleep diary. Essential information to collect during the interview includes the presentation and daytime impact of the sleep complaint, the development of the sleep complaint within the context of their cancer diagnosis, a differential diagnosis with particular attention paid to the potential for other comorbid sleep and psychological disorders, and the influence of other medical conditions and/or current medications. It is also important to also ask the patient to identify what their goals for treatment are in the first session. This can help to either tailor their treatment plan accordingly or begin the process of adjusting an unrealistic expectation. The collective information gained from the clinical interview and sleep diary is essential to explain how the treatment plan has been tailored to address the unique features of their insomnia. It is also helpful to have the patient note in their sleep diary any cancer-related symptoms which may impact their sleep (e.g., other medications, pain, hot flashes, nocturia). In the case of concomitant steroid use during chemotherapy or other treatments, education should be provided on how these medications can impact sleep.

Sleep restriction and stimulus control

Patient understanding of the treatment rationale for using sleep restriction and stimulus control, the safety of these for use in cancer survivors, and how these techniques will work to address their specific sleep concerns is essential. The therapist should spend time explaining the two-process model of sleep, the impact of arousal, and the 3P model of insomnia using examples from the patient's experience. After ensuring patient understanding, the therapist should review the patient's sleep diary and discuss how to implement sleep restriction based on their total sleep time and circadian preference. Using a collaborative approach means that the therapist should start by having the patient suggest a preferred wake-up time and then calculate a time to bed based on that. This initial bedtime can be unappealing to the patient, which leads them to suggest an earlier wake-up time. Having the patient make these determinations with the expert guidance of the therapist encourages adherence.

Using a sleep efficiency cutoff of greater than or equal to 90% as the indicator for increasing the sleep window may not be a realistic goal for many cancer survivors. By nature of their condition, they may have multiple chronic comorbidities that interfere with sleep. As a result, a sleep efficiency of 85% may be more appropriate for use in cancer survivors. Further, the therapist may choose to increase the sleep window in 30-min increments as opposed to 15. This serves the purpose of efficiently increasing total sleep time as a means of improving daytime function. Should a 30-min increase result in worse sleep efficiency, remaining at the previous weeks' sleep window for another week, or increasing the sleep window by 15 min may be considered. A sleep efficiency between 80% and 84% suggests that the patient may benefit from another week at the prescribed sleep window whereas a sleep efficiency of less than 80% suggests a tighter sleep restriction should be considered. Considering the often-compromised physical health of people diagnosed with cancer, a total time in bed of 5 h is the minimum amount recommended for the sleep window.

The traditional recommendation of eliminating naps may also need to be revised if the individual is currently undergoing cancer treatment. In this case, naps should be limited, taken in the bed, and performed early in the day. The duration of the nap may need to be individually tailored depending on where the individual is in their treatment cycles. If the goal is to consolidate sleep over the 24 h, naps and daytime sleep should be taken into account when determining patient total sleep time to set time in bed restriction. For example, 6 h sleep at night but 1-h nap during the day would be consolidated into a TIB of 7 h. If daytime naps are helpful to retain, this should not be considered when determining a nighttime sleep window.

Sleep compression may be preferred for individuals who are undergoing cancer treatment, have significant impairment from comorbid conditions, or have a great deal of anxiety when presented with sleep restriction instructions. It is important that the patient be willing to engage with stimulus control during the sleep compression period to minimize further reinforcing the bed's association with wakefulness. The therapist should explain that this gentler process may increase the time it takes to see results with the procedures to reduce the likelihood the patient will get discouraged. Efforts to force sleep should be discouraged and instead, treatment should focus on coping with the temporary sleeplessness as an attempt to avoid additional sleep-related anxiety. Short-term use of sleeping medication may be indicated for use during this time.

Cancer-related fatigue and/or cognitive distortions may make sleep restriction more difficult or unappealing. Many cancer survivors find it hard to distinguish fatigue from sleepiness. This lack of definitional clarity is not a surprise considering that a cancer diagnosis and treatment can be a direct cause of both sleepiness and fatigue. Psychoeducation can help cancer survivors conceptualize sleepiness as the propensity to fall asleep and fatigue as low levels of physical or mental energy, both of which require different strategies to mitigate. In the case of a patient who finds sleep restriction too difficult or anxiety-provoking, cognitive restructuring can be used to address the consequences of the fear of a later bedtime with the intention of transitioning to more of a sleep restriction program. A program of energy generation through behavioral activation (i.e., activities that increase feelings of energy) to manage daytime fatigue rather than energy conservation (i.e., managing energy output through scheduling rest, pacing) may be recommended. Behavioral activation can differ by a patient and may include regular moderate exercise, properly timed light exposure, and social support. See Table 2 for a list of potential energy generating activities that you can build on. In addition to informal circadian entrainment with a regular wake up time and other zeitgebers, the use of

TABLE 2 10 suggested energy generation activities.

Energy Generation Activities
1. Go for a brisk walk or do 10 jumping jacks
2. Watch a movie or show that makes you laugh
3. Call a friend who has a positive attitude and ask about their day
4. Get sunlight or exposure to other means of bright light
5. Optimize your diet
6. Do something that will make you feel like you accomplished something
7. Make time to show gratitude to yourself or someone else
8. Drink a glass of water
9. Listen to upbeat music (and sing along)
10. Smile at other people

light therapy in the morning hours has some evidence of efficacy for reducing cancer-related fatigue (Johnson et al., 2018; Redd et al., 2014; Wu et al., 2018), which may have the additional effect of improving mood.

Stimulus control has some unique features in the context of cancer. For some patients, the bed can become associated with feeling unwell if it was where they spent time being sick and recovering from cancer, in addition to being conditioned with wakefulness. This can increase negative feelings or reminders of cancer while in bed. For others, the bed is associated with feeling safe or comforted which can lead patients to spend more time in bed in an effort to cultivate these feelings. In both of these situations, these feelings need to be identified because they can drive counterproductive behaviors. Potential remedies include making changes to the bed and bedroom to make the setting physically different than what it was when the individual was acutely ill and making other areas of the environment more comfortable. For cancer survivors with significant comorbid pain or other health conditions, those currently hospitalized or recovering from acute illness, and those who it may be unsafe to get out of bed at the night, stimulus control may be contraindicated. In this case, it is recommended that the patient make clear behavioral distinctions when they are in bed but not sleeping during the day by staying on top of the blankets, sitting upright, changing into their clothes for the day, and exposing themselves to daylight. At night, instead of getting out of bed, they are asked to remain in dim light but sit up, stop "trying" to sleep, and engage in something pleasant and relaxing until they feel sleepy, at which time they can lay down again.

Cognitive restructuring

Cognitive restructuring is critical in correcting unrealistic expectations and misattributions. Specific cognitive restructuring targets include the reduction of sleep effort, worry, and catastrophic predictions of the impact of insomnia on functioning and health, and helplessness in the face of insomnia. Strategies to address these maladaptive cognitions can include education, collaborative discovery using thought records, Socratic questioning, cost–benefit analyses, and behavioral experiments. The Sleep Diary is an invaluable tool to provide the patient with evidence contrary to their held belief.

Beginning in the first session, the clinician should pay particular attention to the thoughts and behaviors that may indicate increased sleep effort and maladaptive coping strategies, and how these may influence adherence to sleep restriction and stimulus control. These thoughts and behaviors may include a preoccupation with sleep during the day, the avoidance of certain behaviors due to or in anticipation of poor sleep, intrusive thoughts about the impact of sleep on functioning, clock watching, going to bed early in an effort to allow more time for sleep, and spending more time in bed in the morning in an effort to catch up on sleep. Formal measures of sleep effort [i.e., Glasgow Sleep Effort Scale (Broomfield & Espie, 2005)] or dysfunctional sleep beliefs [i.e., Dysfunctional Beliefs and Attitudes about Sleep (Morin, Vallieres, & Ivers, 2007)] can complement the informal assessment of maladaptive sleep beliefs and behaviors that are amenable to cognitive restructuring.

One of the most challenging beliefs that cancer survivors may express is a fear that poor sleep may increase the chances that their cancer will re-occur or get worse. A recent study, adapting the Dysfunctional Beliefs and Attitudes about Sleep scale for cancer survivors, added two cancer-specific items (Youn et al., 2020). These specific cancer-related sleep beliefs are: "My immune system will have serious problems if I don't go to sleep at a certain time" and "If I don't sleep well at night, my cancer may recur or metastasize" (Chung, Youn, & Choi, 2017). The difficulty with challenging these beliefs is that there may be some merit in this concern. While there is still more we have to learn about the relationship between insomnia and cancer and not all research is consistent, evidence is accumulating that insomnia may be a risk factor for the development of cancer (Fang, Miao, Chen, Sithole, & Chung, 2015; Sen et al., 2017), the aggressiveness of the disease (Liang et al., 2020; Wiggins et al., 2020), and may negatively influence recovery (Bach, Kalder, & Kostev, 2020; Ge et al., 2019; Palesh et al., 2014). The message that sleep is essential for health is reinforced by other healthcare providers and the media encouraging cancer survivors to "get enough sleep." Unfortunately, for someone with insomnia, these messages only serve to increase sleep and health-related anxiety and efforts to force sleep which ultimately reinforces insomnia. When engaging in Socratic questioning and the downward arrow technique to discover sleep-related fears, one might find that a fear of cancer recurrence may be at the core of their sleep-related worries. It is best to validate this concern while carefully introducing the suggestion that there are many other health behaviors that the patient has more control over that influence cancer incidence and recovery, such as levels of physical activity and nutrition. It can also be helpful to use this concern to encourage engagement with the CBT-I techniques. This requires that the patient agree that the short-term discomfort associated with sleep restriction and stimulus control is necessary to ensure that insomnia does not remain a factor that may influence their long-term health.

It is also not uncommon for cancer survivors to use busyness and distraction during the day to actively avoid engaging with difficult emotions, particularly fears of cancer recurrence. Unfortunately, these feelings tend to reoccur when the patient is trying to sleep or awake during the night. This can create extra emotional arousal and prompt them to engage in distraction techniques while in bed (e.g., device use, watching TV) which can further perpetuate insomnia. It may be helpful to work with the patient to develop the skills to process their cancer experience, which can include designating a time during the day as a "clear your head time," during which they address their worries so they do not interfere with sleep at night.

It is also important to challenge the belief in the benefits of "rest" versus "sleep." Many cancer survivors will remain in bed if awake during the night because of a belief that "at least the body is resting." This belief can be identified as irrational considering that there is no reason that resting in bed would be more restorative than resting in other locations. Further, the patient may have a fear that if they get out of bed, it will make it even less likely that they will be able to return to sleep. This fear is typically driven by past experiences where the patient got out of bed but instead of engaging in pleasant, sedentary, and relaxing activities in dim light, they may have engaged in arousal-producing activities that promoted wakefulness. These experiences serve to reinforce their belief that getting out of bed will result in sleeplessness. The belief in the benefits of staying in bed to "rest" may be best challenged using a behavioral experiment wherein they agree to get out of bed on certain nights and remain in bed on others to evaluate the comparative impact. It may also be addressed using cognitive restructuring to explore the accuracy of perceiving the experience to be restful when in reality they are likely feeling frustrated and/or defeated, calculating the number of hours until they have to get up for the day, or perhaps falling in and out of light and restless sleep.

Relaxation strategies

An important component of CBT-I in cancer survivors is the implementation of a prebed "buffer zone." This is 60–90 min before the designated sleep window where the patient is instructed to engage in activities that are pleasant, relaxing, sedentary, and can be performed in dim light. The patient and therapist collaboratively develop these recommended activities when planning the sleep window. These activities need to be individualized based on the interests of the patient but may include: reading a book on something other than a backlit device, doing puzzles or crosswords, or engaging in self-care activities (e.g., taking a bath, painting nails). Listening to music, an audiobook, or a podcast has the added benefit of being able to be performed with one's eyes closed, which can enhance their capacity to enhance relaxation. Many patients, although initially reluctant, grow to value the buffer zone as the protected time that they have been told they can use for things that they enjoy as opposed to feeling pressure to use the time in the service of others.

Some patients also benefit from practicing some form of relaxation as a way to reduce arousal before bed or if they wake up during the night, though this is not recommended as a standalone treatment. In addition to physical relaxation, this can serve the purpose of distracting the mind from habitual activity, worries, etc. Progressive muscle relaxation or autogenic training can be used to promote relaxation; however, it may be contraindicated in those cancer survivors who have peripheral neuropathy or lymphedema caused by cancer treatments. Similarly, diaphragmatic breathing may be stress-inducing for lung cancer because of the potential limited ability to take a deep breath and feelings of oxygen desaturation or suffocation. Working with the patient to develop a guided imagery scene from a pleasant memory can also be practiced for the purpose of promoting relaxation. Such a scene is potentiated when it includes aspects that engage as many senses as possible (visual, tactile, auditory, olfactory, and gustatory). The therapist may want to have the patient develop a script that can be reviewed and revised with the therapist and then practiced until the scene can be brought to mind easily. Patients may have some familiarity with other meditation or body scan techniques that can be incorporated into the buffer zone or when awake in bed. Any of these relaxation techniques can be incorporated into the stimulus control instructions provided that the patient can use the relaxation procedures in bed to promote sleep. All of the strategies work by decreasing physical and cognitive arousal, so if the patient experiences increased stress by focusing on the body part impacted by cancer, they can choose alternate techniques (PMR, breathing, visualization, body scan). If the relaxation techniques do not help facilitate sleep, they should be practiced outside of the bed for the purpose of reducing arousal and not facilitating sleep.

Relapse prevention

Cancer is considered a chronic disease as a result of the increases in survival time and the number of patients who will live longer with the disease. The chronicity of cancer increases the potential risk for a relapse of insomnia. With time, the patient may begin to relax some of the routines that helped improve their sleep. This is expected. However, the patient should be encouraged to continue to get bright light in the morning and darkness at night, avoid backlit devices in the prebed hours, keep their wakeup time consistent, and never, ever "try" to sleep. These behaviors, if kept, will reduce the likelihood of an insomnia relapse.

The time leading up to cancer-related scans or testing procedures may be triggers for increased anxiety which can lead to trouble sleeping. Helping patients anticipate these times and providing them with strategies to manage their anxiety and cope with short-term sleep disruption may reduce the likelihood of an insomnia relapse. Further to this, the therapist can remind the patient that they now have the skills and knowledge to prevent a relapse of insomnia or reapply the techniques should the bout of insomnia last longer than 5 or so days.

Summary

Nearly half of cancer survivors experience problems with sleep before diagnosis, which can worsen during treatment, and for the remaining survivors, a cancer diagnosis and treatment can serve as the precipitant for insomnia. We have good evidence that CBT-I is an effective intervention for cancer survivors and there are many ways to adapt it for use in patients who are currently undergoing cancer treatment and/or unable to access a provider. While cancer can (and does) bring additional considerations and complications to the treatment of insomnia, providers should feel confident that CBT-I can, and should, be delivered to individuals with cancer as a way to improve their overall physical and emotional recovery.

References

American Cancer Society. (2019). *Cancer treatment & survivorship facts & figures 2019–2021* (Retrieved from Atlanta). American Cancer Society.

Ancoli-Israel, S. (2009). Recognition and treatment of sleep disturbances in cancer. *Journal of Clinical Oncology, 27*(35), 5864–5866.

Ancoli-Israel, S., Liu, L., Rissling, M., Natarajan, L., Neikrug, A. B., Palmer, B. W., et al. (2014). Sleep, fatigue, depression, and circadian activity rhythms in women with breast cancer before and after treatment: A 1-year longitudinal study. *Support Care Cancer, 22*(9), 2535–2545. https://doi.org/10.1007/s00520-014-2204-5.

Arndt, V., Merx, H., Stegmaier, C., Ziegler, H., & Brenner, H. (2005). Persistence of restrictions in quality of life from the first to the third year after diagnosis in women with breast cancer. *Journal of Clinical Oncology, 23*(22), 4945–4953.

Aydın Sayılan, A., Kulakaç, N., & Sayılan, S. (2020). The effects of noise levels on pain, anxiety, and sleep in patients. *Nursing in Critical Care*. https://doi.org/10.1111/nicc.12525 (1478-5153 (electronic)).

Bach, L., Kalder, M., & Kostev, K. (2020). Depression and sleep disorders are associated with early mortality in women with breast cancer in the United Kingdom. *Journal of Psychiatric Research*. https://doi.org/10.1016/j.jpsychires.2020.11.036 (1879-1379 (electronic)).

Balachandran, D. D., Faiz, S., Bashoura, L., & Manzullo, E. (2013). Cancer-related fatigue and sleep disorders. *Sleep Medicine Clinics, 8*(2), 229–234.

Banks, S., & Dinges, D. F. (2007). Behavioral and physiological consequences of sleep restriction. *Journal of Clinical Sleep Medicine, 3*(5), 519–528. Retrieved from https://www.ncbi.nlm.nih.gov/pmc/articles/PMC1978335/pdf/jcsm.3.5.519.pdf.

Banthia, R., Malcarne, V. L., Ko, C. M., Varni, J. W., & Sadler, G. R. (2009). Fatigued breast cancer survivors: The role of sleep quality, depressed mood, stage and age. *Psychology & Health, 24*(8), 965–980. https://doi.org/10.1080/08870440802110831.

Barsevick, A. M., Irwin, M. R., Hinds, P., Miller, A., Berger, A., Jacobsen, P., et al. (2013). Recommendations for high-priority research on cancer-related fatigue in children and adults.

Journal of the National Cancer Institute, 105(19), 1432–1440. https://doi.org/10.1093/jnci/djt242.

Beck, S. L., Berger, A. M., Barsevick, A. M., Wong, B., Stewart, K. A., & Dudley, W. N. (2010). Sleep quality after initial chemotherapy for breast cancer. *Support Care Cancer, 18*(6), 679–689. https://doi.org/10.1007/s00520-009-0662-y.

Blask, D. E., Hill, S. M., Dauchy, R. T., Xiang, S., Yuan, L., Duplessis, T., et al. (2011). Circadian regulation of molecular, dietary, and metabolic signaling mechanisms of human breast cancer growth by the nocturnal melatonin signal and the consequences of its disruption by light at night. *Journal of Pineal Research, 51*(3), 259–269.

Bower, J. E. (2014). Cancer-related fatigue—Mechanisms, risk factors, and treatments. *Nature Reviews. Clinical Oncology, 11*(10). https://doi.org/10.1038/nrclinonc.2014.127.

Broomfield, N. M., & Espie, C. A. (2005). Towards a valid, reliable measure of sleep effort. *Journal of Sleep Research, 14*(4), 401–407. https://doi.org/10.1111/j.1365-2869.2005.00481.x.

Burse, N. R., Bhuiyan, N., Mama, S. K., & Schmitz, K. H. (2020). Physical activity barriers and resources among black women with a history of breast and endometrial cancer: A systematic review. *Journal of Cancer Survivorship, 14*(4), 556–577. https://doi.org/10.1007/s11764-020-00873-z.

Caplette-Gingras, A., Savard, J., Savard, M.-H., & Ivers, H. (2013). Is insomnia associated with cognitive impairments in breast cancer patients? *Behavioral Sleep Medicine, 11*(4), 239–257.

Casault, L., Savard, J., Ivers, H., & Savard, M. H. (2015). A randomized-controlled trial of an early minimal cognitive-behavioural therapy for insomnia comorbid with cancer. *Behaviour Research and Therapy, 67*, 45–54. https://doi.org/10.1016/j.brat.2015.02.003.

Casault, L., Savard, J., Ivers, H., Savard, M. H., & Simard, S. (2012). Utilization of hypnotic medication in the context of cancer: Predictors and frequency of use. *Support Care Cancer, 20*(6), 1203–1210. https://doi.org/10.1007/s00520-011-1199-4.

Cash, E., Sephton, S., Chagpar, A., Spiegel, D., Rebholz, W., Zimmaro, L., et al. (2015). Circadian disruption and biomarkers of tumor progression in breast cancer patients awaiting surgery. *Brain, Behavior, and Immunity, 48*, 102–114.

Chen, M. L., Yu, C. T., & Yang, C. H. (2008). Sleep disturbances and quality of life in lung cancer patients undergoing chemotherapy. *Lung Cancer, 62*(3), 391–400. https://doi.org/10.1016/j.lungcan.2008.03.016.

Chung, S., Youn, S., & Choi, B. (2017). Assessment of cancer-related dysfunctional beliefs about sleep for evaluating sleep disturbance in cancer patients. *Sleep Medicine Research, 8*(2), 98–101. https://doi.org/10.17241/smr.2017.00073.

Cillessen, L., Johannsen, M., Speckens, A. E. M., & Zachariae, R. (2019). Mindfulness-based interventions for psychological and physical health outcomes in cancer patients and survivors: A systematic review and meta-analysis of randomized controlled trials. *Psychooncology, 28*(12), 2257–2269. https://doi.org/10.1002/pon.5214.

Davidson, J. R., MacLean, A. W., Brundage, M. D., & Schulze, K. (2002). Sleep disturbance in cancer patients. *Social Science & Medicine, 54*(9), 1309–1321. https://doi.org/10.1016/s0277-9536(01)00043-0.

Desai, K., Mao, J. J., Su, I., Demichele, A., Li, Q., Xie, S. X., et al. (2013). Prevalence and risk factors for insomnia among breast cancer patients on aromatase inhibitors. *Support Care Cancer, 21*(1), 43–51. https://doi.org/10.1007/s00520-012-1490-z.

Dimsdale, J. E., Norman, D., DeJardin, D., & Wallace, M. S. (2007). The effect of opioids on sleep architecture. *Journal of Clinical Sleep Medicine, 3*, 33–36 (1550-9389 (print)).

Drake, C. L., Pillai, V., & Roth, T. (2014). Stress and sleep reactivity: A prospective investigation of the stress-diathesis model of insomnia. *Sleep, 37*(8), 1295–1304. https://doi.org/10.5665/sleep.3916.

Dzierzewski, J. M., Dautovich, N., & Ravyts, S. (2018). Sleep and cognition in older adults. *Sleep Medicine Clinics, 13*(1), 93–106. https://doi.org/10.1016/j.jsmc.2017.09.009.

Enderlin, C. A., Coleman, E. A., Cole, C., Richards, K. C., Hutchins, L. F., & Sherman, A. C. (2010). Sleep across chemotherapy treatment: A growing concern for women older than 50 with breast cancer. *Oncology Nursing Forum, 37*(4), 461–A463. https://doi.org/10.1188/10.ONF.461-468.

Engstrom, C. A., Strohl, R. A., Rose, L., Lewandowski, L., & Stefanek, M. E. (1999). Sleep alterations in cancer patients. *Cancer Nursing, 22*(2), 143–148. Retrieved from https://www.ncbi.nlm.nih.gov/pubmed/10217030.

Espie, C. A., Fleming, L., Cassidy, J., Samuel, L., Taylor, L. M., White, C. A., et al. (2008). Randomized controlled clinical effectiveness trial of cognitive behavior therapy compared with treatment as usual for persistent insomnia in patients with cancer. *Journal of Clinical Oncology, 26*(28), 4651–4658. https://doi.org/10.1200/JCO.2007.13.9006.

Fang, H.-F., Miao, N.-F., Chen, C.-D., Sithole, T., & Chung, M.-H. (2015). Risk of cancer in patients with insomnia, parasomnia, and obstructive sleep apnea: A Nationwide nested case-control study. *Journal of Cancer, 6*(11), 1140–1147. https://doi.org/10.7150/jca.12490.

Filipski, E., King, V. M., Li, X., Granda, T. G., Mormont, M.-C., Claustrat, B., et al. (2003). Disruption of circadian coordination accelerates malignant growth in mice. *Pathologie Biologie, 51*(4), 216–219.

Filipski, E., Li, X. M., & Lévi, F. (2006). Disruption of circadian coordination and malignant growth. *Cancer Causes & Control, 17*(4), 509–514.

Fleming, L., Gillespie, S., & Espie, C. A. (2010). The development and impact of insomnia on cancer survivors: A qualitative analysis. *Psychooncology, 19*(9), 991–996. https://doi.org/10.1002/pon.1652.

Fleming, L., Randell, K., Harvey, C. J., & Espie, C. A. (2014). Does cognitive behaviour therapy for insomnia reduce clinical levels of fatigue, anxiety and depression in cancer patients? *Psychooncology, 23*(6), 679–684. https://doi.org/10.1002/pon.3468.

Fuller, J. T., Hartland, M. C., Maloney, L. T., & Davison, K. (2018). Therapeutic effects of aerobic and resistance exercises for cancer survivors: A systematic review of meta-analyses of clinical trials. *British Journal of Sports Medicine, 52*(20), 1311. https://doi.org/10.1136/bjsports-2017-098285.

Garland, S. N., Barg, F. K., Cakouros, B., Gehrman, P., DuHamel, K. N., & Mao, J. J. (2018). A qualitative examination of the factors related to the development and maintenance of insomnia in cancer survivors. *Palliative & Supportive Care*, 1–6. https://doi.org/10.1017/S1478951518000135.

Garland, S. N., Roscoe, J. A., Heckler, C. E., Barilla, H., Gehrman, P., Findley, J. C., et al. (2016). Effects of armodafinil and cognitive behavior therapy for insomnia on sleep continuity and daytime sleepiness in cancer survivors. *Sleep Medicine, 20*, 18–24. https://doi.org/10.1016/j.sleep.2015.12.010.

Garland, S. N., Vargas, I., Grandner, M. A., & Perlis, M. L. (2018). Treating insomnia in patients with comorbid psychiatric disorders: A focused review. *Canadian Psychology/Psychologie Canadienne, 59*(2), 176–186. https://doi.org/10.1037/cap0000141.

Ge, L., Guyatt, G., Tian, J., Pan, B., Chang, Y., Chen, Y., et al. (2019). Insomnia and risk of mortality from all-cause, cardiovascular disease, and cancer: Systematic review and meta-analysis of prospective cohort studies. *Sleep Medicine Reviews.* https://doi.org/10.1016/j.smrv.2019.101215 (1532-2955 (electronic)).

Global Burden of Disease Cancer Collaboration, Fitzmaurice, C., Allen, C., Barber, R. M., Barregard, L., Bhutta, Z. A., et al. (2017). Global, regional, and National Cancer Incidence, mortality, years of life lost, years lived with disability, and disability-adjusted life-years for 32 Cancer groups, 1990 to 2015: A systematic analysis for the global burden of disease study. *JAMA Oncology, 3*(4), 524–548. https://doi.org/10.1001/jamaoncol.2016.5688.

Goldman, S. E., Hall, M., Boudreau, R., Matthews, K. A., Cauley, J. A., Ancoli-Israel, S., et al. (2008). Association between nighttime sleep and napping in older adults. *Sleep, 31*(5), 733–740. https://doi.org/10.1093/sleep/31.5.733.

Gonzalez, B. D., Small, B. J., Cases, M. G., Williams, N. L., Fishman, M. N., Jacobsen, P. B., et al. (2018). Sleep disturbance in men receiving androgen deprivation therapy for prostate cancer: The role of hot flashes and nocturia. *Cancer, 124*(3), 499–506. https://doi.org/10.1002/cncr.31024.

Gooneratne, N. S., Dean, G. E., Rogers, A. E., Nkwuo, J. E., Coyne, J. C., & Kaiser, L. R. (2007). Sleep and quality of life in long-term lung cancer survivors. *Lung Cancer, 58*(3), 403–410. https://doi.org/10.1016/j.lungcan.2007.07.011.

Gottfried, T., Kamer, I., Salant, I., Urban, D., Lawrence, Y. R., Onn, A., et al. (2020). Self-reported sleep quality as prognostic for survival in lung cancer patients. *Cancer Management and Research, 12*, 313–321. https://doi.org/10.2147/CMAR.S234523.

Graham, K., Ogbuji, G., Williams, Z., Crain, M., Rolin, B., Juala, J., et al. (2020). Challenges of implementing the choosing wisely guideline to promote sleep and rest at night for hospitalized patients. *Journal of Nursing Care Quality*. https://doi.org/10.1097/NCQ.0000000000000494.

Gress, K. L., Charipova, K., Kaye, A. D., Viswanath, O., & Urits, I. (2020). An overview of current recommendations and options for the Management of Cancer Pain: A comprehensive review. *Oncology and Therapy, 8*(2), 251–259. https://doi.org/10.1007/s40487-020-00128-y.

Harrington, C. B., Hansen, J. A., Moskowitz, M., Todd, B. L., & Feuerstein, M. (2010). It's not over when it's over: Long-term symptoms in cancer survivors—A systematic review. *International Journal of Psychiatry in Medicine, 40*(2), 163–181. https://doi.org/10.2190/PM.40.2.c.

Hartman, S. J., Marinac, C. R., Natarajan, L., & Patterson, R. E. (2015). Lifestyle factors associated with cognitive functioning in breast cancer survivors. *Psychooncology, 24*(6), 669–675. https://doi.org/10.1002/pon.3626.

Harvey, C.-J., Gehrman, P., & Espie, C. A. (2014). Who is predisposed to insomnia: A review of familial aggregation, stress-reactivity, personality and coping style. *Sleep Medicine Reviews, 18*(3), 237–247. https://doi.org/10.1016/j.smrv.2013.11.004.

Heckler, C. E., Garland, S. N., Peoples, A. R., Perlis, M. L., Shayne, M., Morrow, G. R., et al. (2016). Cognitive behavioral therapy for insomnia, but not armodafinil, improves fatigue in cancer survivors with insomnia: A randomized placebo-controlled trial. *Support Care Cancer, 24*(5), 2059–2066. https://doi.org/10.1007/s00520-015-2996-y.

Henderson, F. M., Cross, A. J., & Baraniak, A. R. (2019). 'A new normal with chemobrain': Experiences of the impact of chemotherapy-related cognitive deficits in long-term breast cancer survivors. *Health Psychology Open, 6*(1). https://doi.org/10.1177/2055102919832234, 2055102919832234.

Henry, N. L., Azzouz, F., Desta, Z., Li, L., Nguyen, A. T., Lemler, S., et al. (2012). Predictors of aromatase inhibitor discontinuation as a result of treatment-emergent symptoms in early-stage breast cancer. *Journal of Clinical Oncology: Official Journal of the American Society of Clinical Oncology, 30*(9), 936–942. https://doi.org/10.1200/JCO.2011.38.0261.

Hoang, H. T. X., Molassiotis, A., Chan, C. W., Nguyen, T. H., & Liep Nguyen, V. (2019). New-onset insomnia among cancer patients undergoing chemotherapy: Prevalence, risk factors, and its correlation with other symptoms. *Sleep & Breathing*. https://doi.org/10.1007/s11325-019-01839-x.

Hoogland, A. I., Bulls, H. W., Gonzalez, B. D., Small, B. J., Liu, L., Pidala, J., et al. (2019). Circadian rhythmicity as a predictor of quality of life in allogeneic hematopoietic cell transplant patients. *Journal of Pain and Symptom Management, 57*(5), 952–960. e951 https://doi.org/10.1016/j.jpainsymman.2019.01.015.

Howell, D., Keller-Olaman, S., Oliver, T. K., Hack, T. F., Broadfield, L., Biggs, K., et al. (2013). A pan-Canadian practice guideline and algorithm: Screening, assessment, and supportive care of adults with cancer-related fatigue. *Current Oncology, 20*(3), e233–e246. https://doi.org/10.3747/co.20.1302.

Howell, D., Oliver, T. K., Keller-Olaman, S., Davidson, J., Garland, S., Samuels, C., et al. (2013). A Pan-Canadian practice guideline: Prevention, screening, assessment, and treatment of sleep disturbances in adults with cancer. *Support Care Cancer, 21*(10), 2695–2706. https://doi.org/10.1007/s00520-013-1823-6.

Howell, D., Oliver, T. K., Keller-Olaman, S., Davidson, J. R., Garland, S., Samuels, C., et al. (2014). Sleep disturbance in adults with cancer: A systematic review of evidence for best practices in assessment and management for clinical practice. *Annals of Oncology, 25*(4), 791–800. https://doi.org/10.1093/annonc/mdt506.

Innominato, P. F., Focan, C., Gorlia, T., Moreau, T., Garufi, C., Waterhouse, J., et al. (2009). Circadian rhythm in rest and activity: A biological correlate of quality of life and a predictor of survival in patients with metastatic colorectal cancer. *Cancer Research, 69*(11), 4700–4707.

Innominato, P. F., Spiegel, D., Ulusakarya, A., Giacchetti, S., Bjarnason, G. A., Levi, F., et al. (2015). Subjective sleep and overall survival in chemotherapy-naive patients with metastatic colorectal cancer. *Sleep Medicine, 16*(3), 391–398. https://doi.org/10.1016/j.sleep.2014.10.022.

Ismail, M. F., Lavelle, C., & Cassidy, E. M. (2017). Steroid-induced mental disorders in cancer patients: A systematic review. *Future Oncology, 13*(29), 2719–2731. https://doi.org/10.2217/fon-2017-0306.

Janelsins, M. C., Kesler, S. R., Ahles, T. A., & Morrow, G. R. (2014). Prevalence, mechanisms, and management of cancer-related cognitive impairment. *International Review of Psychiatry, 26*(1), 102–113. Retrieved from https://www.ncbi.nlm.nih.gov/pmc/articles/PMC4084673/pdf/nihms-568444.pdf.

Jarrin, D. C., Morin, C. M., Rochefort, A., Ivers, H., Dauvilliers, Y. A., Savard, J., et al. (2017). Familial aggregation of insomnia. *Sleep, 40*(2). https://doi.org/10.1093/sleep/zsw053.

Jason, L. A., Evans, M., Brown, M., & Porter, N. (2010). What is fatigue? Pathological and non-pathological fatigue. *PM & R: The Journal of Injury, Function, and Rehabilitation, 2*(5), 327–331. https://doi.org/10.1016/j.pmrj.2010.03.028.

Jean-Pierre, P., Grandner, M. A., Garland, S. N., Henry, E., Jean-Louis, G., & Burish, T. G. (2015). Self-reported memory problems in adult-onset cancer survivors: Effects of cardiovascular disease and insomnia. *Sleep Medicine, 16*(7), 845–849. https://doi.org/10.1016/j.sleep.2015.02.531.

Jim, H. S., Jacobsen, P. B., Phillips, K. M., Wenham, R. M., Roberts, W., & Small, B. J. (2013). Lagged relationships among sleep disturbance, fatigue, and depressed mood during chemotherapy. *Health Psychology, 32*(7), 768–774. https://doi.org/10.1037/a0031322.

Johnson, J. A., Garland, S. N., Carlson, L. E., Savard, J., Simpson, J. S. A., Ancoli-Israel, S., et al. (2018). Bright light therapy improves cancer-related fatigue in cancer survivors: A randomized controlled trial. *Journal of Cancer Survivorship, 12*(2), 206–215. https://doi.org/10.1007/s11764-017-0659-3.

Johnson, J. A., Rash, J. A., Campbell, T. S., Savard, J., Gehrman, P. R., Perlis, M., et al. (2016). A systematic review and meta-analysis of randomized controlled trials of cognitive behavior therapy for insomnia (CBT-I) in cancer survivors. *Sleep Medicine Reviews, 27*, 20–28. https://doi.org/10.1016/j.smrv.2015.07.001.

Kamdar, B. B., King, L. M., Collop, N. A., Sakamuri, S., Colantuoni, E., Neufeld, K. J., et al. (2013). The effect of a quality improvement intervention on perceived sleep quality and cognition in a medical ICU. *Critical Care Medicine, 41*(3), 800–809. https://doi.org/10.1097/CCM.0b013e3182746442.

Kaplan, M., Mahon, S. M., Lubejko, B. G., & Ginex, P. K. (2020). Hot flashes: Clinical summary of the ONS guidelines™ for cancer treatment-related hot flashes in women with breast cancer and men with prostate cancer. *Clinical Journal of Oncology Nursing, 24*(4), 430–433. https://doi.org/10.1188/20.CJON.430-433.

LeBlanc, M., Merette, C., Savard, J., Ivers, H., Baillargeon, L., & Morin, C. M. (2009). Incidence and risk factors of insomnia in a population-based sample. *Sleep, 32*(8), 1027–1037. Retrieved from https://www.ncbi.nlm.nih.gov/pubmed/19725254.

Leysen, L., Lahousse, A., Nijs, J., Adriaenssens, N., Mairesse, O., Ivakhnov, S., et al. (2019). Prevalence and risk factors of sleep disturbances in breast cancer survivors: Systematic review and meta-analyses. *Support Care Cancer, 27*(12), 4401–4433. https://doi.org/10.1007/s00520-019-04936-5.

Li, N., Otomaru, T., & Taniguchi, H. (2017). Sleep quality in long-term survivors of head and neck cancer: Preliminary findings. *Support Care Cancer, 25*(12), 3741–3748. https://doi.org/10.1007/s00520-017-3804-7.

Liang, X., Harris, H., Hendryx, M., Shadyab, A. H., Hale, L., Li, Y., et al. (2020). Sleep characteristics and risk of ovarian cancer among postmenopausal women. *Cancer Prevention Research*. https://doi.org/10.1158/1940-6207.CAPR-20-0174.

Lowery-Allison, A. E., Passik, S. D., Cribbet, M. R., Reinsel, R. A., O'Sullivan, B., Norton, L., et al. (2018). Sleep problems in breast cancer survivors 1-10 years posttreatment. *Palliative & Supportive Care, 16*(3), 325–334. https://doi.org/10.1017/S1478951517000311.

Maguire, R., Drummond, F. J., Hanly, P., Gavin, A., & Sharp, L. (2019). Problems sleeping with prostate cancer: Exploring possible risk factors for sleep disturbance in a population-based sample of survivors. *Supportive Care in Cancer*. https://doi.org/10.1007/s00520-018-4633-z.

Matthews, E., Carter, P., Page, M., Dean, G., & Berger, A. (2018). Sleep-wake disturbance: A systematic review of evidence-based interventions for management in patients with cancer. *Clinical Journal of Oncology Nursing, 22*(1), 37–52. https://doi.org/10.1188/18.CJON.37-52.

Mercier, J., Ivers, H., & Savard, J. (2018). A non-inferiority randomized controlled trial comparing a home-based aerobic exercise program to a self-administered cognitive-behavioral therapy for insomnia in cancer patients. *Sleep, 41*(10). https://doi.org/10.1093/sleep/zsy149.

Miaskowski, C., & Lee, K. A. (1999). Pain, fatigue, and sleep disturbances in oncology outpatients receiving radiation therapy for bone metastasis: A pilot study. *Journal of Pain and Symptom Management, 17*(5), 320–332. Retrieved from https://www.ncbi.nlm.nih.gov/pubmed/10355211.

Minton, O., Berger, A., Barsevick, A., Cramp, F., Goedendorp, M., Mitchell, S. A., et al. (2013). Cancer-related fatigue and its impact on functioning. *Cancer, 119*(Suppl 11), 2124–2130. https://doi.org/10.1002/cncr.28058.

Moore, T. A., Berger, A. M., & Dizona, P. (2011). Sleep aid use during and following breast cancer adjuvant chemotherapy. *Psychooncology, 20*(3), 321–325. https://doi.org/10.1002/pon.1756.

Morin, C. M. (2017). Issues and challenges in implementing clinical practice guideline for the management of chronic insomnia. *Journal of Sleep Research, 26*(6), 673–674. https://doi.org/10.1111/jsr.12639.

Morin, C. M., & Jarrin, D. C. (2013). Epidemiology of insomnia: Prevalence, course, risk factors, and public health burden. *Sleep Medicine Clinics, 8*(3), 281–297. https://doi.org/10.1016/j.jsmc.2013.05.002.

Morin, C. M., Vallieres, A., & Ivers, H. (2007). Dysfunctional beliefs and attitudes about sleep (DBAS): Validation of a brief version (DBAS-16). *Sleep, 30*(11), 1547–1554. Retrieved from https://www.ncbi.nlm.nih.gov/pubmed/18041487.

Moscetti, L., Agnese, F. M., Sperduti, I., Fabrizio, N., Frittelli, P., Massari, A., et al. (2015). Adjuvant aromatase inhibitor therapy in early breast cancer: What factors lead patients to discontinue treatment? *Tumori, 101*(5), 469–473. https://doi.org/10.5301/tj.5000376.

Mouch, C. A., Baskin, A. S., Yearling, R., Miller, J., & Dossett, L. A. (2020). Sleep patterns and quality among inpatients recovering from elective surgery: A mixed-method study. *The Journal of Surgical Research, 254*, 268–274.

Otte, J. L., Carpenter, J. S., Russell, K. M., Bigatti, S., & Champion, V. L. (2010). Prevalence, severity, and correlates of sleep-wake disturbances in long-term breast cancer survivors. *Journal of Pain and Symptom Management, 39*(3), 535–547. https://doi.org/10.1016/j.jpainsymman.2009.07.004.

Owens, J. F., Buysse, D. J., Hall, M., Kamarck, T. W., Lee, L., Strollo, P. J., et al. (2010). Napping, nighttime sleep, and cardiovascular risk factors in mid-life adults. *Journal of Clinical Sleep Medicine, 6*(4), 330–335. Retrieved from https://www.ncbi.nlm.nih.gov/pubmed/20726280.

Palesh, O., Aldridge-Gerry, A., Zeitzer, J. M., Koopman, C., Neri, E., Giese-Davis, J., et al. (2014). Actigraphy-measured sleep disruption as a predictor of survival among women with advanced breast cancer. *Sleep, 37*(5), 837–842. https://doi.org/10.5665/sleep.3642.

Palesh, O. G., Collie, K., Batiuchok, D., Tilston, J., Koopman, C., Perlis, M. L., et al. (2007). A longitudinal study of depression, pain, and stress as predictors of sleep disturbance among women with metastatic breast cancer. *Biological Psychology, 75*(1), 37–44. https://doi.org/10.1016/j.biopsycho.2006.11.002.

Palesh, O., Peppone, L., Innominato, P. F., Janelsins, M., Jeong, M., Sprod, L., et al. (2012). Prevalence, putative mechanisms, and current management of sleep problems during chemotherapy for cancer. *Natural Science Sleep, 4*, 151–162. https://doi.org/10.2147/NSS.S18895.

Palesh, O. G., Roscoe, J. A., Mustian, K. M., Roth, T., Savard, J., Ancoli-Israel, S., et al. (2010). Prevalence, demographics, and psychological associations of sleep disruption in patients with cancer: University of Rochester Cancer Center-Community Clinical Oncology Program. *Journal of Clinical Oncology, 28*(2), 292–298. https://doi.org/10.1200/JCO.2009.22.5011.

Palesh, O., Scheiber, C., Kesler, S., Gevirtz, R., Heckler, C., Guido, J. J., et al. (2019). Secondary outcomes of a behavioral sleep intervention: A randomized clinical trial. *Health Psychology, 38*(3), 196–205. https://doi.org/10.1037/hea0000700.

Palesh, O., Scheiber, C., Kesler, S., Janelsins, M. C., Guido, J. J., Heckler, C., et al. (2018). Feasibility and acceptability of brief behavioral therapy for cancer-related insomnia: Effects on insomnia and circadian rhythm during chemotherapy: A phase II randomised multicentre controlled trial. *British Journal of Cancer, 119*(3), 274–281. https://doi.org/10.1038/s41416-018-0154-2.

Palesh, O., Solomon, N., Hofmeister, E., Jo, B., Shen, H., Cassidy-Eagle, E., et al. (2020). A novel approach to management of sleep-associated problems in patients with breast cancer (MOSAIC) during chemotherapy: A pilot study. *Sleep, 43*(10). https://doi.org/10.1093/sleep/zsaa070.

Paltiel, O., Marzec-Boguslawska, A., Soskolne, V., Massalha, S., Avitzour, M., Pfeffer, R., et al. (2004). Use of tranquilizers and sleeping pills among cancer patients is associated with a poorer quality of life. *Quality of Life Research, 13*(10), 1699–1706. https://doi.org/10.1007/s11136-004-8745-1.

Payne, J., Piper, B., Rabinowitz, I., & Zimmerman, B. (2006). Biomarkers, fatigue, sleep, and depressive symptoms in women with breast cancer: A pilot study. *Oncology Nursing Forum, 33*(4), 775–783. https://doi.org/10.1188/06.ONF.775-783.

Peoples, A. R., Garland, S. N., Perlis, M. L., Savard, J., Heckler, C. E., Kamen, C. S., et al. (2017). Effects of cognitive behavioral therapy for insomnia and armodafinil on quality of life in cancer survivors: A randomized placebo-controlled trial. *Journal of Cancer Survivorship, 11*(3), 401–409. https://doi.org/10.1007/s11764-017-0597-0.

Peoples, A. R., Garland, S. N., Pigeon, W. R., Perlis, M. L., Wolf, J. R., Heffner, K. L., et al. (2019). Cognitive behavioral therapy for insomnia reduces depression in cancer survivors. *Journal of Clinical Sleep Medicine, 15*(1), 129–137. https://doi.org/10.5664/jcsm.7586.

Poort, H., Peters, M., van der Graaf, W. T. A., Nieuwkerk, P. T., van de Wouw, A. J., Nijhuis-van der Sanden, M. W. G., et al. (2020). Cognitive behavioral therapy or graded exercise therapy compared with usual care for severe fatigue in patients with advanced cancer during treatment: A randomized controlled trial. *Annals of Oncology*, *31*(1), 115–122. https://doi.org/10.1016/j.annonc.2019.09.002.

Portenoy, R. K., Thaler, H. T., Kornblith, A. B., Lepore, J. M., Friedlander-Klar, H., Coyle, N., et al. (1994). Symptom prevalence, characteristics and distress in a cancer population. *Quality of Life Research*, *3*(3), 183–189. Retrieved from https://www.ncbi.nlm.nih.gov/pubmed/7920492.

Qu, D., Zhang, Z., Yu, X., Zhao, J., Qiu, F., & Huang, J. (2016). Psychotropic drugs for the management of cancer-related fatigue: A systematic review and meta-analysis. *European Journal of Cancer Care*, *25*(6), 970–979. https://doi.org/10.1111/ecc.12397.

Quesnel, C., Savard, J., Simard, S., Ivers, H., & Morin, C. M. (2003). Efficacy of cognitive-behavioral therapy for insomnia in women treated for nonmetastatic breast cancer. *Journal of Consulting and Clinical Psychology*, *71*(1), 189–200.

Redd, W. H., Valdimarsdottir, H., Wu, L. M., Winkel, G., Byrne, E. E., Beltre, M. A., et al. (2014). Systematic light exposure in the treatment of cancer-related fatigue: A preliminary study. *Psychooncology*, *23*(12), 1431–1434. https://doi.org/10.1002/pon.3553.

Reynolds-Cowie, P., & Fleming, L. (2020). Living with persistent insomnia after cancer: A qualitative analysis of impact and management. *British Journal of Health Psychology*. https://doi.org/10.1111/bjhp.12446, e12446.

Roscoe, J. A., Garland, S. N., Heckler, C. E., Perlis, M. L., Peoples, A. R., Shayne, M., et al. (2015). Randomized placebo-controlled trial of cognitive behavioral therapy and armodafinil for insomnia after cancer treatment. *Journal of Clinical Oncology*, *33*(2), 165–171. https://doi.org/10.1200/JCO.2014.57.6769.

Roscoe, J. A., Kaufman, M. E., Matteson-Rusby, S. E., Palesh, O. G., Ryan, J. L., Kohli, S., et al. (2007). Cancer-related fatigue and sleep disorders. *The Oncologist*, *12*(Suppl 1), 35–42. https://doi.org/10.1634/theoncologist.12-S1-35.

Santoso, A. M. M., Jansen, F., de Vries, R., Leemans, C. R., van Straten, A., & Verdonck-de Leeuw, I. M. (2019). Prevalence of sleep disturbances among head and neck cancer patients: A systematic review and meta-analysis. *Sleep Medicine Reviews*, *47*, 62–73. https://doi.org/10.1016/j.smrv.2019.06.003.

Savard, J., Ivers, H., Savard, M. H., & Morin, C. M. (2014). Is a video-based cognitive behavioral therapy for insomnia as efficacious as a professionally administered treatment in breast cancer? Results of a randomized controlled trial. *Sleep*, *37*(8), 1305–1314. https://doi.org/10.5665/sleep.3918.

Savard, J., Ivers, H., Savard, M. H., & Morin, C. M. (2015). Cancer treatments and their side effects are associated with aggravation of insomnia: Results of a longitudinal study. *Cancer*, *121*(10), 1703–1711. https://doi.org/10.1002/cncr.29244.

Savard, J., Ivers, H., Savard, M. H., & Morin, C. M. (2016). Long-term effects of two formats of cognitive behavioral therapy for insomnia comorbid with breast Cancer. *Sleep*, *39*(4), 813–823. https://doi.org/10.5665/sleep.5634.

Savard, J., Ivers, H., Villa, J., Caplette-Gingras, A., & Morin, C. M. (2011). Natural course of insomnia comorbid with cancer: An 18-month longitudinal study. *Journal of Clinical Oncology*, *29*(26), 3580–3586. https://doi.org/10.1200/JCO.2010.33.2247.

Savard, J., & Morin, C. M. (2001). Insomnia in the context of cancer: A review of a neglected problem. *Journal of Clinical Oncology*, *19*(3), 895–908.

Savard, J., & Savard, M.-H. (2013). Insomnia and cancer: Prevalence, nature, and nonpharmacologic treatment. *Sleep Medicine Clinics*, *8*(3), 373–387. https://doi.org/10.1016/j.jsmc.2013.04.006.

Savard, M. H., Savard, J., Trudel-Fitzgerald, C., Ivers, H., & Quesnel, C. (2011). Changes in self-reported hot flashes and their association with concurrent changes in insomnia symptoms among women with breast cancer. *Menopause*, *18*(9), 985–993. https://doi.org/10.1097/gme.0b013e31820db6a1.

Savard, J., Simard, S., Hervouet, S., Ivers, H., Lacombe, L., & Fradet, Y. (2005). Insomnia in men treated with radical prostatectomy for prostate cancer. *Psychooncology, 14*(2), 147–156. https://doi.org/10.1002/pon.830.

Savard, J., Villa, J., Ivers, H., Simard, S., & Morin, C. M. (2009). Prevalence, natural course, and risk factors of insomnia comorbid with cancer over a 2-month period. *Journal of Clinical Oncology, 27*(31), 5233–5239. https://doi.org/10.1200/JCO.2008.21.6333.

Schieber, K., Niecke, A., Geiser, F., Erim, Y., Bergelt, C., Buttner-Teleaga, A., et al. (2019). The course of cancer-related insomnia: don't expect it to disappear after cancer treatment. *Sleep Medicine, 58*, 107–113. https://doi.org/10.1016/j.sleep.2019.02.018.

Schmidt, M. E., Wiskemann, J., & Steindorf, K. (2018). Quality of life, problems, and needs of disease-free breast cancer survivors 5 years after diagnosis. *Quality of Life Research: an International Journal of Quality of Life Aspects of Treatment, Care and Rehabilitation, 27*(8), 2077–2086. https://doi.org/10.1007/s11136-018-1866-8.

Sen, A., Opdahl, S., Strand, L. B., Vatten, L. J., Laugsand, L. E., & Janszky, I. (2017). Insomnia and the risk of breast Cancer: The HUNT study. *Psychosomatic Medicine, 79*(4), 461–468. https://doi.org/10.1097/PSY.0000000000000417.

Sharma, N., Hansen, C. H., O'Connor, M., Thekkumpurath, P., Walker, J., Kleiboer, A., et al. (2012). Sleep problems in cancer patients: Prevalence and association with distress and pain. *Psychooncology, 21*(9), 1003–1009. https://doi.org/10.1002/pon.2004.

Shi, Q., Giordano, S. H., Lu, H., Saleeba, A. K., Malveaux, D., & Cleeland, C. S. (2013). Anastrozole-associated joint pain and other symptoms in patients with breast cancer. *The Journal of Pain, 14*(3), 290–296. https://doi.org/10.1016/j.jpain.2012.11.010.

Siegel, R., Naishadham, D., & Jemal, A. (2012). Cancer statistics, 2012. *CA: A Cancer Journal for Clinicians, 62*(1), 10–29. https://doi.org/10.3322/caac.20138.

Slade, A. N., Waters, M. R., & Serrano, N. A. (2019). Long-term sleep disturbance and prescription sleep aid use among cancer survivors in the United States. *Supportive Care in Cancer*. https://doi.org/10.1007/s00520-019-04849-3.

Stepanski, E. J., Walker, M. S., Schwartzberg, L. S., Blakely, L. J., Ong, J. C., & Houts, A. C. (2009). The relation of trouble sleeping, depressed mood, pain, and fatigue in patients with cancer. *Journal of Clinical Sleep Medicine, 5*(2), 132–136. Retrieved from https://www.ncbi.nlm.nih.gov/pubmed/19968046.

Trudel-Fitzgerald, C., Savard, J., & Ivers, H. (2013). Which symptoms come first? Exploration of temporal relationships between cancer-related symptoms over an 18-month period. *Annals of Behavioral Medicine, 45*(3), 329–337. https://doi.org/10.1007/s12160-012-9459-1.

Van Onselen, C., Paul, S. M., Lee, K., Dunn, L., Aouizerat, B. E., West, C., et al. (2013). Trajectories of sleep disturbance and daytime sleepiness in women before and after surgery for breast cancer. *Journal of Pain and Symptom Management, 45*(2), 244–260. https://doi.org/10.1016/j.jpainsymman.2012.02.020.

Von Ah, D., & Tallman, E. F. (2015). Perceived cognitive function in breast cancer survivors: Evaluating relationships with objective cognitive performance and other symptoms using the functional assessment of cancer therapy-cognitive function instrument. *Journal of Pain and Symptom Management, 49*(4), 697–706. https://doi.org/10.1016/j.jpainsymman.2014.08.012.

Wiggins, E. A.-O., Oyekunle, T., Howard, L. E., Markt, S. C., Mucci, L. A., Bliwise, D. L., et al. (2020). Sleep quality and prostate cancer aggressiveness: Results from the REDUCE trial. *The Prostate, 80*, 1304–1313. https://doi.org/10.1002/pros.24052.

Wu, L. M., Amidi, A., Valdimarsdottir, H., Ancoli-Israel, S., Liu, L., Winkel, G., et al. (2018). The effect of systematic light exposure on sleep in a mixed Group of Fatigued Cancer Survivors. *Journal of Clinical Sleep Medicine, 14*(1), 31–39. https://doi.org/10.5664/jcsm.6874.

Xu, S., Thompson, W., Ancoli-Israel, S., Liu, L., Palmer, B., & Natarajan, L. (2018). Cognition, quality-of-life, and symptom clusters in breast cancer: Using Bayesian networks to elucidate complex relationships. *Psychooncology, 27*(3), 802–809. https://doi.org/10.1002/pon.4571.

Youn, S., Kim, C., Lee, J., Yeo, S., Suh, S., & Chung, S. (2020). Development of dysfunctional beliefs and attitude about sleep scale for cancer patients. *Behavioral Sleep Medicine*, *18*(3), 287–297. https://doi.org/10.1080/15402002.2019.1578773.

Zachariae, R., Amidi, A., Damholdt, M. F., Clausen, C. D. R., Dahlgaard, J., Lord, H., et al. (2018). Internet-delivered cognitive-behavioral therapy for insomnia in breast cancer survivors: A randomized controlled trial. *Journal of the National Cancer Institute*, *110*(8), 880–887. https://doi.org/10.1093/jnci/djx293.

Zhang, B., & Wing, Y. K. (2006). Sex differences in insomnia: A meta-analysis. *Sleep*, *29*(1), 85–93. https://doi.org/10.1093/sleep/29.1.85.

Zhou, E. S., Clark, K., Recklitis, C. J., Obenchain, R., & Loscalzo, M. (2018). Sleepless from the get go: Sleep problems prior to initiating cancer treatment. *International Journal of Behavioral Medicine*, *25*(5), 502–516. https://doi.org/10.1007/s12529-018-9715-2.

Zhou, E. S., Partridge, A. H., Syrjala, K. L., Michaud, A. L., & Recklitis, C. J. (2017). Evaluation and treatment of insomnia in adult cancer survivorship programs. *Journal of Cancer Survivorship*, *11*(1), 74–79. https://doi.org/10.1007/s11764-016-0564-1.

CHAPTER

13

CBT-I in patients with a history of traumatic brain injury

Erin A. Almklov[a], *Guadalupe L. Rivera*[b], *and Henry Orff*[a,c]

[a]VA San Diego Healthcare System-Center of Excellence for Stress and Mental Health (CESAMH), San Diego, CA, United States, [b]VA San Diego Healthcare System, San Diego, CA, United States, [c]Clinical Health Sciences, Department of Psychiatry, UCSD, San Diego, CA, United States

Prevalence and societal costs of traumatic brain injury (TBI)

TBI is a common injury and a leading cause of disability in the United States. Each year an estimated 1.5 million Americans sustain a TBI. As a consequence of these injuries, 230,000 people are hospitalized and survive; 50,000 people die; and 80,000–90,000 people experience the onset of long-term disability. An estimated 5.3 million men, women, and children are living with a permanent TBI-related disability in the United States today. While TBIs occur in all age groups, the risk is highest among adolescents, young adults, and people older than 75 years. The risk of TBI among males is twice that of females. The major causes of TBI are motor vehicle accidents, violence, and falls (Cassidy et al., 2004). Motor vehicle accidents are the leading cause of TBI-related hospitalization. Violence, especially suicidal behavior and assaults that involve firearms, is the primary cause of TBI-related death. Falls are the main cause of TBI among the elderly (Amyot et al., 2015).

Adapting Cognitive Behavioral Therapy for Insomnia
https://doi.org/10.1016/B978-0-12-822872-2.00009-8

TBI is also observed in higher prevalence in certain subsections of the general population. Sports and recreational activities account for approximately 10% of TBIs. Among children and adolescents, sports and recreational activities contribute to over 21% of all TBI and are a leading cause of TBI-related emergency department visits. Sustaining an injury while playing sports can range from a mild physical trauma such as a scalp contusion or laceration to severe TBI with concurrent bleeding in the brain or coma. Concussions frequently affect athletes in both contact and noncontact sports and are considered to be diffuse brain injuries that induce alterations of mental status. A concussion may result from shaking the brain within the skull and, if severe, can cause shearing injuries to nerve fibers and neurons. It is estimated that as many as 3.8 million sports and recreation-related concussions occur in the United States annually, yet as many as 50% may go unreported. Repeat injury also is more likely among sports participants, and athletes are particularly vulnerable to second impact syndrome—an acute, sometimes fatal, brain swelling that occurs when a second concussion is sustained before complete recovery from a previous concussion. TBI is also more prevalent among military service members. TBI was identified as the "signature wound" of the Iraq and Afghanistan Wars, with increased rates of TBI attributed to blast-related injuries (Gondusky & Reiter, 2005). About 19% of returning service members report having experienced a TBI while deployed (Tanielian & Jaycox, 2008). Other investigations have suggested that over 60% of service members exposed to a blast may have had a TBI (Warden, 2006), and approximately 67% of post-9/11 veterans seen in polytrauma settings show evidence of possible persistent postconcussive symptoms secondary to a TBI (Lew et al., 2009). With regard to injury severity, the reported incidence of mild, moderate, and severe TBIs in these veterans has varied among investigations. According to the Defense and Veterans Brain Injury Center, 266,810 TBI cases were documented from 2000 to 2012, 82.4% of which were mild, 8.2% of which were moderate, and 1% of which were severe (DVBIC, 2013).

TBI can have both short-term and long-term effects. The annual economic burden in the United States is approximately $48 billion. For the millions of Americans who live with a TBI-related disability, the financial cost is only part of the burden. The long-term impairments and disabilities associated with TBI can be substantial. However, unlike a broken leg, TBI-related disabilities are often not readily apparent to the public. Thus, TBI has become known as the invisible epidemic. These disabilities, arising from damage to cognitive, emotional, sensory, and motor systems often permanently alter a person's vocational aspirations and have profound effects on social functioning, family relationships, and quality of life.

How to recognize and diagnose TBI

TBI is an alteration in brain function or other brain pathology due to the impact of contact forces, including rapid acceleration, deceleration, or collision, manifesting as an altered state of consciousness, neurological deficits, and/or amnesia (Katz, Cohen, & Alexander, 2015). Based on factors assessed at the time of injury [e.g., level of responsiveness, duration of loss of consciousness, and duration of posttraumatic amnesia], as well as findings on neuroimaging, TBIs are classified as mild (mTBI or concussion), moderate, or severe (Bryan, 2013). Injury severity is traditionally based on Glasgow Coma Scale (GCS), duration of loss of consciousness (LOC) or alteration of consciousness (AOC), posttraumatic amnesia (PTA), and brain imaging results. While different definitions exist, mild TBI (mTBI) is often characterized by GCS of 13–15, brief AOC or LOC, and PTA for less than 1h. In patients with typical mTBI, standard acute structural imaging studies such as head computed tomography scans do not show hemorrhage or other overt structural abnormalities, although specialized imaging techniques may show evidence of diffuse axonal injury (Amyot et al., 2015). Of the annual cases of traumatic brain injury, the World Health Organization estimates that 70%–90% of those are mild TBI (Cassidy et al., 2004). mTBI is a remarkably heterogeneous condition with varying degrees of clinical manifestations and severity. In addition, patient-level characteristics such as age, sex, premorbid headaches, and psychiatric conditions likely influence resilience and vulnerability to mTBI sequelae, as well as the persistence of postconcussive symptoms. mTBI can lead to a wide array of cognitive, emotional, and somatic symptoms (Bergersen, Halvorsen, Tryti, Taylor, & Olsen, 2017). Common symptoms associated with mTBI include headache, dizziness, nausea/vomiting, impaired balance and coordination, tinnitus, vision changes, memory impairment, concentration deficits, fatigue, and sleep disturbance (Ling, Hardy, & Zetterberg, 2015; Viola-Saltzman & Watson, 2012). The majority of patients achieve complete resolution of symptoms quickly after a mTBI, but 10%–20% may develop persisting symptoms (Bergersen et al., 2017). Moderate TBI is diagnosed when GCS is 9–12, LOC is 1–24h, PTA for 1–24h of the TBI, and abnormal brain imaging results. Moderate injuries are characterized by more serious effects, which may include the inability to communicate, partial paralysis, and diminished cognitive skills. Patients with moderate brain injuries are more likely to recover than those with a more severe prognosis and may benefit from rehabilitation therapy. Severe TBI can be defined as GCS of 3–8, LOC or coma for more than 24h, and abnormal brain imaging. Such injuries are more likely to result in longstanding disability. Some common concepts for clinicians to know include:

Types of injury: Forces causing brain injury include the head being struck by an object, the head striking an object, the brain undergoing an acceleration/deceleration movement without direct external trauma to the head, a foreign body penetrating the brain, and forces generated from events such as a blast or explosion.

Open Versus *Closed TBI:* A TBI resulting from something passing through the skull into the brain, such as a bullet or fragments from an explosion, is called a penetrating or open head injury. A TBI that results from either an object hitting the head or from the head hitting something forcefully, such as the dashboard of a car, is referred to as a nonpenetrating or closed head injury.

Focal Lesions: These occur primarily in moderate to severe TBI and include hematoma, hemorrhage, and cortical contusion.

Diffuse Axonal Injury (DAI): This results from rotational acceleration–deceleration forces or blast waves (e.g., IED blast). The axonal injury occurs from shearing forces causing microhemorrhages, cerebral edema, increased intracranial pressure, and/or changes in cerebral blood flow leading to hypoxia or anoxia.

Blast injuries: These occur as a result of rocket-propelled grenades, improvised explosive devices, explosively formed projectiles, land mines, artillery, rocket and mortar shells, and aerial bombs. Brain injury is common following blasts and can occur from multiple mechanisms—possibly from direct exposure to the over-pressurization wave, from the impact of blast-energized debris (both penetrating and nonpenetrating), from the individual being physically thrown into environmental hazards or from motor vehicle accidents triggered by the blast, and from inhalation of gases and vapors, or from anoxic injuries. Nonpenetrating concussive injuries may go undiagnosed and untreated as attention is focused on the more "visible" injuries.

Primary Versus *Secondary Injury:* Primary injury occurs during the initial trauma and results from mechanical injury. Secondary injury is caused by the physiologic responses to the initial injury. It often occurs more gradually and may include altered cellular, neurochemical, and metabolic responses.

Repeat Injury: Repeated mTBIs occurring over an extended period of time can result in cumulative neurological and cognitive deficits; and those occurring within a short period of time (i.e., hours, days, or weeks) can be catastrophic or fatal.

TBI Sequelae: Sequelae of TBI may resolve quickly, within minutes to hours after the event, or may persist longer. Some sequelae of TBI, particularly after moderate or severe injury may be permanent. Most signs and symptoms will manifest immediately following the event, but following more severe injury, other symptoms or complications may be delayed. There are many symptoms of TBI that can affect all aspects of functioning:

Emotional: Depression, anxiety, hopelessness, helplessness, lack of drive or initiation, irritability, emotional numbness, reduced confidence, and fear. The same exposures (e.g., combat or other traumatic events) that cause TBI may also result in other comorbidities, such as posttraumatic stress disorder (PTSD), pain conditions, acute stress reactions, and substance use/abuse.

Behavioral: Impatience, anger, frustration, confrontational behaviors, impulsivity, avoidance of situations or activities that feel uncomfortable, and withdrawal.

Physical: Headaches, chronic pain, fatigue, weakness or numbness, changes in vision, changes in hearing, other sensory changes (touch, taste, smell), vertigo, nausea, impairments in fine motor speed, balance, and coordination, and in sexual functioning.

Cognitive: Changes in attention, diminished memory, slowing down of mental processing, confusion, disorientation, changes in decision making, alterations in judgment, changes in the ability to plan and organize, changes in visual processing, difficulties with language comprehension or production, and increased distractibility. TBI can also increase the risk for conditions, such as Alzheimer's disease, Parkinson's disease, and other brain disorders, and can lead to serious health conditions such as epilepsy and sleep disorders.

Social: Changes in relationships, changed the ability to engage in hobbies and leisure activities, decreased ability to perform work or school, isolation/alienation from others.

Sleep: Notably, disturbed sleep is one of the most common complaints following TBI and worsens morbidity and long-term sequelae.

Individuals who experience mTBI are typically expected to show full recovery, with 80%–90% returning to preinjury levels of functioning in less than 90 days. This said, approximately 10%–20% of patients with mTBI do not recover within 90 days and develop what is typically referred to as postconcussive symptoms or syndrome (PCS). This group may continue to report symptoms (such as those listed above) for several months or years after their injury, often at levels of severity or in areas of functioning that are difficult to correlate with the nature, location, and severity of the original injury. While it is difficult to predict who will suffer from PCS, research suggests that women and older adults are at greater risk than men and younger individuals. In addition, repeated concussions and general medical history can affect PCS risk. Deterioration over time after mild TBI is uncommon, and in situations where patients have worsening complaints, psychological or social stressors should be evaluated. mTBI patients are more likely to develop insomnia than moderate/severe TBI patients and are therefore more likely to be encountered by a sleep

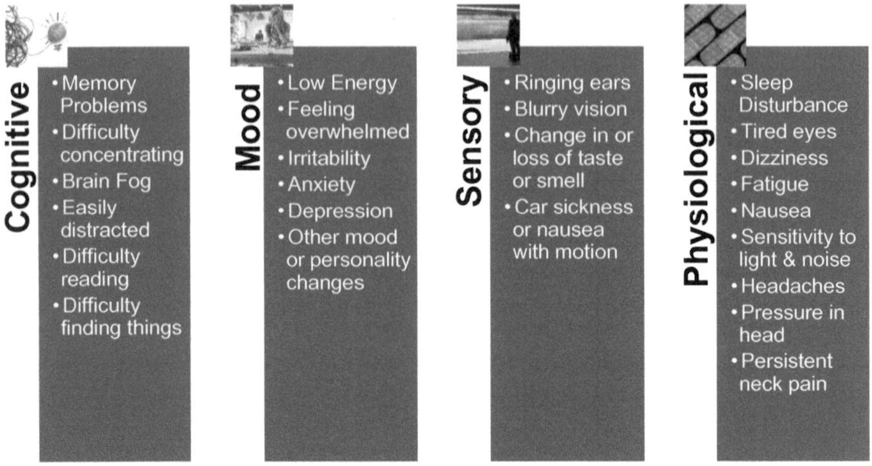

FIG. 1 Common postconcussive symptoms.

clinician in an outpatient clinic setting. Examples of common postconcussive symptoms can be found in Fig. 1.

Relationship of TBI and sleep disorders

One of the significant problems arising from TBI is that the biological rhythm of sleep is disrupted. Sleep–wake disturbances are among the most prevalent and persistent symptoms following TBI (Castriotta et al., 2007; Duclos et al., 2014; Orff, Ayalon, & Drummond, 2009; Sandsmark, Elliott, & Lim, 2017) with 30%–70% of individuals reporting difficulty in sleeping, altered sleep pattern, or need to sleep an unusually long amount following injury (Aoun, Rawal, Attarian, & Sahni, 2019; Castriotta et al., 2007). Sleep disturbance complicates recovery and the resolution of symptoms. Problems with sleep can result in symptoms similar to those caused by TBI itself and can also aggravate existing TBI symptoms. In addition, depression, anxiety, PTSD, and pain are common TBI comorbidities with substantial influence on sleep. For example, those with mTBI and PTSD tend to have greater sleep disturbances compared to those without PTSD.

Two types of TBI negatively impact sleep: contact injuries causing focal brain damage and acceleration/deceleration injuries causing more generalized brain damage. The type of sleep disturbance resulting from a closed head injury depends on the location of injury within sleep-regulating brain regions. Posttraumatic hypersomnia is seen when areas involving the maintenance of wakefulness are damaged. These regions include the brainstem reticular formation, posterior hypothalamus, and the area surrounding the third ventricle. High cervical cord lesions have also been known to cause sleepiness and obstructive sleep apnea (OSA).

Low cerebral spinal fluid (CSF) hypocretin-1 levels are found in most cases of narcolepsy with cataplexy. Most patients with moderate-to-severe TBI have low or intermediate hypocretin-1 levels in the acute injury phase. Hypocretin levels tend to normalize 6 months following the injury, which may explain why post-TBI sleepiness resolves in many over time. Coup (i.e., an injury resulting from a moving object impacting a stationary head)-contrecoup (i.e., an injury resulting from a moving head striking a stationary object) brain injury following head trauma occurs most frequently at the base of the skull in areas of bony irregularities (especially the sphenoid ridges), with consequent damage to the inferior frontal and anterior temporal regions, including the basal forebrain (an area involved in sleep initiation). As a result, insomnia is a common symptom following injuries of this mechanism. Closed head injury can also involve the suprachiasmatic nucleus (the body's biological clock) and/or its output tracts leading to disturbance of circadian rhythmicity with concomitant hypersomnia and insomnia. A variety of genes involved in inflammation, glial function, neuronal plasticity, immunity, and circadian rhythm are thought to have implications on sleep disturbance post-TBI as well (Imbach et al., 2015; Zeitzer, Friedman, & O'Hara, 2009). In addition, individuals with TBI tend to use more medications than the general population, including medications that cross the blood–brain barrier, such as antidepressants (Grima, Ponsford, Rajaratnam, Mansfield, & Pase, 2016; Yasseen, Colantonio, & Ratcliff, 2008), which may contribute to sleep deficits observed in those with TBI. Other secondary complications following TBI, such as medical and psychiatric comorbidities, may also contribute to sleeping difficulties (Gilbert, Kark, Gehrman, & Bogdanova, 2015; Lavigne, Khoury, Chauny, & Desautels, 2015; Tan et al., 2009; Wickwire et al., 2016).

Poor sleep may develop acutely following injury or emerge later during recovery (Mantua et al., 2018); it can last several years postinjury and is often described as one of the most debilitating consequences (Orff et al., 2009; Zhou & Greenwald, 2018). Predictors of persistent sleep disturbance following TBI included female gender, poor preinjury sleep quality, and symptoms of poor sleep or cognition within 2 weeks after injury (Sandsmark et al., 2017). Untreated sleep disturbances contribute to longer hospital stays, higher cost of rehabilitation, disability (Aoun et al., 2019; Thomas & Greenwald, 2018), morbidity, and long-term sequelae (Mathias & Alvaro, 2012; Wickwire et al., 2016) including memory and cognitive complaints, chronic pain, and psychological distress (Beetar, Guilmette, & Sparadeo, 1996; Boakye et al., 2016; Lavigne et al., 2015; Mahmood, Rapport, Hanks, & Fichtenberg, 2004; Martindale et al., 2017; Sandsmark et al., 2017; Theadom et al., 2016). Unfortunately, comorbid sleep disturbance has often been viewed as a symptom of mTBI, rather than as a modifiable factor that can potentially affect the rate and extent of recovery (Wickwire et al., 2016). In reality, many postconcussive symptoms, such as anxiety, headaches, fatigue, and irritability, can result from and exacerbate sleep disturbances in a vicious cycle (Wickwire et al., 2016).

Some research suggests that sleep problems are not dependent on injury severity. For example, sleep–wake disturbances have been reported in approximately 30%–70% of individuals with mild, moderate, or severe TBI up to 3 years postinjury (Sandsmark et al., 2017). However, several studies have shown that mTBI is associated with more sleep disturbances and complaints compared to moderate to severe TBI (Aoun et al., 2019; Bryan, 2013; Grima et al., 2016; Ouellet, Beaulieu-Bonneau, & Morin, 2006; Parcell, Ponsford, Rajaratnam, & Redman, 2006) possibly because those with mild TBI retain more self-awareness (Grima et al., 2016; Ponsford et al., 2012) or because those with severe TBI may perceive sleep disturbances as minor compared to other TBI sequelae (Aoun et al., 2019). Others have postulated that lesion location may be more important than TBI severity in predicting sleep outcomes, with damage to the sleep–wake centers causing the most sleep disturbance (Aoun et al., 2019; Grima et al., 2016; Ponsford et al., 2012).

Physiology: Sleep is central to learning and memory consolidation, brain development and restoration, and neuronal synaptic plasticity by eliminating weak connections and preserving strong connections within the synapses (Cirelli, 2012; Wickwire et al., 2016). Recent evidence demonstrates the importance of sleep for neural growth and plasticity (Cirelli, 2012; Wickwire et al., 2016). Moreover, sleep likely has a unique and neuroprotective role through the elimination of neurotoxic waste products that does not occur during wakefulness (Wickwire et al., 2016; Xie et al., 2013).

In virtually all mammalian species, sleep is composed of two distinct states: rapid eye movement (REM; in adult humans about 20% of the night) and non-REM (NREM; in adult humans about 80% of the night) sleep (Wickwire et al., 2016). NREM sleep is characterized by a progressive synchronization of electroencephalography (EEG) activity (NREM stages 1, 2, and 3) in parallel with an increase in arousal threshold. In contrast, REM sleep is characterized by EEG activation, rapid eye movements, and skeletal muscle atonia. These distinct states are hypothesized to perform independent and complementary physiologic and mental restorative functions (Assefa, Diaz-Abad, Wickwire, & Scharf, 2015; Wickwire et al., 2016). Observed changes of sleep in mTBI patients include increased stages 1 and 2 sleep (light sleep), decreased REM sleep (Lucke-Wold et al., 2015; Schreiber et al., 2008; Wilkinson et al., 2012; Zhou & Greenwald, 2018), longer sleep onset latencies, shorter total duration of sleep, and more nighttime awakenings than controls (Aoun et al., 2019).

Types of Sleep Disturbances: TBI is strongly associated with several clinically recognized sleep–wake disturbances. The most common sleep–wake disturbances are insomnia and hypersomnia/pleiosomnia (increased need for sleep), followed by sleep-related breathing disorder, circadian rhythm disorder, and parasomnia/movement disorders (Sandsmark et al., 2017). A recent meta-analysis of patients with TBI of mixed severity revealed that 50% of patients reported sleep complaints, and approximately 30% were diagnosed with a clinical sleep disorder (Mathias & Alvaro, 2012; Wickwire et al., 2016). Specifically, patients with TBI experienced high rates of insomnia (29%), hypersomnia (28%), and sleep apnea (25%) (Aoun et al., 2019).

Insomnia and TBI

Insomnia is characterized by poor sleep quantity or quality in the forms of delayed sleep onset, nocturnal awakenings with difficulty returning to sleep, waking too early, and not feeling rested despite adequate sleep opportunity. A required criterion for diagnosing insomnia of any form is that it leads to distress and subjective impairment during the day (Bolge, Doan, Kannan, & Baran, 2009; Zhou & Greenwald, 2018). Insomnia is important to address as it can have widespread effects on health and wellness and impede a patient's return to normal functioning. Insomnia has been associated with increased disability and delayed recovery from brain injury in workers independent of age, gender, and other psychiatric comorbidities (Aoun et al., 2019; Mollayeva et al., 2016). Insomnia symptoms are among the most commonly reported sleep complaints following TBI of all severities (Aoun et al., 2019; Bryan, 2013; Ouellet et al., 2006; Sandsmark et al., 2017) although it is more common following milder injury (Clinchot, Bogner, Mysiw, Fugate, & Corrigan, 1998; Collen, Orr, Lettieri, Carter, & Holley, 2012; Farrell-Carnahan et al., 2015; Ohayon, 2002; Ouellet et al., 2006; Ouellet, Savard, & Morin, 2004; Sandsmark et al., 2017; Theadom et al., 2015; Wickwire et al., 2016; Zhou & Greenwald, 2018). Estimates suggest 50% of TBI patients report symptoms and 29% meet diagnostic criteria for insomnia disorder, with sleep onset insomnia is especially prevalent among TBI patients (Fichtenberg, Putnam, Mann, Zafonte, & Millard, 2001; Fichtenberg, Zafonte, Putnam, Mann, & Millard, 2002; Kalmbach et al., 2018; Ouellet et al., 2006). The type of insomnia might also vary according to the number of TBIs. Following a first TBI, the most commonly reported complaint is sleep onset insomnia (Aoun et al., 2019). Following an additional TBI, sleep maintenance insomnia intensifies (Aoun et al., 2019; Bryan, 2013). In military personnel, the number of lifetime TBIs was found to be a significant predictor of insomnia severity even when controlling for depression, PTSD, and severity of concussion symptoms (Aoun et al., 2019; Bryan, 2013; Sandsmark et al., 2017).

A popular model of insomnia contains two components, a general predisposition to developing insomnia followed by an acute stressor (Zhou & Greenwald, 2018). There are various interpretations on how this model applies to TBI. In one interpretation, those suffering from insomnia post-TBI may have had previous episodes of insomnia or family history. The acute stressor would therefore be the TBI itself (Zhou & Greenwald, 2018). Another interpretation surmises that both aspects of the model may be affected by TBI because pathophysiological changes of the brain create a predisposition for insomnia while acute stressors come in the forms of comorbidities such as pain, depression, and anxiety (Viola-Saltzman & Musleh, 2016; Zeitzer et al., 2009; Zhou & Greenwald, 2018). TBI patients will also often experience multiple psychosocial stressors simultaneously such as inability to return to work, financial difficulties, redefined familial roles, and strained social relationships. Increased familial discord, marital problems, and litigation procedures have been documented with TBI patients and are obvious sources of significant stress (Ouellet et al., 2004; Zhou & Greenwald, 2018).

In addition to insomnia, many individuals exhibit hypersomnia or an increased need for sleep following TBI (Sandsmark et al., 2017; Sommerauer, Valko, Werth, & Baumann, 2013). For example, at 6 months post-TBI, individuals required 1–2 h more sleep (compared to healthy controls as measured by actigraphy), which positively correlated with injury severity (Imbach et al., 2015; Sandsmark et al., 2017); in another study, individuals also reported requiring 2 more hours of sleep in a 24-h period as compared to preinjury (Baumann, Werth, Stocker, Ludwig, & Bassetti, 2007; Sandsmark et al., 2017). Obstructive sleep apnea also occurs at substantially higher rates in patients with TBI than in the general population. Studies have reported OSA in 35%–61% of patients with TBI (Collen et al., 2012; Masel, Scheibel, Kimbark, & Kuna, 2001; Wickwire et al., 2016). In addition, patients with TBI with comorbid OSA experience greater neurocognitive impairments in memory and attention than those with similar TBI severity who do not have OSA (Wickwire et al., 2016; Wilde et al., 2007). Circadian rhythm sleep disturbances, most commonly identified by delayed sleep phase syndrome and irregular sleep–wake pattern, maybe especially prominent in the acute phase after TBI (Sandsmark et al., 2017).

Prognosis of mTBI is typically good with one study finding that almost all previously healthy adults (96%) return to work/normal activities within 1-year post-mTBI (Losoi et al., 2016; Zhou & Greenwald, 2018). Despite this prognosis, a large prospective cohort study discovered a that significant minority of patients after mild TBI, around 20%, are not functionally recovered even by 1 year postinjury (Imbach et al., 2015; McMahon et al., 2014). Sleep difficulty is one of the postconcussive symptoms that is assumed to resolve spontaneously over time. However, a study found that for veterans with mTBI, poor sleep quality lasted on average 6years postinjury and was independent of combat exposure, PTSD, mood disorders, anxiety, and substance use (Imbach et al., 2015; Martindale et al., 2017).

A growing body of research suggests that sleep health is associated with recovery of function after TBI. Patients in whom sleep–wake disturbances persist beyond the acute recovery period tend to have worse outcomes when followed longitudinally (Sandsmark et al., 2017). Studies have also shown that severity of sleep disturbances are associated with broad cognitive impairment (Kalmbach et al., 2018; Nakase-Richardson et al., 2016), posttraumatic amnesia (Kalmbach et al., 2018; Makley et al., 2009; Nakase-Richardson et al., 2013), postconcussion symptoms (Kalmbach et al., 2018; Kostyun, Milewski, & Hafeez, 2015), and global disability (Kalmbach et al., 2018; Mollayeva, Mollayeva, Shapiro, Cassidy, & Colantonio, 2016). TBI patients with aberrant sleep are more likely to suffer from headaches (Chaput, Giguère, Chauny, Denis, & Lavigne, 2009; Kalmbach et al., 2018) neurobehavioral deficits (Bloomfield, Espie, & Evans, 2010; Dean & Sterr, 2013; Kalmbach et al., 2018), and depression and other mood alterations (Kalmbach et al., 2018; Kempf, Werth, Kaiser, Bassetti, & Baumann, 2010; Ouellet & Morin, 2006). Notably, while sleep and mental health are interrelated, several studies suggest that sleep–wake disturbances impact clinical outcomes independent of associated mental health conditions (Sandsmark et al., 2017).

It needs to be emphasized that TBI is an event, not an illness. Whether TBI is directly causal to subsequent PCS or whether the path to PCS is mediated by other factors has been an ongoing debate in the field. In the traditional injury/illness model, the mTBI-PCS relationship is seen as a direct path with the injury being causally related to PCS. Conceptually, mTBI itself therefore would result in the impairment(s) observed in the concussed individual (see Fig. 2). In this model, therefore, mTBI would be the principal cause for the onset of insomnia (e.g., (Martindale et al., 2017).

Alternatively, Hoge et al. (2008), in an influential paper, determined that most if not all PCS are mediated by pain or PTSD symptoms resulting from mTBI. This model (see Fig. 3) has impacted the field in the way many

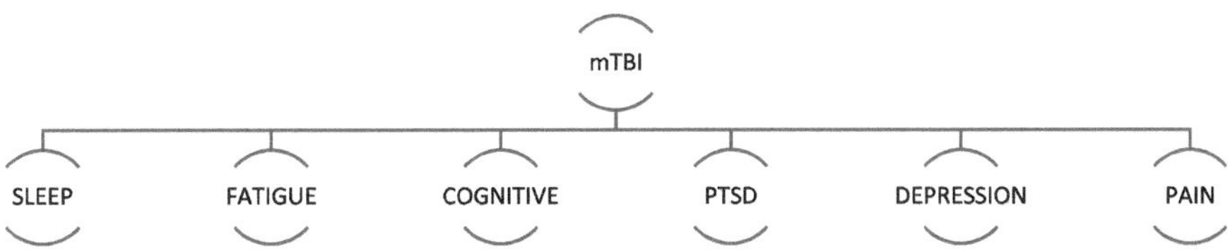

FIG. 2 Causal model of the relationship between mTBI and postconcussive symptoms.

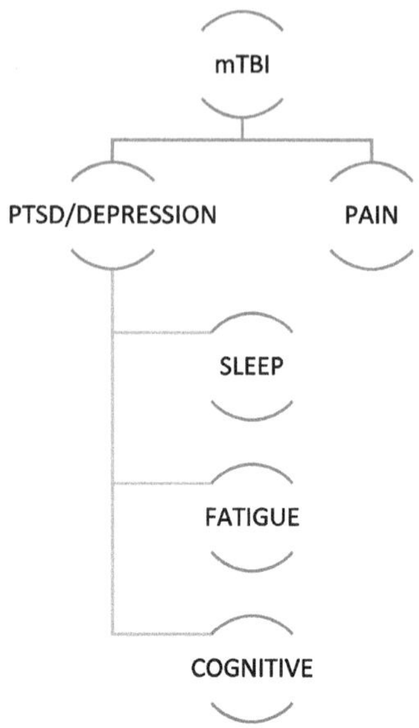

FIG. 3 Mediation model of the relationship between mTBI and postconcussive symptoms.

clinicians approach treatment of insomnia, viewing sleep problems as "secondary" to other "primary" concerns (especially PTSD). This model predicts that if one treats the "primary" disorder then concurrent improvement in the "secondary" should occur.

Finally, it should be noted that most studies of mTBI and PCS are cross-sectional and retrospective in nature. As such these investigations suffer from reporting and history biases, and it is often not possible to truly determine the cause–effect relationship between mTBI and any later development of PCS symptoms and/or whether such symptoms bore any relationship to the injury at all (e.g., sleep problems may have existed before the injury or developed in response to other stressors at a later time that were unrelated to the injury). It is not unsurprising therefore that the scientific literature has found conflicting results and associated models, given the often heterogeneous nature of the samples from which the data are drawn.

CBT-I in patients with TBI

Although CBT-I has demonstrated efficacy in several clinical populations (e.g., depression, pain), to date there is only one published case report (Ouellet & Morin, 2007) demonstrating the possible advantages of utilizing CBT-I in the context of mTBI. Other investigations using elements of CBT-I in the context of structured therapies for sleep problems in patients with mild–severe TBI have also shown promise for use of CBT-I in patients with a history of (Nguyen et al., 2017; Theadom et al., 2018; Wiseman-Hakes et al., 2013) TBI. Although the evidence points to CBT-I holding great potential to assist individuals with sleep problems, further clinical trials of CBT-I are needed to determine the efficacy of this treatment approach in mTBI and to explore the potential mental and physical health benefits that may result from improved sleep.

Modifications to CBT-I that may improve CBT-I treatment outcomes in patients with TBI

Given the complexity of medical and psychiatric comorbidities with which patients with mTBI might present to the clinic, a detailed summary of all potential modifications to CBT-I, which might need to be considered to enhance treatment outcomes would be challenging. To streamline these recommendations, PCS comorbidities described previously have been categorized into three main areas of clinical focus: Cognitive Deficits, Pain Symptoms, and Mental Health.

Note that since these topics are covered in greater detail in other chapters in this text, the following recommendations are abbreviated in nature. Also, note that CBT-I is very likely to be effective in treating insomnia in patients with a history of mTBI without modification(s), so the recommendations proposed may only be needed in specific and/or atypical cases where treatment response to traditional CBT-I appears muted or identified and significant barriers to treatment exist.

Cognitive deficits and TBI

Research shows a clear association between moderate to severe TBI and impaired cognitive functioning, with less of the association noted for mTBI and cognitive deficits (>6months postinjury) (Dikmen et al., 2009). Individuals with moderate/severe TBI often show greater problems with memory/attention and motor impairments (Testa, Malec, Moessner, & Brown, 2006) following injury. Research on patients with mTBI has found that at baseline, more than 20% showed deficits on tests of executive ability, complex attention, and cognitive flexibility (Barker-Collo et al., 2015). Additionally, up to 39% of mTBI patients may experience cognitive complaints 6months postinjury (Stulemeijer, Vos, Bleijenberg, & Van der Werf, 2007), mostly in areas of processing speed and executive functioning (Hall, Hall, & Chapman, 2005; King, 2003). In sum, sleep has been shown to mediate the relationship between severity of injury and recovery of cognitive function (Chiu, Lo, Chiang, & Tsai, 2014).

In instances where cognitive deficits are present, strategies to mitigate the impact of memory and/or concentration difficulties on CBT-I treatment will need to be prioritized. A patient recall is considered to be a key component of treatment adherence (Dong, Lee, & Harvey, 2017; Kessels, 2003) and as patients accurately recall only about one-third of the recommendations made during a CBT session (Lee & Harvey, 2015), the use of memory support strategies should help improve patient retention of health-related information (Dillon, 2012) and enhance treatment adherence (Cox, Tisdelle, & Culbert, 1988; Dong et al., 2017). Research has demonstrated that the incorporation of cognitive assistive strategies may enhance CBT-I treatment outcomes. For example, in one investigation of independent living seniors meeting diagnostic criteria for insomnia and mild cognitive impairment, adaptations to CBT-I were successfully employed (Cassidy-Eagle, Siebern, Unti, Glassman, & O'Hara, 2018). These adaptations included: adjustments to content, decreasing the amount of content covered and providing a brief, focused rationale for the treatment components leaving time for review and repetition of content covered, utilization of learning and memory aids to enhance understanding and retention, ensuring sufficient time and opportunity to review material and ask questions, adjusting the pace to account for changes in information processing, repeating key material and adding troubleshooting, and reminder calls between intervention session. Overall, seniors in the modified treatment condition showed a significant improvement in sleep (and select areas of cognitive performance). These results are encouraging and suggest that formal interventions such as Cognitive Symptom Management and Rehabilitation Therapy (CogSMART) could be integrated into CBT-I for individuals who require compensatory strategies to improve learning, memory, attention, and executive functioning in the context of treatment for sleep disturbance (Twamley, Jak, Delis, Bondi, & Lohr, 2014). CogSMART has been shown to improve cognition, functional capacity, neurobehavioral symptom severity, and quality of life in individuals with cognitive impairment associated with psychiatric illness and TBI (Caplan et al., 2015). Although cognitive support strategies should be helpful in the setting of more mild impairment(s), for individuals with more moderate to severe injuries, additional support for treatment such as involvement of the health care team and/or caregivers may be beneficial. In cases where the patient is unable to track sleep accurately with diaries, the use of assistive technologies such as apps and/or wearable devices might be employed to monitor sleep. Overall, cognitive support strategies may be particularly helpful to individuals with cognitive challenges following TBI; however, these techniques may also be useful for any patient who needs more structure or organizational support while receiving CBT-I.

Pain symptoms and TBI

Chronic pain is a common symptom related to TBI, even for mild injuries. 75.3% of patients with mTBI and 32.1% of those with moderate to severe TBI report pain symptoms (Nampiaparampil, 2008). Late-onset pain syndrome can also be associated with TBI, with symptoms appearing 6 months or more after the injury (Ofek & Defrin, 2007). Headache pain is reported in 57.8%–81% of adults (Nampiaparampil, 2008; Smith-Seemiller, Fow, Kant, & Franzen, 2003) and up to 87% of children (Kwan, Vo, Noel, & Yeates, 2018) following a TBI. Musculoskeletal pain is also a frequent concern (Lucas, 2015). The intensity of pain has also been shown to increase with comorbid mental illness (especially PTSD) and sleep disturbance (Balba et al., 2018).

Modifications to CBT-I in patients with pain may include incorporation of other empirically supported psychological interventions including Acceptance and Commitment Therapy (ACT) and traditional Cognitive-Behavioral Therapy (CBT). Complementary approaches may include acupuncture, mindfulness-based stress reduction, tai chi, yoga, progressive relaxation, biofeedback, and spinal manipulation, all of which have independent sleep-promoting benefits. The use of medications to manage pain will be common in this patient population, and many pain medications may cause drowsiness (e.g., antihistamines, muscle relaxants, antidepressants, Topiramate, beta-blockers, narcotics, and benzodiazepines). Appropriate timing of medication administration may be helpful in supporting or promoting sleep routines prescribed during CBT-I. Behaviorally, patients with pain will typically report a need to rest more frequently, so proper management of rest schedules (i.e., planned and time-limited naps) and rest settings (i.e., avoiding resting in bed as much as possible) will be necessary. As well, environmental adaptations to the bed or bedroom environment may be helpful to provide more comfort for sleeping (e.g., adjustable bed, extra pillows). Finally, in cases where stimulus control is needed, modifications might be required to allow patients to engage in out of bedtime in a chair or lounger in the bedroom, as opposed to requiring the patient travel to a separate room when in pain at night.

Mental health symptoms and TBI

Patients with a history of TBI who present at a sleep clinic will often have one or more comorbid psychiatric disorders. Research suggests that 31% of patients with TBI report a psychiatric disorder, and up to 22% are diagnosed with a newly developed a psychiatric disorder at 12-months postinjury (Bryant et al., 2010). This same report determined that depression, generalized anxiety disorder, PTSD, and agoraphobia were the most commonly diagnosed concerns (9%, 9%, 6%, and 6%, respectively). In another study of postinjury TBI patients, 65% received at least 1 psychiatric diagnosis. In this sample, 46% were diagnosed with depression and 38% with anxiety (72% of those with depression and 74% of those with anxiety were newly diagnosed) (Whelan-Goodinson, Ponsford, Schönberger, & Johnston, 2010). The rates of comorbid psychiatric disturbance are even higher in veterans. It is well-established that veterans with a history of TBI are more likely to have depression and PTSD than those without (Maguen, Lau, Madden, & Seal, 2012; Murphy et al., 2015; Testa et al., 2006). In fact, one study determined that 70% of Veterans with mTBI met the criteria for PTSD, and of those veterans, 45.8% also experienced depression (Seal, Bertenthal, & Kumar, 2016). Research has also shown a significant association between TBI and suicidal ideation (Gradus et al., 2015). Given the high rates of insomnia in TBI patients and the high levels of comorbidity with psychiatric disturbance, treatment of sleep in individuals with postinjury mental health issues is essential. Potential modifications to CBT-I for mental health issues are provided below.

PTSD

In addition to CBT, specialized trauma-based interventions (e.g., Prolonged Exposure and Cognitive Processing Therapy) are commonly employed for the treatment of individuals with PTSD. Combined therapies involving the use of PTSD-specific treatments and CBT-I would have significant benefits to patients as they may allow patients to address both symptoms of PTSD/insomnia within a shortened timeframe and enhance PTSD outcomes by addressing PTSD/insomnia-related factors that interfere with PTSD treatment. Other conditionally supported treatments such as Eye Movement Desensitization and Reprocessing Therapy and Narrative Exposure Therapy may also be helpful (but more so for PTSD symptomatology than insomnia). For those individuals with PTSD whose sleep is perturbed by significant nightmare frequency or intensity, incorporation of Image Rehearsal Therapy into treatment may be advisable. SSRIs such as sertraline, paroxetine, or fluoxetine and antidepressants such as venlafaxine are approved for the treatment of PTSD and may also independently benefit sleep. As well, complementary treatments such as relaxation and meditation may be used as a sleep aid in this clinical population. This said, perhaps the most challenging feature of PTSD is a physiological and psychological hyperarousal that perpetuates and supports insomnia. Addressing arousal in the context of PTSD is likely essential to success with CBT-I, so integrated or modified therapies may be most useful and/or necessary for this patient population.

Mood

Although depression is a common PCS, very few randomized controlled trials (RCTs) evaluating treatment outcomes have been performed. One systematic review concluded that CBT for depression (CBT-D), along with SSRIs, appeared to show evidence of the greatest efficacy in treating depression following TBI (Fann, Hart, & Schomer, 2009); however, this review noted that substantially more research into evidence-based treatments for depression following TBI is needed (see also Tsaousides, Ashman, & Gordon, 2013). Of the empirically supported choices, CBT-D would be the option most conducive to incorporation into a modified CBT-I treatment plan. CBT-D helps patients develop strategies to modify dysfunctional cognitions and maladaptive behaviors to assist in resolving depressive symptomatology. CBT-D helps break the downward spiral of depression by teaching patients that for factors such as thoughts, activities, and social interactions, and there are aspects of each that can be individually managed and changed. Increased behavioral activation and reduced negative cognitions would be beneficial adjuncts to sleep interventions, and therefore, combining sleep and depression treatments into a single intervention should help maximize rehabilitation outcomes, improve quality of life, and decrease the need for healthcare utilization over time.

Anxiety

CBT is the most commonly used therapy for anxiety disorders, and it has been shown to be effective in the treatment of panic disorders, generalized anxiety disorders, phobias, and social anxiety disorders. A recent Cochrane review examining CBT for patients with mTBI found evidence for the effectiveness of CBT for the treatment of acute stress disorder and CBT (combined with neurorehabilitation) for general anxiety disorder (Soo & Tate, 2007). Other psychological treatments such as exposure therapy, systematic desensitization, response prevention are frequently used in the management of anxiety. Each of these therapies has common features with components of CBT-I including conditioning, relaxation, and stimulus control and could easily be integrated into CBT-I treatment plan. Like pain conditions (above) medications (e.g., benzodiazepines) and complementary approaches to anxiety could be used in an ancillary fashion to support CBT-I treatment. The cognitive component of CBT-I may take on a particularly significant role in the treatment of patients with anxiety as sleep-related fears, worries, stress, and catastrophizing are reliable factors that maintain insomnia, and addressing these issues more robustly in the context of sleep therapy could have broader mental health benefits (Table 1).

TABLE 1 Adaptation of CBT-I for traumatic brain injury patient.

CBT-I components	Standard practice	Adaptations for individuals with TBI
Sleep education	3-P model, 2-process model of sleep regulation, sleep stages	– Incorporate education regarding relationship between TBI and insomnia – For mild TBI emphasize that expectation should be full recovery to premorbid level of functioning – Address contribution of physical and cognitive limitations as well as comorbid psychiatric concerns on insomnia and CBT-I treatment outcomes
Sleep restriction	Improve sleep efficiency by limiting time in bed to the amount of time sleeping then expanding slowly as long as sleep efficiency is preserved	– If standard sleep restriction is not indicated or cannot be tolerated then attempt sleep compression therapy (i.e., restrict time in bed gradually by 15–30 min each week until sleep efficiency $\geq$85% is reached) – Emphasize that resting is not the same or as beneficial to recovery as consolidated sleep – Establish reminder cues for sleep timing in patients with cognitive difficulties
Stimulus control	Associate bed/bedroom solely as a cue for sleep by eliminating nonsleep activities from the bedroom. Instruction to get out of bed at night if awake >15 min.	– For individuals with mobility or vestibular issues try to accommodate stimulus control instructions by allowing patients to sit up in bed and/or move a short distance to a chair (as opposed to leaving the room) – Try to avoid sleeping and/or napping outside of the bed/bedroom

Napping/daytime sleep	Discontinue or restrict daytime napping to 30 min	– In patients who require rest breaks due to fatigue and/or pain set a schedule for timed rest/activity periods during the day – Limit napping, but when necessary, have a scheduled and time-limited nap
Sleep hygiene education	Address daytime habits and sleep environment interfering with sleep	– Encourage physical activity consistent with medical rehabilitation – Adjust bed/bedroom environment to accommodate potential barriers to good sleep (e.g., use more pillows or obtain an adjustable bed to allow for more comfort when dealing with nighttime pain)
Cognitive therapy	Challenge patient's dysfunctional beliefs interfering with sleep and misconceptions about sleep. Replace/restructure to more helpful and realistic thoughts about sleep	– Work with patient to help alleviate concerns regarding insomnia and possible implications for recovery in other areas of functioning – Incorporate stress management strategies if needed – In patients with actual cognitive deficits, use this component of treatment to provide cognitive support strategies designed to assist in the treatment
Relapse prevention	Discuss practicing less rigid sleep plan over time and what do to prevent sleep disturbance from turning into another episode of insomnia in the future	– Review success established with insomnia treatment and use that message to encourage and support other ongoing post-TBI recovery efforts – Remind patient to use successful sleep strategies should insomnia symptoms return
Sleep diaries	Establish baseline sleep patterns, track progress, reinforce appropriate behavior change, problem-solve obstacles to adherence	– Provide patients with reminders to complete diary – Use electronic diaries or apps if helpful – Allow patient to track sleep with wearable tech if filling out diaries is not possible due to limitations

Circadian disruption in patients with TBI

Several older studies examining patients with TBI have noted evidence for circadian rhythm disruption (Nagtegaal, Kerkhof, Smits, Swart, & Van Der Meer, 1997; Smits & Nagtegaal, 2000), particularly delayed sleep phase preference. One study also found that up to 36% of patients with TBI history had either delayed or advanced sleep phase (Ayalon, Borodkin, Dishon, Kanety, & Dagan, 2007), and others have found evidence for lower melatonin production in post-TBI patients (Grima et al., 2016; Shekleton et al., 2010). Although this work is compelling, the relationship between TBI and circadian disruption is somewhat limited, and even in the context of the existing published work, it is unknown whether the observed circadian changes occurred before or postinjury. Nonetheless, as circadian issues may present in cases of TBI, sleep clinicians should be aware of and screen for this disorder when evaluating patients. In cases where a circadian advance or delay is suspected, CBT-I can be supplemented with behavioral modifications, light therapy, and melatonin. These approaches have been used with some success in patients with TBI in cases reports and small studies (Kemp, Biswas, Neumann, & Coughlan, 2004; Nagtegaal et al., 1997).

Conclusions

TBI is a prevalent and clinically relevant event that can produce significant and lasting medical and psychiatric concerns. Fortunately, most individuals with more mild forms of TBI will experience a full recovery, though for 10%–20% of patients problems with PCS may cause disruption in normal activities and lead to decreased quality of life. Whether occurring as a direct result of the injury itself or as a by-product of other medial/psychosocial factors, one of the most commonly reported PCS is insomnia. Although RCTs evaluating the efficacy of using CBT-I to treat insomnia in this clinical population are lacking, CBT-I Is still the treatment of choice for sleep clinicians who see patients with a history of TBI (Ford et al., 2020). In addition to insomnia, many post-TBI patients will present with one or more comorbidities that may present a challenge to successful treatment. Broadly speaking, these comorbidities include issues with cognitive deficits, pain, and mental health symptomatology. For each of these areas of impairment, effective cognitive-behavioral, complementary/alternative, cognitive skills training, and/or pharmacological interventions are available, which may be integrated with CBT-I to enhance treatment response and outcomes. Overall, for sleep clinicians, awareness and understanding of the complexities of TBI and resulting PCS are essential components of training and practice, as improving sleep in patients with TBI can have a dramatic impact on reducing long-term disability while promoting more complete recovery of normal functioning.

References

Amyot, F., Arciniegas, D. B., Brazaitis, M. P., Curley, K. C., Diaz-Arrastia, R., Gandjbakhche, A., et al. (2015). A review of the effectiveness of neuroimaging modalities for the detection of traumatic brain injury. *Journal of Neurotrauma, 32*(22), 1693–1721.

Aoun, R., Rawal, H., Attarian, H., & Sahni, A. (2019). Impact of traumatic brain injury on sleep: An overview. *Nature and science of sleep, 11*, 131.

Assefa, S. Z., Diaz-Abad, M., Wickwire, E. M., & Scharf, S. M. (2015). The functions of sleep. *AIMS Neuroscience, 2*(3), 155–171.

Ayalon, L., Borodkin, K., Dishon, L., Kanety, H., & Dagan, Y. (2007). Circadian rhythm sleep disorders following mild traumatic brain injury. *Neurology, 68*(14), 1136–1140.

Balba, N. M., Elliott, J. E., Weymann, K. B., Opel, R. A., Duke, J. W., Oken, B. S., et al. (2018). Increased sleep disturbances and pain in veterans with comorbid traumatic brain injury and posttraumatic stress disorder. *Journal of Clinical Sleep Medicine, 14*(11), 1865–1878.

Barker-Collo, S., Jones, K., Theadom, A., Starkey, N., Dowell, A., McPherson, K., et al. (2015). Neuropsychological outcome and its correlates in the first year after adult mild traumatic brain injury: A population-based New Zealand study. *Brain Injury, 29*(13–14), 1604–1616.

Baumann, C. R., Werth, E., Stocker, R., Ludwig, S., & Bassetti, C. L. (2007). Sleep–wake disturbances 6 months after traumatic brain injury: A prospective study. *Brain, 130*(7), 1873–1883.

Beetar, J. T., Guilmette, T. J., & Sparadeo, F. R. (1996). Sleep and pain complaints in symptomatic traumatic brain injury and neurologic populations. *Archives of Physical Medicine and Rehabilitation, 77*(12), 1298–1302.

Bergersen, K., Halvorsen, J.Ø., Tryti, E. A., Taylor, S. I., & Olsen, A. (2017). A systematic literature review of psychotherapeutic treatment of prolonged symptoms after mild traumatic brain injury. *Brain Injury, 31*(3), 279–289.

Bloomfield, I. L., Espie, C. A., & Evans, J. J. (2010). Do sleep difficulties exacerbate deficits in sustained attention following traumatic brain injury? *Journal of the International Neuropsychological Society, 16*(1), 17–25.

Boakye, P. A., Olechowski, C., Rashiq, S., Verrier, M. J., Kerr, B., Witmans, M., et al. (2016). A critical review of neurobiological factors involved in the interactions between chronic pain, depression, and sleep disruption. *The Clinical Journal of Pain, 32*(4), 327–336.

Bolge, S. C., Doan, J. F., Kannan, H., & Baran, R. W. (2009). Association of insomnia with quality of life, work productivity, and activity impairment. *Quality of Life Research, 18*(4), 415.

Bryan, C. J. (2013). Repetitive traumatic brain injury (or concussion) increases severity of sleep disturbance among deployed military personnel. *Sleep, 36*(6), 941–946.

Bryant, R. A., O'donnell, M. L., Creamer, M., McFarlane, A. C., Clark, C. R., & Silove, D. (2010). The psychiatric sequelae of traumatic injury. *American Journal of Psychiatry, 167*(3), 312–320.

Caplan, B., Bogner, J., Brenner, L., Twamley, E. W., Thomas, K. R., Gregory, A. M., et al. (2015). CogSMART compensatory cognitive training for traumatic brain injury: Effects over 1 year. *The Journal of Head Trauma Rehabilitation, 30*(6), 391–401.

Cassidy, J. D., Carroll, L., Peloso, P., Borg, J., Von Holst, H., Holm, L., et al. (2004). Incidence, risk factors and prevention of mild traumatic brain injury: Results of the WHO collaborating centre task force on mild traumatic brain injury. *Journal of Rehabilitation Medicine, 36*(0), 28–60.

Cassidy-Eagle, E., Siebern, A., Unti, L., Glassman, J., & O'Hara, R. (2018). Neuropsychological functioning in older adults with mild cognitive impairment and insomnia randomized to CBT-I or control group. *Clinical Gerontologist, 41*(2), 136–144.

Castriotta, R. J., Wilde, M. C., Lai, J. M., Atanasov, S., Masel, B. E., & Kuna, S. T. (2007). Prevalence and consequences of sleep disorders in traumatic brain injury. *Journal of Clinical Sleep Medicine, 3*(4), 349–356.

Chaput, G., Giguère, J.-F., Chauny, J.-M., Denis, R., & Lavigne, G. (2009). Relationship among subjective sleep complaints, headaches, and mood alterations following a mild traumatic brain injury. *Sleep Medicine, 10*(7), 713–716.

Chiu, H.-Y., Lo, W.-C., Chiang, Y.-H., & Tsai, P.-S. (2014). The effects of sleep on the relationship between brain injury severity and recovery of cognitive function: A prospective study. *International Journal of Nursing Studies, 51*(6), 892–899.

Cirelli, C. (2012). Brain plasticity, sleep and aging. *Gerontology, 58*(5), 441–445.

Clinchot, D. M., Bogner, J., Mysiw, W. J., Fugate, L., & Corrigan, J. (1998). Defining sleep disturbance after brain Injury1. *American Journal of Physical Medicine & Rehabilitation, 77*(4), 291–295.

Collen, J., Orr, N., Lettieri, C. J., Carter, K., & Holley, A. B. (2012). Sleep disturbances among soldiers with combat-related traumatic brain injury. *Chest, 142*(3), 622–630.

Cox, D. J., Tisdelle, D. A., & Culbert, J. P. (1988). Increasing adherence to behavioral homework assignments. *Journal of Behavioral Medicine, 11*(5), 519–522.

Dean, P. J. A., & Sterr, A. (2013). Long-term effects of mild traumatic brain injury on cognitive performance. *Frontiers in Human Neuroscience, 7*, 30.

Dikmen, S. S., Corrigan, J. D., Levin, H. S., Machamer, J., Stiers, W., & Weisskopf, M. G. (2009). Cognitive outcome following traumatic brain injury. *The Journal of Head Trauma Rehabilitation, 24*(6), 430–438.

Dillon, P. J. (2012). Assessing the influence of patient participation in primary care medical interviews on recall of treatment recommendations. *Health Communication, 27*(1), 58–65.

Dong, L., Lee, J. Y., & Harvey, A. G. (2017). Memory support strategies and bundles: A pathway to improving cognitive therapy for depression? *Journal of Consulting and Clinical Psychology, 85*(3), 187.

Duclos, C., Dumont, M., Wiseman-Hakes, C., Arbour, C., Mongrain, V., Gaudreault, P.-O., et al. (2014). Sleep and wake disturbances following traumatic brain injury. *Pathologie Biologie, 62*(5), 252–261.

DVBIC. (2013). *DoD worldwide numbers for TBI*. Retrieved from http://www.dvbic.org/sites/default/files/uploads/dod-tbi-worldwide-2000-2012-as-of-130213.pdf.

Fann, J. R., Hart, T., & Schomer, K. G. (2009). Treatment for depression after traumatic brain injury: A systematic review. *Journal of Neurotrauma, 26*(12), 2383–2402.

Farrell-Carnahan, L., Barnett, S., Lamberty, G., Hammond, F. M., Kretzmer, T. S., Franke, L. M., et al. (2015). Insomnia symptoms and behavioural health symptoms in veterans 1 year after traumatic brain injury. *Brain Injury, 29*(12), 1400–1408.

Fichtenberg, N. L., Putnam, S. H., Mann, N. R., Zafonte, R. D., & Millard, A. E. (2001). Insomnia screening in postacute traumatic brain injury: Utility and validity of the Pittsburgh sleep quality index. *American Journal of Physical Medicine & Rehabilitation, 80*(5), 339–345.

Fichtenberg, N. L., Zafonte, R. D., Putnam, S., Mann, N. R., & Millard, A. E. (2002). Insomnia in a post-acute brain injury sample. *Brain Injury, 16*(3), 197–206.

Ford, M. E., Groet, E., Daams, J. G., Geurtsen, G. J., Van Bennekom, C. A., & Van Someren, E. J. (2020). Non-pharmacological treatment for insomnia following acquired brain injury: A systematic review. *Sleep Medicine Reviews, 50*, 101255.

Gilbert, K. S., Kark, S. M., Gehrman, P., & Bogdanova, Y. (2015). Sleep disturbances, TBI and PTSD: Implications for treatment and recovery. *Clinical Psychology Review, 40*, 195–212.

Gondusky, J. S., & Reiter, M. P. (2005). Protecting military convoys in Iraq: An examination of battle injuries sustained by a mechanized battalion during operation Iraqi freedom II. *Military Medicine, 170*(6), 546–549.

Gradus, J. L., Wisco, B. E., Luciano, M. T., Iverson, K. M., Marx, B. P., & Street, A. E. (2015). Traumatic brain injury and suicidal ideation among US operation enduring freedom and operation Iraqi freedom veterans. *Journal of Traumatic Stress*, *28*(4), 361–365.

Grima, N., Ponsford, J., Rajaratnam, S. M., Mansfield, D., & Pase, M. P. (2016). Sleep disturbances in traumatic brain injury: A meta-analysis. *Journal of Clinical Sleep Medicine*, *12*(3), 419–428.

Hall, R. C., Hall, R. C., & Chapman, M. J. (2005). Definition, diagnosis, and forensic implications of postconcussional syndrome. *Psychosomatics*, *46*(3), 195–202.

Hoge, C. W., McGurk, D., Thomas, J. L., Cox, A. L., Engel, C. C., & Castro, C. A. (2008). Mild traumatic brain injury in US soldiers returning from Iraq. *New England Journal of Medicine*, *358*(5), 453–463.

Imbach, L. L., Valko, P. O., Li, T., Maric, A., Symeonidou, E.-R., Stover, J. F., et al. (2015). Increased sleep need and daytime sleepiness 6 months after traumatic brain injury: A prospective controlled clinical trial. *Brain*, *138*(3), 726–735.

Kalmbach, D. A., Conroy, D. A., Falk, H., Rao, V., Roy, D., Peters, M. E., et al. (2018). Poor sleep is linked to impeded recovery from traumatic brain injury. *Sleep*, *41*(10), zsy147.

Katz, D. I., Cohen, S. I., & Alexander, M. P. (2015). Mild traumatic brain injury. In *Vol. 127. Handbook of clinical neurology* (pp. 131–156). Elsevier.

Kemp, S., Biswas, R., Neumann, V., & Coughlan, A. (2004). The value of melatonin for sleep disorders occurring post-head injury: A pilot RCT. *Brain Injury*, *18*(9), 911–919.

Kempf, J., Werth, E., Kaiser, P. R., Bassetti, C. L., & Baumann, C. R. (2010). Sleep–wake disturbances 3 years after traumatic brain injury. *Journal of Neurology, Neurosurgery & Psychiatry*, *81*(12), 1402–1405.

Kessels, R. P. (2003). Patients' memory for medical information. *Journal of the Royal Society of Medicine*, *96*(5), 219–222.

King, N. S. (2003). Post-concussion syndrome: Clarity amid the controversy? *The British Journal of Psychiatry*, *183*(4), 276–278.

Kostyun, R. O., Milewski, M. D., & Hafeez, I. (2015). Sleep disturbance and neurocognitive function during the recovery from a sport-related concussion in adolescents. *The American Journal of Sports Medicine*, *43*(3), 633–640.

Kwan, V., Vo, M., Noel, M., & Yeates, K. (2018). A Scoping review of pain in children after traumatic brain injury: is there more than headache? *J. Neurotrauma.*, *35*(7), 877–888. https://doi.org/10.1089/neu.2017.5281.

Lavigne, G., Khoury, S., Chauny, J.-M., & Desautels, A. (2015). Pain and sleep in post-concussion/mild traumatic brain injury. *Pain*, *156*, S75–S85.

Lee, J. Y., & Harvey, A. G. (2015). Memory for therapy in bipolar disorder and comorbid insomnia. *Journal of Consulting and Clinical Psychology*, *83*(1), 92.

Lew, H. L., Otis, J. D., Tun, C., Kerns, R. D., Clark, M. E., & Cifu, D. X. (2009). Prevalence of chronic pain, posttraumatic stress disorder, and persistent postconcussive symptoms in OIF/OEF veterans: Polytrauma clinical triad. *Journal of Rehabilitation Research and Development*, *46*(6), 697–702.

Ling, H., Hardy, J., & Zetterberg, H. (2015). Neurological consequences of traumatic brain injuries in sports. *Molecular and Cellular Neuroscience*, *66*, 114–122.

Losoi, H., Silverberg, N. D., Wäljas, M., Turunen, S., Rosti-Otajärvi, E., Helminen, M., et al. (2016). Recovery from mild traumatic brain injury in previously healthy adults. *Journal of Neurotrauma*, *33*(8), 766–776.

Lucas, S. (2015). Posttraumatic headache: Clinical characterization and management. *Current Pain and Headache Reports*, *19*(10), 48.

Lucke-Wold, B. P., Smith, K. E., Nguyen, L., Turner, R. C., Logsdon, A. F., Jackson, G. J., et al. (2015). Sleep disruption and the sequelae associated with traumatic brain injury. *Neuroscience & Biobehavioral Reviews*, *55*, 68–77.

Maguen, S., Lau, K. M., Madden, E., & Seal, K. (2012). Relationship of screen-based symptoms for mild traumatic brain injury and mental health problems in Iraq and Afghanistan veterans: Distinct or overlapping symptoms? *Journal of Rehabilitation Research and Development, 49*(7), 1115–1126.

Mahmood, O., Rapport, L. J., Hanks, R. A., & Fichtenberg, N. L. (2004). Neuropsychological performance and sleep disturbance following traumatic brain injury. *The Journal of Head Trauma Rehabilitation, 19*(5), 378–390.

Makley, M. J., Johnson-Greene, L., Tarwater, P. M., Kreuz, A. J., Spiro, J., Rao, V., et al. (2009). Return of memory and sleep efficiency following moderate to severe closed head injury. *Neurorehabilitation and Neural Repair, 23*(4), 320–326.

Mantua, J., Grillakis, A., Mahfouz, S. H., Taylor, M. R., Brager, A. J., Yarnell, A. M., et al. (2018). A systematic review and meta-analysis of sleep architecture and chronic traumatic brain injury. *Sleep Medicine Reviews, 41*, 61–77.

Martindale, S. L., Farrell-Carnahan, L. V., Ulmer, C. S., Kimbrel, N. A., McDonald, S. D., & Rowland, J. A. (2017). Sleep quality in returning veterans: The influence of mild traumatic brain injury. *Rehabilitation Psychology, 62*(4), 563.

Masel, B. E., Scheibel, R. S., Kimbark, T., & Kuna, S. T. (2001). Excessive daytime sleepiness in adults with brain injuries. *Archives of Physical Medicine and Rehabilitation, 82*(11), 1526–1532.

Mathias, J., & Alvaro, P. (2012). Prevalence of sleep disturbances, disorders, and problems following traumatic brain injury: A meta-analysis. *Sleep Medicine, 13*(7), 898–905.

McMahon, P. J., Hricik, A., Yue, J. K., Puccio, A. M., Inoue, T., Lingsma, H. F., et al. (2014). Symptomatology and functional outcome in mild traumatic brain injury: Results from the prospective TRACK-TBI study. *Journal of Neurotrauma, 31*(1), 26–33.

Mollayeva, T., Mollayeva, S., Shapiro, C. M., Cassidy, J. D., & Colantonio, A. (2016). Insomnia in workers with delayed recovery from mild traumatic brain injury. *Sleep Medicine, 19*, 153–161.

Mollayeva, T., Pratt, B., Mollayeva, S., Shapiro, C. M., Cassidy, J. D., & Colantonio, A. (2016). The relationship between insomnia and disability in workers with mild traumatic brain injury/concussion: Insomnia and disability in chronic mild traumatic brain injury. *Sleep Medicine, 20*, 157–166.

Murphy, D., Palmer, E., Wessely, S., Oddy, M., Ramos, S., Forescue, D., et al. (2015). Prevalence and associations between traumatic brain injury and mental health difficulties within UK veterans accessing support for mental health difficulties. *Psychological Research, 11*, 613–623.

Nagtegaal, J., Kerkhof, G., Smits, M., Swart, A., & Van Der Meer, Y. (1997). Traumatic brain injury-associated delayed sleep phase syndrome. *Functional Neurology, 12*(6), 345–348.

Nakase-Richardson, R., Holcomb, E. M., Towns, S., Kamper, J. E., Barnett, S. D., Sherer, M., et al. (2016). The relationship between sleep-wake cycle disturbance and trajectory of cognitive recovery during acute traumatic brain injury. *The Journal of Head Trauma Rehabilitation, 31*(2), 108–116.

Nakase-Richardson, R., Sherer, M., Barnett, S. D., Yablon, S. A., Evans, C. C., Kretzmer, T., et al. (2013). Prospective evaluation of the nature, course, and impact of acute sleep abnormality after traumatic brain injury. *Archives of Physical Medicine and Rehabilitation, 94*(5), 875–882.

Nampiaparampil, D. E. (2008). Prevalence of chronic pain after traumatic brain injury: A systematic review. *JAMA, 300*(6), 711–719.

Nguyen, S., McKay, A., Wong, D., Rajaratnam, S. M., Spitz, G., Williams, G., et al. (2017). Cognitive behavior therapy to treat sleep disturbance and fatigue after traumatic brain injury: A pilot randomized controlled trial. *Archives of Physical Medicine and Rehabilitation, 98*(8), 1508–1517. e1502.

Ofek, H., & Defrin, R. (2007). The characteristics of chronic central pain after traumatic brain injury. *Pain, 131*(3), 330–340.

Ohayon, M. M. (2002). Epidemiology of insomnia: What we know and what we still need to learn. *Sleep Medicine Reviews, 6*(2), 97–111.

Orff, H. J., Ayalon, L., & Drummond, S. P. (2009). Traumatic brain injury and sleep disturbance: A review of current research. *The Journal of Head Trauma Rehabilitation*, *24*(3), 155–165.

Ouellet, M.-C., Beaulieu-Bonneau, S., & Morin, C. M. (2006). Insomnia in patients with traumatic brain injury: Frequency, characteristics, and risk factors. *The Journal of Head Trauma Rehabilitation*, *21*(3), 199–212.

Ouellet, M.-C., & Morin, C. M. (2006). Subjective and objective measures of insomnia in the context of traumatic brain injury: A preliminary study. *Sleep Medicine*, *7*(6), 486–497.

Ouellet, M.-C., & Morin, C. M. (2007). Efficacy of cognitive-behavioral therapy for insomnia associated with traumatic brain injury: A single-case experimental design. *Archives of Physical Medicine and Rehabilitation*, *88*(12), 1581–1592.

Ouellet, M.-C., Savard, J., & Morin, C. M. (2004). Book review: Insomnia following traumatic brain injury: A review. *Neurorehabilitation and Neural Repair*, *18*(4), 187–198.

Parcell, D. L., Ponsford, J. L., Rajaratnam, S. M., & Redman, J. R. (2006). Self-reported changes to nighttime sleep after traumatic brain injury. *Archives of Physical Medicine and Rehabilitation*, *87*(2), 278–285.

Ponsford, J. L., Ziino, C., Parcell, D. L., Shekleton, J. A., Roper, M., Redman, J. R., et al. (2012). Fatigue and sleep disturbance following traumatic brain injury—Their nature, causes, and potential treatments. *The Journal of Head Trauma Rehabilitation*, *27*(3), 224–233.

Sandsmark, D. K., Elliott, J. E., & Lim, M. M. (2017). Sleep-wake disturbances after traumatic brain injury: Synthesis of human and animal studies. *Sleep*, *40*(5), 1–18.

Schreiber, S., Barkai, G., Gur-Hartman, T., Peles, E., Tov, N., Dolberg, O. T., et al. (2008). Long-lasting sleep patterns of adult patients with minor traumatic brain injury (mTBI) and non-mTBI subjects. *Sleep Medicine*, *9*(5), 481–487.

Seal, K. H., Bertenthal, D., & Kumar, S. (2016). Association between mild traumatic brain injury and mental health problems and self-reported cognitive dysfunction in Iraq and Afghanistan veterans. *Journal of Rehabilitation Research and Development*, *53*(2), 185.

Shekleton, J., Parcell, D. L., Redman, J. R., Phipps-Nelson, J., Ponsford, J., & Rajaratnam, S. M. (2010). Sleep disturbance and melatonin levels following traumatic brain injury. *Neurology*, *74*(21), 1732–1738.

Smith-Seemiller, L., Fow, N. R., Kant, R., & Franzen, M. D. (2003). Presence of post-concussion syndrome symptoms in patients with chronic pain vs mild traumatic brain injury. *Brain Injury*, *17*(3), 199–206.

Smits, M., & Nagtegaal, J. (2000). Post-traumatic delayed sleep phase syndrome. *Neurology*, *55*(6), 902–903.

Sommerauer, M., Valko, P. O., Werth, E., & Baumann, C. R. (2013). Excessive sleep need following traumatic brain injury: A case–control study of 36 patients. *Journal of Sleep Research*, *22*(6), 634–639.

Soo, C., & Tate, R. L. (2007). Psychological treatment for anxiety in people with traumatic brain injury. *Cochrane Database of Systematic Reviews*, (3), CD005239.

Stulemeijer, M., Vos, P. E., Bleijenberg, G., & Van der Werf, S. P. (2007). Cognitive complaints after mild traumatic brain injury: Things are not always what they seem. *Journal of Psychosomatic Research*, *63*(6), 637–645.

Tan, G., Fink, B., Dao, T. K., Hebert, R., Farmer, L. S., Sanders, A., et al. (2009). Associations among pain, PTSD, mTBI, and heart rate variability in veterans of operation enduring and Iraqi freedom: A pilot study. *Pain Medicine*, *10*(7), 1237–1245.

Tanielian, T., & Jaycox, L. H. (2008). *Invisible wounds of war: Psychological and cognitive injuries, their consequences, and services to assist recovery*. CA: Retrieved from Santa Monica.

Testa, J. A., Malec, J. F., Moessner, A. M., & Brown, A. W. (2006). Predicting family functioning after TBI: Impact of neurobehavioral factors. *The Journal of Head Trauma Rehabilitation*, *21*(3), 236–247.

Theadom, A., Barker-Collo, S., Jones, K., Dudley, M., Vincent, N., & Feigin, V. (2018). A pilot randomized controlled trial of on-line interventions to improve sleep quality in adults after mild or moderate traumatic brain injury. *Clinical Rehabilitation*, *32*(5), 619–629.

Theadom, A., Cropley, M., Parmar, P., Barker-Collo, S., Starkey, N., Jones, K., et al. (2015). Sleep difficulties one year following mild traumatic brain injury in a population-based study. *Sleep Medicine, 16*(8), 926–932.

Theadom, A., Rowland, V., Levack, W., Starkey, N., Wilkinson-Meyers, L., & McPherson, K. (2016). Exploring the experience of sleep and fatigue in male and female adults over the 2 years following traumatic brain injury: A qualitative descriptive study. *BMJ Open, 6*(4).

Thomas, A., & Greenwald, B. D. (2018). Nonpharmacological management of sleep disturbances after traumatic brain injury. *NeuroRehabilitation, 43*(3), 355–360.

Tsaousides, T., Ashman, T. A., & Gordon, W. A. (2013). Diagnosis and treatment of depression following traumatic brain injury. *Brain Impairment, 14*(1), 63–76.

Twamley, E. W., Jak, A. J., Delis, D. C., Bondi, M. W., & Lohr, J. B. (2014). Cognitive symptom management and rehabilitation therapy (CogSMART) for veterans with traumatic brain injury: Pilot randomized controlled trial. *Journal of Rehabilitation Research and Development, 51*(1), 59–70.

Viola-Saltzman, M., & Musleh, C. (2016). Traumatic brain injury-induced sleep disorders. *Neuropsychiatric Disease and Treatment, 12*, 339.

Viola-Saltzman, M., & Watson, N. F. (2012). Traumatic brain injury and sleep disorders. *Neurologic Clinics, 30*(4), 1299–1312.

Warden, D. (2006). Military TBI during the Iraq and Afghanistan wars. *The Journal of Head Trauma Rehabilitation, 21*(5), 398–402.

Whelan-Goodinson, R., Ponsford, J. L., Schönberger, M., & Johnston, L. (2010). Predictors of psychiatric disorders following traumatic brain injury. *The Journal of Head Trauma Rehabilitation, 25*(5), 320–329.

Wickwire, E. M., Williams, S. G., Roth, T., Capaldi, V. F., Jaffe, M., Moline, M., et al. (2016). Sleep, sleep disorders, and mild traumatic brain injury. What we know and what we need to know: Findings from a national working group. *Neurotherapeutics, 13*(2), 403–417.

Wilde, M. C., Castriotta, R. J., Lai, J. M., Atanasov, S., Masel, B. E., & Kuna, S. T. (2007). Cognitive impairment in patients with traumatic brain injury and obstructive sleep apnea. *Archives of Physical Medicine and Rehabilitation, 88*(10), 1284–1288.

Wilkinson, C. W., Pagulayan, K. F., Petrie, E. C., Mayer, C. L., Colasurdo, E. A., Shofer, J. B., et al. (2012). High prevalence of chronic pituitary and target-organ hormone abnormalities after blast-related mild traumatic brain injury. *Frontiers in Neurology, 3*, 11.

Wiseman-Hakes, C., Murray, B., Moineddin, R., Rochon, E., Cullen, N., Gargaro, J., et al. (2013). Evaluating the impact of treatment for sleep/wake disorders on recovery of cognition and communication in adults with chronic TBI. *Brain Injury, 27*(12), 1364–1376.

Xie, L., Kang, H., Xu, Q., Chen, M. J., Liao, Y., Thiyagarajan, M., et al. (2013). Sleep drives metabolite clearance from the adult brain. *science, 342*(6156), 373–377.

Yasseen, B., Colantonio, A., & Ratcliff, G. (2008). Prescription medication use in persons many years following traumatic brain injury. *Brain Injury, 22*(10), 752–757.

Zeitzer, J. M., Friedman, L., & O'Hara, R. (2009). Insomnia in the context of traumatic brain injury. *Journal of Rehabilitation Research and Development, 46*(6), 827–836.

Zhou, Y., & Greenwald, B. D. (2018). Update on insomnia after mild traumatic brain injury. *Brain Sciences, 8*(12), 223.

PART 5

CBT-I across the lifespan

CHAPTER

14

CBT-I for adolescents

Melisa E. Moore[a] *and Alison R. Hartman*[b]

[a]Department of Child and Adolescent Psychiatry and Behavioral Sciences, Children's Hospital of Philadelphia, Philadelphia, PA, United States, [b]Department of Psychology, Drexel University, Philadelphia, PA, United States

Insomnia in adolescents

Adolescent sleep has historically been characterized by difficulty falling asleep, insufficient sleep, and late bedtimes. The causes of these sleep difficulties are multifactorial and are influenced by normal physiology, psychological and social factors, and habits that interfere with sleep. While many adolescents experience sleep problems, insomnia is one of the most common sleep disorders of adolescence. The prevalence of *diagnosed* adolescent insomnia is, in large part, dependent on diagnostic criteria and ranges from 13.6% to 23.6% (Hysing et al., 2013). In studies of insomnia *symptoms,* the prevalence is as high as 68.5% (Johnson et al., 2006). Fortunately, the most recent versions of the International Classification of Sleep Disorders (ICSD-3) (American Academy of Sleep Medicine, 2014) and the Diagnostic and Statistical Manual of Mental Disorders (DSM-5) (American Psychiatric Association, 2013) have broadened their definitions and are now more consistent, which should be useful in conducting and interpreting research. The key components of both diagnostic systems are (1) a subjective complaint of sleep quantity or quality, (2) difficulty initiating or maintaining sleep or early morning waking, (3) the sleep problems cause impairment in daytime functioning, and (4) these symptoms occur in the presence of adequate sleep opportunity.

Not only is insomnia common, but it is also persistent. Insomnia is a thread that can continue from early childhood through adulthood (Combs et al., 2016). Hysing et al. showed that for approximately 1/3 of 7- to 9-year-olds with insomnia, insomnia remained at 16–19 years of age (Sivertsen et al., 2017). Insomnia was also found to be stable in about

Adapting Cognitive Behavioral Therapy for Insomnia
https://doi.org/10.1016/B978-0-12-822872-2.00010-4

50% of adolescents age 16–18 who were evaluated again at ages 22–25 (Hysing et al., 2020). Taken together, this highlights the importance of intervening early and developing empirically supported treatments for insomnia that are specific to children and adolescents.

Adolescent insomnia is associated with myriad deleterious effects and comorbidities, including psychopathology, medical, and behavioral concerns (Combs et al., 2016). A large body of research suggests a bidirectional relationship between insomnia and psychopathology by which insomnia may contribute to the development or exacerbation of disorders such as depression, anxiety, ADHD, and anorexia nervosa (Allison, Spaeth, & Hopkins, 2016; Gregory & Sadeh, 2016; Owens et al., 2013; Roberts & Duong, 2013). While the relationship between insomnia and depression is at least partially bidirectional in nature, longitudinal studies have suggested that insomnia is a strong risk factor for depression in adolescents: those with insomnia are up to four times more likely to develop subsequent depression than those without (Johnson, Roth, & Breslau, 2006). This suggests that insomnia may be prodromal to depression in adolescents, and/or

TABLE 1 Adaptation of CBT-I for Adolescents.

CBT-I Components	Standard practice	Adaptations for adolescents
Sleep education	3-P model, 2-process model of sleep regulation, sleep stages	– Education about a typical circadian shift in adolescents – Education about impact & persistence of insomnia
Sleep restriction	Improve sleep efficiency by limiting time in bed to the amount of time sleeping then expanding slowly as long as sleep efficiency is preserved	– Utilize more naturalistic ways of restricting sleep: bedtime closer to the time the adolescent is currently falling asleep, consistent wake time, avoid daytime napping
Stimulus control	Associate bed/bedroom solely as a cue for sleep by eliminating nonsleep activities from the bedroom. Instruction to get out of bed at night if awake >15 min.	– If unable to sleep in 15–20 min, get out of bed and do something boring (not electronics) – Problem-solve around potential boring activities – Don't do homework, eat, play video games, watch tv, be on the computer or phone in bed – Don't sleep outside of the bed, sleep only in bed
Napping/ daytime sleep	Discontinue or restrict daytime napping to 30 min	– Avoid napping whenever possible

TABLE 1 Adaptation of CBT-I for Adolescents—cont'd

CBT-I Components	Standard practice	Adaptations for adolescents
Sleep hygiene education	Address daytime habits and sleep environment interfering with sleep	– Encourage physical activity, especially during usual napping times – Avoid caffeine after lunch – Avoid electronics 30–60 min before bedtime – Have a bedtime routine – Weekend schedules should be no more than 2 h later than weekday schedules
Cognitive therapy	Challenge patient's dysfunctional beliefs interfering with sleep and misconceptions about sleep. Replace/restructure to more helpful and realistic thoughts about sleep	– Challenge beliefs that poor sleep will be catastrophic to school performance and/or social activities – Challenge idea that poor sleep is catastrophic to future outcomes (college, career, etc.) – Encourage typical daily activities regardless of sleep quality and discuss how adolescent has been able to do this in the past
Relapse Prevention	Discuss practicing less rigid sleep plan over time and what do to prevent sleep disturbance from turning into another episode of insomnia in the future	– Encourage maintenance of healthy sleep habits – Discuss less rigid sleep plan during vacations, holidays and discuss risks of relapse especially during summer – Include caregiver in the plan for relapse prevention
Sleep diaries	Establish baseline sleep patterns, track progress, reinforce appropriate behavior change, problem-solve obstacles to adherence	– Consider an online sleep diary – Identify whether caregiver or adolescent will be completing sleep diary

that insomnia may contribute to the etiology of depression in this population. Poor sleep quality and insomnia in adolescence have been associated with increased risk for self-harm and suicidal ideation (Wong, Brower, & Zucker, 2011), and sleep disturbance appears to be an independent risk factor for suicidality in this population (Wong, Brower, & Craun, 2016).

Adolescents with insomnia or disturbed sleep are at increased risk for behavioral concerns, including substance use (de Zambotti et al., 2018) and drunk driving (O'Brien & Mindell, 2005). Poor sleep quality, short sleep duration, and daytime sleepiness in adolescence are associated with decreased school performance (Dewald et al., 2010), as measured by objective (i.e., standardized test scores, GPA) and subjective (i.e., teacher, parent, and self-report) assessments. These behavioral concerns may be partially explained by the deficits in executive functioning that have been observed in adolescents with poor sleep quality (Kuula et al., 2015). Chronic insomnia of adolescence, or insomnia that persists for more than 12 months, has been associated with subsequent risk for somatic and psychological health concerns, interpersonal difficulties, and problems performing daily activities (Roberts, Roberts, & Duong, 2008).

Clearly, the scope, impact, and persistence of adolescent insomnia make treatment essential. Treatments for adolescent insomnia have included medications, sleep education, and cognitive behavioral therapy for insomnia (CBT-I), the latter being the current first-line treatment for insomnia in adults (Morgenthaler, Kramer, Alessi, & Friedman, 2006). Randomized-controlled trials investigating the efficacy of CBT-I for the treatment of adolescent insomnia have delivered promising results, though relatively few empirical studies have been published to date (Dewald-Kaufmann, de Bruin, & Michael, 2019).

Modifications to treatment of adolescent insomnia

Treatment of adolescent insomnia can be challenging, as developmental considerations necessitate modifications to standard cognitive-behavioral treatments for adult insomnia. Some components of CBT-I such as mindfulness are easily applied and have empirical support. For example, a recent randomized controlled trial by de Bruin and colleagues (de Bruin, Meijer, & Bögels, 2020) investigated whether a body scan mindfulness meditation added to CBT-I improved treatment outcomes for adolescents with insomnia. Results demonstrated that both traditional CBT-I and CBT-I with a mindfulness component were effective in reducing symptoms of insomnia and improving multiple objective and subjective measures of sleep. However, the addition of a body scan mindfulness meditation also led to objective improvements in nighttime awakenings after sleep onset and subjective improvements in sleep duration and daytime irritation, which were not observed in the group that received traditional CBT-I. This suggests that mindfulness training may be a helpful addition to traditional CBT-I with adolescents (Table 1).

Given the pervasive use of caffeine and electronics in adolescents, focusing on the impact of caffeine and blue light on sleep is especially important to review when discussing sleep hygiene (Calamaro, Mason, & Ratcliffe, 2009). Both daytime and bedtime use of electronics has been associated with an increased risk of short sleep duration, long sleep onset latency, and increased sleep deficiency and demonstrates a dose–response relationship (Hysing et al., 2015).

Other components of CBT-I such as sleep restriction are more difficult to apply, as the impact on the developing brain is less well known. Typically in CBT-I with adolescents, sleep restriction is conducted in a more naturalistic way: By moving bedtime closer to the time, the adolescent is actually falling asleep, moving wake times earlier, and eliminating daytime napping. These strategies, similar to traditional sleep restriction, are designed to increase sleep pressure to promote the onset of sleep in an easier, earlier way. There are few studies that have investigated the impact of sleep restriction on the adolescent brain; however, one recent study demonstrated that experimental sleep restriction can cause an increase in somatic symptoms (Krietsch, King, & Beebe, 2020). To investigate the impact of sleep restriction on somatic complaints in adolescents, Krietsch and colleagues (Krietsch et al., 2020) compared adolescents who had slept 6.5 h per night for the previous five nights to those who had slept 9.5 h per night for the same amount of time. The researchers found that sleep restriction led to an increase in somatic complaints, specifically headaches and low back pain, in healthy adolescents.

The adolescent's level of independence also impacts treatment recommendations. Depending on current caregiver involvement and the adolescent's level of self-sufficiency, the goals and recommendations at the end of each session may include caregivers. Questions to ask include: What additional interventions are needed for the adolescent to be successful at following a prescribed sleep schedule? Can the adolescent get out of bed independently to enact stimulus control safely? Adding visual cues, as well as setting alarms on watches and phones to increase autonomy, can be useful. In addition, managing the potential resistance of parents to certain recommendations, such as a later bedtime, can be a factor. One way to address this is to explicitly lay out the goals: the first goal is to get your child to fall asleep faster while the second goal is to increase total sleep time. Emphasize that there will be a stepwise approach that does not necessarily include a later bedtime as a permanent solution.

Another important consideration specific to *internet* delivery of CBT-I for adolescents is therapist communication. One dismantling study (de Bruin & Meijer, 2017) investigated the specific aspects of therapist involvement that were important to internet-delivered CBT-I outcomes in adolescents. Weekly written therapeutic feedback was coded, and four factors emerged from the therapists' communication: Forging a therapeutic alliance (supportive comments, reflection, complements, tips), forging therapy integrity (goal setting, clarification of deviations from goals, homework), forging a positive attitude (explanation, expressing an understanding of difficulties, positive reframing), and sleep expertise (calculation of sleep efficiency, instructions for the time in bed). Only sleep expertise was found to be significant, relating both to increased sleep efficiency post-treatment and decreased insomnia symptoms at 2 months follow up. Conversely, forging therapy integrity, forging a positive attitude, and a number of words were negatively related to both total sleep time and sleep efficiency. Taken together, this suggests that feedback less directly targeted to the subject's sleep efficiency and schedule may not be helpful when applying internet-based CBT-I.

Finally, addressing the circadian delay common to adolescence is a critical consideration in CBT-I. The physiological circadian shift toward a preference for eveningness (Gradisar, Gardner, & Dohnt, 2011; Hagenauer, Perryman, Lee, et al., 2011) leads to a propensity for later bedtimes and waketimes and, in large part due to early school start times, insufficient sleep. Because this circadian preference may override the effects of increased sleep pressure induced by sleep restriction, it should be a critical focus in CBT-I for adolescents. Exposure to sunlight as well as maintaining active daytime functioning (including physical exercise, regular mealtimes, and avoiding naps) should be encouraged. The TranS-C (Harvey & Buysse, 2018) approach subsequently described in this chapter, addresses this natural eveningness preference.

Specific adaptations for core components of CBT-I in adolescents

Stimulus control

Stimulus control, or the pairing of a stimulus (bed) with a conditioned response (sleep), is a core component of CBT-I. In adolescents, it is recommended that the adolescent only sleep in their bed and not engage in activities such as homework or videogames in bed. Given that adolescence is a time of growing independence, teens often like to have their own space, which often ends up being their room and specifically their bed by default. If the adolescent has a space to sit other than their bed, such as a beanbag, comfortable chair, or even a nest of blankets, this is an option for practicing stimulus control by being out of bed. If this is not an option, collaboration with families to determine a private space for the adolescent for certain parts of the day may circumvent the desire to spend large quantities of time in bed.

Sleep restriction

Sleep restriction is considered the other core "active ingredient" in CBT-I. Sleep restriction aims to increase sleep efficiency by decreasing time spent awake in bed. Because the impact of sleep restriction on the developing brain is unknown, often a more naturalistic approach is taken, where the adolescent's bedtime is moved closer to when they are actually falling asleep. Other ways to implement sleep restriction include setting a consistent wake time with a wake time less than 2h later on weekends and eliminating all daytime naps after waking for the day. As sleep efficiency increases throughout treatment, bedtime can gradually be moved earlier in 15-min increments (Spielman, Yang, & Glovinsky, 2016).

Sleep education

Sleep hygiene education, while not considered a standalone treatment for insomnia, is an important component of CBT-I and should include factors specific to adolescence. Many families do not know that a biological predisposition to a later sleep schedule is present in adolescents across the globe. Although the emphasis in sleep hygiene is often on caffeine and electronics, given the prevalence of use in adolescents, psychoeducation should include a review of "best practices" for sleep, including avoiding alcohol, tobacco, and vaping and modifying the sleep environment to be dark, quiet, temperate, and comfortable (Posner & Gehrman, 2011).

Cognitive restructuring

Cognitive restructuring or thought challenging, originally developed by Beck and colleagues in the 1970s for the treatment of depression (Beck, 1979), has been widely adapted by researchers and clinicians to treat a range of psychopathologies in adolescents. When it comes to adolescent insomnia, the cognitive aspect is often not as salient as the behavioral components. When adolescents do hold beliefs such as, "If I don't get 8h of sleep, I won't get into college," or "I can't sleep so I might as well just go on social media because that helps me relax."

Relaxation and mindfulness

Relaxation strategies may also be helpful adjunctive components in CBT-I, particularly for patients who report somatic complaints or somaticized anxiety. Relaxation techniques vary (Lichstein, 1988) and can include progressive muscle relaxation, diaphragmatic breathing, calming imagery, and biofeedback. For example, de Bruin and colleagues (de Bruin et al., 2020) found that a body scan mindfulness meditation added to CBT-I led not only to improvements in insomnia symptoms but also to improvements in mood that were above and beyond the group receiving traditional CBT-I.

Transdiagnostic approach

Harvey and Buysse's transdiagnostic approach (TranS-C) (Harvey & Buysse, 2018; Harvey et al., 2018) brings together typical components of CBT-I and addresses evening circadian preference as well as other co-occurring symptoms such as worry and racing thoughts. *tranS*-C consists of four modules that apply to all sessions: case formulation, patient education on sleep and circadian rhythms, motivation and behavior change related to sleep habits, and goal setting. While typically introduced in the first three sessions, they are generally revisited in all subsequent sessions.

In addition to the four cross-cutting modules, there are four core modules that are typically utilized: setting regular sleep/wake times, improving daytime functioning independent of nighttime sleep, challenging unhelpful beliefs about sleep, and maintaining behavior change. There are seven additional modules, which are optional and are applied depending on the patient's symptoms, comorbidities, and the factors that perpetuate their sleep difficulties. Module 3 addresses the phase shift common to adolescents by addressing the timing and intensity of zeitgebers (environmental signals to the body, which impact the timing of the circadian clock), use of electronics, and gradually shifting bedtimes and waketimes earlier. To minimize resistance from the adolescent and family, it is critical to build rapport with *both* parent and child and to collaboratively develop recommendations that are likely to be followed. Recommendations need to be specifically tailored and may be easier for the adolescent to follow on their own. Often a first target is a consistent wake time, even if it is much later than ideal and avoiding all daytime napping after waking for the day. It can also be advantageous to plan interventions around motivating activities for the adolescent such as summer camp, where the rise time is earlier or weekends when they may have a preferred school activity.

One study of TranS-C vs Psychoeducation in youth ages 10–18 found that TranS-C was not associated with greater total sleep time or an earlier bedtime on weeknights; however, it was associated with a reduction in evening circadian preference, earlier endogenous circadian phase, less weeknight–weekend discrepancy, less daytime sleepiness, and better self-reported sleep via youth and parent report (Harvey et al., 2018). This suggests that it is possible to modify the evening circadian preference germane to adolescence to more effectively treat insomnia.

Modes of delivery

To meet demand and increase accessibility, CBT-I has been adapted from the original individual, in-person format to accommodate other modes of delivery. A growing body of research suggests that internet-delivered

CBT-I is as effective as in-person CBT-I in reducing insomnia symptoms in adults (Seyffert et al., 2016). Similarly, group format CBT-I appears to be a highly efficacious treatment for insomnia (Koffel, Koffel, & Gehrman, 2015) and may provide insomnia sufferers with an increased sense of community. Recent years have seen the emergence of automated digital CBT-I applications such as Sleepio (Espie et al., 2012) and SHUTi (Ritterband et al., 2009). While the efficacy of these and other applications warrant further investigation, preliminary results are promising.

Alternative modes of delivery may be of benefit to adolescents in particular. Research suggests that adolescents may be reluctant to seek mental health services and that adolescents may find online treatment formats more acceptable (Havas et al., 2011). One randomized-controlled trial found that both group and internet-delivered CBT-I were effective at reducing multiple symptoms of insomnia in adolescents, reporting medium to large effect sizes, compared to a control condition (de Bruin et al., 2015a). Both group and internet-delivered CBT-I were acceptable to adolescents and improvements were sustained over time in both group and internet-delivered conditions; however, a follow-up investigation determined that internet-delivered CBT-I was more cost-effective than group format (De Bruin, Van Steensel, & Meijer, 2016). There is preliminary evidence to suggest that digital CBT-I (Sleepio) may be acceptable to adolescents and may be an effective intervention for adolescent insomnia (Cliffe et al., 2020), though further investigations are warranted.

When feasible, evidence has increasingly suggested that internet-delivered, group format, and application-based CBT-I can be highly effective tools for treating insomnia in adolescents. Specific aspects of therapeutic feedback delivered via internet CBT-I (previously discussed) should also be considered (de Bruin & Meijer, 2017).

CBT-I and comorbidities

Insomnia may be caused by or occur with myriad possible comorbidities including mood disorders, pain, cancer, asthma, and traumatic brain injuries (Roberts, Roberts, & Duong, 2008; Short et al., 2011). Nonetheless, there are few studies of CBT-I for insomnia in adolescents with such comorbid conditions (Law et al., 2018; Moore, Phillips, Palermo, & Lah, 2021; Palermo et al., 2017).

The high comorbidity rate of insomnia and mood disorders, which may interfere with CBT-I in both adults and adolescents (Clarke & Harvey, 2012), warrants specific intervention. Because insomnia and mood disorders may share a genetic component (Gehrman et al., 2011), the likelihood of those conditions co-occurring is high. Promising research has suggested that in adolescents with comorbid depression and insomnia, the addition of CBT-I to standard CBT for depression improves both depression and insomnia outcomes compared to the addition of a lower-intensity sleep intervention (Clarke et al., 2015). Strategies for treating adolescents with comorbid insomnia and depression include increasing engagement of the patient and their strengths and including parents or other caregivers in treatment (Orchard et al., 2020). Evidence from the adult population suggests that traditional CBT-I may be more efficacious than self-help CBT-I for patients with comorbid insomnia and depression (Ashworth et al., 2015).

In terms of anxiety symptoms, one of the optional modules in the TranS-C approach addresses sleep-related worry and vigilance (Harvey & Buysse, 2018). Strategies include having a wind-down period (a bedtime routine), employing mindfulness exercises, identifying and managing automatic thoughts, and changing unhelpful beliefs about sleep and worry.

While only studied in typically developing adolescents, CBT-I may be helpful in adolescents with deficits in executive functioning. De Bruin and colleagues examined executive functioning in adolescents following six guided, self-help online CBT-I sessions compared with a waitlist control group (de Bruin et al., 2015b). Following CBT-I, the treatment group showed significant improvements in sleep efficiency and insomnia symptoms. In terms of executive functioning, individuals in the treatment group showed gains in visuospatial processing, selective attention, phonological working memory. This study is one of the first in adolescents to demonstrate that changes in sleep via CBT-I may be related to changes in cognitive functioning.

CBT-I is an effective intervention in adolescents with a variety of comorbidities. CBT-I has been found to improve outcomes across many categories of adolescent psychopathology, including affective, anxiety, somatic, ADHD, and oppositional defiant problems (de Bruin et al., 2018), as well as substance abuse problems (Bootzin & Stevens, 2005). CBT-I may also improve health-related quality of life and psychological complaints in adolescents with physical or psychiatric comorbidities (Palermo et al., 2017).

Conclusion

Insomnia disorder, characterized by persistent difficulty falling asleep, maintaining sleep, or early waking that adversely affects daytime functioning, is common in adolescence. Insomnia disorder in adolescence is associated with a multitude of deleterious effects, including increased risk for psychopathology, somatic health complaints, and behavioral and school-related problems. Importantly, insomnia in adolescence frequently persists into adulthood. Cognitive-behavioral therapy for insomnia

(CBT-I), an intervention that combines behavioral, psychoeducational, cognitive, and relaxation/mindfulness techniques, is recommended as the first line of treatment for insomnia disorder in adults.

Although there is a paucity of research examining the efficacy of CBT-I for the treatment of insomnia in adolescents, a growing body of literature suggests that this is an efficacious intervention. Adolescents report a preference for online treatment, which may be an efficacious and cost-effective mode of delivery for this population. A number of modifications have been recommended when delivering CBT-I to adolescents. These include addressing the normative circadian shift toward eveningness that occurs in adolescence, monitoring somatic symptoms in the context of sleep restriction, selectively involving parents or other caregivers in treatment, including mindfulness components, and providing feedback that demonstrates the clinician's expertise. Further, CBT-I can be effectively delivered to adolescents with a range of comorbidities, and may also improve outcomes in domains other than sleep. These promising outcomes may be related to changes in cognitive functioning that occur as a result of CBT-I.

While current research on the efficacy of CBT-I in adolescents and the adaptation treatment principles for optimal delivery in this population is promising, more research in this area is greatly needed.

References

Allison, K. C., Spaeth, A., & Hopkins, C. M. (2016). Sleep and eating disorders. *Current Psychiatry Reports, 18*(10), 92.

American Academy of Sleep Medicine. (2014). *International classification of sleep disorders* (3rd ed.). Darien, IL: American Academy of Sleep Medicine.

American Psychiatric Association. (2013). *Diagnostic and statistical manual of mental disorders* (5 ed.). Arlington, VA: American Psychiatric Association.

Ashworth, D. K., et al. (2015). A randomized controlled trial of cognitive behavioral therapy for insomnia: An effective treatment for comorbid insomnia and depression. *Journal of Counseling Psychology, 62*(2), 115.

Beck, A. T. (1979). *Cognitive therapy of depression*. Guilford press.

Bootzin, R. R., & Stevens, S. J. (2005). Adolescents, substance abuse, and the treatment of insomnia and daytime sleepiness. *Clinical Psychology Review, 25*(5), 629–644.

Calamaro, C. J., Mason, T. B. A., & Ratcliffe, S. J. (2009). Adolescents living the 24/7 lifestyle: Effects of caffeine and technology on sleep duration and daytime functioning. *Pediatrics, 123*(6), e1005–e1010.

Clarke, G., & Harvey, A. G. (2012). The complex role of sleep in adolescent depression. *Child and Adolescent Psychiatric Clinics of North America, 21*(2), 385–400.

Clarke, G., et al. (2015). Cognitive-behavioral treatment of insomnia and depression in adolescents: A pilot randomized trial. *Behaviour Research and Therapy, 69*, 111–118.

Cliffe, B., et al. (2020). Digital cognitive behavioral therapy for insomnia for adolescents with mental health problems: Feasibility open trial. *JMIR Mental Health, 7*(3), e14842.

Combs, D., et al. (2016). Insomnia, health-related quality of life and health outcomes in children: A seven year longitudinal cohort. *Scientific Reports, 6*, 27921.

de Bruin, E. J., & Meijer, A. M. (2017). The impact of online therapeutic feedback on outcome measures in internet-CBTI for adolescents with insomnia. *Sleep Medicine*, *29*, 68–75.

de Bruin, E. J., Meijer, A., & Bögels, S. M. (2020). The contribution of a body scan mindfulness meditation to effectiveness of internet-delivered CBT for insomnia in adolescents. *Mindfulness*, *11*(4), 872–882.

De Bruin, E. J., Van Steensel, F. J. A., & Meijer, A. M. (2016). Cost-effectiveness of group and internet cognitive behavioral therapy for insomnia in adolescents: Results from a randomized controlled trial. *Sleep*, *39*(8), 1571–1581.

de Bruin, E. J., et al. (2015a). Efficacy of cognitive behavioral therapy for insomnia in adolescents: A randomized controlled trial with internet therapy, group therapy and a waiting list condition. *Sleep*, *38*(12), 1913–1926.

de Bruin, E. J., et al. (2015b). Differential effects of online insomnia treatment on executive functions in adolescents. *Sleep Medicine*, *16*(4), 510–520.

de Bruin, E. J., et al. (2018). Improvements of adolescent psychopathology after insomnia treatment: Results from a randomized controlled trial over 1 year. *Journal of Child Psychology and Psychiatry*, *59*(5), 509–522.

de Zambotti, M., et al. (2018). Insomnia disorder in adolescence: Diagnosis, impact, and treatment. *Sleep Medicine Reviews*, *39*, 12–24.

Dewald, J. F., et al. (2010). The influence of sleep quality, sleep duration and sleepiness on school performance in children and adolescents: A meta-analytic review. *Sleep Medicine Reviews*, *14*(3), 179–189.

Dewald-Kaufmann, J., de Bruin, E., & Michael, G. (2019). Cognitive behavioral therapy for insomnia (CBT-i) in school-aged children and adolescents. *Sleep Medicine Clinics*, *14*(2), 155–165.

Espie, C. A., et al. (2012). A randomized, placebo-controlled trial of online cognitive behavioral therapy for chronic insomnia disorder delivered via an automated media-rich web application. *Sleep*, *35*(6), 769–781.

Gehrman, P. R., et al. (2011). Heritability of insomnia symptoms in youth and their relationship to depression and anxiety. *Sleep*, *34*(12), 1641–1646.

Gradisar, M., Gardner, G., & Dohnt, H. (2011). Recent worldwide sleep patterns and problems during adolescence: A rveiw and meta-analysis of age, region, and sleep. *Sleep Medicine*, *12*(2), 110–118.

Gregory, A. M., & Sadeh, A. (2016). Annual research review: Sleep problems in childhood psychiatric disorders–a review of the latest science. *Journal of Child Psychology and Psychiatry*, *57*(3), 296–317.

Hagenauer, M. H. P., Perryman, J. I., Lee, T. M., et al. (2011). Adolescent changes in the homeostatic and circadian regulation of sleep. *Developmental Neuroscience*, *31*(4), 276–284.

Harvey, A. G., & Buysse, D. (2018). *Treating sleep problems: A transdiagnostic approach*. New York: Guilford Press.

Harvey, A. G., et al. (2018). Modifying the impact of eveningness chronotype ("night-owls") in youth: A randomized controlled trial. *Journal of the American Academy of Child and Adolescent Psychiatry*, *57*(10), 742–754.

Havas, J., et al. (2011). Adolescents' views about an internet platform for adolescents with mental health problems. *Health Education*, *111*, 164–176.

Hysing, M., et al. (2013). Sleep patterns and insomnia among adolescents: A population-based study. *Journal of Sleep Research*, *22*(5), 549–556.

Hysing, M., et al. (2015). Sleep and use of electronic devices in adolescence: Results from a large population-based study. *BMJ Open*, *5*(1), e006748.

Hysing, M., et al. (2020). Trajectories of sleep problems from adolescence to adulthood. Linking two population-based studies from Norway. *Sleep Medicine*, *75*, 411–417.

Johnson, E. O., Roth, T., & Breslau, N. (2006). The association of insomnia with anxiety disorders and depression: Exploration of the direction of risk. *Journal of Psychiatric Research*, *40*(8), 700–708.

Johnson, E. O., et al. (2006). Epidemiology of DSM-IV insomnia in adolescence: Lifetime prevalence, chronicity, and an emergent gender difference. *Pediatrics, 117*(2), e247–e256.
Koffel, E. A., Koffel, J. B., & Gehrman, P. R. (2015). A meta-analysis of group cognitive behavioral therapy for insomnia. *Sleep Medicine Reviews, 19*, 6–16.
Krietsch, K. N., King, C. D., & Beebe, D. W. (2020). Experimental sleep restriction increases somatic complaints in healthy adolescents. *Sleep Medicine, 73*, 213–216.
Kuula, L., et al. (2015). Poor sleep and neurocognitive function in early adolescence. *Sleep Medicine, 16*(10), 1207–1212.
Law, E. F., et al. (2018). Hybrid cognitive-behavioral therapy intervention for adolescents with co-occurring migraine and insomnia: A single-arm pilot trial. *Headache, 58*(7), 1060–1073.
Lichstein, K. L. (1988). *Clinical relaxation strategies*. John Wiley & Sons.
Moore, T., Phillips, N., Palermo, T., & Lah, S. (2021). Acceptability, feasibility, and usability of a manualized cognitive behavioural programme for treatment of insomnia in children who sustained traumatic brain injury: A service providers' perspective. *Neuropsychological Rehabilitation, 31*(4), 583–600.
Morgenthaler, T., Kramer, M., Alessi, C., & Friedman, L. (2006). Practice parameters for the psychological and behavioral treatment of insomnia: an update. An American Academy of sleep medicine report. *Sleep, 29*(11), 1415–1419.
O'Brien, E. M., & Mindell, J. A. (2005). Sleep and risk-taking behavior in adolescents. *Behavioral Sleep Medicine, 3*(3), 113–133.
Orchard, F., et al. (2020). Adapting brief CBT-I for depressed adolescents: A case illustration of the sleeping better program. *Cognitive and Behavioral Practice, 27*(3), 336–346.
Owens, J., et al. (2013). Future research directions in sleep and ADHD: Report of a consensus working group. *Journal of Attention Disorders, 17*(7), 550–564.
Palermo, T. M., et al. (2017). A single arm pilot trial of brief cognitive behavioral therapy for insomnia in adolescents with physical and psychiatric comorbidities. *Journal of Clinical Sleep Medicine, 13*(3), 401–410.
Posner, D., & Gehrman, P. R. (2011). Sleep hygiene. In *Behavioral treatments for sleep disorders* (pp. 31–43). Elsevier.
Ritterband, L. M., et al. (2009). Efficacy of an internet-based behavioral intervention for adults with insomnia. *Archives of General Psychiatry, 66*(7), 692–698.
Roberts, R. E., & Duong, H. T. (2013). Depression and insomnia among adolescents: A prospective perspective. *Journal of Affective Disorders, 148*(1), 66–71.
Roberts, R. E., Roberts, C. R., & Duong, H. T. (2008). Chronic insomnia and its negative consequences for health and functioning of adolescents: A 12-month prospective study. *Journal of Adolescent Health, 42*(3), 294–302.
Seyffert, M., et al. (2016). Internet-delivered cognitive behavioral therapy to treat insomnia: A systematic review and meta-analysis. *PLoS One, 11*(2), e0149139.
Short, M. A., et al. (2011). Time for bed: Parent-set bedtimes associated with improved sleep and daytime functioning in adolescents. *Sleep, 34*(6), 797–800.
Sivertsen, B., et al. (2017). Trajectories of sleep problems from childhood to adolescence: A population-based longitudinal study from Norway. *Journal of Sleep Research, 26*(1), 55–63.
Spielman, A. J., Yang, C.-M., & Glovinsky, P. B. (2016). 25 insomnia: Sleep restriction therapy. *Diagnosis and Treatment*, 277.
Wong, M. M., Brower, K. J., & Craun, E. A. (2016). Insomnia symptoms and suicidality in the national comorbidity survey–adolescent supplement. *Journal of Psychiatric Research, 81*, 1–8.
Wong, M. M., Brower, K. J., & Zucker, R. A. (2011). Sleep problems, suicidal ideation, and self-harm behaviors in adolescence. *Journal of Psychiatric Research, 45*(4), 505–511.

CHAPTER

15

CBT-I in pregnancy

Anna L. MacKinnon[a], *Ivan D. Sedov*[b], *and Lianne M. Tomfohr-Madsen*[a]

[a]Department of Psychology, University of Calgary, Calgary, AB, Canada
[b]Alberta Health Services, Calgary, AB, Canada

Sleep changes during pregnancy

Sleep disturbances and poor sleep quality are common in pregnancy and may develop into insomnia disorder. As reported by many women and supported by empirical research, sleep changes during pregnancy. A number of factors appear to underlie the changes in the sleep of pregnant women. During pregnancy, women experience a series of physiologic and emotional changes, ranging from alterations of hormonal secretions, physical discomfort, and pain, to fear of childbirth and worries about parenthood. These changes can cause a range of somatic symptoms including sleep disturbances. As early as the first trimester, pregnant women experience changes in their hormone levels, which result in increased levels of sleepiness (Freeman, Crissman, Louw, Butcher, & Inskeep, 1970; Lancel, Faulhaber, Holsboer, & Rupprecht, 1996). Subsequently, the developing fetus begins to apply pressure to the bladder, reducing functional capacity and resulting in women needing to wake up more frequently throughout the night (Mindell & Jacobson, 2000). The risk for sleep disorders such as restless leg syndrome (RLS), frequent snoring, and obstructive sleep apnea (OSA) also increases during pregnancy (Facco, Kramer, Ho, Zee, & Grobman, 2010; Nodine & Matthews, 2013). A meta-analysis by our research group indicated a high prevalence (45.7%) of poor sleep quality reported among pregnant women, worsening from the second to third trimester (Sedov, Cameron, Madigan, & Tomfohr-Madsen, 2018). Finally, stress and anxiety have been noted as important concerns during pregnancy (Dunkel Schetter & Tanner, 2012) and higher levels of stress and anxiety have been linked to changes in

Adapting Cognitive Behavioral Therapy for Insomnia
https://doi.org/10.1016/B978-0-12-822872-2.00013-X

sleep (Âkerstedt, 2006; Hicks & Garcia, 1987). Across pregnancy, women consistently rate their thoughts as one of the leading causes for difficulties in either falling or staying asleep (Mindell & Jacobson, 2000).

A number of researchers have examined pregnant women's sleep using polysomnography (PSG) (Brunner et al., 1994; Coble et al., 1994; Hertz et al., 1992; Izci-Balserak et al., 2018; Wilson & Donachie, 2018). PSG yields standard sleep parameters such as total time spent sleeping, number of awakenings during sleep, and time spent awake after falling asleep. Findings from this cross-sectional line of research have indicated that relative to nonpregnant controls, pregnant women spend more time awake after falling asleep, obtain less rapid-eye-movement (REM) sleep, spend more time in lighter stages of sleep (non-REM 1), and experience a decrease in deeper (slow-wave) stages of sleep (Hertz et al., 1992; Wilson et al., 2011). Furthermore, longitudinal studies have reported that late pregnancy (e.g., 27–39 weeks) is characterized by less total sleep time, more time spent in light stages of sleep, less time in deep sleep and REM sleep, and more time spent awake after falling asleep relative to early pregnancy (e.g., 8–14 weeks) (Brunner et al., 1994; Izci-Balserak et al., 2018). Overall, the research evidence suggests that pregnancy is a time of less restorative and more disturbed sleep characterized by restlessness.

These extensively studied changes provide important information regarding the sleep of pregnant women. Yet, sleep parameters alone provide little information regarding women's perceptions of their sleep, and therefore, little information regarding insomnia, which is characterized as dissatisfaction with the quantity or quality of one's sleep (American Psychiatric Association, 2013). These subjective perceptions are highly important as distress related to sleep is a likely motivator to seek help, and is strongly linked to adverse perinatal outcomes, including increased risk of preterm birth (Felder, Baer, Rand, Jelliffe-Pawlowski, & Prather, 2017). As such, an understanding of insomnia disorder as it occurs during pregnancy is of high importance to both researchers and clinicians working with pregnant women.

Insomnia during pregnancy

The development of insomnia is characterized by a stress-diathesis model of predisposing, precipitating, and perpetuating factors (Spielman, Caruso, & Glovinsky, 1987). The theory and data suggest that individuals who are high in stress reactivity (Harvey, Gehrman, & Espie, 2014) and undergo a period of stress, particularly related to family (e.g., separation and marital problems) and health (e.g., pain and medical problems) (Bastien, Vallieres, & Morin, 2004), are most at risk of experiencing insomnia. Undeniably, pregnancy can constitute a period of such stress.

Estimates of insomnia prevalence during pregnancy range from 13% to 62% in the samples tested (Dørheim, Bjorvatn, & Eberhard-Gran, 2012; Okun, Buysse, & Hall, 2015), likely due to differences in the timing of data collection and instruments used to measure insomnia. A meta-analysis of 24 studies with 15,564 total participants conducted by our research group in 2020 found the overall prevalence of insomnia symptoms (above the clinical cut-off suggestive of insomnia) during pregnancy to be 38.2% (Sedov, Anderson, Dhillon, & Tomfohr-Madsen, 2021). Interestingly, a longitudinal evaluation found significant increases in insomnia from early (38%) to late (54%) pregnancy (Facco et al., 2010). Such estimates should raise serious concerns for both researchers and healthcare providers; as a 13% prevalence rate is what would be expected in the general population (American Psychiatric Association, 2013), while higher rates may be indicative of pregnancy constituting a time of insomnia-vulnerability.

The timing and progression of insomnia during pregnancy have also been explored in the literature. Some authors reported that insomnia prevalence is elevated relative to the general population across all months of pregnancy (Mindell, Cook, & Nikolovski, 2015) and that the entire period may be considered a time of high risk for the development or re-emergence of insomnia. Other authors have reported that the third trimester is associated with worse insomnia symptoms (Facco et al., 2010; Kızılırmak, Timur, & Kartal, 2012; Román-Gálvez et al., 2018). A recent trajectory analysis of 142 women conducted by our research team identified three distinct patterns: a no-insomnia group (42.2%) with consistently low symptoms, a subclinical insomnia group (44.3%) with a brief increase in symptom severity in the third trimester, and a clinical insomnia group (13.4%) with consistently elevated symptoms across the perinatal period (Sedov & Tomfohr-Madsen, 2021). These findings suggest that symptoms of insomnia are relatively stable across pregnancy, such that women who sleep well in early pregnancy can expect to sleep well throughout, while those few who report severe insomnia at the beginning will continue to. However, it seems that many women will experience some symptoms of insomnia early in pregnancy, which then increases in late pregnancy.

Anxiety and depression have been highlighted as important correlates of insomnia during pregnancy (Osnes et al., 2020; Polo-Kantola, Aukia, Karlsson, Karlsson, & Paavonen, 2017; Swanson, Pickett, Flynn, & Armitage, 2011; van der Zwan et al., 2017; Volkovich, Tikotzky, & Manber, 2016) such that women with sleep disturbance are also more likely to be anxious and/or depressed. This relationship has been documented extensively in nonpregnant samples (Alvaro, Roberts, & Harris, 2013) and is an important area of research and clinical attention, given the robust body of work documenting the effects of anxiety and depression during pregnancy on the health of the mother and developing fetus (Dunkel Schetter & Glynn, 2011; Guardino & Dunkel Schetter, 2014; Gurung, Dunkel Schetter, Collins, Rini, & Hobel, 2005). The limited number of studies on longitudinal relationships between anxiety and sleep in pregnant women has produced mixed results such that some authors have reported anxiety predicting subsequent decreases in sleep duration (van der Zwan et al., 2017) and others have reported no relationship over time between anxiety symptoms and sleep disturbances such as self-reported insomnia and poor sleep quality (Polo-Kantola et al., 2017; Tham et al., 2016). A recent study by our research group demonstrated that higher symptoms of generalized anxiety and depression in early pregnancy (before 19 weeks gestation) predicted consistently elevated symptoms of insomnia across the perinatal period (Sedov & Tomfohr-Madsen, 2021). These results suggest that anxiety and depression early in pregnancy have important implications for the later severity of insomnia symptoms. Maternal mental health is recognized as a global public health priority (World Health Organization, 2021) and several agency guidelines, including the ACOG (American College of Obstetricians Gynecologists, 2018) and SOGC (Society of Obstetricians and Gynecologists of Canada), recommend screening for depression, anxiety, and psychosocial factors that impact mental health during the perinatal period (Austin, Highet, & The Expert Working Group, 2017)—insomnia should be considered in this constellation of screening.

Consequences of insomnia on maternal and infant outcomes

Insomnia during pregnancy has consequences for maternal and child health. For example, insomnia and sleep disturbances in pregnancy have been associated with numerous pregnancy complications including preeclampsia, growth retardation, preterm birth, longer labor, and cesarean delivery (Chang, Pien, Duntley, & Macones, 2010; Lee & Gay, 2004; Naghi, Keypour, Ahari, Tavalai, & Khak, 2011). Experiencing poor sleep quality in pregnancy has been shown to predict maternal suicidal ideation (Gelaye et al., 2015) and symptoms of postpartum depression (Okun, Hanusa, Hall, & Wisner, 2009; Park, Meltzer-Brody, & Stickgold, 2013; Tomfohr, Buliga, Letourneau, Campbell, & Giesbrecht, 2015). In fact, experiencing a sleep trajectory characterized by consistently poor sleep quality in the perinatal period or development of poor sleep quality in the third trimester of pregnancy has been associated with 10 to 20-fold increases in the risk of experiencing symptoms indicative of postpartum depression, even after controlling for robust predictors of postpartum depression such as depression in pregnancy and socioeconomic status (Tomfohr et al., 2015). Postpartum depression is itself associated with numerous negative child outcomes (Stein et al., 2014). Emerging evidence also suggests that mothers' sleep disturbances, particularly sleep restriction, during pregnancy may negatively impact their children's sleep (Lyu et al., 2020; Pires et al., 2020).

Assessment of insomnia in pregnancy

Sleep beliefs and expectations vary by culture. Transitioning to parenthood itself constitutes entry into a new role with its own beliefs about sleep. Cultural considerations are an important part of good therapeutic assessment and feedback, and this is no different for insomnia. Although outside the bounds of this chapter, we recommend that providers follow best practices in cultural considerations for the group they are assessing. In pregnancy, we often see clients who believe in the importance of breastfeeding/feeding to sleep or bedsharing/cosleeping with infants and small children. Breastfeeding practices at night may also differ by culture. Therapists who do not understand and respect cultural differences or who pathologize them as part of the assessment, run the risk of losing credibility and trust.

Assessment of insomnia and sleep difficulties is important for accurately understanding a patient's presentation and experience in the context of pregnancy, as well as for tracking or evaluating progress in response to treatment. Self-report questionnaires can be easily administered for screening insomnia symptomatology. However, few scales have been validated for use during pregnancy. We recommend the 7-item Insomnia Severity Index (ISI) (Morin, Belleville, Bélanger, & Ivers, 2011), which corresponds to the criteria for insomnia disorder in the Diagnostic and Statistical Manual of Mental Disorders (DSM) (Bastien, Vallières, & Morin, 2001). A clinical cut-off score of 10 on the ISI indicates insomnia (Morin et al., 2011). The ISI has been reliably used to assess insomnia during pregnancy and has been shown to be sensitive to change in insomnia severity in response to CBT-I treatment during pregnancy, by ours and other research groups (Manber et al., 2019; Swanson, Flynn, Adams-Mundy, Armitage, & Arnedt, 2013; Tomfohr-Madsen, Clayborne, Rouleau, & Campbell, 2017).

In terms of monitoring sleep problems more broadly, the Pittsburgh Sleep Quality Index (PSQI) (Buysse, Reynolds, Monk, Berman, & Kupfer, 1989) is a useful 19-item questionnaire. A general cut-off score of 5 and above is used to indicate poor subjective sleep quality (Buysse et al., 1989). However, a recent meta-analysis conducted by our research group (Sedov et al., 2018) found that the average PSQI score among pregnant women was 6.07, with 45.7% scoring above the >5 cut-off. This finding suggests that the PSQI would identify the average pregnant woman as a poor sleeper, and thus, the general cut-off score may be inappropriate for the pregnant population. A higher score may be required to differentiate pregnant women in need of further assessment and treatment; therefore, we suggest a cut-off score of 7 and above during pregnancy as used in other studies (Okun et al., 2009). The PSQI has been validated against polysomnography and used reliably among pregnant women (Qiu et al., 2016; Skouteris, Wertheim, Germano, Paxton, & Milgrom, 2009;

Zhong, Gelaye, Sánchez, & Williams, 2015). The Patient-Reported Outcomes Measurement Information System (PROMIS) Sleep Disturbance—Short Form 4a and Sleep-Related Impairment—Short Form 4a (Yu et al., 2012) also provide brief, four-item screening options that have been used reliably in maternal samples (Mersky, Lee, Gilbert, & Goyal, 2020). As with other PROMIS® measures, raw scores are converted to T-scores; where T-scores ranging from 60 to 69.9 are indicative of moderate problems and scores at or above 70 are considered severely elevated.

A clinical diagnostic interview, such as the Structured Clinical Interview for DSM-5 (SCID-5; First, Williams, Karg, & Spitzer, 2016), is the gold standard for determining the diagnosis of an insomnia disorder during pregnancy. The SCID-5 Sleep Disorders Module has demonstrated excellent reliability for insomnia in general adult samples (Taylor et al., 2018). The Duke Structured Interview for Sleep Disorders (Edinger et al., 2004) has also been reliably used as a screening tool for insomnia in pregnant women (Manber et al., 2019). It is important to note that while pregnancy is often a trigger for insomnia (i.e., due to hormones, bladder, etc.), the symptoms and maintenance factors (e.g., napping, dysfunctional cognitions) are similar to those in other times of life.

Given the increased prevalence of OSA and RLS (i.e., due to hormonal changes and weight gain) in pregnancy (Facco et al., 2010; Nodine & Matthews, 2013), if either of these is screened in (e.g., on the SCID-5), we recommend referring to the family physician for further assessment including a sleep study as well as a discussion about a potential treatment for RLS (e.g., often high dose oral or infusion iron depending on what ferritin testing reveals).

Treatment of insomnia in pregnancy

Treating insomnia in pregnancy with pharmacotherapy has been shown to improve sleep quality and confers a protective benefit against the onset of postpartum depression (Khazaie, Ghadami, Knight, Emamian, & Tahmasian, 2013); however, recent best practice guidelines advise against the use of sleep medications in pregnancy due to potential teratogenicity (Abbott, Attarian, & Zee, 2014). Additionally, data suggest that the majority of pregnant women are reluctant to take prescription medications due to their perception of risk (Arch, 2014; Dimidjian & Goodman, 2014). Results from a recent study conducted by our research group, assessing patient perceptions, found that when presented with descriptions of pharmacotherapy versus cognitive behavioral therapy for insomnia (CBT-I), pregnant women rated CBT-I as significantly more credible and indicated that it was a preferable treatment for insomnia experienced in pregnancy when compared to pharmacotherapy (Sedov, Goodman, & Tomfohr-Madsen, 2017). In concordance with reports from pregnant women, their partners also indicated a preference for CBT-I to treat maternal insomnia during pregnancy (Sedov, Madsen, Goodman, & Tomfohr-Madsen, 2019).

CBT-I in the perinatal period

Pregnant women have historically been excluded from intervention research and insomnia treatment is no exception, prompting calls for further development of interventions to treat insomnia in pregnancy and postpartum (Sharkey, 2013). There has been one open pilot of CBT-I for women with insomnia and comorbid postpartum depression (Swanson et al., 2013). Results indicated that participation in five sessions of individual CBT-I was associated with improvements in maternal sleep efficiency and quality, reduced fatigue, insomnia severity, and symptoms of depression. To date, there have been four studies (Felder, Epel, Neuhaus, Krystal, & Prather, 2020; Kalmbach et al., 2020; Manber et al., 2019; Tomfohr-Madsen et al., 2017) examining the effectiveness of in-person or online CBT-I in pregnancy specifically, the first of which was an open pilot conducted by our research group at the University of Calgary in Alberta, Canada.

The Sleeping for Two intervention was delivered to thirteen pregnant women with insomnia and results suggested that CBT-I was effective in reducing both subjective symptoms of insomnia and improving objective indices of sleep quality (Tomfohr-Madsen et al., 2017). Additionally, the intervention was acceptable to participants with 100% of women who began treatment successfully completing the five-session group protocol. The majority of women entered the study reporting elevated depressive symptoms, and, consistent with previous findings observed in other populations (Swanson et al., 2013; Tsuno, Besset, & Ritchie, 2005), they experienced a significant decline in depressive symptoms in the follow-up period. These results are encouraging, as recent trajectory analyses from our group show that without intervention, disturbed sleep and depressive symptoms are relatively stable or increasing in the perinatal period (Sedov & Tomfohr-Madsen, 2021; Tomfohr et al., 2015). Group treatment with five sessions of CBT-I also significantly improved subjective sleep quality, even as the pregnancy progressed.

Another research group, from Stanford University in California, conducted a multisite randomized controlled trial (RCT) of CBT-I with an ethnically diverse sample of treatment-naive women meeting the criteria for insomnia disorder, but not depression, during pregnancy

(Manber et al., 2019). The intervention consisted of five individual therapy sessions during pregnancy. Results indicated significantly greater reductions in insomnia severity among pregnant women, with 62% attaining remission, and faster (median 31 days), than those in the control group (52% in 48 days). CBT-I intervention also led to significant reductions in self-reported total wake time and symptoms of depression.

Two studies have examined the efficacy of CBT-I in pregnancy delivered online (Felder et al., 2020; Kalmbach et al., 2020). Digital or eHealth adaptations are valuable options to reach the largest number of pregnant women, especially those living in remote or rural areas or for whom transportation, childcare, and/or work hours present as barriers to accessing treatment (Dennis & Chung-Lee, 2006; Flynn, Henshaw, O'Mahen, & Forman, 2010; Kim et al., 2010; Smith, Lawrence, Sadler, & Easter, 2019). The digital CBT-I program Sleepio (Big Health Inc.) has demonstrated effectiveness for reducing insomnia severity and significantly improving sleep duration, efficiency, and quality, as well as decreasing symptoms of anxiety and depression (Felder et al., 2017; Kalmbach et al., 2020).

Together, the research to date demonstrates the effectiveness of adapting CBT-I as a nonpharmacologic treatment for women experiencing insomnia during pregnancy.

Sleeping for two: A five-session protocol for CBT-I in pregnancy

As part of treatment, we recognize that sleep norms around timing and location vary by culture. Exploring beliefs with clients and cocreating a shared conceptualization of the presenting sleep problem and negotiating a mutually agreed-upon treatment plan is key to achieving success with diverse clients. The principles of culturally adapted treatment (Domenech Rodríguez & Bernal, 2012) are as important for CBT-I in pregnancy as they are for other presenting disorders.

The Sleeping for Two adaptation for CBT-I in pregnancy consists of five weekly 90-min individual or group therapy sessions. Patients are asked to use a daily sleep diary for self-monitoring and receive a manual containing readings summarizing the material being taught in session. The manual was adapted from a treatment protocol previously validated for oncology patients with comorbid insomnia (Garland et al., 2014). In adapting the CBT-I protocol for use with pregnant women, we followed steps outlined in the ORBIT Model (Czajkowski et al., 2015; Walker & Czajkowski, 2019) for developing behavioral therapies to treat or prevent chronic diseases and enhance health-promoting behaviors (e.g., sleep): Phase I (i.e., defined the question), Phase IIa (i.e., created a fixed treatment package; see Appendix 1 in Tomfohr-Madsen et al., 2017 for group curriculum), Phase IIb (i.e., pilot tested the intervention), and Phase III (i.e., a randomized controlled trial; RCT) which is currently underway testing individual sessions delivered either in person or online depending on public health social distancing guidelines. Interim analysis of our pre-post data indicated large effect sizes for improving insomnia, with a 16 × higher remission rate, among pregnant women who received CBT-I (manuscript in preparation). Moreover, telehealth (i.e., videoconferencing) delivery was as effective as in-person sessions, even during the context of the COVID-19 pandemic.

During this five-session intervention, patients are familiarized with the self-management approach for insomnia (e.g., active vs. passive coping strategies). First, patients are oriented to CBT-I (e.g., use of daily sleep diaries) and set individualized treatment goals (Session 1). The remaining sessions consist of weekly review of sleep diaries, psychoeducation about sleep and sleep consolidation (Session 2), stimulus control (Session 3), cognitive strategies to examine attitudes and beliefs about sleep (Session 4), and problem-solving to cope with sleep disturbances and relapse prevention (Session 5). A more detailed description of the Sleeping for Two protocol adaptations for CBT-I in pregnancy is provided below (see Table 1).

TABLE 1 Adaptation for CBT-I in pregnancy.

CBT-I components	Standard practice	Modifications/adaptions
Sleep education	3-P model, 2-process model of sleep regulation, sleep stages	Recognize and understand the controllable and uncontrollable factors that affect sleep, including physiologic and emotional changes during pregnancy, such as hormonal alterations, that can affect sleep quality and quantity
Sleep restriction	Improve sleep efficiency by limiting time in bed to the amount of time sleeping then expanding slowly as long as sleep efficiency is preserved	Initial time in bed recommendations equal to average total sleep time plus 30 min, but never less than 5 h of total sleep time during pregnancy
Stimulus control	Associate bed/bedroom solely as a cue for sleep by eliminating nonsleep activities from the bedroom. Instruction to get out of bed at night if awake >15 min	Address family arrangements (e.g., partner watching TV, breastfeeding in bed) and physical discomfort issues related to pregnancy (e.g., pain, bladder control) preventing sleeping in bed

Continued

TABLE 1 Adaptation for CBT-I in pregnancy—cont'd

CBT-I components	Standard practice	Modifications/adaptions
Napping/daytime sleep	Discontinue or restrict daytime napping to 30 min	Daytime napping and sleeping are discouraged. However, given some women experience an increased need for sleep during pregnancy, some flexibility is offered, so long as naps are in the morning to avoid starting the sleep period early
Sleep hygiene education	Address daytime habits and sleep environment interfering with sleep	Discuss and problem-solve family environment and sleep routines (e.g., use of baby monitors, cosleeping with other children) that could be interfering with sleep Reinforce the positive benefits of physical activity for sleep. Guidelines recommend 150 min of moderate or strenuous activity per week during pregnancy
Cognitive therapy	Challenge patient's dysfunctional beliefs interfering with sleep and misconceptions about sleep. Replace/restructure to more helpful and realistic thoughts about sleep	Address fears about the amount of sleep or sleep position affecting fetal development In preparation for the postpartum period, review common cognitive distortions about infant sleep
Relapse prevention	Discuss practicing less rigid sleep plan over time and what to do prevent sleep disturbance from turning into another episode of insomnia in the future	Discuss effective ways to cope with relapse, especially in the postpartum period, and acknowledge that sleep disruptions are likely after bringing baby home Discuss infant sleep and how to best establish healthy habits for infants in the postpartum period
Sleep diaries	Establish baseline sleep patterns, track progress, reinforce appropriate behavior change, problem-solve obstacles to adherence	Monitor any external factors related to the family environment (partner, children) that might impact sleep. Encourage tracking infant sleep for a few days after birth to help identify infant sleep needs

Understanding sleep problems in the context of pregnancy

Therapists start by gathering a brief history of patients' sleeping difficulties and presleep routines, taking into account their stage of pregnancy and the related somatic symptoms and physical discomforts (e.g., back pain, overactive bladder), employment and maternity leave status, as well as sleep arrangements with partners and other children that may impact sleep.

Pregnancy-specific materials are used to help patients understand and reflect on the manifestations of insomnia they may be experiencing. For example, in the first session patients read a common case story of a pregnant woman struggling with insomnia (see Box 1) and are asked to determine which symptoms relate to their experience.

Pregnant individuals are encouraged to reflect on their sleep problems within the system of their family (Tracy & Troxel, 2019), and to work with the therapist to identify barriers to changing sleep (e.g., a toddler with sleep problems, a partner who likes to watch TV in the bedroom) (Table 2). When discussing goals for the treatment program, the following point can also be made:

> Did you know that factors that promote good maternal sleep are also good predictors of infant, child and adolescent sleep? Our hope is that what you learn in this program will translate into better sleep for your whole family.

Pregnant individuals are also encouraged to engage a support person in the treatment program, to review materials with each week, and to support them in making sleep-related behavior changes. Indeed, social support is associated with better sleep (Kent de Grey, Uchino, Trettevik, Cronan, & Hogan, 2018; Troxel, 2010), as well as better adherence and

---

BOX 1

A common story.

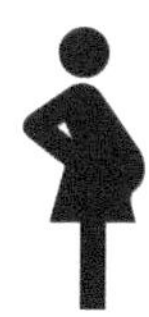

Jane is a 33-year-old woman who is 28 weeks pregnant. Before being pregnant, Jane had little trouble with sleep, despite sometimes waking up during the night to use the washroom. Now she finds sleep to be very frustrating. She tosses and turns all night and wakes up exhausted and irritated. Jane tries to nap during the day to feel better but then finds that she can't sleep at night. Her sleeping problems have not gotten any better and she worries about how they might affect her pregnancy and mood.

TABLE 2 Examples of common pregnancy-related and family-level barriers to changing sleep.

Barriers	Recommendations
Pregnancy	
Fatigue	Pacing out activities during the day
Frequent urination	Reducing liquid intake (2h) before bed
Aches and pains	A warm bath before bed, positional pillow
Worries about sleep impacting baby	Cognitive restructuring to challenge thoughts
Partner	
Snoring or restless sleeping	Assessment, earplugs, separate rooms
Likes to watch TV in the bedroom	Different location, before buffer zone
Different work schedules/ wake-up times	Coordinate, quieter alarms
Children	
	In all cases of concurrent child sleep problems, we recommend the involment of a partner (if present in the home) to arrive at systemic solutions
Nighttime feedings	Gradually wean as increasing daytime calories
A baby monitor that causes frequent awakenings	Reduce volume, leave the door open instead
Toddler/child with sleep problems	Address sleep associations, talk to a pediatrician to make an evidence-based sleep plan for the child
Falling asleep with children at bedtime	Develop a new routine, transfer bedtime and/or night responsibility to partner (if possible)

response (e.g., decreased insomnia severity) to CBT-I (Kamen et al., 2019). In particular, partner alliance or involvement in CBT-I is purported to increase treatment adherence and completion (Ellis, Deary, & Troxel, 2015; Mellor et al., 2019), because partners can act as agents of social control who monitor and promote health and sleep-related behaviors (Rogojanski, Carney, & Monson, 2013). If buy-in or agreement to change sleep routines or help with nighttime childcare is low, having partners attend sessions is often helpful.

Psychoeducation about sleep in pregnancy

Psychoeducation includes a review of the biology (i.e., sleep stages, awakenings) and function (i.e., restoration, survival) of sleep, controllable (i.e., routine) and uncontrollable (i.e., circadian) factors that influence sleep, as well as providing information specific to sleep during pregnancy to help validate and normalize patients' experience of insomnia. For example, in the second session, the following points are highlighted:

- There is a high prevalence of insomnia among pregnant women (30%–60%, depending on the survey); use this to demonstrate patients are not alone.
- Objectively, sleep seems to decline by about 20 min from the beginning to end of pregnancy.
- The most common sleep complaints among pregnant women are delayed time to fall asleep, reduced sleep time, repeated awakenings to go to the bathroom, and poor sleep quality. People may differ in how they experience these symptoms.
- Alterations of hormonal secretions during pregnancy cause physiologic changes which affect sleep. For example, progesterone levels decrease the amount of REM sleep and reduce the latency to non-REM sleep. Progesterone is also responsible for the induced smooth muscle relaxation, which causes frequent urination, heartburn, pregnancy rhinitis, and possibly raises body temperature that disrupts sleep quality. Hormonal changes cause other symptoms such as leg cramps, shortness of breath, breast tenderness, backache, and itching, which can explain multiple awakenings.
- The average healthy person wakes up 5 to 15 times; use this to emphasize that it is normal for someone to wake up several times throughout the night. Point out the adaptive functions of cyclic awakenings (e.g., parents need to hear children's cries).
- Other common reasons contributing to sleep problems in pregnancy are fears about labor and delivery, the anticipation of parenthood, financial concerns and worries about work position after maternity leave, or anxiety about changing relationships with partners, which can all affect the ability to fall or stay asleep. This is especially more common among first-time mothers.

Sleep restriction

Sleep restriction procedures are introduced in the second session. Consistent with standard CBT-I, the initial time in bed recommendation equals the average total sleep time plus 30 min. However, pregnant patients are instructed to not restrict their sleep to less than the number of hours they report getting before beginning treatment or to less than 5h per night, whichever number is greater. Research evidence suggests that pregnant women with sleep deprivation (less than 5h) are at higher risk for preterm birth (Micheli et al., 2011), which is where this number was drawn from initially. Although the National Sleep Foundation recommends an average sleep duration of ≥7h per night as adequate for adults (Hirshkowitz et al., 2015), pregnant women report needing an average of 8.2h of sleep to feel rested (Mindell & Jacobson, 2000). Time spent waking up to engage in childcare or feeding at night is counted as a time not sleeping (e.g., waking after sleep onset), and as time out of bed unless these activities occur in the parent's bed. Time is added to the sleep window to account for this, acknowledging that potentially 60min of the night will be spent engaging in childcare/feeding.

Stimulus control

Stimulus control procedures are introduced in the third session. Patients are asked to get out of bed if they can't fall asleep within 15–20min. This applies to their initial bedtime, after nighttime awakenings (e.g., due to discomfort or using the bathroom), and trying to fall asleep after engaging in childcare or feeding at night. If patients report frequent awakenings due to bladder control, therapists may suggest a behavioral experiment to test how much urine is produced each time (e.g., to challenge the need to go to the bathroom) and to try out if they can fall back asleep after contracting muscles to hold the urge. If bladder control complaints persist or worsen, we recommend client's consult with their family physician for assessment of possible causes (e.g., gestational diabetes) and discussion of potential treatments or recommendations.

Another stimulus control procedure asks patients not to use the bed or bedroom for any activity other than sleep or sex. Many pregnant women report sleeping on the couch, or somewhere other than their bed, usually due to physical discomfort or a partner interrupting their sleep in the bedroom. In these cases, we encourage therapists to have an open discussion exploring possible adjustments that could be made to increase comfort in the bed (e.g., extra pillows, weighted blankets) and decrease partner disruptions (e.g., coordinating sleep/wake-up times, earplugs, moving or turning down the volume of alarms, removing screens, or sleeping separately).

Napping and daytime sleeping

Avoiding daytime napping is difficult for many pregnant women, especially in the last trimester of pregnancy. Indeed, research suggests women take more (and longer) daytime naps during 35–38weeks gestation (Mindell & Jacobson, 2000). Women often report that as the day wears on, their fatigue increases with activity, making a nap in the afternoon "feel necessary." However, there are strategies, such as pacing (e.g., spreading out activities into manageable chunks) or finding alternative activities incompatible with sleeping (e.g., going for a walk outside), that can be used to prevent a build-up of fatigue caused by too much activity at one time. Patients are encouraged not to nap in their bed, and to try to schedule naps before noon to avoid reducing sleep pressure. It is helpful to engage in a frank discussion about napping and sleep pressure, with the goal of building self-efficacy and transferring control to the client—so they can make their own decision about whether they want to interrupt their sleep pressure. For maximum gain, we do recommend keeping napping to a minimum. Clients are reminded that it is dangerous to drive a motor vehicle or operate heavy equipment while feeling tired, and if they find themselves in such cases where safety is a concern, a nap may be warranted.

Sleep hygiene and lifestyle factors

Sleep hygiene is also reviewed in Session 3. Therapists reinforce the positive benefits of physical activity for sleep, particularly during pregnancy when guidelines recommend engaging in at least 150 min of moderate or strenuous activity per week (Mottola et al., 2018). Patients are also informed that activity of any kind is known to increase slow-wave sleep and therefore deepen sleep. In terms of diet, pregnant individuals may also experience increased heartburn or food sensitivities that impair sleep. In this case, it is suggested that patients track their food and medication intake to observe any links with their sleep patterns. We recommend establishing good communication with a client's maternity care team, especially since women are seeing their providers more during pregnancy, regarding any recommendations or treatments related to physical discomfort such as pain (e.g., positional pillows, sleeping on an incline) or digestive issues such as acid reflux/GERD (e.g., the timing of meals, eating a light snack before bed that metabolizes slowly).

Therapists also encourage an open discussion and problem-solving around any family environment and sleep routines (e.g., use/volume of baby monitors, cosleeping with other children) that could be interfering with maternal sleep. For example, it is common to explore whether a partner could help with other children's presleep routines or night awakenings, and often we find that simple recommendations about lowering baby monitor volume used for other children reduces maternal awakenings. It is often helpful to challenge the common misconception of "sleeping like a baby," or the belief that (good) sleep should be silent and motionless, by discussing how infants and young children are actually *not* quiet sleepers. In fact, during active (REM) sleep it is *normal* for infants to make a range of sounds (e.g., sigh, coo, groan, whimper, etc.) and movements (e.g., smile, breath heavily, open eyes partially, move arms or legs) (Mindell, 2010). Therefore, it is not necessary to listen for or check on these little sounds or small movements, and instead parents could try turning off or reducing baby monitor volume, as the *loud persistent* sounds that indicate infants are distressed and need help soothing (e.g., hard, continuous crying) are likely to cause parents to wake up on their own. This information can alleviate worry, decrease hypervigilance, and reduce reliance on baby monitors, which can all disrupt parents' sleep.

Notably, there are large cultural variations in sleep norms for infants and children and these should be explored and respected as the therapist works collaboratively with the client to conceptualize their sleep problems and cocreate sustainable solutions for the family.

Cognitive restructuring

Cognitive restructuring is introduced in Session 4. Examples that are relevant to pregnancy and the postpartum period are provided (see Table 3). It is also important to address fears or unrealistic thoughts about whether the amount of sleep or sleep position can negatively affect fetal development. For example, expectant mothers might think "I need more sleep than before pregnancy" or "My lack of sleep will harm my baby." Clients are asked to identify the assumptions (e.g., unrealistic expectations

TABLE 3 Examples of cognitive restructuring for negative sleep-related thoughts in pregnancy and the postpartum.

Category of negative self-talk	Actual evidence and alternative explanations	Positive self-statements you can use instead
Misunderstanding the cause of disturbed sleep—"Worry wakes me up"	Many pregnant women do have good nights of sleep.	"Just because I am pregnant, that doesn't mean that I will suffer from poor sleep every night"
Unrealistic Expectations about Sleep—"I need 8h of sleep every night"	People differ in the amount of sleep they need; the range is from 4 to 10h in the general population	"I used to get by on less sleep before I became pregnant"
Magnifying the negative consequences of sleep disturbances—"My baby is not getting enough sleep and their brain will not develop properly."	Infants tend to get the sleep they require. Just like adults, infants differ in the amount of sleep they need.	"My baby is developing normally." "Just because my friend's baby sleeps 12h at night, doesn't mean my baby will"

about sleep) and thinking biases/cognitive distortions (e.g., jumping to conclusions) of this self-talk, and then challenge it by evaluating the accuracy of evidence for (e.g., I've been having strange pains/cramps) and against (e.g., my check-ups all indicate normal growth and development, my diary shows I'm getting more sleep than I realized, lots of people have mild sleep problems or some nights of poor sleep). Then, we try to help clients generate more accurate/realistic self-statements, such as "It's not how much I sleep that is important, it is the quality of my sleep" or "I am doing many good things to take care of mine and my baby's health while pregnant," and try out how that feels.

Another example, pregnant women might think "Sleeping on my back is dangerous for my baby!" as they often hear that they should not sleep on their back during pregnancy because it could lead to stillbirth or fetal growth restriction (Fox & Oster, 2019), and become anxious about shifting positions while they sleep. To challenge this assumption (e.g., magnifying the negative consequences of sleep disturbances) and distorted thinking (e.g., catastrophizing), therapists can provide patients with an overview of the current state of the actual evidence. Indeed, the validity of the extant research about this topic is unclear, as most studies have been small, retrospective, and not randomized (Gordon et al., 2015; Heazell et al., 2018; McCowan et al., 2017; Owusu et al., 2013; Stacey et al., 2011); therefore, caution is warranted in drawing definitive conclusions. Results from a recently published prospective study of 8706 women indicated that objective assessment of sleeping in the supine or right lateral position was *not* associated with stillbirth, low or small-for-gestational-age birthweights, nor hypertensive disorders of pregnancy (Silver et al., 2019). However, pregnant women who sleep on their backs may be those who experience snoring or sleep apnea, both of which could affect maternal sleep and delivery outcomes (Bin, Cistulli, & Ford, 2016; O'Brien et al., 2013). Sleeping on one's back may become more uncomfortable as pregnancy progresses due to increasing weight. After a discussion of the facts, patients are asked to generate self-statements they can use instead, such as "Sleeping on my back sometimes is okay." Patients can also be encouraged to discuss any outstanding concerns with their maternity care provider.

Relaxation strategies

Relaxation techniques are also introduced in Session 4. Patients are presented to paced breathing, progressive or deep muscle relaxation, imagery-induced relaxation, and self-hypnosis. At least one technique of the patient's choice is practiced in session. Given the physical discomfort often experienced in pregnancy, patients are encouraged to try all the techniques, practice when they are not stressed, and find at least one that is helpful for them. For example, if paced breathing leads to increased stress (e.g., because of difficulty breathing deeply in the third trimester, feelings of not getting enough air), or if progressive muscle relaxation leads to increased pain (e.g., back pain), you can recommend trying a different relaxation technique. Several general techniques for managing stress-related bedtime thoughts are also provided, including concentrating on one problem at a time, setting aside "worrying time," thinking the worst (i.e., catastrophizing) and then developing a plan to deal with it, doing worrying on paper instead of in your head, and distraction.

Relapse prevention

In the fifth and final session, participants are provided information about how to maintain gains in the postpartum period, as well as information on infant sleep (see Table 4) and the importance of mutual regulation which was adapted from evidenced-based behavioral-education programs (Stremler et al., 2013) and consultation with infant sleep experts. The following points are highlighted:

- Remind the client that bringing the baby home will likely cause some sleep disruptions.
- The tips learned throughout the course of treatment can all be applied to child sleep (e.g., good sleep hygiene, creating bedtime routines, challenging distorted cognitions about sleep).
- Make a sleep plan for the baby. Reinforce how important this is to discuss with those at home who may be helping with sleep routines. It is easier to make a coparenting plan before the baby is born.
- Infants have 6 different sleep states: crying > active alert > quiet alert > drowsy > light sleep > deep sleep, and often require help to move from one to another (mutual regulation).
- Over the first few years, infants and young children gradually learn to move through these states independently (self-regulation), including how to fall and stay asleep. This does not mean leaving the baby alone to soothe themself, but to "pause, watch, and wonder" how your baby tells you they are in distress and needs assistance or if they need a bit more time to try to self-soothe. When your baby needs your assistance to fall asleep or be soothed, try to start with the lowest "level" of help (i.e., the sound of your voice, gentle patting, rocking) and gradually move to more "intensive" strategies (i.e., feeding, rocking, or bouncing). It is also recommended to try to end feeding before infants fall asleep, and if they do, to can gently wake them before putting them down to fall asleep.
- The most effective treatment for infant sleep problems is to establish set bedtime routines and to not reinforce frequent awakenings of the child.

Stage	Sleep characteristics and changes	Tips for parents
Gestation	• REM sleep starts at 6–7 mos, non-REM sleep shortly after • Sleep patterns established at 8 mos	• Regular sleeping, eating, and activity routines in late pregnancy may help infants develop sleep patterns more quickly • Develop a plan (with a partner, if in the house) for when the baby arrives
0–3 months	• 50% active (REM) and 50% quiet (non-REM) sleep • Sleep throughout day and night in shorter cycles (2–4 h blocks) • At 8 weeks a diurnal/nocturnal pattern develops (night > day) • Crying/colic peaks at 8–10 weeks	• Newborns often need help falling asleep with soothing strategies • Try to end feedings before baby falls asleep • Waking at the same time each day can help infants get into a routine • Remember: every baby is different
3–6 months	• Stage 2 spindles (rapid brain activity) begin to occur • 50% of infants take 3+ naps/day • Sleep associations begin to form (e.g., relying on parent delivered strategies such as rocking or feeding to fall asleep; or others such as white noise, pacifier)	• Try waiting a few minutes after baby wakes to see if they can settle themselves back to sleep • Start practicing the sleep associations that you would like your baby to use to fall asleep • Start introducing regular routines • Put to sleep drowsy but awake
6–12 months	• 30% active (REM) and 70% quiet (non-REM) sleep • Develop the 4 distinct stages of non-REM sleep • Spontaneous k-complexes (large, slow brain waves) begin to occur • 60% of infants take 2 naps/day at set times (morning and afternoon) • Develop a pattern to their days • No longer need night feedings (getting calories during daytime)	• Linking activities (e.g., first feeding in a bright room, walk in the morning, lunch before nap, bath before bed) helps teach infants what to expect • 15–20 min bedtime routine; activities you both enjoy, start with last feeding, end where baby sleeps • 3–5 min naptime routine, with 2–3 activities from bedtime routine (e.g., change the diaper, cuddle, lullaby) • Try to wean off night feedings
1–3 years	• Most take 1 nap/day by 18mos • Many transition from crib to bed • Some resist bedtime/get up at night • Some start having fears/nightmares	• Maintain regular daily schedule and consistent bedtime routine • Set and consistently enforce limits • Keep same bedroom environment • Transitional objects (e.g., blanket, stuffed animal) help to settle on own
3–6 years	• Need 11–13 h of sleep • Most sleep at night (between 7:00–9:00 pm to 6:30–8:00 am) • Some take an afternoon nap at 3–4 yrs. • Many try to stall bedtime	• Maintain regular daily schedule and consistent bedtime routine • Set and consistently enforce limits • Cool, dark, quiet, comfortable room • Have child fall asleep independently

This is sometimes known as the "cry it out" method, or "Ferberizing." Parents may have strong feelings about this and it is important to discuss and acknowledge them while helping to problem-solve around infant sleep disruption.

Conclusion

Although insomnia symptoms are common in pregnancy and postpartum, a preponderance of research evidence and our own clinical experience suggests that symptoms are very responsive to treatment using cognitive behavioral therapy for insomnia (CBT-I) and associated intervention techniques for children. Our experience suggests that taking treatment preferences into account is important. Collaborative decision-making regarding treatment strategies and child sleep, inclusion of key support people, and addressing shifting roles related to sleep should be considered when treating sleep problems in this period. As is the case with all effective psychotherapy, consideration of cultural norms and cocreation of problem conceptualization and treatment planning remains standard when treating individuals with insomnia during the perinatal period.

References

Abbott, S. M., Attarian, H., & Zee, P. C. (2014). Sleep disorders in perinatal women. *Best Practice & Research. Clinical Obstetrics & Gynaecology, 28*(1), 159–168.

Âkerstedt, T. (2006). Psychosocial stress and impaired sleep. *Scandinavian Journal of Work, Environment & Health, 32*(6), 493–501.

Alvaro, P. K., Roberts, R. M., & Harris, J. K. (2013). A systematic review assessing bidirectionality between sleep disturbances, anxiety, and depression. *Sleep, 36*(7), 1059–1068.

American College of Obstetricians Gynecologists. (2018). ACOG Committee Opinion No. 757: Screening for perinatal depression. *Obstetrics and Gynecology, 132*, e208–e212.

American Psychiatric Association. (2013). *Diagnostic and statistical manual of mental disorders (DSM-5®)*. American Psychiatric Pub.

Arch, J. J. (2014). Cognitive behavioral therapy and pharmacotherapy for anxiety: Treatment preferences and credibility among pregnant and non-pregnant women. *Behaviour Research and Therapy, 52*, 53–60.

Austin, M.-P., Highet, N., & The Expert Working Group. (2017). *Mental health care in the perinatal period: Australian clinical practice guideline*. Centre of Perinatal Excellence.

Bastien, C. H., Vallières, A., & Morin, C. M. (2001). Validation of the Insomnia Severity Index as an outcome measure for insomnia research. *Sleep Medicine, 2*(4), 297–307.

Bastien, C. H., Vallieres, A., & Morin, C. M. (2004). Precipitating factors of insomnia. *Behavioral Sleep Medicine, 2*(1), 50–62.

Bin, Y. S., Cistulli, P. A., & Ford, J. B. (2016). Population-based study of sleep apnea in pregnancy and maternal and infant outcomes. *Journal of Clinical Sleep Medicine, 12*(6), 871–877.

Brunner, D. P., Münch, M., Biedermann, K., Huch, R., Huch, A., & Borbély, A. A. (1994). Changes in sleep and sleep electroencephalogram during pregnancy. *Sleep, 17*(7), 576–582.

Buysse, D. J., Reynolds, C. F., Monk, T. H., Berman, S. R., & Kupfer, D. J. (1989). The Pittsburgh sleep quality index: A new instrument for psychiatric practice and research. *Psychiatry Research, 28*(2), 193–213.

Chang, J. J., Pien, G. W., Duntley, S. P., & Macones, G. A. (2010). Sleep deprivation during pregnancy and maternal and fetal outcomes: Is there a relationship? *Sleep Medicine Reviews, 14*(2), 107–114.

Coble, P. A., Reynolds, C. F., III, Kupfer, D. J., Houck, P. R., Day, N. L., & Giles, D. E. (1994). Childbearing in women with and without a history of affective disorder. II. Electroencephalographic sleep. *Comprehensive Psychiatry, 35*(3), 215–224.

Czajkowski, S. M., Powell, L. H., Adler, N., Naar-King, S., Reynolds, K. D., Hunter, C. M., et al. (2015). From ideas to efficacy: The ORBIT model for developing behavioral treatments for chronic diseases. *Health Psychology, 34*(10), 971–982. https://doi.org/10.1037/hea0000161.

Dennis, C.-L., & Chung-Lee, L. (2006). Postpartum depression help-seeking barriers and maternal treatment preferences: A qualitative systematic review. *Birth, 33*(4), 323–331.

Dimidjian, S., & Goodman, S. H. (2014). Preferences and attitudes toward approaches to depression relapse/recurrence prevention among pregnant women. *Behaviour Research and Therapy, 54*, 7–11.

Domenech Rodríguez, M. M., & Bernal, G. (2012). Frameworks, models, and guidelines for cultural adaptation. In G. Bernal, & M. M. Domenech Rodríguez (Eds.), *Cultural adaptations: Tools for evidence-based practice with diverse populations* (pp. 23–44). American Psychological Association. https://doi.org/10.1037/13752-000.

Dørheim, S. K., Bjorvatn, B., & Eberhard-Gran, M. (2012). Insomnia and depressive symptoms in late pregnancy: A population-based study. *Behavioral Sleep Medicine, 10*(3), 152–166.

Dunkel Schetter, C., & Glynn, L. M. (2011). Stress in pregnancy: Empirical evidence and theoretical issues to guide interdisciplinary research. In R. J. Contrada & A. Baum (Eds.), *The handbook of stress science: Biology, psychology, and health* (pp. 321–347). Springer Publishing Company.

Dunkel Schetter, C., & Tanner, L. (2012). Anxiety, depression and stress in pregnancy: Implications for mothers, children, research, and practice. *Current Opinion in Psychiatry, 25*(2), 141–148. https://doi.org/10.1097/YCO.0b013e3283503680.

Edinger, J., Kirby, A., Lineberger, M., Loiselle, M., Wohlgemuth, W., & Means, M. (2004). *The Duke structured interview for sleep disorders.* Durham: University Medical Center.

Ellis, J. G., Deary, V., & Troxel, W. M. (2015). The role of perceived partner alliance on the efficacy of CBT-I: Preliminary findings from the Partner Alliance in Insomnia Research Study (PAIRS). *Behavioral Sleep Medicine, 13*(1), 64–72.

Facco, F. L., Kramer, J., Ho, K. H., Zee, P. C., & Grobman, W. A. (2010). Sleep disturbances in pregnancy. *Obstetrics & Gynecology, 115*(1), 77–83.

Felder, J. N., Baer, R. J., Rand, L., Jelliffe-Pawlowski, L. L., & Prather, A. A. (2017). Sleep disorder diagnosis during pregnancy and risk of preterm birth. *Obstetrics & Gynecology, 130*(3), 573–581.

Felder, J. N., Epel, E. S., Neuhaus, J., Krystal, A. D., & Prather, A. A. (2020). Efficacy of digital cognitive behavioral therapy for the treatment of insomnia symptoms among pregnant women: A randomized clinical trial. *JAMA Psychiatry, 77*(5), 484–492.

Felder, J. N., Segal, Z., Beck, A., Sherwood, N. E., Goodman, S. H., Boggs, J., et al. (2017). An open trial of web-based mindfulness-based cognitive therapy for perinatal women at risk for depressive relapse. *Cognitive and Behavioral Practice, 24*(1), 26–37. https://doi.org/10.1016/j.cbpra.2016.02.002.

First, M. B., Williams, J. B., Karg, R. S., & Spitzer, R. L. (2016). *User's guide for the SCID-5-CV structured clinical interview for DSM-5® disorders: Clinical version.* American Psychiatric Publishing, Inc.

Flynn, H. A., Henshaw, E., O'Mahen, H., & Forman, J. (2010). Patient perspectives on improving the depression referral processes in obstetrics settings: A qualitative study. *General Hospital Psychiatry*, *32*(1), 9–16.
Fox, N. S., & Oster, E. F. (2019). The advice we give to pregnant women: Sleep on it. *Obstetrics & Gynecology*, *134*(4), 665–666.
Freeman, M., Crissman, J., Jr., Louw, G., Butcher, R., & Inskeep, E. (1970). Thermogenic action of progesterone in the rat. *Endocrinology*, *86*(4), 717–720.
Garland, S. N., Carlson, L. E., Stephens, A. J., Antle, M. C., Samuels, C., & Campbell, T. S. (2014). Mindfulness-based stress reduction compared with cognitive behavioral therapy for the treatment of insomnia comorbid with cancer: A randomized, partially blinded, noninferiority trial. *Journal of Clinical Oncology*, *32*(5), 449–457.
Gelaye, B., Barrios, Y. V., Zhong, Q.-Y., Rondon, M. B., Borba, C. P., Sánchez, S. E., et al. (2015). Association of poor subjective sleep quality with suicidal ideation among pregnant Peruvian women. *General Hospital Psychiatry*, *37*(5), 441–447.
Gordon, A., Raynes-Greenow, C., Bond, D., Morris, J., Rawlinson, W., & Jeffery, H. (2015). Sleep position, fetal growth restriction, and late-pregnancy stillbirth: The Sydney stillbirth study. *Obstetrics & Gynecology*, *125*(2), 347–355.
Guardino, C. M., & Dunkel Schetter, C. (2014). Understanding pregnancy anxiety: Concepts, correlates, and consequences. *Zero to Three*, *34*(4), 12–21.
Gurung, R. A., Dunkel Schetter, C., Collins, N., Rini, C., & Hobel, C. J. (2005). Psychosocial predictors of prenatal anxiety. *Journal of Social and Clinical Psychology*, *24*(4), 497–519.
Harvey, C.-J., Gehrman, P., & Espie, C. A. (2014). Who is predisposed to insomnia: A review of familial aggregation, stress-reactivity, personality and coping style. *Sleep Medicine Reviews*, *18*(3), 237–247.
Heazell, A. E., Li, M., Budd, J., Thompson, J., Stacey, T., Cronin, R. S., et al. (2018). Association between maternal sleep practices and late stillbirth–findings from a stillbirth case-control study. *BJOG: An International Journal of Obstetrics & Gynaecology*, *125*(2), 254–262.
Hertz, G., Fast, A., Feinsilver, S. H., Albertario, C. L., Schulman, H., & Fein, A. M. (1992). Sleep in normal late pregnancy. *Sleep*, *15*(3), 246–251.
Hicks, R. A., & Garcia, E. R. (1987). Level of stress and sleep duration. *Perceptual and Motor Skills*, *64*(1), 44–46.
Hirshkowitz, M., Whiton, K., Albert, S. M., Alessi, C., Bruni, O., DonCarlos, L., et al. (2015). National Sleep Foundation's updated sleep duration recommendations. *Sleep Health*, *1*(4), 233–243.
Izci-Balserak, B., Keenan, B. T., Corbitt, C., Staley, B., Perlis, M., & Pien, G. W. (2018). Changes in sleep characteristics and breathing parameters during sleep in early and late pregnancy. *Journal of Clinical Sleep Medicine*, *14*(7), 1161–1168.
Kalmbach, D. A., Cheng, P., O'Brien, L. M., Swanson, L. M., Sangha, R., Sen, S., et al. (2020). A randomized controlled trial of digital cognitive behavioral therapy for insomnia in pregnant women. *Sleep Medicine*, *72*, 82–92.
Kamen, C., Garland, S. N., Heckler, C. E., Peoples, A. R., Kleckner, I. R., Cole, C. L., et al. (2019). Social support, insomnia, and adherence to cognitive behavioral therapy for insomnia after cancer treatment. *Behavioral Sleep Medicine*, *17*(1), 70–80.
Kent de Grey, R. G., Uchino, B. N., Trettevik, R., Cronan, S., & Hogan, J. N. (2018). Social support and sleep: A meta-analysis. *Health Psychology*, *37*(8), 787.
Khazaie, H., Ghadami, M. R., Knight, D. C., Emamian, F., & Tahmasian, M. (2013). Insomnia treatment in the third trimester of pregnancy reduces postpartum depression symptoms: A randomized clinical trial. *Psychiatry Research*, *210*(3), 901–905.
Kim, J. J., La Porte, L. M., Corcoran, M., Magasi, S., Batza, J., & Silver, R. K. (2010). Barriers to mental health treatment among obstetric patients at risk for depression. *American Journal of Obstetrics and Gynecology*, *202*(3), 312.e311–312.e315.

Kızılırmak, A., Timur, S., & Kartal, B. (2012). Insomnia in pregnancy and factors related to insomnia. *The Scientific World Journal, 2012*, 197093–197098. https://doi.org/10.1100/2012/197093.

Lancel, M., Faulhaber, J., Holsboer, F., & Rupprecht, R. (1996). Progesterone induces changes in sleep comparable to those of agonistic GABAA receptor modulators. *American Journal of Physiology-Endocrinology and Metabolism, 271*(4), E763–E772.

Lee, K. A., & Gay, C. L. (2004). Sleep in late pregnancy predicts length of labor and type of delivery. *American Journal of Obstetrics and Gynecology, 191*(6), 2041–2046.

Lyu, J., Ye, X., Chen, Y., Xia, Y., Zhu, J., Tong, S., et al. (2020). Children's sleep may depend on maternal sleep duration during pregnancy: A retrospective study. *Nature and Science of Sleep, 12*, 197.

Manber, R., Bei, B., Simpson, N., Asarnow, L., Rangel, E., Sit, A., et al. (2019). Cognitive behavioral therapy for prenatal insomnia: A randomized controlled trial. *Obstetrics and Gynecology, 133*(5), 911.

McCowan, L. M., Thompson, J. M., Cronin, R. S., Li, M., Stacey, T., Stone, P. R., et al. (2017). Going to sleep in the supine position is a modifiable risk factor for late pregnancy stillbirth; Findings from the New Zealand multicentre stillbirth case-control study. *PLoS ONE, 12*(6), e0179396.

Mellor, A., Hamill, K., Jenkins, M. M., Baucom, D. H., Norton, P. J., & Drummond, S. P. (2019). Partner-assisted cognitive behavioural therapy for insomnia versus cognitive behavioural therapy for insomnia: A randomised controlled trial. *Trials, 20*(1), 262.

Mersky, J. P., Lee, C. P., Gilbert, R. M., & Goyal, D. (2020). Prevalence and correlates of maternal and infant sleep problems in a low-income US sample. *Maternal and Child Health Journal, 24*(2), 196–203.

Micheli, K., Komninos, I., Bagkeris, E., Roumeliotaki, T., Koutis, A., Kogevinas, M., et al. (2011). Sleep patterns in late pregnancy and risk of preterm birth and fetal growth restriction. *Epidemiology, 22*(5), 738–744.

Mindell, J. A. (2010). *Sleeping through the night: How infants, toddlers, and parents can get a good night's sleep* (Revised Ed.). Harper Collins.

Mindell, J. A., Cook, R. A., & Nikolovski, J. (2015). Sleep patterns and sleep disturbances across pregnancy. *Sleep Medicine, 16*(4), 483–488.

Mindell, J. A., & Jacobson, B. J. (2000). Sleep disturbances during pregnancy. *Journal of Obstetric, Gynecologic, and Neonatal Nursing, 29*(6), 590–597.

Morin, C. M., Belleville, G., Bélanger, L., & Ivers, H. (2011). The insomnia severity index: Psychometric indicators to detect insomnia cases and evaluate treatment response. *Sleep, 34*(5), 601–608.

Mottola, M. F., Davenport, M. H., Ruchat, S. M., Davies, G. A., Poitras, V. J., Gray, C. E., et al. (2018). 2019 Canadian guideline for physical activity throughout pregnancy. *British Journal of Sports Medicine, 52*(21), 1339–1346. https://doi.org/10.1136/bjsports-2018-100056.

Naghi, I., Keypour, F., Ahari, S. B., Tavalai, S. A., & Khak, M. (2011). Sleep disturbance in late pregnancy and type and duration of labour. *Journal of Obstetrics and Gynaecology, 31*(6), 489–491. https://doi.org/10.3109/01443615.2011.579196.

Nodine, P. M., & Matthews, E. E. (2013). Common sleep disorders: Management strategies and pregnancy outcomes. *Journal of Midwifery & Women's Health, 58*(4), 368–377.

O'Brien, L. M., Bullough, A. S., Owusu, J. T., Tremblay, K. A., Brincat, C. A., Chames, M. C., et al. (2013). Snoring during pregnancy and delivery outcomes: A cohort study. *Sleep, 36*(11), 1625–1632.

Okun, M. L., Buysse, D. J., & Hall, M. H. (2015). Identifying insomnia in early pregnancy: Validation of the insomnia symptoms questionnaire (ISQ) in pregnant women. *Journal of Clinical Sleep Medicine, 11*(6), 645–654.

Okun, M. L., Hanusa, B. H., Hall, M., & Wisner, K. L. (2009). Sleep complaints in late pregnancy and the recurrence of postpartum depression. *Behavioral Sleep Medicine*, *7*(2), 106–117.

Osnes, R. S., Eberhard-Gran, M., Follestad, T., Kallestad, H., Morken, G., & Roaldset, J. O. (2020). Mid-pregnancy insomnia and its association with perinatal depressive symptoms: A prospective cohort study. *Behavioral Sleep Medicine*, *19*(3), 285–302.

Owusu, J. T., Anderson, F. J., Coleman, J., Oppong, S., Seffah, J. D., Aikins, A., et al. (2013). Association of maternal sleep practices with pre-eclampsia, low birth weight, and stillbirth among Ghanaian women. *International Journal of Gynecology & Obstetrics*, *121*(3), 261–265.

Park, E. M., Meltzer-Brody, S., & Stickgold, R. (2013). Poor sleep maintenance and subjective sleep quality are associated with postpartum maternal depression symptom severity. *Archives of Women's Mental Health*, *16*(6), 539–547.

Pires, G. N., Benedetto, L., Cortese, R., Gozal, D., Gulia, K. K., Kumar, V. M., et al. (2020). Effects of sleep modulation during pregnancy in the mother and offspring: Evidences from preclinical research. *Journal of Sleep Research*, *30*(3), e13135.

Polo-Kantola, P., Aukia, L., Karlsson, H., Karlsson, L., & Paavonen, E. J. (2017). Sleep quality during pregnancy: Associations with depressive and anxiety symptoms. *Acta Obstetricia et Gynecologica Scandinavica*, *96*(2), 198–206.

Qiu, C., Gelaye, B., Zhong, Q.-Y., Enquobahrie, D. A., Frederick, I. O., & Williams, M. A. (2016). Construct validity and factor structure of the Pittsburgh Sleep Quality Index among pregnant women in a Pacific-Northwest cohort. *Sleep & Breathing*, *20*(1), 293–301.

Rogojanski, J., Carney, C. E., & Monson, C. M. (2013). Interpersonal factors in insomnia: A model for integrating bed partners into cognitive behavioral therapy for insomnia. *Sleep Medicine Reviews*, *17*(1), 55–64.

Román-Gálvez, R., Amezcua-Prieto, C., Salcedo-Bellido, I., Martínez-Galiano, J., Khan, K., & Bueno-Cavanillas, A. (2018). Factors associated with insomnia in pregnancy: A prospective cohort study. *European Journal of Obstetrics & Gynecology and Reproductive Biology*, *221*, 70–75.

Sedov, I. D., Cameron, E. E., Madigan, S., & Tomfohr-Madsen, L. M. (2018). Sleep quality during pregnancy: A meta-analysis. *Sleep Medicine Reviews*, *38*, 168–176.

Sedov, I. D., Goodman, S. H., & Tomfohr-Madsen, L. M. (2017). Insomnia treatment preferences during pregnancy. *Journal of Obstetric, Gynecologic & Neonatal Nursing*, *46*(3), e95–e104.

Sedov, I., Anderson, N., Dhillon, A., & Tomfohr-Madsen, L. (2021). Insomnia symptoms during pregnancy: A meta-analysis. *Journal of Sleep Research*, *30*(1), e13207. https://doi.org/10.1111/jsr.13207.

Sedov, I., Madsen, J. W., Goodman, S. H., & Tomfohr-Madsen, L. M. (2019). Couples' treatment preferences for insomnia experienced during pregnancy. *Families, Systems & Health*, *37*(1), 46.

Sedov, I. D., & Tomfohr-Madsen, L. M. (2021). Trajectories of insomnia symptoms and associations with mood and anxiety from early pregnancy to the postpartum. *Behavioral Sleep Medicine*, *19*(3), 395–406.

Sharkey, K. M. (2013). Time to treat problematic sleep disturbance in perinatal women. *Behavioral Sleep Medicine*, *11*(4), 308–310.

Silver, R. M., Hunter, S., Reddy, U. M., Facco, F., Gibbins, K. J., Grobman, W. A., et al. (2019). Prospective evaluation of maternal sleep position through 30 weeks of gestation and adverse pregnancy outcomes. *Obstetrics & Gynecology*, *134*(4), 667–676.

Skouteris, H., Wertheim, E. H., Germano, C., Paxton, S. J., & Milgrom, J. (2009). Assessing sleep during pregnancy: A study across two time points examining the Pittsburgh Sleep Quality Index and associations with depressive symptoms. *Women's Health Issues*, *19*(1), 45–51.

Smith, M. S., Lawrence, V., Sadler, E., & Easter, A. (2019). Barriers to accessing mental health services for women with perinatal mental illness: Systematic review and meta-synthesis of qualitative studies in the UK. *BMJ Open*, *9*(1), e024803.

Spielman, A. J., Caruso, L. S., & Glovinsky, P. B. (1987). A behavioral perspective on insomnia treatment. *Psychiatric Clinics of North America*, *10*(4), 541–553.

Stacey, T., Thompson, J. M., Mitchell, E. A., Ekeroma, A. J., Zuccollo, J. M., & McCowan, L. M. (2011). Association between maternal sleep practices and risk of late stillbirth: A case-control study. *BMJ*, *342*, d3403.

Stein, A., Pearson, R. M., Goodman, S. H., Rapa, E., Rahman, A., McCallum, M., et al. (2014). Effects of perinatal mental disorders on the fetus and child. *The Lancet*, *384*(9956), 1800–1819.

Stremler, R., Hodnett, E., Kenton, L., Lee, K., Weiss, S., Weston, J., et al. (2013). Effect of behavioural-educational intervention on sleep for primiparous women and their infants in early postpartum: Multisite randomised controlled trial. *BMJ*, *346*, f1164.

Swanson, L. M., Flynn, H., Adams-Mundy, J. D., Armitage, R., & Arnedt, J. T. (2013). An open pilot of cognitive-behavioral therapy for insomnia in women with postpartum depression. *Behavioral Sleep Medicine*, *11*(4), 297–307.

Swanson, L. M., Pickett, S. M., Flynn, H., & Armitage, R. (2011). Relationships among depression, anxiety, and insomnia symptoms in perinatal women seeking mental health treatment. *Journal of Women's Health*, *20*(4), 553–558.

Taylor, D. J., Wilkerson, A. K., Pruiksma, K. E., Williams, J. M., Ruggero, C. J., Hale, W., et al. (2018). Reliability of the structured clinical interview for DSM-5 sleep disorders module. *Journal of Clinical Sleep Medicine*, *14*(3), 459–464.

Tham, E. K., Tan, J., Chong, Y.-S., Kwek, K., Saw, S.-M., Teoh, O.-H., et al. (2016). Associations between poor subjective prenatal sleep quality and postnatal depression and anxiety symptoms. *Journal of Affective Disorders*, *202*, 91–94.

Tomfohr, L. M., Buliga, E., Letourneau, N. L., Campbell, T. S., & Giesbrecht, G. F. (2015). Trajectories of sleep quality and associations with mood during the perinatal period. *Sleep*, *38*(8), 1237–1245.

Tomfohr-Madsen, L. M., Clayborne, Z. M., Rouleau, C. R., & Campbell, T. S. (2017). Sleeping for two: An open-pilot study of cognitive behavioral therapy for insomnia in pregnancy. *Behavioral Sleep Medicine*, *15*(5), 377–393.

Tracy, E. L., & Troxel, W. M. (2019). Family relationships in the context of sleep. In D. T. Duncan, I. Kawachi, & S. Redline (Eds.), *The social epidemiology of sleep* (pp. 325–350). Oxford University Press.

Troxel, W. M. (2010). It's more than sex: Exploring the dyadic nature of sleep and implications for health. *Psychosomatic Medicine*, *72*(6), 578.

Tsuno, N., Besset, A., & Ritchie, K. (2005). Sleep and depression. *The Journal of Clinical Psychiatry*, *66*(10), 1254–1269. https://doi.org/10.4088/jcp.v66n1008.

van der Zwan, J. E., de Vente, W., Tolvanen, M., Karlsson, H., Buil, J. M., Koot, H. M., et al. (2017). Longitudinal associations between sleep and anxiety during pregnancy, and the moderating effect of resilience, using parallel process latent growth curve models. *Sleep Medicine*, *40*, 63–68.

Volkovich, E., Tikotzky, L., & Manber, R. (2016). Objective and subjective sleep during pregnancy: Links with depressive and anxiety symptoms. *Archives of Women's Mental Health*, *19*(1), 173–181.

Walker, L. O., & Czajkowski, S. M. (2019). Designing interventions to improve the health of women using the ORBIT model. *Journal of Obstetric, Gynecologic & Neonatal Nursing*, *48*(2), 197–204.

Wilson, D. L., Barnes, M., Ellett, L., Permezel, M., Jackson, M., & Crowe, S. F. (2011). Decreased sleep efficiency, increased wake after sleep onset and increased cortical arousals in late pregnancy. *Australian and New Zealand Journal of Obstetrics and Gynaecology, 51*(1), 38–46.

Wilson, H., & Donachie, A. L. (2018). Evaluating the effectiveness of a dialectical behaviour therapy (DBT) informed programme in a community perinatal team. *Behavioural and Cognitive Psychotherapy, 46*(5), 541–553. https://doi.org/10.1017/S1352465817000790.

World Health Organization. (2021). *Maternal mental health*. https://www.who.int/mental_health/maternal-child/maternal_mental_health/en/.

Yu, L., Buysse, D. J., Germain, A., Moul, D. E., Stover, A., Dodds, N. E., et al. (2012). Development of short forms from the PROMIS™ sleep disturbance and sleep-related impairment item banks. *Behavioral Sleep Medicine, 10*(1), 6–24.

Zhong, Q.-Y., Gelaye, B., Sánchez, S. E., & Williams, M. A. (2015). Psychometric properties of the Pittsburgh Sleep Quality Index (PSQI) in a cohort of Peruvian pregnant women. *Journal of Clinical Sleep Medicine, 11*(8), 869–877.

CHAPTER

16

CBT-I for perimenopause and postmenopause

Jessica M. Meers[a], *Darius B. Dawson*[b], *and Sara Nowakowski*[b,c]

[a]Department of Psychology, University of Houston, Houston, TX, United States, [b]Department of Medicine, Baylor College of Medicine, Houston, TX, United States, [c]Center for Innovation in Quality, Effectiveness and Safety, Michael E DeBakey VA Medical Center, Houston, TX, United States

Introduction

The end of a woman's reproductive years is often accompanied by a number of physiological and psychological complaints, such as hot flashes, mood changes, and weight gain. Insomnia is one of the most distressing of these symptoms, affecting 39%–60% of women in peri- and postmenopause (Kravitz et al., 2003; Kravitz, Zhao, & Bromberger, 2008; NIH, 2005). In fact, sleep disturbance was identified as a core symptom of menopause by the National Institutes of Health (NIH) in their 2005 State-of-the-Science Conference panel report on Menopause (NIH, 2005). Peri- and postmenopausal women are up to twice as likely to report dissatisfaction with their sleep, compared to their premenopausal counterparts (Young, Rabago, Zgierska, Austin, & Finn, 2003). Their most common complaint is difficulty falling asleep, but nighttime awakenings and daytime sleepiness are also reported (Glazer, Zeller, Delumba, et al., 2002; Kravitz et al., 2003; Ohayon, 2006; Regestein, Friebely, Shifren, et al., 2004; Soares, 2005).

Adapting Cognitive Behavioral Therapy for Insomnia
https://doi.org/10.1016/B978-0-12-822872-2.00011-6

Overview of menopause

Menopause, defined as the permanent cessation of a woman's menstrual cycle, is either due to natural aging or induced by surgery, chemotherapy, or radiation (World Health Organization WHO, 1996). Menopause can be categorized into two stages: the menopausal transition (variable menstrual cycle length 7 days different from the normal cycle or more than two skipped menstrual cycles) and postmenopause (amenorrhea greater than 12 months) (Soules, Sherman, Parrott, et al., 2001). Occurring during this time is the degeneration of follicles in the ovaries and increased variability and decline of the production of sex hormones, including estrogen and progesterone. For most Western women, menopause occurs between the ages 50 and 52, although this range can vary according to race, ethnicity, and lifestyle factors (Gold, 2011). For most women, the menopausal transition lasts between seven and eight years, with postmenopause extending for the duration of the lifetime, often beyond 30 years. Criteria developed by the Stages of Reproductive Aging Workshop (STRAW) in an effort to standardize the definitions of menstrual stages (Soules et al., 2001).

The change in the hormonal milieu of menopause results in symptoms that are disruptive and distressing to many women. Vasomotor symptoms (hot flashes) are one of the most commonly reported complaints, occurring in an estimated 60%–80% of women and persisting for upwards of 4–5 years (Col, Guthrie, Politi, & Dennerstein, 2009; Politi, Schleinitz, & Col, 2008). Hot flashes are thought to be due to the effects of decreased estrogen on the thermoregulatory functioning of the central nervous system (Freedman, 2001). For most women, a hot flash is experienced as a sudden sensation of heat, usually in the upper body, that reaches its peak within the first several minutes and gradually dissipates over the course of a quarter of an hour (Freedman, 2001). When occurring during the night, hot flashes often disrupt sleep, although not every nocturnal hot flash is associated with an awakening (Thurston, Chang, Buysse, Hall, & Matthews, 2019). Those who report more severe hot flashes are more likely to report chronic insomnia (Ohayon, 2006). The fact that those with hot flashes are also more sensitive to changes in temperature is likely a contributing factor. Women who report severe hot flashes tend to exhibit general thermoregulatory dysfunction, where even a small rise in temperature can trigger a hot flash and a small drop in temperature can elicit shivering (Freedman, 2014). This swing between the two can be particularly disruptive to sleep.

Further compounding these issues is the gradual withdrawal of hormones thought to be directly and indirectly protective of sleep, namely estrogen and progesterone. The decline in reproductive hormones appears to increase susceptibility to sleep disruption through thermoregulatory, respiratory, circadian, and mood disruption (Eichling & Sahni,

2005). Insomnia is not the only sleep-related disorder linked to menopause. Rates of sleep-disordered breathing, such as obstructive sleep apnea (OSA), increases dramatically with the transition into menopause. OSA is relatively rare among premenopausal women, but by the time a woman reaches postmenopause, she is 3.5 times more likely than premenopausal women to have moderate or severe OSA, even after age and body mass index are accounted for (Dancey, Hanly, Soong, Lee, & Hoffstein, 2001; Young, Finn, Austin, & Peterson, 2003). Estrogen and progesterone are thought to be protective for OSA through the enhancement of the upper airway dilator function and respiratory control during sleep, and therefore, rates increase as production of these hormones decline (Driver et al., 2005; Popovic & White, 1998). Although not the sole cause for increased rates of OSA, weight gain during the menopausal transition is a known contributor, increasing neck circumference and other risk factors. Weight gain is considered a function of not only changes in the hormonal milieu but likely also a consequence of sleep disruptions among other factors. Disrupted sleep or chronic sleep loss is known to increase hunger drive and disrupt metabolic functioning (Bass & Turek, 2005; Kravitz, Kazlauskaite, & Joffe, 2018). Thus, it is important to assess for symptoms of OSA (e.g., snoring, gasping for breath, witnessed apneic events, waking with a morning headache, dry mouth, and/or sore throat) during the initial intake and make a referral to a sleep medicine clinic for a polysomnographic (PSG) sleep study or home sleep test if the patient endorses untreated OSA symptoms.

A woman's well-being is often influenced by her menopausal status. Susceptibility to mood disorders increases dramatically in those reporting menopausal symptoms (Freeman, 2010). The fluctuation of reproductive hormones can lead to an increase in mood-related symptoms in predisposed women, but environmental and lifestyle factors interact with these processes in a unique way during this time of transition in women (Bromberger & Epperson, 2018). The "domino" theory of sleep disruption is often used to explain menopausal depression, in which sleep is thought to be disrupted by hot flashes and other menopausal symptoms. This, in turn, leads to chronic insomnia, which can eventually result in depression (Campbell & Whitehead, 1977). The role of key life events that typically occur with significant transitions in a woman's life, however, cannot be ignored. During midlife, women may be at the peak of their careers and dealing with stressors associated with leadership positions and various role responsibilities. Women are frequently balancing caregiving responsibilities, caring for their children, and/or caring for aging parents or other family members. Caregiver stress independently increases the risk for depression and reduced quality of life (Li, Lin, Xu, & Zhou, 2018; Miller, Lindquist, Olsen, et al., 2019). As women age, they also have an increased risk of their ailing health; including increased risk of breast cancer, osteoarthritis, low bone/muscle density, and cardiac and metabolic disorders. It is unsurprising, then, that health-related stress and anxiety increase in older adults (Balsamo, Cataldi, Carlucci, & Fairfield, 2018). Finally, sexual dysfunction affects women at higher rates during this time, caused by vaginal dryness, low libido, and mood disruptions related to shifts in hormones (Nappi & Lachowsky, 2009). This can impact both relationship satisfaction as well as the general quality of life, further increasing stress during this period of a woman's life (Robinson & Molzahn, 2007).

It is clear, then, that there is no single precipitating factor for menopausal insomnia. Instead, the presence of insomnia during the menopausal transition can most often be attributed to a host of physiological, psychological, and environmental factors. It is therefore important to keep in mind the complexity of a woman's presentation when she presents for insomnia evaluation and treatment. The following sections address how these factors can be conceptualized in the context of cognitive-behavioral therapy for insomnia (CBT-I) and how they can be addressed in treatment.

Conceptualizing insomnia in menopausal women

Spielman's Three Factor Model is a general approach taken to case conceptualization in CBT-I (Spielman, Caruso, & Glovinsky, 1987) and can aid in the systematic approach to adapting CBT-I for use with midlife women. Speilman proposes three factors including predisposing factors, precipitating events, and perpetuating mechanisms, which contribute to chronic insomnia (see Table 1). Below is an example of how one might conceptualize menopausal women for each of the three factors.

TABLE 1 3-P Model of insomnia for menopausal women.

Predisposing factors	**Precipitating factors**	**Perpetuating factors**
Factors that increase risk for insomnia disorder	Events that lead to sleep disruption	Factors that sustain poor sleep over time
• Elevated risk for developing insomnia • Hormonal fluctuation • Childhood or interpersonal trauma • Personal or family history for mental health conditions	• Vasomotor symptoms • Depression • Health conditions • Other sleep disorders • Sexual dysfunction • Social or interpersonal life stressors (e.g., caregiver responsibility, marital discord, job responsibilities)	• Irregular sleep/wake schedule • Hypervigilance • Maladaptive beliefs (poor sleep and hot flashes are unbearable) • Maladaptive coping (napping, alcohol, caffeine use, avoiding situations due to hot flashes)

Predisposing factors

Spielman conceptualized predisposing factors as those that increase an individual's vulnerability to insomnia, typically as a result of dysfunction in biological or arousal-based functioning. The changes in hormonal functioning and resulting symptoms in this stage of a woman's life as discussed above can be considered powerful predisposing factors. Aging is associated with shorter, lighter, and more fragmented sleep naturally (Latreille et al., 2019). For women, in particular, the decline in sleep-promoting hormones also increases vulnerability to sleep disruption particularly for those who experience hot flashes. Additional predisposing factors may include childhood or interpersonal trauma, and personal or family history for mental health disorders. These natural, biological factors lower the threshold for insomnia onset.

Precipitating factors

It is often the case that predisposing and precipitating factors are not entirely mutually exclusive (Spielman, 1986). This is particularly true as it relates to menopausal insomnia. Disrupted sleep patterns resulting from newly emerging physical symptoms are stressful for many women. The onset of hot flashes and night sweats as well as a reduced ability to maintain sleep is distressing. This is particularly true as women are concurrently coming to terms with the changes occurring in their bodies and reproductive functionality. A woman's perceptions of her menopausal experiences can therefore precipitate sleep difficulties. Women often feel out of control over their physiological functioning, which increases sleep-related stress. In fact, women who perceive more control over their reactions to hot flashes report fewer and less problematic hot flashes (Hunter & Liao, 1995; Hunter & Mann, 2010; Reynolds, 1997). In the predisposed woman, changes in physical and mental health status (e.g., onset of mood disorder), job or caregiver stress, and changes in social roles (e.g., empty nest syndrome) are often more than enough to elevate a women's risk above the insomnia threshold.

Perpetuating factors

Perpetuating factors are those maladaptive strategies employed in an attempt to compensate for the loss of sleep. Increased sleep effort, excessive time in bed, napping during the day, and irregular bed and wake times are not unique to menopausal women. Poor coping skills for addressing both sleep disturbance and hot flashes, however, may have an additive effect. For instance, alcohol's initial drowsiness-inducing effects may cause women to believe that a drink or two before bed helps with their sleep; however, alcohol is known to increase both sleep disruption and hot flash symptoms (Colrain, Nicholas, & Baker, 2014; Sievert, Obermeyer, & Price, 2006). Sleep interfering thoughts, such as "No matter what I do, I'll never get a full night's sleep again," or "I just can't handle these hot flashes" may also perpetuate insomnia and keep women from implementing more helpful coping strategies, such as changing her bedroom temperature, clothing, or maintaining a regular sleep schedule and employing other stress-reduction strategies.

Evidence for CBT-I in midlife women

Evidence for standard CBT-I

CBT-I has been implemented in midlife women, with several randomized clinical trials (RCTs) demonstrating efficacy. McCurry et al. (2016) delivered a telephone-based CBT-I intervention to 106 *peri* or postmenopausal women, comparing it to a psychoeducation-based control. It included six, 20–30-min sessions over eight weeks addressing sleep restriction, stimulus control, sleep hygiene, and cognitive restructuring using standard CBT-I with no adaptions for menopause. Women who received CBT-I saw significant reductions in self-reported insomnia symptoms, sleep quality, and sleep efficiency compared to women who received menopause education control at 8 weeks and these effects were maintained at the 24-week follow-up.

Four RCTs conducted by Guthrie et al. (2018), coined The Menopause Strategies: Finding Lasting Answers for Symptoms and Health (MsFLASH) Trials, provided evidence of the efficacy of CBT-I for menopause. The trials aimed to test the effects of pharmacologic and nonpharmacologic interventions on insomnia and sleep quality for women with hot flashes. Two compared active pharmacological treatments to a placebo (i.e., an SSRI and an SNRI). One study compared yoga and aerobic exercise separately to a usual activity control group, and simultaneously compare Omega-3 fatty acid supplementation to placebo. The last RCT compared telephone-delivered CBT-I to a menopause education control. The MsFLASH team concluded that the CBT-I condition produced the greatest reduction in insomnia, followed by the exercise and SNRI conditions, while the other conditions yielded only small decreases in insomnia. Participants in the CBT-I showed the greatest improvement in sleep quality.

A study by Drake et al. (2019) also showed promise for CBT-I in a menopausal population. This randomized clinical trial compared the full CBT-I protocol to a sleep restriction therapy (SRT)-only protocol and a sleep hygiene control condition. The CBT-I protocol included 6 weekly in-person sessions whereas the sleep restriction group received one in-person session and four follow-up sessions. The control condition consisted of weekly emails addressing general sleep and menopause-related information delivered across six weeks. Both CBT-I and SRT resulted in a reduction of insomnia symptoms, with CBT-I outperforming sleep hygiene in long-term sleep maintenance outcomes. Additionally, depressive symptoms were reduced in both CBT-I and SRT conditions, with large improvements in dysfunctional beliefs about sleep (Kalmbach et al., 2019). CBT-I and SRT produced weak effects on presleep cognitive arousal, rumination, and worry. Finally, this team concluded that quality of life and daytime functioning were also improved by CBT-I and SRT. Broadly, both treatments provided improvements in fatigue, energy, sleepiness, and work function. The CBT-I group reported better quality of life attributed to improvements in emotional wellbeing and resiliency to physical and emotional problems.

Evidence for adapted CBT-I

Nowakowski et al. (2017) demonstrated efficacy in an adapted CBT for insomnia and nocturnal hot flashes. Forty women (mean age $=55\pm6.2$-years) self-described as peri- or postmenopausal who reported $\geq$1 nocturnal hot flash/night and those who met diagnostic criteria for insomnia disorder were randomized to adapted CBT for insomnia and nocturnal hot flashes or an education control condition. CBT treatment included four individual 50-min sessions over eight weeks delivered by social workers in gynecology clinics. Adaption included education on menopause and hot flashes, and how it impacts sleep; providing daytime and nighttime coping strategies for hot flashes, monitoring and identifying hot flash triggers, and cognitive restructuring for both sleep and hot flashes. The control condition was introduced as a self-help intervention and included a 1-h meeting to discuss menopausal health symptoms and sleep hygiene. The control condition also provided educational material and a nondirective suggestion to "make any behavioral changes as desired." Results revealed significant improvement in insomnia severity, objective and subjective sleep disturbance, and sleep efficiency. Depression severity also declined.

Adapting CBT-I for menopause

In CBT-I, the psychoeducation component is of particular importance. The psychoeducational component increases the patient's ability to understand the rationale behind behavioral recommendations and elicits patient buy-in to motivate behavioral change. Research demonstrates increased efficacy and better outcomes if treatment is tailored to specific patient-generated problems and goals (Constantino, Arnkoff, Glass, Ametrano, & Smith, 2017). When considering how to tailor CBT-I to midlife women, it can be helpful to explain predisposing and precipitating factors in the context of midlife and menopausal symptoms described above. In particular, discussing the natural age-related changes on sleep, i.e., that the average sleep duration changes across the lifespan, can be helpful in addressing unrealistic expectations about sleep. For women experiencing nocturnal hot flashes, a description of the physiology of a hot flash (that it peaks within five minutes and core body temperature decreases slowly across a 20-min period) might also be helpful. Furthermore, discussing the common changes in mood, anxiety, and life stress that co-occur with the menopause transition may be normalizing and destigmatizing for women. When providing a rationale for the treatment, providers can emphasize that improvements in sleep consolidation obtained through stimulus control and sleep restriction strategies may increase a woman's ability to sleep through hot flashes or return to sleep more quickly.

Sleep hygiene education focused on habits that interfere with sleep and increase hot flashes can be helpful. For example, consumption of alcohol, caffeine, and nicotine products not only interferes with sleep but also increases hot flashes. Focus on temperature-related challenges experienced by women with nocturnal hot flashes is also particularly important. In addition to the conventional recommendation to set the thermostat at a cool, comfortable temperature; providers may also recommend using sweat-wicking night attire, sleeping on a towel, and/or having a change of pajamas on hand in case night sweating is an issue. Women may report sleep disruption during the cool-off period after a hot flash due to feeling cold. Providers may encourage layering additional bedding to regulate temperature more easily. Other appropriate sleep environment recommendations include a plan to keep ice water next to the bed for quick access and use of fans or other cooling devices.

Coping successfully with hot flashes during the day can have carryover effects during the night. Similar to nighttime behavioral methods, daytime coping methods include layering clothing, reducing alcohol, caffeine, and nicotine consumption. Building in time in the morning and setting an earlier rise time, along with implementing general time management skills to allow for hot flash recovery have been shown to decrease hot flash severity. Because increased body mass index is also a risk factor for hot flashes, providers may encourage regular physical activity to help reduce hot flash severity and improve sleep. Finally, carrying a frozen water bottle or using a cooling device applied to cooling points of the body (such as wrists, chest/sternum, or the back of the neck) can be helpful.

Anxiety triggers the autonomic nervous system and increases symptoms similar to hot flashes such as racing heart, increased body temperature, sweating, and flushing. Related experiences can interact to increase hot flash severity and exacerbate insomnia symptoms and sleep disruption. Providers can integrate relaxation techniques into CBT-I to help with hot flash severity and sleep disturbance. For example, slowed breathing techniques and meditation practices relax the nervous system, lower the stress response, and decrease hot flash severity.

Cognitive restructuring of sleep-related and hot flash-related thoughts can be a useful component within CBT-I for menopausal women. Studies have demonstrated that a woman's perception of her hot flashes and feelings of control are critical components to target. Reframing inaccurate or negative thoughts associated with hot flashes ("everyone can tell I am having a hot flash") has been shown to prevent cascading physiological symptoms such as racing heart and feelings of embarrassment and self-consciousness that increase perceived bother and severity of hot flashes. Similar to the cognitive restructuring of unhelpful sleep beliefs, changing women's perception of hot flashes and teaching them to function despite experiencing symptoms, can change a woman's perception of intensity and bother of the hot flash. For example, providers can encourage more positive and accurate self-talk such as "This is okay, many women experience this" or "This too shall pass." Providers can consider the use of a hot flash log to help patients identify triggers that bring on hot flashes. These logs examine the situation and context associated with the hot flash (e.g., location, time, activity, are others present), internal thoughts surrounding the situation, and physiological symptoms experienced when having a hot flash. Providers should encourage women to not completely avoid having a hot flash but learn how to cope with hot flashes and build tolerance in experiencing negative symptoms; see Table 2.

TABLE 2 Adaptations of CBT-I for peri- and postmenopausal women.

CBT-I components	Standard practice	Modifications for women in menopause
Sleep education	3-P model, 2-process model of sleep regulation, sleep stages	– Education about normal age-related changes to sleep – Education about menopausal symptoms, the impact of the menopausal transition on sleep – Education on hot flash physiology – Education on stages of sleep and thermoregulatory effect of REM sleep

Continued

TABLE 2 Adaptations of CBT-I for peri- and postmenopausal women—cont'd

CBT-I components	Standard practice	Modifications for women in menopause
Sleep restriction	Improve sleep efficiency by limiting time in bed to the amount of time sleeping then expanding slowly as long as sleep efficiency is preserved	– Emphasize improving sleep quality may aid in the ability to sleep through arousal/awakening due to hot flashes – May build in additional 15 min of earlier wake/rise time to avoid rushing in the morning to reduce morning hot flashes (if rushing is the trigger)
Stimulus control	Associate bed/bedroom solely as a cue for sleep by eliminating nonsleep activities from the bedroom. Instruction to get out of bed at night if awake >15 min	– No change to stimulus control instructions
Napping/daytime sleep	Discontinue or restrict daytime napping to 30 min	– No changes to limiting napping and daytime sleep.
Sleep hygiene education	Address daytime habits and sleep environment interfering with sleep	– Limit caffeine, nicotine alcohol for effects on sleep and hot flashes. – Greater emphasis on cool ambient temperature, use of a fan, layering blankets. – Consider towel, sweat-wicking pjs, and change of pjs nearby if excessive night sweating. – Brainstorm daytime hot flash coping strategies.
Cognitive therapy	Challenge patient's dysfunctional beliefs interfering with sleep and misconceptions about sleep. Replace/restructure to more helpful and realistic thoughts about sleep	– Identifying & altering response to possible hot flash triggers thereby increasing the sense of control over reaction to hot flashes. – Identifying & structuring negative beliefs about sleep and menopausal symptoms. – Adopting an objective nonjudgmental awareness of hot flashes from beginning to end can reduce catastrophic thoughts, improve self-image, as well as bother and perceived hot flash interference.

TABLE 2 Adaptations of CBT-I for peri- and postmenopausal women—cont'd

CBT-I components	Standard practice	Modifications for women in menopause
Relaxation and meditation techniques	Relaxation can help reduce racing thoughts/tension that accompanies lying in bed awake, and may include: deep breathing, progressive muscle relaxation, guided imagery, biofeedback, hypnosis, autogenic training, and meditation practices	– In addition to using relaxation and meditation to reduce arousal and aid sleep, provide training to promote the calm observance of the hot flash, without trying to escape; designed to change how a woman relates to her hot flash experience
Relapse Prevention	Discuss practicing less rigid sleep plan over time and what do to prevent sleep disturbance from turning into another episode of insomnia in the future	– Discuss how to get sleep back on track after health or life events beyond the menopausal transition
Sleep diaries	Establish baseline sleep patterns, track progress, reinforce appropriate behavior change, problem-solve obstacles to adherence	– May consider adding an item to track hot flash symptom severity and bother at night; and awakenings due to hot flashes versus other reasons

Conclusions

Mid-life women experience a unique risk for sleep complaints. Sleep can be disrupted by fluctuating hormones, hot flashes, and stress; and maladaptive coping strategies increase risk. Even still, the core components of CBT-I have been found to be effective in the treatment of menopause-related insomnia, even without significant adaptations. What may be most important is developing an appropriate case conceptualization that considers the relevant predisposing, precipitating, and perpetuating factors relevant to menopause and contextualizing psychoeducation and problem-solving to the specific presentation of the menopausal women. For instance, psychoeducation can include information about normative menopausal changes as they relate to sleep, sleep hygiene education might focus on reducing hot flash triggers, while cognitive and relaxation might focus on acceptance and taking a nonjudgmental stance toward hot flashes and reducing hyperarousal. These strategies add no additional time to treatment and have the additional benefit of providing women with additional support and validation during this transition period.

References

Balsamo, M., Cataldi, F., Carlucci, L., & Fairfield, B. (2018). Assessment of anxiety in older adults: A review of self-report measures. *Clinical Interventions in Aging*. https://doi.org/10.2147/CIA.S114100.

Bass, J., & Turek, F. W. (2005). Sleepless in America: A pathway to obesity and the metabolic syndrome? *Archives of Internal Medicine*. https://doi.org/10.1001/archinte.165.1.15.

Bromberger, J. T., & Epperson, C. N. (2018). Depression during and after the perimenopause: Impact of hormones, genetics, and environmental determinants of disease. *Obstetrics and Gynecology Clinics of North America*. https://doi.org/10.1016/j.ogc.2018.07.007.

Campbell, S., & Whitehead, M. (1977). Oestrogen therapy and the menopausal syndrome. *Clinics in Obstetrics and Gynaecology*, *4*(1), 31–47.

Col, N. F., Guthrie, J. R., Politi, M., & Dennerstein, L. (2009). Duration of vasomotor symptoms in middle-aged women: A longitudinal study. *Menopause*. https://doi.org/10.1097/gme.0b013e31818d414e.

Colrain, I. M., Nicholas, C. L., & Baker, F. C. (2014). Alcohol and the sleeping brain. *Handbook of Clinical Neurology*, *125*, 415–431. https://doi.org/10.1016/B978-0-444-62619-6.00024-0.

Constantino, M. J., Arnkoff, D. B., Glass, C. R., Ametrano, R. M., & Smith, J. Z. (2017). Expectations. *Journal of Clinical Psychology*, *67*, 184–192. https://doi.org/10.1002/jclp.20754.

Dancey, D. R., Hanly, P. J., Soong, C., Lee, B., & Hoffstein, V. (2001). Impact of menopause on the prevalence and severity of sleep apnea. *Chest*. https://doi.org/10.1378/chest.120.1.151.

Drake, C. L., Kalmbach, D. A., Arnedt, J. T., Cheng, P., Tonnu, C. V., Cuamatzi-Castelan, A., et al. (2019). Treating chronic insomnia in postmenopausal women: A randomized clinical trial comparing cognitive-behavioral therapy for insomnia, sleep restriction therapy, and sleep hygiene education. *Sleep*, *42*(2), zsy217. https://doi.org/10.1093/sleep/zsy217.

Driver, H. S., McLean, H., Kumar, D. V., Farr, N., Day, A. G., & Fitzpatrick, M. F. (2005). The influence of the menstrual cycle on upper airway resistance and breathing during sleep. *Sleep*. https://doi.org/10.1093/sleep/28.4.449.

Eichling, P. S., & Sahni, J. (2005). Menopause related sleep disorders. *Journal of Clinical Sleep Medicine*. https://doi.org/10.5664/jcsm.26347.

Freedman, R. R. (2001). Physiology of hot flashes. *American Journal of Human Biology*. https://doi.org/10.1002/ajhb.1077.

Freedman, R. R. (2014). Menopausal related hot flashes: Mechanisms, endocrinology and treatment. *The Journal of Steroid Biochemistry and Molecular Biology*, *142*, 115–120. https://doi.org/10.14440/jbm.2015.54.A.

Freeman, E. W. (2010). Associations of depression with the transition to menopause. *Menopause*. https://doi.org/10.1097/gme.0b013e3181db9f8b.

Glazer, G., Zeller, R., Delumba, L., et al. (2002). The Ohio midlife women's study. *Health Care for Women International*. https://doi.org/10.1080/07399330290107377.

Gold, E. B. (2011). The timing of the age at which natural menopause occurs. *Obstetrics and Gynecology Clinics of North America*. https://doi.org/10.1016/j.ogc.2011.05.002.

Guthrie, K. A., Larson, J. C., Ensrud, K. E., Anderson, G. L., Carpenter, J. S., Freeman, E. W., et al. (2018). Effects of pharmacologic and nonpharmacologic interventions on insomnia symptoms and self-reported sleep quality in women with hot flashes: A pooled analysis of individual participant data from four MsFLASH trials. *Sleep*, *41*(1), zsx190. https://doi.org/10.1093/sleep/zsx190.

Hunter, M. S., & Liao, K. L. (1995). A psychological analysis of menopausal hot flushes. *The British Journal of Clinical Psychology*, *34*(Pt. 4), 589–599.

Hunter, M. S., & Mann, E. (2010). A cognitive model of menopausal hot flushes and night sweats. *Journal of Psychosomatic Research*, *69*(5), 491–501.

Kalmbach, D. A., Cheng, P., Arnedt, J. T., Cuamatzi-Castelan, A., Atkinson, R. L., Fellman-Couture, C., et al. (2019). Improving daytime functioning, work performance, and quality of life in postmenopausal women with insomnia: Comparing cognitive behavioral therapy for insomnia, sleep restriction therapy, and sleep hygiene education. *Journal of Clinical Sleep Medicine, 15*(7), 999–1010. https://doi.org/10.5664/jcsm.7882.

Kravitz, H. M., Ganz, P. A., Bromberger, J., Powell, L. H., Sutton-Tyrrell, K., & Meyer, P. M. (2003). Sleep difficulty in women at midlife: A community survey of sleep and the menopausal transition. *Menopause, 10*, 19–28. https://doi.org/10.1097/00042192-200310010-00005.

Kravitz, H. M., Kazlauskaite, R., & Joffe, H. (2018). Sleep, health, and metabolism in midlife women and menopause: Food for thought. *Obstetrics and Gynecology Clinics of North America*. https://doi.org/10.1016/j.ogc.2018.07.008.

Kravitz, H. M., Zhao, X., & Bromberger, J. T. (2008). Sleep disturbance during the menopausal transition in a multi-ethnic community sample of women. *Sleep, 31*(7), 979–990. https://doi.org/10.5665/sleep/31.7.979.

Latreille, V., Gaubert, M., Dubé, J., Lina, J. M., Gagnon, J. F., & Carrier, J. (2019). Age-related cortical signatures of human sleep electroencephalography. *Neurobiology of Aging, 76*, 106–114. https://doi.org/10.1016/j.neurobiolaging.2018.12.012.

Li, Q., Lin, Y., Xu, Y., & Zhou, H. (2018). The impact of depression and anxiety on quality of life in Chinese cancer patient-family caregiver dyads, a cross-sectional study. *Health and Quality of Life Outcomes*. https://doi.org/10.1186/s12955-018-1051-3.

McCurry, S. M., Guthrie, K. A., Morin, C. M., Woods, N. F., Landis, C. A., Ensrud, K. E., et al. (2016). Telephone-based cognitive behavioral therapy for insomnia in perimenopausal and postmenopausal women with vasomotor symptoms: A MsFLASH randomized clinical trial. *JAMA Internal Medicine, 176*(7), 913–920. https://doi.org/10.1001/jamainternmed.2016.1795.

Miller, K. E. M., Lindquist, J. H., Olsen, M. K., et al. (2019). Invisible partners in care: Snapshot of well-being among caregivers receiving comprehensive support from Veterans Affairs. *Health Science Reports*. https://doi.org/10.1002/hsr2.112.

Nappi, R. E., & Lachowsky, M. (2009). Menopause and sexuality: Prevalence of symptoms and impact on quality of life. *Maturitas*. https://doi.org/10.1016/j.maturitas.2009.03.021.

NIH. (2005). National Institutes of Health state-of-the-science conference statement: Management of menopause-related symptoms. *Annals of Internal Medicine, 142*, 1003–1013. https://doi.org/10.7326/0003-4819-142-12_part_1-200506210-00117.

Nowakowski, S., Thurston, R. C., Meers, J. M., Stout-Aguilar, J., Sadruddin, S. M., Hayman, J. M., et al. (2017). Cognitive behavioral therapy for menopausal insomnia in midlife women with insomnia and nocturnal hot flashes. *Sleep, 40*, A125.

Ohayon, M. M. (2006). Severe hot flashes are associated with chronic insomnia. *Archives of Internal Medicine*. https://doi.org/10.1001/archinte.166.12.1262.

Politi, M. C., Schleinitz, M. D., & Col, N. F. (2008). Revisiting the duration of vasomotor symptoms of menopause: A meta-analysis. *Journal of General Internal Medicine*. https://doi.org/10.1007/s11606-008-0655-4.

Popovic, R. M., & White, D. P. (1998). Upper airway muscle activity in normal women: Influence of hormonal status. *Journal of Applied Physiology*. https://doi.org/10.1152/jappl.1998.84.3.1055.

Regestein, Q. R., Friebely, J., Shifren, J. L., et al. (2004). Self-reported sleep in postmenopausal women. *Menopause*. https://doi.org/10.1097/01.GME.0000097741.18446.3E.

Reynolds, F. A. (1997). Perceived control over menopausal hot flushes: Exploring the correlates of a standardized measure. *Maturitas, 27*(3), 215–221.

Robinson, J. G., & Molzahn, A. E. (2007). Sexuality and quality of life. *Journal of Gerontological Nursing*. https://doi.org/10.3928/00989134-20070301-05.

Sievert, L. L., Obermeyer, C. M., & Price, K. (2006). Determinants of hot flashes and night sweats. *Annals of Human Biology, 33*(1), 4–16. https://doi.org/10.1080/03014460500421338.
Soares, C. N. (2005). Insomnia in women: An overlooked epidemic? *Archives of Women's Mental Health*. https://doi.org/10.1007/s00737-005-0100-1.
Soules, M. R., Sherman, S., Parrott, E., et al. (2001). Executive summary: Stages of reproductive aging workshop (STRAW). *Climacteric*. https://doi.org/10.1080/cmt.4.4.267.272.
Spielman, A. J. (1986). Assessment of insomnia. *Clinical Psychology Review, 6*, 11–23.
Spielman, A. J., Caruso, L. S., & Glovinsky, P. B. (1987). A behavioral perspective on insomnia treatment. *The Psychiatric Clinics of North America, 10*(4), 541–553. PMID: 3332317.
Thurston, R. C., Chang, Y., Buysse, D. J., Hall, M. H., & Matthews, K. A. (2019). Hot flashes and awakenings among midlife women. *Sleep, 42*(9), 1–7. https://doi.org/10.1093/sleep/zsz131.
World Health Organization (WHO) (1996). *Research on the menopause in the 1990s. Report of a WHO Scientific Group. (Vol. 866)*. Switzerland: WHO.
Young, T., Finn, L., Austin, D., & Peterson, A. (2003). Menopausal status and sleep-disordered breathing in the Wisconsin Sleep Cohort Study. *American Journal of Respiratory and Critical Care Medicine*. https://doi.org/10.1164/rccm.200209-1055OC.
Young, T., Rabago, D., Zgierska, A., Austin, D., & Finn, L. (2003). Objective and subjective sleep quality in premenopausal, perimenopausal, and postmenopausal women in the wisconsin sleep cohort study. *Sleep*. https://doi.org/10.1093/sleep/26.6.667.

CHAPTER

17

CBT-I for older adults

Jaime M. Hughes[a] *and Jennifer L. Martin*[b]

[a]Department of Population Health Sciences, School of Medicine, Duke University, Health Services Research & Development, Durham VA Healthcare System, Durham, NC, United States, [b]Geriatric Research, Education, and Clinical Center, VA Greater Los Angeles Healthcare System, David Geffen School of Medicine at the University of California Los Angeles, Los Angeles, CA, United States

Insomnia in older adults

Studies have historically demonstrated an increase in rates of insomnia with age, suggesting insomnia disorder is most prevalent in older patient groups; however, more recent data suggest that some of what was originally considered age effects may be more accurately described as cohort effects (Foley, Monjan, Simonsick, Wallace, & Blazer, 1999; Gislason, Reynisdottir, Kristbjarnarson, & Benediktsdottir, 1993; Monjan & Foley, 1995). In recent data, it appears that insomnia is more common in young- or middle-aged populations compared to older adults (Grandner et al., 2012; Martin et al., 2017).

Clinical insomnia disorder is diagnosed when an individual has frequent (at least three nights per week) sleep-related complaints that are accompanied by daytime impairments or consequences and persist for over 3 months (see Table 1) (American Academy of Sleep Medicine, 2005; American Psychiatric Association, 2013). A key challenge in establishing the prevalence of insomnia disorder in older adults is the attribution of daytime impairments to difficulties with sleep, and age-related expectations about sleep itself. In older adults with medical comorbidities, for example, they may attribute daytime symptoms to other conditions, rather than to poor sleep.

Adapting Cognitive Behavioral Therapy for Insomnia
https://doi.org/10.1016/B978-0-12-822872-2.00005-0

TABLE 1 Core diagnostic criteria for insomnia disorder.

Criterion	Age-related considerations
A: trouble falling asleep, maintaining sleep, and waking up earlier than desired	Older adults are more likely to experience difficulties with sleep maintenance and early morning awakenings
B: Daytime symptoms related to nighttime sleep difficulties: fatigue/malaise; attention, concentration, or memory impairments; impaired functioning or performance; mood disturbance/irritability; daytime sleepiness; behavioral problems; reduced motivation/energy/accidents; concerns about or dissatisfaction with sleep	Many older adults suffer from multiple chronic conditions and may attribute daytime symptoms to nonsleep factors. It can be helpful to ask about variation in daytime symptoms and variations in sleep to assess whether there is a link between daytime consequences and sleep difficulties Daytime napping patterns (timing, duration, frequency) should also be addressed
C: The complaint cannot be explained by an inadequate opportunity or circumstances for sleep	The residential setting should be taken into consideration as the built environment of assisted living or skilled nursing facilities may not be conducive to restorative, quality sleep
Frequency: Symptoms occur at least 3 times per week	
Duration: Symptoms persist for at least 3months	Older adults may be poor historians of sleep problems. In some cases, eliciting input from family members can be helpful in identifying symptom onset
Comorbidities: Sleep difficulties are not better explained by another sleep disorder, mental health condition, medical condition, or medication	As mentioned above, older adults often suffer from multiple chronic conditions and it can be difficult to determine the relative contribution of each factor. A chronological history regarding changes in health status, variation in symptoms, and sleep difficulties can be helpful

Older adults may also have "low expectations" when it comes to sleep (Hughes & Martin, 2015). Some may expect that poor sleep is simply part of normal aging, and in some cultures, seeing older adults sleeping during the day is considered socially acceptable (Li, Vitiello, & Gooneratne, 2018).

Evidence for CBT-I in older adults

Healthy older adults with limited cognitive or functional impairments can successfully participate in, and benefit from, traditional CBT-I (Irwin, Cole, & Nicassio, 2006; Rybarczyk, Lund, Garroway, & Mack, 2013).

However, for some select groups of older adults, it is important to take several considerations into account when adapting and delivering CBT-I. These patient-centered adaptations can enhance the ability of older adults with comorbidities and impairments to engage in CBT-I, adhere to recommended behavior changes, and benefit from treatment of their insomnia. Some of these considerations are described below.

Medical complexity. More than three-quarters of older Americans have multiple chronic conditions (Gertis et al., 2014), which can result in challenges around managing the medical and psychological symptoms of these various conditions. Although many chronic medical conditions should be treated promptly when they are identified (e.g., hypertension, hyperlipidemia, diabetes), the presence of such conditions should not preclude or delay the treatment of insomnia disorder. In fact, treating underlying sleep problems may improve older adults' health, daytime function, mood, and quality of life, which may, in turn, aid in adhering to other health behavior recommendations and chronic disease management regimens.

Chronic pain. In addition, chronic pain is also endorsed by roughly one-half of older adults (Patel, Guralnik, Dansie, & Turk, 2013) and may be related to chronic conditions such as osteoarthritis or neuropathic pain associated with diabetes. Sleep disturbances are more common in older adults with chronic pain (Lunde, Pallesen, Krangnes, & Nordhus, 2010) and poor sleep may exacerbate pain symptoms, further increasing the clinical challenges around pain management in older adult populations. Acknowledging this potential bidirectional nature between poor sleep and chronic pain (Smith & Haythornthwaite, 2004; Smith, Quartana, Okonkwo, & Nasir, 2009) may be especially critical for older adults. For example, chronic pain may negatively impact an older adult's nighttime sleep quality while also limiting one's ability to engage in daytime activities, including physical activity. Reductions in daytime activity may then contribute to increased sedentary time which can both worsen pain and contribute to unintentional daytime napping. Together, these factors can contribute to poor nighttime sleep.

Medications. Medication use should also be acknowledged in the course of insomnia assessment and treatment. The prevalence of polypharmacy, or the use of multiple medications, continues to rise among adults (Wastesson, Morin, Tan, & Johnell, 2018). In addition to polypharmacy, medication side effects, drug–drug interactions, and the use of inappropriate medications (American Geriatrics Society Beers Criteria Update Expert Panel, 2015; Steinman et al., 2006) should also be taken into consideration. Furthermore, the timing and dosage of medications, including those that have either sedating or alerting effects, may also impact an older adult's sleep–wake patterns. Attention should be made that alerting medications are taken in the morning, or during the day, while sedating medications are taken in the evening.

Functional and sensory impairments. Both normative and non-normative aging processes can contribute to an increase in functional and sensory impairments.

Functional impairments are typically classified as difficulty completing activities of daily living (e.g., dressing, grooming, getting in and out of bed) and instrumental activities of daily living (e.g., preparing meals, managing finances, housework). However, more global functional capacity, including general mobility (e.g., walking, sitting, and standing with minimal assistance) may be particularly relevant to older adults' sleep and activity patterns. Older adults with limited mobility may have difficulty engaging in regular daytime activity and are, thus, more likely to spend extended periods of time in daytime sedentary activities. This reduction in daytime activity may, in turn, contribute to unintentional daytime napping. Older adults with functional limitations are also at increased risk of falls, which may be particularly consequential during the middle of the night.

Common sensory impairments include changes to both vision and hearing with as many as one-third of older adults reporting vision and/or hearing impairments (Correia et al., 2016). Sleep complaints are common among older adults with visual impairments and may be due to changes in both exposure to, and regulation of, natural light and circadian rhythms (Zizi et al., 2002). Visual and hearing impairments may also impact an older adults' ability to interact with treatment materials, including completion of nightly sleep diaries. Sensory impairments may also be associated with reduced daytime activities, which can further dysregulate sleep–wake schedules.

Cognitive impairment. Some aspects of older adults' cognitive capacity and performance naturally decline as a part of normal part of aging (e.g., attention, memory, processing speed, reasoning, visuospatial skills) (Drag & Bieliauskas, 2010; Salthouse, 2010). More significant changes in cognitive performance may be a result of Alzheimer's Disease and related dementias. Mild Cognitive Impairment (MCI), classified by subjective complaints in cognitive impairment without noticeable impacts on functional independence (Plassman et al., 2008), maybe a precursor to more advanced forms of dementia. Neurological changes, including those related to Alzheimer's and other dementias, include disruptions or alterations in circadian rhythms. Other symptoms related to poor sleep can include sundowning (i.e., increased agitation or problematic behaviors in the evening) and daytime fatigue or napping.

Cognitive impairment may impact an older adult's ability to initiate and complete behavioral treatment. Examples may include difficulty following directions, diminished motivation and/or ability to make decisions around daytime activities or routines, poor perseveration, and some sensory impairments. Despite some of these challenges, CBT-I interventions can be adapted so that these challenges are minimized and that older adults' ability to fully participate in an intervention is maximized. Our team's prior experience suggests that older adults with cognitive impairment are able to fully participate in a brief sleep intervention and experience improvements in sleep that are similar to their cognitively intact peers (unpublished data).

Physical environment and residential status. Older adults live in a range of different settings, including single-family homes, planned senior living communities, continuing care retirement communities, assisted living facilities, and skilled nursing facilities. Both the physical environment and social opportunities of each setting can influence an older adult's sleep. For example, older adults' daytime activity levels may depend on availability of, and access to, structured activity programs and/or access to safe, walkable neighborhoods. The degree to which older adults experience social isolation and/or engagement can also impact daytime activity levels and, in turn, evening behaviors and nighttime sleep quality. However, for many older adults living in a residential or skilled nursing facility, the physical characteristics of the built environment may be outside their control. Common challenges within residential facilities include limited exposure to natural light, shared rooms, and noise and light disruptions across a 24-h period, including at night (Martin & Ancoli-Israel, 2008; Ye & Richards, 2018).

Mental health. Although rates of mental health disorders are often lower in older persons compared to younger adults (Karlin, Duffy, & Gleaves, 2008), the prevalence is expected to rise as the population continues to age (Karel, Gatz, & Smyer, 2012). For many older adults, mental health disorders may be comorbid with one or more physical health conditions. As discussed elsewhere in this volume, understanding how mental health conditions impact sleep and ensuring that patients receive appropriate treatment for both insomnia and other mental health disorders is important. Finally, older adults with chronic insomnia may be at greater risk for developing incident depression (Perlis et al., 2006) and/or exacerbating existing depressive symptoms (Pigeon, Unutzer, & Perlis, 2008), providing further support that early detection and treatment of insomnia in older adults is critical.

Below, we summarize strategies for adapting CBT-I for special populations of older adults. One example of an adapted version of CBT-I for frail older adults attending Adult Day Health Care is shown in Table 3.

Targeted adaptations of CBT-I components for older adults

As noted above, CBT-I can and should be used as the first-line treatment of insomnia disorder in older adults. However, for some specific subpopulations of older adults, treatment components can, and should, be modified, taking into consideration the health status of each patient. Below, and in Table 2, we summarize the most common adaptations to CBT-I components for select groups of older adults.

Sleep restriction therapy

Sleep restriction therapy is a multistep approach in which sleep diaries are used to adjust the patient's time in bed to match their total sleep time. At first, patients are often sleep-deprived, but as time in bed increases, this short-term issue resolves. There are two main reasons why implementation of standard sleep restriction therapy can be challenging in older adults. First, some older adults spend extended time in bed due to lack of sufficient daytime stimulation making it very difficult to adhere to a significantly reduced time in bed period. For example, an older adult who habitually goes to bed at 8:00 pm, and stays in bed until 8:00 am, but sleeps only 6.5 h may find it difficult to identify activities to fill an additional 5.5 h each day. Second, some older adults experience daytime sleepiness and/or fatigue due to comorbid conditions, and the additional temporary increase in sleepiness can be intolerable for the patient or even unsafe. For example, older adults who have to drive a long distance to clinical appointments, or who are caregivers for someone else who requires supervision (e.g., a spouse with dementia) may not be able to tolerate increased sleepiness, even for a short period of time, because of safety concerns.

Total sleep time ± 30 min: One common modification is to use the patient's total sleep time plus an additional 30 min for the time in the bed window. This minor modification can be used with many patients as a starting point. If sleep efficiency does not sufficiently improve, time in bed can be reduced by 15-min increments.

Sleep compression: In sleep compression, the process begins with the patient's current time in bed (based on sleep diaries), which is then gradually reduced (in 15 or 30 min increments) until sleep efficiency increases to 85% or higher. This can be a useful approach both for patients who begin with a long time in bed and those who cannot tolerate a temporary increase in sleepiness.

Account for napping/dozing during the day: Some older adults spend extended periods of time sleeping during the day, and this should be considered in calculating their baseline total sleep time. For example, an older adult may sleep only 5 h at night, but then take a 2-h nap each afternoon making their total sleep time 7 h per 24-h period. In this case, a brief planned nap while "shifting" most of the daytime sleeping to the nighttime sleep window can prevent extreme sleepiness. Rather than restricting time in bed at night to 5 h and eliminating the nap entirely, the clinician can consider shifting some or all of the daytime sleeping into the nighttime

TABLE 2 Adaptations of specific CBT-I components for older adult populations.

CBT-I component	Populations	Adaptations
Sleep restriction therapy	Comorbid sleep disorders (e.g., sleep apnea) that increase sleepiness High fall risk Functional limitations Social isolation	Consider time spent sleeping during the day in calculating TST (e.g., nap time + nighttime TST). Incorporate short daytime nap into sleep plan Use sleep compression (begin with TIB rather than TST and gradually reduce TIB until SE increases)
Stimulus control	High fall risk Functional limitations	Adhere to stimulus control during the daytime (i.e., not spending time in bed during the day) Omit instruction to get out of bed at night Instruct patient to stay in bed, but engage in activity that does not relate to trying to fall asleep
Napping/daytime sleep	All, including patients with chronic pain	Limit daytime naps, if possible. As needed, schedule and restrict daytime nap to 30-min maximum
Sleep hygiene	All	Metabolism of caffeine, alcohol, and nicotine may be impacted by age and may need to be eliminated earlier in the day Encourage time outdoors or in brightly lit indoor areas to increase light exposure during the day
Counterarousal/ relaxation	All	Consider patient preferences in relaxing activities
Cognitive therapy	Cognitive impairment	Use written prompts and reminders
Behavioral activation/activity scheduling	Social isolation Limited activity engagement	Use when the range of daytime activities is restricted or when an older adult is socially isolated to increase daytime activity level and avoid accidental dozing
Relapse prevention	All	Discuss strategies for getting back on track after stressful health or life event (e.g., use sleep diary to monitor sleep, consistent schedule, daytime routines, seek help if needed)
Sleep diary	Visual impairments Cognitive impairments	Simplified formatting and instructions Large printing, automated telephone diaries, or other adaptations may be needed

TST, total sleep time; *TIB*, time in bed; *SE*, sleep efficiency.

sleep period. For example, the initial schedule could include a planned 30-min daytime nap, plus 6.5h in bed at night.

For some older adults with chronic pain and/or chronic medical conditions, eliminating all daytime naps may not be desirable or feasible. For these patients, naps should be prescribed as part of the weekly sleep–wake schedule. In collaboration with the patient, the clinician suggests a scheduled time for a daily nap (preferably no later than early afternoon) and encourages the patient to limit the nap to no more than 30min. Encouraging patients to utilize an alarm clock and nap in the bed can also be useful. For patients with chronic pain, the clinician can encourage daytime "resting" away from the bed or bedroom, if possible.

Stimulus control

Stimulus control involves a set of instructions that intend to break the association between the bed (or sleep environment more generally) and alertness/anxiety, and instead create an association between the bed and falling asleep quickly. This typically involves eliminating nonsleep activities while in bed and getting out of bed at night if struggling with sleep. For some older patients, this presents safety concerns (e.g., nighttime fall risk). Also, older adults frequently sleep in locations outside of their bedroom, and this factor may also contribute to a lack of an association between the bed and sleep. For older adults with family caregivers, it also can be disruptive to the caregivers' sleep to have the patient out of bed during the night. In such instances, it is critical that the caregiver understands the rationale for stimulus control, and perhaps identifies safe ideas on what the patient can do during the night rather than struggling with sleep in the bed. In some instances, the best option for the patient–caregiver dyad may be using one of the adaptations described below.

One alternative approach is the use of *counter-control*. Counter-control is a modification that involves keeping the patient in bed when awake at night but having them engage in a relaxing activity that is not related to falling asleep. For example, rather than worry about the consequences of not sleeping well, the patient can read, listen to music, or meditate. This approach is useful for patients who cannot safely and/or independently transfer in and out of bed at night. In this case, the remaining stimulus control instructions are still followed. The patient should continue to avoid using the bed for nonsleep activities during the daytime.

When administering stimulus control, it is important to consider both sides of the issue: avoid wakefulness in bed *and* avoid sleeping outside of the bed. Many older adults struggle to maintain wakefulness throughout the day, and as a result, fall asleep in locations other than their sleeping bed. This can lead to other locations becoming associated with sleep such as a sofa or recliner. Additional efforts and strategies to limit daytime sleeping outside of the nighttime sleep environment may be needed. For example, if the patient tends to doze off in the evening while watching TV from the family room sofa, it is important to incorporate strategies to increase alerting activities. Examples of such activities include walking outdoors, standing at regular intervals, or engaging in social activities such as playing card games with others. In some cases, the patient may need to avoid the situation where they habitually fall asleep entirely. In this example, the patient may need to sit in a different place to watch TV in the evening, as the family room sofa may have become an inappropriate cue for sleeping.

Sleep hygiene

Basic sleep hygiene instructions focused on sleep environment, timing of meals, intake of substances, and daytime activities can be a useful addition to insomnia treatments. Special considerations for older adults include slower metabolism of substances such as caffeine and alcohol, which may necessitate a longer substance-free window before bedtime. In addition, because pain conditions are more common in older adults, the sleeping surface may be important to avoiding discomfort at night. Correcting sleep hygiene issues is seldom sufficient to address a long-standing insomnia problem at any age, and for this reason, it is not recommended as a stand-alone approach (Edinger et al., 2021).

Cognitive therapy and relaxation techniques

Other components of CBT-I can include relaxation techniques or other counter-arousal measures and cognitive therapy techniques. These treatment components can generally be delivered in their usual way, considering patient preferences and cognitive abilities. In some instances, relaxation techniques that include muscle tension and relaxation must be adjusted to account for physical limitations, and using methods that do not require such techniques (e.g., diaphragmatic breathing, mindfulness) may be preferable. In patients with mild cognitive impairments, cognitive therapy exercises can be challenging as these experiences often require patients to engage in complex thinking tasks such as holding both evidence for and against a given belief in working memory. In these cases, using simple strategies such as "flashcards" that display helpful, or healthy, thoughts can be a useful adaptation.

Sleep diaries

Maintaining a daily sleep diary is an important aspect of delivering CBT-I, but completion can be a challenge for older patients. Some paper-and-pencil diaries are printed in small text and instructions are complex, making it difficult for older adults to write on them. Some older adults are uncomfortable with technology and may not be comfortable completing a diary electronically. In these cases, clinicians can include only the key essential elements on the diary, including bedtime and rise time, plus targeted sleep symptoms. When it is not possible to obtain sufficient information to compute sleep efficiency, a threshold for improvement can be set. For example, the sleep diary can be used to track bedtime, rise time, and total time awake at night. Sleep diaries may also capture levels of daytime energy and/or fatigue which can be useful in adjusting a patient's sleep schedule during the course of treatment. Finally, given high rates of visual impairment, using large-print diaries (14—point font or larger) and simple formats (e.g., high-contrast text) can make it easier for older adults to complete diaries daily. When patients are not able to complete diaries on their own, assistance from caregivers on aspects that are directly observable can be informative. Caregivers may be able to reliably describe bedtime and rise times and daytime sleeping; however, it depends upon whether the caregiver is awake when these behaviors occur. When the caregiver cannot accurately reflect the patients' behavior, it may be necessary to use alternative approaches, such as wrist actigraphy, for evaluating sleep-wake patterns.

Addition of behavioral activation to CBT-I

Due to social isolation and reduced physical activity, it is sometimes necessary to incorporate additional activating strategies to address daytime considerations. Behavioral activation and activity scheduling during the day, similar to what is used in the treatment of depression (Orgeta, Brede, & Livingston, 2017), can be incorporated into insomnia treatments. These additional strategies can have the added benefits of elevating mood while also helping older adults to sustain wakefulness during the day. Without explicitly addressing daytime behaviors, older adults may find it difficult to avoid daytime napping and/or reduce time in bed in the evenings.

Along these lines, a specific plan for evening activities that are sufficiently engaging to prevent dozing should be included in the treatment plan. Aging is associated with a "phase advance" in circadian rhythms (Duffy & Czeisler, 2002), which leads to earlier sleep tendency. Older adults therefore may find it difficult to delay bedtime because of this normal age-related alteration in the circadian timing system. In some instances, this phase advance may be severe enough that the patient cannot adjust their sleep times without targeted circadian interventions. In such instances, it can be helpful to use evidence-based treatment for advanced sleep–wake phase disorder such as bright light therapy (Auger et al., 2015).

Examples of CBT-I for special populations of older adults

Older adults who require caregiving at home

Many older adults, due to cognitive impairments or functional limitations, require assistance from paid caregivers, informal family caregivers, or both. In these instances, engaging the caregiver in the treatment of insomnia from the very beginning is critical. Caregivers must understand the importance of healthy sleep for sustaining independence and overall health in addition to appreciating the rationale for the components of CBT-I. In providing CBT-I to individuals with cognitive impairment, it is also important to note that family caregivers frequently suffer from sleep issues of their own (McCurry, Song, & Martin, 2015), including interruption of their sleep because of nighttime behavioral disturbances. As a result, it is often necessary to develop strategies that improve the health of both members of the dyad. There is preliminary evidence that a dyadic approach for patients with dementia can lead to improvement in symptoms for both patients and their family caregivers (Song et al., 2019).

CBT-I in community-based programs

Our team previously developed and tested a brief, four-session sleep intervention for frail older Veterans utilizing VA Adult Day Health Care (ADHC), an outpatient program designed for older Veterans at risk for social isolation, poor medical management, or premature institutionalization (Veterans Health Administration, 2009). On average, program participants were 70 years old, had a significant number of comorbidities documented in the medical record (mean = 24.3), functional impairments, and demonstrated some cognitive impairment (average MMSE score = 25.9) (Hughes & Martin, 2015). Although characteristics of poor sleep were high, only a fraction endorsed poor sleep quality. ADHC participants attended the day program 2–5 days per week where they participated in individual and group exercise, health education groups, and social activities.

Primary considerations for program adaptation in this population included competing cognitive and functional impairments. Key adaptations to nighttime treatment components included modified stimulus

Monday morning	What time did you go to bed last night?	Did it take more than 30 minutes to fall asleep?	Were you awake for more than 30 minutes during the night?	What time did you get up this morning?	Rate your sleep quality last night
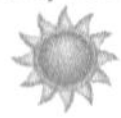	__:__ am / pm	Yes / No	Yes / No	__:__ am / pm	__ better than usual __ same as usual __ worse than usual
Monday night	Did you take any naps or doze off today?				
	Yes / No		If yes, how long? ______ minutes		

FIG. 1 Sleep diary used with Adult Day Health Care participants.

control (e.g., avoid recommendations to get out of bed at night due to fall risks), employing sleep compression therapy rather than sleep restriction, tailored sleep hygiene (e.g., healthy daytime and evening routines), and a simplified sleep diary (see Fig. 1). Key adaptations to daytime treatment components including scheduled naps when elimination of naps was not feasible or desired, and inclusion of daytime routines and activities. Table 3 displays the content across each of our four sessions. In a randomized controlled trial of this adapted intervention, all participants randomized to the brief sleep intervention ($N = 21$) successfully completed all four sessions with intervention staff recording patients' high engagement and comprehension throughout the program (Martin et al., 2017).

CBT-I informed recommendations for long-term care

Many older adults require levels of care that cannot be provided in their own homes and therefore reside in nursing homes or similar long-term care facilities. In these settings, poor sleep is nearly universal (Martin et al., 2006; Skottheim, Lövheim, Isaksson, Sandman, & Gustafsson, 2018). This is a result of a combination of factors, including both resident characteristics and environmental conditions. Residents typically suffer from multiple medical issues and many are cognitively impaired, making engagement in traditional behavioral therapies challenging. Furthermore, residents have only limited control over their sleep–wake schedules. Meals are typically served at specific times, and out of necessity, care is provided according to staffing schedules rather than resident preferences. Given the dependence of nursing home residents on staff to meet their basic daily needs, it is essential that staff members are educated about the importance of sleep, in terms of improving key outcomes for nursing home residents. For example, studies show that poor sleep is associated with the risk of falls (Stone et al., 2014) as is the use of sedative–hypnotic medications (Maust, Kales, Wiechers, Blow, & Olfson, 2016). Addressing sleep issues, therefore, requires a different approach; however, the core

TABLE 3 The 4-session sleep intervention program: session by session content and at-home activities.

Session and topics covered	At-home Activities
Session 1: How sleep works	
• Program overview • *Education*: Healthy sleep, sleep stages, circadian clock (rationale for regular schedule) • *Stimulus control*: limiting nonsleep activities in the bed (note: no instruction to get out of bed at night given due to fall risk) • *Education*: Daily light exposure and regular daytime activities; impact of daytime napping on nighttime sleep quality • *Sleep compression*: Initial sleep schedule (bedtime and rise time) established based on preferred routine and current time in bed • Instruction in the use of daily sleep diary • Summary and Review	• Follow sleep schedule • Move nonsleep activities out of bed • Complete sleep diary
Session 2: Steps to getting sleep	
• Session overview • Check-in and review sleep diary • *Education*: sleep drive (rationale for sleep compression) • *Sleep compression*: Reduce time in bed by 30 min and adjust sleep schedule accordingly, avoid naps or limit to <30 min before 5 pm • *Behavioral activation*: Identify engaging activities for the evening hours to maintain wakefulness until scheduled bedtime • 1–2 individualized sleep-hygiene related recommendations • *Sleep compression*: Revised sleep schedule (if indicated) • Reminder to complete the daily sleep dairy • Summary and Review	• Follow sleep schedule • Keep nonsleep activities out of bed • Implement 1–2 sleep hygiene practices • Complete sleep diary
Session 3: Healthy Habits for Healthy Sleep	
• Session overview • Check-in and review sleep diary • *Sleep Compression*: Reduce time in bed by 15–30 min and adjust sleep schedule accordingly • Bedtime routine: Identify activities for the last hour before bedtime (engaging but not activating)	• Follow sleep schedule • Keep nonsleep activities out of bed • Follow sleep-hygiene practices • Complete sleep diary

Continued

TABLE 3 The 4-session sleep intervention program: session by session content and at-home activities—cont'd

Session and topics covered	At-home Activities
• *Sleep hygiene principles*: physical activity, light exposure, social activities during the day • *Sleep hygiene principles*: diet, liquids near bedtime, alcohol, smoking, sleep environment • *Sleep Compression*: Revision of planned sleep schedule (if indicated) • Summary and Review	
Session 4: Preventing the return of chronic insomnia	

• Session overview
• Check-in and review sleep diary
• *Long-term strategies*:
  ○ If sleeping well, discuss a regular but less rigid sleep schedule
  ○ If not sleeping well, discuss continued sleep compression
  ○ Discuss how to get sleep back on track after health or life events
• *Education*: When to contact a healthcare provider about sleep
• *Sleep Compression*: Revision of planned sleep schedule (if indicated) to align with a long-term sleep plan
• Summary and Review
	• Recommend following sleep schedule (with some flexibility)
	• Recommend keeping nonsleep activities out of bed
	• Recommend continuing to follow good sleep-hygiene practices
	• Complete sleep diary
	• Recommend continuing to follow sleep-hygiene related recommendations

principles of CBT-I can still be applied, and studies show that residents sleep can be improved with nonpharmacological approaches (Alessi et al., 2005; Bloom et al., 2009; Capezuti et al., 2018). Table 4 provides a summary of key strategies that can be used to address sleep issues in long-term care environments.

First and foremost, early studies show that sleep and wakefulness are distributed throughout the 24-h day (Jacobs, Ancoli-Israel, Parker, & Kripke, 1989), and sleep difficulties should be approached as a 24-h issue. During the day, interventions should focus on having residents out of bed and active as much as possible, and nighttime interventions should focus on spending an appropriate amount of time in bed and creating a nighttime environment that is conducive to consolidated sleep. There is some evidence that interventions to increase light exposure at specific times during the day have beneficial impacts on sleep (Ancoli-Israel et al., 2003; Ancoli-Israel, Martin, Kripke, Marler, & Klauber, 2002); however, these interventions, which typically involve exposure to artificial light, are difficult to sustain within routine care in nursing homes. Encouraging and supporting daytime activities that are social and interactive, such as

TABLE 4 CBT-I informed strategies to improve sleep in long-term care settings.

	Daytime strategies	Nighttime strategies
Environmental factors	Increase light levels indoors When possible, encourage residents to spend time outdoors Support in-person or virtual visits with family and friends to increase alertness and socialization	Reduce nighttime light levels in resident rooms. Use dim lights when providing nighttime care Reduce nighttime noise levels in resident rooms. Turn down the volume on televisions, close room doors when safe, limit staff conversations in or near resident rooms
Resident factors	Identify and encourage each resident's preferred daytime activities Address comorbid mental health problems including depression and anxiety as these conditions can exacerbate sleep difficulties	Evaluate and treat sleep disorders such as sleep apnea, restless legs syndrome, and REM behavior disorder
Facility and staffing factors	Serve meals out of bed, ideally in common areas with socialization during mealtimes Use brightly lit areas for meals and daytime activities Educate staff regarding the importance of sleep for improving key outcomes for residents	Avoid placing noisy equipment in resident sleeping areas Dim lights if safe Have a facility-wide "quiet hours" policy at night Structured screening for sleep difficulties and symptoms of sleep disorders

games and physical activities. When residents need assistance with transferring in and out of bed, this presents a challenge for staff. Furthermore, the bedroom is typically the resident's only private space, and they may wish to spend time there during the day. When this is the case, efforts to make the room bright and engaging and providing a comfortable chair where the resident can spend time during the day can be helpful. Equally important, the sleeping rooms should be quiet and dimly lit during the nighttime hours. Together, these adjustments to environmental characteristics can help to improve daytime activity and nighttime sleep patterns.

Future directions

In our team's prior work with older Veterans using VA Healthcare services, we found that as many as two-thirds complained of insomnia-like symptoms while one-half met diagnostic criteria for Insomnia Disorder (Hughes & Martin, 2015; Ryden et al., 2019). Despite the high prevalence, access to CBT-I remains limited. Unfortunately, these challenges exist in non-VA settings as well. To improve access to CBT-I for older adults, several major gaps must be addressed, including (1) brief, accurate assessments; (2) guidance on how to refer older adults to accessible, appropriate treatment options; (3) expanding access to CBT-I; and (4) further understanding of how CBT-I may impact nonsleep outcomes, including overall health, quality of life, and physical function. Each is addressed in greater detail below.

Screening and assessment. Identifying brief, accurate methods to identify poor sleeping older adults is critical for early detection and treatment. In our team's prior work, we found notable discrepancies between older adults' sleep quality ratings and the presence of poor sleep characteristics (Hughes et al., 2018). As alluded to above, more than two-thirds endorsed insomnia-like symptoms, including trouble falling or staying asleep and/or daytime consequences resulting from poor nighttime sleep. However, when asked to describe their sleep, only one-quarter rated their sleep quality as "poor" (Hughes & Martin, 2015). Additional research to understand how older adults evaluate their sleep quality and endorse sleep problems is critical. As brief insomnia measures are developed and validated for older adults, care should also be given to how, where, and when such measures should be deployed. For instance, should older adults be routinely screened for sleep problems by primary care providers at regular intervals or might sleep be assessed in rehabilitation or specialty settings?

Expanding access to CBT-I. In recent years, there have been several efforts to expand access to CBT-I. Some of these efforts have included self-management programs (Cheung, Jarrin, Ballot, Bharwani, & Morin, 2019), mobile health applications or web-based treatments (Seyffert et al., 2016; Zachariae, Lyby, Ritterband, & O'Toole, 2016), and stepped care models (Mack & Rybarczyk, 2011). For the most part, these efforts have not focused on older adults and special considerations that are needed for this population. For example, some older adults may not have access to web-based programs and the self-guided approach of self-management may not be appropriate for patients with comorbidities and/or cognitive or functional limitations. Identifying where, when, and how older adults prefer to receive CBT-I will be critical in expanding access.

Older adults obtain care for the health and social needs across a diverse set of services including primary care, specialty services, and home and community-based services (e.g., senior centers, Adult Day Health Care, home-based primary care). Integrating CBT-I into these different settings may expand access. Exploring which type of provider is best suited to deliver CBT-I (e.g., physician, psychologist, nurse, social worker) within each of these settings is also critical as well as identifying what, if any, additional training is needed to prepare providers to implement and sustain such programs.

Mechanisms and outcomes of CBT-I in older adults. Although the body of literature demonstrating the positive effects of CBT-I in older adults is growing, additional questions about the mechanisms and outcomes of CBT-I remain. First, is CBT-I effective in complex patients with multiple chronic conditions? If so, how, and to what extent, might improvements in insomnia symptoms contribute to improvements in other conditions? Second, for which subgroups of older adults is CBT-I most effective? Third, how does CBT-I impact older adults' physical function, quality of life, and resilience? Which outcomes matter most to older adults? To address these questions, future trials should employ broad eligibility criteria that include older adults with multiple chronic conditions, functional impairments, and cognitive limitations. Future studies should also utilize engaged methods that formulate research questions, develop study procedures, analyze data, and disseminate findings in collaboration with older adults, caregivers, and other key stakeholders.

Conclusion

Poor sleep is common among older adults and, left untreated, is associated with a range of negative consequences. As the population of older adults continues to expand significantly, it is essential that effective insomnia screening tools and treatment options are developed and disseminated for this population. Older adults can successfully participate in, and benefit from, CBT-I when adapted in response to comorbid conditions, functional challenges, or residential settings.

References

Alessi, C. A., Martin, J. L., Webber, A. P., Kim, E. C., Harker, J. O., & Josephson, K. R. (2005). Randomized, controlled trial of a nonpharmacological intervention to improve abnormal sleep/wake patterns in nursing home residents. *Journal of the American Geriatrics Society, 53*, 803–810.

American Academy of Sleep Medicine. (2005). Insomnia. In *Vol. 2nd. International classification of sleep disorders* (pp. 1–31). Chicago, IL: American Academy of Sleep Medicine. Reprinted from: NOT IN FILE.

American Geriatrics Society Beers Criteria Update Expert Panel. (2015). American geriatrics society 2015 updated beers criteria for potentially inappropriate medication use in older adults. *Journal of the American Geriatrics Society, 63*(11), 2227–2246. https://doi.org/10.1111/jgs.13702.

American Psychiatric Association. (2013). *Diagnostic and statistical manual of mental disorders*. Arlington, VA: American Psychiatric Association.

Ancoli-Israel, S., Gehrman, P., Martin, J. L., Shochat, T., Marler, M., Corey-Bloom, J., et al. (2003). Increased light exposure consolidates sleep and strengthens circadian rhythms in severe Alzheimer's disease patients. *Behavioral Sleep Medicine, 1*(1), 22–36. https://doi.org/10.1207/s15402010bsm0101_4.

Ancoli-Israel, S., Martin, J. L., Kripke, D. F., Marler, M., & Klauber, M. R. (2002). Effect of light treatment on sleep and circadian rhythms in demented nursing home patients. *Journal of the American Geriatrics Society, 50*(2), 282–289. https://doi.org/10.1046/j.1532-5415.2002.50060.x.

Auger, R. R., Burgess, H. J., Emens, J. S., Deriy, L. V., Thomas, S. M., & Sharkey, K. M. (2015). Clinical practice guideline for the treatment of intrinsic circadian rhythm sleep-wake disorders: Advanced sleep-wake phase disorder (ASWPD), delayed sleep-wake phase disorder (DSWPD), non-24-hour sleep-wake rhythm disorder (N24SWD), and irregular sleep-wake rhythm disorder (ISWRD). An update for 2015: An American Academy of Sleep Medicine clinical practice guideline. *Journal of Clinical Sleep Medicine, 11*(10), 1199–1236. https://doi.org/10.5664/jcsm.5100.

Bloom, H. G., Ahmed, I., Alessi, C. A., Ancoli-Israel, S., Buysse, D. J., Kryger, M. H., et al. (2009). Evidence-based recommendations for the assessment and management of sleep disorders in older persons. *Journal of the American Geriatrics Society, 57*(5), 761–789. https://doi.org/10.1111/j.1532-5415.2009.02220.x.

Capezuti, E., Sagha Zadeh, R., Pain, K., Basara, A., Jiang, N. Z., & Krieger, A. C. (2018). A systematic review of non-pharmacological interventions to improve nighttime sleep among residents of long-term care settings. *BMC Geriatrics, 18*(1), 143. https://doi.org/10.1186/s12877-018-0794-3.

Cheung, J. M. Y., Jarrin, D. C., Ballot, O., Bharwani, A. A., & Morin, C. M. (2019). A systematic review of cognitive behavioral therapy for insomnia implemented in primary care and community settings. *Sleep Medicine Reviews, 44*, 23–36. https://doi.org/10.1016/j.smrv.2018.11.001.

Correia, C., Lopez, K. J., Wroblewski, K. E., Huisingh-Scheetz, M., Kern, D. W., Chen, R. C., et al. (2016). Global sensory impairment in older adults in the United States. *Journal of the American Geriatrics Society, 64*(2), 306–313. https://doi.org/10.1111/jgs.13955.

Drag, L. L., & Bieliauskas, L. A. (2010). Contemporary review 2009: Cognitive aging. *Journal of Geriatric Psychiatry and Neurology, 23*(2), 75–93. https://doi.org/10.1177/0891988709358590.

Duffy, J. F., & Czeisler, C. A. (2002). Age-related change in the relationship between circadian period, circadian phase, and diurnal preference in humans. *Neuroscience Letters, 318*(3), 117–120. https://doi.org/10.1016/s0304-3940(01)02427-2.

Edinger, J. D., Arnedt, J. T., Bertisch, S. M., Carney, C. E., Harrington, J. J., Lichstein, K. L., et al. (2021). Behavioral and psychological treatments for chronic insomnia disorder in adults: An American Academy of sleep medicine clinical practice guideline. *Journal of Clinical Sleep Medicine*. https://doi.org/10.5664/jcsm.8986. jcsm.8986.

Foley, D. J., Monjan, A., Simonsick, E. M., Wallace, R. B., & Blazer, D. G. (1999). Incidence and remission of insomnia among elderly adults: An epidemiologic study of 6,800 persons over three years. *Sleep, 22*(Suppl.2), S366–S372.

Gertis, J., Izrael, D., Deitz, D., LeRoy, L., Ricciardi, R., Miller, T., et al. (2014). *Multiple chronic conditions chartbook. (Q14–0038)*. Rockville, MD: AHRQ Publications.

Gislason, T., Reynisdottir, H., Kristbjarnarson, H., & Benediktsdottir, B. (1993). Sleep habits and sleep disturbances among the elderly—An epidemiological survey. *Journal of Internal Medicine, 234*(1), 31–39.

Grandner, M. A., Martin, J. L., Patel, N. P., Jackson, N. J., Gehrman, P. R., Pien, G., et al. (2012). Age and sleep disturbances among American men and women: Data from the U.S. behavioral risk factor surveillance system. *Sleep, 35*(3), 395–406. https://doi.org/10.5665/sleep.1704.

Hughes, J. M., & Martin, J. L. (2015). Sleep characteristics in veterans affairs adult day health care participants. *Behavioral Sleep Medicine, 13*(3), 197–207.

Hughes, J. M., Song, Y., Fung, C. H., Dzierzewski, J. M., Mitchell, M. N., Jouldjian, S., et al. (2018). Measuring sleep in vulnerable older adults: A comparison of subjective and objective sleep measures. *Clinical Gerontologist, 41*(2), 145–157.

Irwin, M. R., Cole, J. C., & Nicassio, P. M. (2006). Comparative meta-analysis of behavioral interventions for insomnia and their efficacy in middle-aged adults and in older adults 55+ years of age. *Health Psychology, 25*(1), 3–14.

Jacobs, D., Ancoli-Israel, S., Parker, L., & Kripke, D. F. (1989). Twenty-four-hour sleep-wake patterns in a nursing home population. *Psychology and Aging, 4*(3), 352–356. https://doi.org/10.1037//0882-7974.4.3.352.

Karel, M. J., Gatz, M., & Smyer, M. A. (2012). Aging and mental health in the decade ahead: What psychologists need to know. *American Psychologist, 67*(3), 184–198. https://doi.org/10.1037/a0025393.

Karlin, B. E., Duffy, M., & Gleaves, D. H. (2008). Patterns and predictors of mental health service use and mental illness among older and younger adults in the United States. *Psychological Services, 5*(3), 275–294. https://doi.org/10.1037/1541-1559.5.3.275.

Li, J., Vitiello, M. V., & Gooneratne, N. S. (2018). Sleep in normal aging. *Sleep Medicine Clinics, 13*(1), 1–11. https://doi.org/10.1016/j.jsmc.2017.09.001.

Lunde, L.-H., Pallesen, S., Krangnes, L., & Nordhus, I. H. (2010). Characteristics of sleep in older persons with chronic pain: A study based on actigraphy and self-reporting. *The Clinical Journal of Pain, 26*(2), 132–137. https://doi.org/10.1097/AJP.0b013e3181b61923.

Mack, L. J., & Rybarczyk, B. (2011). Behavioral treatment of insomnia: A proposal for a stepped-care approach to promote public health. *Nature and Science of Sleep, 3*, 87–99.

Martin, J. L., & Ancoli-Israel, S. (2008). Sleep disturbances in long-term care. *Clinics in Geriatric Medicine, 24*(1), 39–vi. https://doi.org/10.1016/j.cger.2007.08.001.

Martin, J. L., Schweizer, C. A., Hughes, J. M., Fung, C. H., Dzierzewski, J. M., Washington, D. L., et al. (2017). Estimated prevalence of insomnia among women veterans: Results of a postal survey. *Women's Health Issues, 27*(3), 366–373.

Martin, J. L., Song, Y., Hughes, J., Jouldjian, S., Dzierzewski, J. M., Fung, C. H., … Alessi, C. A. (2017). A four-session sleep intervention program improves sleep for older Adult Day Health Care participants: Results of a randomized controlled trial. *Sleep, 40*(8), zsx079.

Martin, J. L., Webber, A. P., Alam, T., Harker, J. O., Josephson, K. R., & Alessi, C. A. (2006). Daytime sleeping, sleep disturbance, and circadian rhythms in the nursing home. *The American Journal of Geriatric Psychiatry, 14*(2), 121–129. https://doi.org/10.1097/01.JGP.0000192483.35555.a3.

Maust, D. T., Kales, H. C., Wiechers, I. R., Blow, F. C., & Olfson, M. (2016). No end in sight: Benzodiazepine use in older adults in the United States. *Journal of the American Geriatrics Society, 64*(12), 2546–2553. https://doi.org/10.1111/jgs.14379.

McCurry, S. M., Song, Y., & Martin, J. L. (2015). Sleep in caregivers: What we know and what we need to learn. *Current Opinion in Psychiatry, 28*(6), 497–503. https://doi.org/10.1097/yco.0000000000000205.

Monjan, A., & Foley, D. (1995). Longitudinal study of chronic insomnia in older persons. *Sleep Research, 24*, 265.

Orgeta, V., Brede, J., & Livingston, G. (2017). Behavioural activation for depression in older people: Systematic review and meta-analysis. *The British Journal of Psychiatry, 211*(5), 274–279. https://doi.org/10.1192/bjp.bp.117.205021.

Patel, K. V., Guralnik, J. M., Dansie, E. J., & Turk, D. C. (2013). Prevalence and impact of pain among older adults in the United States: Findings from the 2011 National Health and aging trends study. *Pain, 154*(12), 2649–2657. https://doi.org/10.1016/j.pain.2013.07.029.

Perlis, M. L., Smith, L. J., Lyness, J. M., Matteson, S. R., Pigeon, W., & R., & Jungquist, C. (2006). Insomnia as a risk factor for onset of depression in the elderly. *Behavioral Sleep Medicine, 4*, 104–113.

Pigeon, W. R., Unutzer, J., & Perlis, M. L. (2008). Is insomnia a perpetuating factor for late-life depression in the IMPACT cohort? *Sleep, 31*(4), 481–488.

Plassman, B., Langa, K. M., Fisher, G., Heeringa, S., Weir, D., Ofstedai, M., et al. (2008). Prevalence of cognitive impairment without dementia in the United States. *Annals of Internal Medicine, 148*(6), 427–434.

Rybarczyk, B., Lund, H. G., Garroway, A. M., & Mack, L. J. (2013). Cognitive behavioral therapy for insomnia in older adults: Background, evidence, and overview of treatment protocol. *Clinical Gerontologist, 36*, 70–93.

Ryden, A. M., Martin, J. L., Matsuwaka, S., Fung, C. H., Dzierzewski, J. M., Song, Y., et al. (2019). Insomnia disorder among older veterans: Results of a postal survey. *Journal of Clinical Sleep Medicine, 15*(04), 543–551. https://doi.org/10.5664/jcsm.7710.

Salthouse, T. A. (2010). Selective review of cognitive aging. *Journal of the International Neuropsychological Society, 16*(5), 754–760. https://doi.org/10.1017/s1355617710000706.

Seyffert, M., Lagisetty, P., Landgraf, J., Chopra, V., Pfeiffer, P. N., Conte, M. L., et al. (2016). Internet-delivered cognitive behavioral therapy to treat insomnia: A systematic review and meta-analysis. *PLoS One, 11*(2). https://doi.org/10.1371/journal.pone.0149139.

Skottheim, A., Lövheim, H., Isaksson, U., Sandman, P. O., & Gustafsson, M. (2018). Insomnia symptoms among old people in nursing homes. *International Psychogeriatrics, 30*(1), 77–85. https://doi.org/10.1017/s1041610217001703.

Smith, M. T., & Haythornthwaite, J. A. (2004). How do sleep disturbance and chronic pain inter-relate? Insights from the longitudinal and cognitive-behavioral clinical trials literature. *Sleep Medicine Reviews, 8*(2), 119–132. https://doi.org/10.1016/S1087-0792(03)00044-3.

Smith, M. T., Quartana, P. J., Okonkwo, R. M., & Nasir, A. (2009). Mechanisms by which sleep disturbance contributes to osteoarthritis pain: A conceptual model. *Current Pain and Headache Reports, 13*(6), 447–454. https://doi.org/10.1007/s11916-009-0073-2.

Song, Y., McCurry, S. M., Lee, D., Josephson, K. R., McGowan, S. K., Fung, C. H., et al. (2019). Development of a dyadic sleep intervention for Alzheimer's disease patients and their caregivers. *Disability and Rehabilitation*, 1–11. https://doi.org/10.1080/09638288.2019.1680748.

Steinman, M. A., Landefeld, C. S., Rosenthal, G. E., Berthenthal, D., Sen, S., & Kaboli, P. J. (2006). Polypharmacy and prescribing quality in older people. *Journal of the American Geriatrics Society, 54*(10), 1516–1523. https://doi.org/10.1111/j.1532-5415.2006.00889.x.

Stone, K. L., Blackwell, T. L., Ancoli-Israel, S., Cauley, J. A., Redline, S., Marshall, L. M., et al. (2014). Sleep disturbances and risk of falls in older community-dwelling men: The outcomes of sleep disorders in older men (MrOS sleep) study. *Journal of the American Geriatrics Society, 62*(2), 299–305. https://doi.org/10.1111/jgs.12649.

Veterans Health Administration. (2009). *Adult day health care (Rep. No. HA Handbook 1141.03)*. Washington, DC: Department of Veterans Affairs.

Wastesson, J. W., Morin, L., Tan, E. C. K., & Johnell, K. (2018). An update on the clinical consequences of polypharmacy in older adults: A narrative review. *Expert Opinion on Drug Safety, 17*(12), 1185–1196. https://doi.org/10.1080/14740338.2018.1546841.

Ye, L., & Richards, K. C. (2018). Sleep and long-term care. *Sleep Medicine Clinics, 13*(1), 117–125.

Zachariae, R., Lyby, M. S., Ritterband, L. M., & O'Toole, M. S. (2016). Efficacy of internet-delivered cognitive-behavioral therapy for insomnia—A systematic review and meta-analysis of randomized controlled trials. *Sleep Medicine Reviews, 30*, 1–10. https://doi.org/10.1016/j.smrv.2015.10.004.

Zizi, F., Jean-Louis, G., Magai, C., Greenidge, K. C., Wolintz, A. H., & Heath-Phillip, O. (2002). Sleep complaints and visual impairment among older Americans: A community-based study. *The Journals of Gerontology. Series A, Biological Sciences and Medical Sciences, 57*(10), M691–M694. https://doi.org/10.1093/gerona/57.10.M691.

PART 6

Other special considerations

CHAPTER

18

CBT-I in the short sleep duration phenotype

Julio Fernandez-Mendoza

Sleep Research and Treatment Center, Department of Psychiatry and Behavioral Health, Penn State Health Milton S. Hershey Medical Center, Penn State University College of Medicine, Hershey, PA, United States

What is the ISSD phenotype?

Insomnia is a disorder diagnosed based on symptoms, that is, based on self-reports of experiencing difficulties initiating, maintaining, or resuming sleep and associated daytime fatigue and other functioning impairment. However, not everyone reporting insomnia symptoms, even severe ones, are found to have an equivalent degree of objective sleep disturbance; in fact, two people with insomnia reporting a similar amount of sleep, or lack thereof, may have very different sleep duration upon objective assessment. This multidimensional (i.e., insomnia symptoms vs. total sleep time) and multimethod (i.e., subjective vs. objective) aspect of insomnia is not captured in its current nosology. This chapter focuses on insomnia with objective short sleep duration (ISSD) phenotype, which uses such multidimensional-multimethod approach to understand the pathophysiology, clinical features, and natural course of insomnia and its impact on health and functioning, particularly cardiometabolic and brain health, by relying on and emphasizing the equal importance of both self-reported (i.e., insomnia symptoms) and objectively measured (i.e., sleep duration) dimensions. We will first provide herein a description of the ISSD phenotype in understanding insomnia heterogeneity, discuss its link to physiologic hyperarousal, and summarize its association with cardiometabolic, neurocognitive, and mental health risk.

Adapting Cognitive Behavioral Therapy for Insomnia
https://doi.org/10.1016/B978-0-12-822872-2.00008-6

Pathophysiology and clinical features

Description

Insomnia is a heterogeneous disorder. This can be expressed in its clinical presentation and etiological factors but also in its phenotypes. For example, two individuals with similar demographic characteristics can report the same severity of nighttime insomnia symptoms, e.g., difficulty initiating or maintaining sleep (DIMS) or early morning awakening (EMA), but differ greatly in the amount of actual time they spend asleep, i.e., objective sleep duration. This issue is not new to insomnia research, as studies dating back to the 1970s already tried to understand why there were individuals with "objective" vs. "subjective" insomnia (Edinger & Krystal, 2003). However, most of those early studies aimed to understand the phenomenology of the experience of "subjective" DIMS despite "normal" objective sleep, which led to the operationalization of "sleep state misperception," but not to a better understanding of the pathophysiology, impact, and course of those potential subtypes. Later subtyping (Edinger et al., 1996) and diagnostic studies showed that the offspring of those "objective" vs. "subjective" subtypes, namely, "psychophysiological insomnia" and "paradoxical insomnia," lacked adequate diagnostic reliability and validity (Edinger et al., 2011), which led to our current nosology with one insomnia disorder, chronic or short-term (American Academy of Sleep Medicine, 2014). It was not until recently that Vgontzas and colleagues formally introduced ISSD as a more biologically severe phenotype of the disorder with specific pathophysiology, clinical features, and health outcomes (Vgontzas, Fernandez-Mendoza, Liao, & Bixler, 2013).

Physiologic hyperarousal

In parallel to the early subtyping efforts, several investigators had been focusing on understanding the association of insomnia heterogeneity with one of the purported pathophysiologic mechanisms of the disorder: "physiologic hyperarousal." Building upon seminal studies in the 1960s, accumulating evidence in the 1990s indicated that indices such as increased daytime alertness, autonomic nervous system (ANS), or hypothalamic-pituitary-adrenal (HPA) axis activity were found in individuals with chronic insomnia, and primarily in those with objective sleep disturbances. Bonnet and Arand early on proposed that "the ability to fall asleep may be determined not only by how long we have been awake (the sleep system) but also by the level of physiological arousal (arousal system)"(Bonnet & Arand, 1997a) and that "objectively-measured sleep ability is a combination of sleep drive and level of central nervous system arousal, where arousal has both state and trait components."(Bonnet & Arand, 2000). At around the same time, Vgontzas and colleagues first proposed that "in chronic insomnia, the activity of both limbs of the stress system (i.e., the HPA axis and the sympathetic system) appears to be directly proportional to the degree of sleep disturbance as objectively measured in the sleep laboratory … and (2) polysomnographic measurements can provide a reliable index of the biological significance and severity of chronic insomnia."(Vgontzas, Bixler, Lin, et al., 2001; Vgontzas, Tsigos, Bixler, et al., 1998) The pathophysiologic mechanism of the ISSD phenotype was, thus, proposed to be physiologic hyperarousal, which reflects a 24-h activation of both limbs of the stress system incompatible with physiologic sleep ability (Vgontzas et al., 2013).

As shown in Fig. 1, 22 studies have found greater indices of physiologic hyperarousal in the ISSD phenotype, such as increased daytime latencies on the multiple sleep latency test (MSLT), impaired cardiac autonomic modulation (CAM), higher noradrenergic output, increased whole-body metabolic rate, hyperactivity of the HPA axis and higher immune system biomarkers (Bonnet & Arand, 1995; Bonnet & Arand, 1997b; Bonnet & Arand, 1998a; Bonnet & Arand, 2000; Castro-Diehl et al., 2015; Castro-Diehl, Diez Roux, Redline, et al., 2016; D'Aurea et al., 2015; Dorsey & Bootzin, 1997; Fernandez-Mendoza et al., 2017; Fernandez-Mendoza, Vgontzas, Calhoun, et al., 2014; Floam et al., 2015; Huang, Goparaju, Chen, & Bianchi, 2018; Jarrin et al., 2018; Li, Vgontzas, Fernandez-Mendoza, et al., 2015; Miller, Bartlett, Mullins, et al., 2016; Mohammadi et al., 2018; Rodenbeck, Huether, Ruther, & Hajak, 2002; Roehrs, Randall, Harris, Maan, & Roth, 2011; Spiegelhalder, Fuchs, Ladwig, et al., 2011; Stepanski, Zorick, Roehrs, Young, & Roth, 1988; Sugerman, Stern, & Walsh, 1985; Tempaku, Hirotsu, Mazzotti, et al., 2018; Vgontzas et al., 1998; Vgontzas et al., 2001; Vgontzas, Zoumakis, Papanicolaou, et al., 2002). A total of 15 of these studies have found that these physiologic indices are not elevated in the insomnia with normal sleep duration (INSD) phenotype (Bonnet & Arand, 1997b; Castro-Diehl et al., 2015; Castro-Diehl et al., 2016; Dorsey & Bootzin, 1997; Fernandez-Mendoza et al., 2014; Fernandez-Mendoza et al., 2017; Li et al., 2015; Miller et al., 2016; Riemann et al., 2002; Roehrs et al., 2011; Spiegelhalder et al., 2011; Sugerman et al., 1985; Tempaku et al., 2018; Vgontzas et al., 2001). Only one study has reported opposite associations between these insomnia phenotypes and the HPA axis; however, it was methodologically flawed by including adolescents (14–62y) and 42% males in those with insomnia compared to good sleeping adults (26–59y) who were 81% males (Mohammadi et al., 2018). In addition, 11 studies have shown that the INSD phenotype does share with the ISSD phenotype the presence of elevated high-frequency cortical activity, and other EEG-measured disruptions, suggesting that such cortical activity

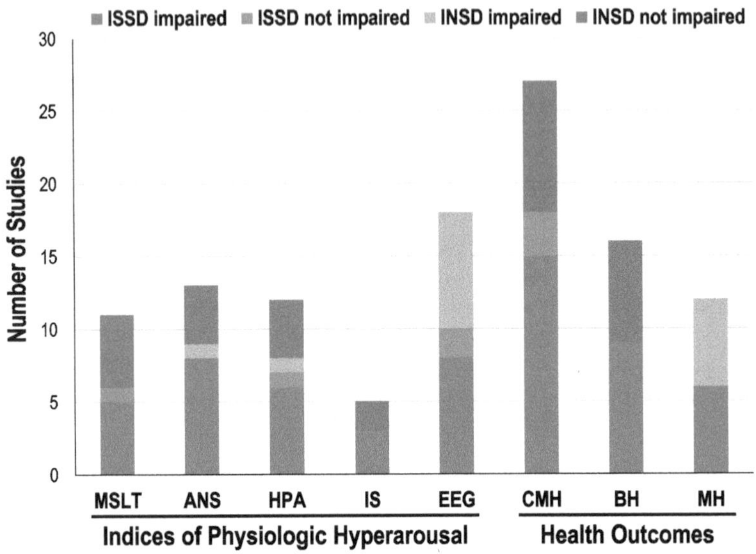

FIG. 1 Summary of the number of positive (impaired) and negative (not impaired) studies on the association of insomnia phenotypes based on objective sleep measures with physiologic hyperarousal and adverse health outcomes. Data are the number of studies that contributed to each finding, not the number of total studies. ANS = autonomic nervous system (including heart rate variability, metabolic rate, norepinephrine levels). BH = brain health (including cognitive performance deficits, cognitive impairment, and neurotransmitter metabolites). CMH = cardiometabolic health (including hypertension, type 2 diabetes, cardiovascular diseases or mortality). EEG = cortical activity of the central nervous system (including spectral electroencephalography activity and evoked-response potential during wake and sleep). HPA = hypothalamic-pituitary-adrenal axis (including cortisol and adrenocorticotropic hormone levels). IS = immune system (including interleukins, tumor necrosis factor-alpha, and c-reactive protein levels). MH = mental health (including prevalent and incident depression, internalizing and externalizing behaviors/traits, dysfunctional beliefs, and coping). MSLT = multiple sleep latency test.

is a marker of cognitive arousal and enhanced information processing during sleep (Bastien, Turcotte, St-Jean, Morin, & Carrier, 2013; Chouvarda, Grassi, Mendez, et al., 2013; Fernandez-Mendoza, Li, Vgontzas, et al., 2016; Krystal, Edinger, Wohlgemuth, & Marsh, 2002; Normand, St-Hilaire, & Bastien, 2016; Parrino, Milioli, De Paolis, Grassi, & Terzano, 2009; Pérusse et al., 2015; Spiegelhalder, Regen, Feige, et al., 2012; St-Jean, Turcotte, & Bastien, 2012; St-Jean, Turcotte, Pérusse, & Bastien, 2013; Turcotte, St-Jean, & Bastien, 2011), which does not necessarily occur in association with other indices of physiologic hyperarousal.

From a clinical impact standpoint, the observed physiologic hyperarousal in the ISSD phenotype, i.e., blunted heart rate variability (CAM), increased catecholamine secretion (ANS), and higher cortisol levels (HPA axis), was proposed as a mechanism linking this phenotype to increased adverse health outcomes and, in particular, cardiovascular and metabolic ones (Vgontzas et al., 1998; Vgontzas et al., 2013).

Clinical characteristics

The ISSD phenotype has not only been characterized as a disorder of physiologic hyperarousal but also by its clinical profile, its persistent, unremitting course and its link with significant morbidity (Vgontzas et al., 2013). Despite the initial studies relying on 4 consecutive nights of 8-h, in-lab PSG (Vgontzas et al., 2001), the first comprehensive description of the ISSD phenotype, as reviewed in the adverse health outcomes section below, was based on several studies in the Penn State Adult Cohort (PSAC) that used one night of 8-h, in-lab PSG to define the presence of objective short sleep duration as a sleep efficiency <75%, equivalent to <6h of sleep (Vgontzas et al., 2013). This threshold of <6h of objective sleep was adopted by other investigators when operationalizing the ISSD phenotype in adults. Although PSG is the gold standard objective measure of sleep, it is expensive, impractical, and most typically restricted to a single night; thus, other recent studies have used actigraphy (ACT) to assess sleep duration over multiple nights in the individual's habitual sleep environment. One study has shown poor concordance between short sleep assessed with a single night of PSG and ACT-assessed habitual short sleep when the same threshold (< 6h) was used in both objective measures (Erwin, Buysse, Hall, Germain, & Kline, 2017). Another study examined the short-term and long-term stability of short sleep assessed by the median in a single night of PSG and showed that those who spent 3 consecutive nights in the lab or who were assessed on two occasions separated by at least 2 years had a >70% concordance in their median short sleep classification from the first night of PSG (Gaines, Vgontzas, Fernandez-Mendoza, et al., 2015). Finally, given the strong association between PSG short sleep duration and increased daytime latencies on the MSLT mentioned above, researchers have used the MSLT, as an index of physiologic hyperarousal, to phenotype insomnia and have shown highly consistent findings with the ISSD phenotype (Bonnet & Arand, 1995; Bonnet & Arand, 1997b; Bonnet & Arand, 2000; Dorsey & Bootzin, 1997; Li et al., 2015; Roehrs et al., 2011; Stepanski et al., 1988; Sugerman et al., 1985). Although the MSLT may be a highly informative tool, it is unlikely that it will make it to clinical scenarios for insomnia phenotyping, given its high costs and need for PSG on a preceding night. Together, these studies suggest that PSG-assessed short sleep may provide a unique physiologic characterization of the ISSD phenotype and that ACT may require its specific threshold to identify short sleep given its ad libitum, ambulatory measurement, and tendency to overestimate total sleep time (Danzig, Wang, Shah, & Trotti, 2020; Withrow, Roth, Koshorek, & Roehrs, 2019).

As it pertains to subjective measures of sleep duration, evidence suggests that they do not reliably capture the degree of physiologic sleep ability, as assessed by PSG, that distinguishes the INSD and ISSD phenotypes. Fernandez-Mendoza and colleagues (Fernandez-Mendoza, Calhoun,

Bixler, et al., 2011) showed that those with the ISSD phenotype, who slept on average 4.7 h in the lab, reported habitually sleeping 6.0 h on average, and 38% of them for <6 h. Similarly, those with the INSD phenotype, who slept on average 6.6 h in the lab, also reported habitually sleeping 5.7 h on average, and 48% of them for <6 h (Fernandez-Mendoza et al., 2011). In fact, about 55% of those with the INSD phenotype showed "sleep misperception," defined as an underestimation of their PSG sleep duration by −1.0 h or more, while only 10% of those with the ISSD phenotype did (Fernandez-Mendoza et al., 2011). Interestingly, when relying on next-morning self-reports upon awakening from the PSG study (i.e., perceived sleep duration), those with the INSD phenotype continued to underestimate their sleep duration (i.e., a discrepancy of about −1.0 h) and 42% of them had "sleep misperception" as defined above, while those with the ISSD phenotype showed higher accuracy (i.e., discrepancy of +0.3 h) with only 15% of them having "sleep misperception."(Fernandez-Mendoza et al., 2011) These findings were consistent with previous data reported by Krystal and Edinger (Krystal et al., 2002) and more recent data reported by Jarrin, Ivers, et al. (2018) among others. These findings are important because they indicate that (1) "sleep misperception", understood as the underestimation of total sleep time, is a clinical feature of those with INSD, a phenotype that includes a much larger number of insomnia cases (50%) that were previously termed "subjective," "sleep state misperception," or "paradoxical" insomnia and regarded to represent only 5% of those with insomnia, (2) habitual and perceived self-reports of sleep duration can diverge between each other but may reflect trait-like features of "sleep misperception" in those with the INSD phenotype, and (3) adults with the INSD vs. ISSD phenotypes report a similar amount of subjective (habitual or perceived) sleep duration, which does not accurately discriminate between the two phenotypes.

Studies also suggest that subjective measures of insomnia symptoms do not capture the same phenotyping of insomnia as PSG sleep duration. No study so far has identified a specific clustering of DIMS, EMA, or reported daytime symptoms that can reliably aid in differentiating the INSD and ISSD phenotypes. Nevertheless, population-based data (Fernandez-Mendoza, 2010) has shown that, while subjects with the INSD and ISSD phenotypes do not differ in the frequency, severity, or duration of their reported DIMS or EMA, those with the INSD phenotype are significantly more likely (85.5%) to report nonrestorative sleep (NRS) and feeling too exhausted or irritable to manage during the day because of their sleep disturbance (60.0%), than those with the ISSD phenotype (50.8% and 28.6%, respectively) (Fernandez-Mendoza, 2010). These are interesting findings when one considers that NRS has been dropped as an essential symptom in the diagnosis of chronic insomnia and that the ISSD phenotype has, in fact, a greater degree of sleep disturbance and performance deficits than the INSD phenotype. Although these clinical features may be suggestive of potential phenotype membership, given their widespread presentation across multiple sleep disorders, they are unlikely to reliably differentiate the two phenotypes as objective measures of sleep do.

As mentioned above, efforts to differentiate insomnia subtypes based on their phenomenology or cognitive-emotional features date back decades ago (Dorsey & Bootzin, 1997; Edinger et al., 1996; Edinger, Fins, Glenn, et al., 2000; Edinger & Krystal, 2003). One of the most influential and methodologically sound studies was "The Eye of the Beholder," in which Edinger and colleagues used 6 consecutive nights of PSG, 3 in-lab and 3 at-home, to subtype individuals with chronic insomnia using a ≥6.5 h threshold to define normal sleep duration, a < 6-h threshold to define short sleep duration, while the remaining individuals sleeping objectively 6.0–6.4 h were reclassified based on age-specific (younger and older than 60 years old) PSG sleep efficiency thresholds (Edinger et al., 2000). These "subjective" and "objective" subtypes were clearly equivalent to what we currently term INSD and ISSD phenotypes, respectively. The study showed that the INSD phenotype had higher mean scores across all but one of the cognitive-emotional scales, indicating that they were more likely to report higher anxiety, lower mood, and more dysfunctional sleep-related beliefs than do those with the ISSD phenotype (Edinger et al., 2000). A series of later studies showed similar findings by relying on very different cognitive-emotional scales, indicating that the INSD phenotype has a profile characterized by elevated anxiety, rumination, depressed mood, introversion and poor coping skills in adults (Fernandez-Mendoza et al., 2011), and externalizing behaviors in children and adolescents (Calhoun et al., 2017; Fernandez-Mendoza, Calhoun, Vgontzas, et al., 2016), while the ISSD phenotype has a profile characterized by somatic concerns, depressed mood and poor health status in adults (Fernandez-Mendoza et al., 2011), and internalizing symptoms in youth (Calhoun et al., 2017; Fernandez-Mendoza, Calhoun, et al., 2016).

Finally, an important clinical feature examined in longitudinal studies has been that of the natural course of insomnia and its phenotypes. Consistent evidence across different population-based studies has shown that individuals reporting poor sleep (e.g., those with insomnia symptoms who do not meet syndrome criteria) experience a full remission rate of about 40%–44%(Fernandez-Mendoza et al., 2012; Morin et al., 2009) and that 14%–17% of them develop chronic insomnia after 3.0–7.5 years of follow-up (Fernandez-Mendoza, Vgontzas, Bixler, et al., 2012; Morin et al., 2009). In contrast, individuals reporting chronic insomnia (e.g., those who meet insomnia syndrome criteria) experience a full remission rate as low as 24%–26% (Morin et al., 2009; Vgontzas et al., 2012) and about 30%–35% partially remit into poor sleep after the same length of follow-up (Morin et al., 2009; Vgontzas et al., 2012). Only three studies to date have provided evidence that the ISSD phenotype has a more persistent, unremitting natural course. Fernandez-Mendoza (Fernandez-Mendoza, Vgontzas, Bixler, et al., 2012) and Vgontzas (Vgontzas et al., 2012) and colleagues showed that adults with poor sleep and shorter PSG sleep duration were 2-times more likely to develop chronic insomnia than poor sleepers with longer sleep duration, and that, once the chronic disorder is developed, the ISSD phenotype is 4.5-times more likely to persist and not fully remit than the INSD phenotype. Commensurate with this persistent natural course observed in a population-based sample, Johann and colleagues showed that adults with the ISSD phenotype reported a longer disorder duration (~13 years) than those with the INSD phenotype (~11 years) in a clinical sample (Johann, Hertenstein, Kyle, et al., 2017).

In summary, the ISSD phenotype has been examined using different approaches, including PSG and ACT, in which a threshold of <6 h has been most consistently used in adults. The ISSD phenotype is more likely to present with a depressive-somatic profile and to have a persistent, unremitting course, while the INSD phenotype is more likely to present with "sleep misperception" and an anxious-ruminative, poor coping skills profile but to have a better long-term prognosis in terms of its likelihood of full remission. Studies have also shown that subjective reports of sleep duration show less precision and incur misclassification when identifying the ISSD phenotype, an issue of particular importance when predicting health risks (Fernandez-Mendoza, 2017).

Adverse health outcomes

Cardiometabolic health

As summarized in Fig. 1, the ISSD phenotype has been associated with adverse cardiometabolic health (CMH) outcomes. One of the first (Vgontzas, Liao, Bixler, Chrousos, & Vela-Bueno, 2009), and most consistent (Bathgate & Fernandez-Mendoza, 2018; Bonnet, Burton, & Arand, 2014; Fernandez-Mendoza, 2017; Hall, Fernandez-Mendoza, Kline, & Vgontzas, 2016; Jarrin et al., 2018), findings is an increased risk of hypertension in the ISSD phenotype, which is supported by 7 studies using PSG- or ACT-assessed sleep duration (Bathgate, Edinger, Wyatt, & Krystal, 2016; Fernandez-Mendoza, Vgontzas, Liao, et al., 2012; Hein, Lanquart, Loas, Hubain, & Linkowski, 2019a; Hein, Lanquart, Loas, Hubain, & Linkowski, 2019b; Huang et al., 2018; Li et al., 2015; Vgontzas, Liao, Bixler, et al., 2009). Vgontzas, Liao, Bixler, et al. (2009) seminal study in the PSAC showed that the ISSD phenotype was associated with a 4-fold increased odds of prevalent hypertension and that this risk showed a dose-response as a function of adults with chronic insomnia sleeping objectively 5–6 h (OR = 3.53) or ≤ 5 h (OR = 5.12); in contrast, the INSD phenotype was not significantly associated with prevalent hypertension (OR = 1.31) when compared to good sleepers. In addition, longitudinal analyses of the PSAC showed that the ISSD phenotype, but not the INSD phenotype (OR = 0.85), was associated with a 3.8-fold increased odds of developing hypertension after 7.5 years of follow-up (Fernandez-Mendoza, Vgontzas, Liao, et al., 2012). These initial findings were replicated in 5 subsequent cross-sectional studies of clinical samples (Bathgate et al., 2016; Hein et al., 2019a; Hein et al., 2019b; Huang et al., 2018; Li et al., 2015), with Bathgate and colleagues showing that the ISSD phenotype had a 3.6-fold increased odds of prevalent hypertension when compared to the INSD phenotype (Bathgate et al., 2016). Only one cross-sectional study using PSG-assessed sleep duration in a clinical sample has not replicated these findings, despite the ISSD phenotype having a 1.8-fold greater prevalence of hypertension (43.5%) than the INSD phenotype (28.5%) in their sample (Johann et al., 2017).

A total of 4 studies have linked the ISSD phenotype to metabolic dysfunction, including increased odds of prevalent type 2 diabetes (OR = 1.81–2.95) (Hein, Lanquart, Loas, Hubain, & Linkowski, 2018; Vgontzas et al., 2009), increased insulin sensitivity (Vasisht, Kessler, Booth III, Imperial, & Penev, 2013), and increased fasting blood glucose levels (D'Aurea et al., 2015). Again, Johann and colleagues could not replicate this finding, despite the ISSD phenotype having a 2.3-fold greater prevalence of type 2 diabetes (7.7%) than the INSD phenotype (2.7%) in their sample (Johann et al., 2017).

Another 3 studies have shown that the ISSD phenotype has an increased risk of cardiovascular disease (CVD), including ultrasound-measured atherosclerosis (Bertisch, Pollock, Mittleman, et al., 2018; Fernandez-Mendoza, He, Liao, Vgontzas, & Bixler, 2018; Nakazaki et al., 2012). In the only longitudinal study to date, Bertisch and colleagues conducted analyses of the Sleep Heart Health Study (SHHS) and showed that the ISSD phenotype, but not the INSD phenotype (OR = 0.99), was associated with a 1.3-fold increased risk of developing CVD after 11.4 years of follow-up (Bertisch et al., 2018). Finally, 3 studies have examined whether the ISSD phenotype is associated with accelerated cellular aging (Tempaku et al., 2018) or increased risk of mortality (Bertisch et al., 2018; Vgontzas, Liao, Pejovic, et al., 2010). While two studies showed that the ISSD phenotype was more likely to have short leukocyte telomere length (Tempaku et al., 2018) or increased odds of all-cause mortality if they were men and had hypertension and/or type 2 diabetes at baseline (Vgontzas et al., 2010), the SHHS could not replicate the increased risk of all-cause mortality (Bertisch et al., 2018).

In summary, most existing studies support that the ISSD phenotype is associated with increased CMH risk, while the INSD phenotype is not. The increased risk of mortality remains inconclusive and deserves further investigation. Of note, the studies reviewed herein had a strong operationalization of insomnia (e.g., chronic disorder) and objective sleep assessment (e.g., PSG, ACT, or MSLT) and did not rely on subjective measures of sleep duration. In fact, 3 studies, including the SHHS, have shown that habitual or sleep diary-assessed sleep duration <6h is not optimal to define the ISSD phenotype and predict CMH risk compared to PSG or ACT-assessed sleep (Bathgate et al., 2016; Bertisch et al., 2018; Jarrin, Ivers, et al., 2018), consistent with previous findings on "sleep misperception" in the INSD phenotype and its high likelihood of reporting <6h of sleep leading to misclassification (Fernandez-Mendoza et al., 2011).

Brain health

Research has also indicated that the ISSD phenotype is associated with adverse brain health (BH) outcomes, including neurocognitive deficits, mild cognitive impairment (MCI), and brain-based biomarkers. As summarized in Fig. 1, a total of 10 studies have reported the presence of cognitive deficits in processing speed, sustained attention, set-switching attention, or working memory in otherwise noncognitively impaired individuals as well as an increased likelihood of prevalent MCI in adults with the ISSD phenotype, but not in those with the INSD phenotype (Biddle et al., 2017; Bonnet & Arand, 1995; Bonnet & Arand, 1997b; Edinger, Means, & Krystal, 2013; Fan, Chen, Shi, et al., 2019; Fernandez-Mendoza et al., 2020; Fernandez-Mendoza, Calhoun, Bixler, et al., 2010; Khassawneh, Bathgate, Tsai, & Edinger, 2018; Miller et al., 2016; Miller, Rae, Green, et al., 2017). Two studies have also shown that shorter PSG-measured sleep duration is associated with lower GABA levels in the anterior cingulate cortex (Spiegelhalder, Regen, Nissen, et al., 2016) and that lower PSG-measured sleep efficiency is associated with greater waking connectivity between the retrosplenial cortex/hippocampus and various nodes of the default mode network in individuals with chronic insomnia (Regen, Kyle, Nissen, et al., 2016). In addition, two recent studies have suggested that the ISSD phenotype is associated with decreased brain-metabolite concentrations (Miller et al., 2017) and brain-derived neurotrophic factor (BDNF) (Fan et al., 2019).

Together, these data are consistent with the proposal that the ISSD phenotype, but not the INSD phenotype, is associated with altered neurocognitive functioning and an increased risk of major neurocognitive disorders (Fernandez-Mendoza, 2017; Vgontzas et al., 2013). Comparatively, however, fewer studies have been performed using BH outcomes as CMH outcomes, and all have been cross-sectional, which highlights the need for longitudinal studies following up individuals with insomnia for cognitive decline using objective measures of sleep and cognition.

Mental health

Poor sleep (i.e., insomnia symptoms) and chronic insomnia (i.e., insomnia disorder) are well-established predictors of adverse mental health (MH) outcomes, including depression, anxiety, and other forms of psychopathology (Hertenstein, Feige, Gmeiner, et al., 2019). Based on such strong previous evidence, the initial characterization of the INSD and ISSD phenotypes hypothesized that both would demonstrate an increased risk for psychopathology (Vgontzas et al., 2013). The sleep EEG cortical arousal observed in both phenotypes (Fig. 1) (Bastien et al., 2013; Chouvarda et al., 2013; Fernandez-Mendoza, Li, et al., 2016; Krystal et al., 2002; Normand et al., 2016; Parrino et al., 2009; Pérusse et al., 2015; Spiegelhalder et al., 2012; St-Jean et al., 2012; St-Jean et al., 2013; Turcotte et al., 2011) was presumed to be one of the shared mechanisms linking both phenotypes to increased MH morbidity (Vgontzas et al., 2013). However, the HPA axis and ANS hyperactivity were also hypothesized to predispose the ISSD phenotype to psychopathology, while the cognitive-emotional factors reviewed above (e.g., coping resources) would predispose the INSD phenotype (Vgontzas et al., 2013). A total of 8 studies have shown that the INSD and ISSD phenotypes are associated with subclinical forms of emotional disturbances as well as prevalent and incident psychopathology (Fig. 1), albeit with specific cognitive-emotional profiles and different underlying mechanisms (Bonnet & Arand, 1995; Bonnet & Arand, 1997b; Calhoun et al., 2017; Dorsey & Bootzin, 1997; Edinger et al., 2000; Fernandez-Mendoza et al., 2011; Fernandez-Mendoza et al., 2015; Fernandez-Mendoza, Calhoun, et al., 2016). As mentioned in the clinical characteristics section above, the ISSD phenotype has been shown to present with a cognitive-emotional profile in adults (Bonnet & Arand, 1997b; Dorsey & Bootzin, 1997; Edinger et al., 2000; Fernandez-Mendoza et al., 2011) and youth (Calhoun et al., 2017; Fernandez-Mendoza, Calhoun, et al., 2016) different than that found in the INSD phenotype, which is characterized by greater anxiety, rumination, maladaptive sleep-related beliefs and poor coping resources in adults (Bonnet & Arand, 1997b; Dorsey & Bootzin, 1997; Edinger et al., 2000; Fernandez-Mendoza et al., 2011), and externalizing behaviors in youth (Calhoun et al., 2017; Fernandez-Mendoza, Calhoun, et al., 2016). Furthermore, in longitudinal analyses of the PSAC, Fernandez-Mendoza and colleagues (Fernandez-Mendoza et al., 2015) showed that the odds of developing depression after 7.5 years of follow-up were significantly increased in both the ISSD phenotype (OR=2.81) and the INSD phenotype (OR=1.80); however, after adjusting for poor coping resources, the risk associated with the INSD phenotype became nonsignificant (OR=1.00), while that associated with the ISSD phenotype remained significantly elevated (OR=2.20). These data suggest that the association of these two insomnia phenotypes with psychopathology is rather strong but potentially determined by specific mechanisms (Fernandez-Mendoza, 2017), which could be the target of different treatment approaches.

Similar to the lack of studies on adverse BH outcomes, there is still a need for longitudinal studies that can help us better understand the mechanisms underlying the association of the INSD and ISSD phenotypes with adverse MH outcomes by including objective sleep testing, behavioral measures, and biomarkers. Furthermore, it does not appear that trait or state measures of cognitive-emotional outcomes can help us reliably differentiated these insomnia phenotypes without the use of objective sleep measures. An updated version of the heuristic phenotyping model reviewed throughout the previous sections is presented in Fig. 2.

Clinical assessment of the ISSD phenotype

This section summarizes any modifications needed in the clinical assessment of chronic insomnia for phenotyping purposes. It also proposes tentative approaches that address the issues reviewed above in the clinical characteristics section.

Diagnostic interview

First things, first. Insomnia is always diagnosed based on the clinical history and reports by the patient: ALWAYS. The diagnostic clinical interview, preferably structured, is an essential tool in establishing a diagnosis of insomnia disorder, which will be based on (1) essential features (i.e., DIMS or EMA despite adequate opportunity for sleep), (2) frequency (i.e., at least 3 nights per week), (3) duration (i.e., at least 3 months to establish chronicity), and (4) daytime impact (i.e., fatigue, mood, occupational) (American Academy of Sleep Medicine, 2014). The patient has to fulfill diagnostic criteria for insomnia disorder based upon clinical history because all phenotypes of insomnia, not matter whether they are or not linked to physiologic hyperarousal or CMH or BH risk, are equally important. This should resolve any doubts if the reader has gotten the impression so far that the ISSD phenotype is "more important," "clinically relevant," or "objective" than the INSD phenotype. This should also resolve any doubts for those readers who have been thinking all along

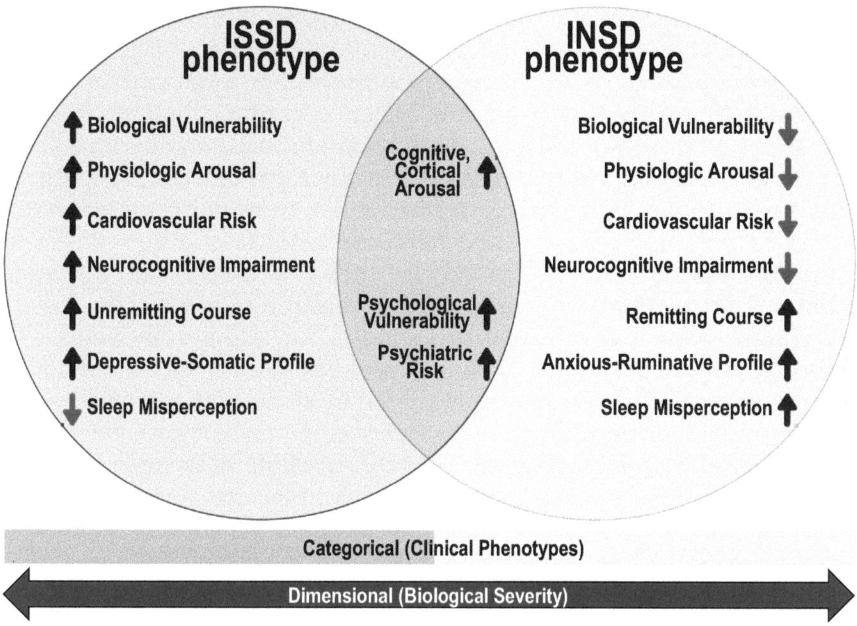

FIG. 2 An updated heuristic model of insomnia phenotypes based on objective sleep duration. Insomnia with short sleep duration (ISSD) phenotype is associated with physiologic hyperarousal, as index by a dysregulated hypothalamic-pituitary-adrenal axis (e.g., cortisol levels), autonomic nervous system (e.g., norepinephrine levels, metabolic rate), and cardiac autonomic modulation (e.g., blunted heart rate variability), with increased cardiometabolic risk (e.g., hypertension, diabetes, heart disease) and neurocognitive impairment (e.g., executive deficits), and its etiology is purported to carry greater biological vulnerability (e.g., genetics, stress reactivity). Individuals with the ISSD phenotype have also been shown to have a persistent, unremitting natural course, to present with a profile characterized by somatic complaints and depressed mood, and to accurately estimate, if not overestimate, their sleep duration (i.e., less sleep misperception). In contrast, insomnia with normal sleep duration (INSD) phenotype is not associated with physiologic hyperarousal, cardiometabolic risk, or neurocognitive impairment. Individuals with the INSD phenotype have been shown to have higher remission rates in their natural course, to present with a profile characterized by anxious-ruminative traits, greater dysfunctional sleep-related beliefs, and poor coping resources, and to underestimate their sleep duration (i.e., sleep misperception). Both phenotypes have been shown to present with cognitive and cortical arousal, as indexed by EEG measures of increased information processing during the presleep period and while asleep, greater psychological vulnerability (i.e., emotional reactivity), and increased psychiatric risk, albeit through different psychobiological mechanisms (e.g., poor coping resources in the INSD phenotype). It is hypothesized that these two insomnia phenotypes may require different treatment approaches.

with this chapter, when referring to the ISSD phenotype, about "short sleepers" (a normal variant) or "insufficient sleep syndrome" (a central disorder of hypersomnolence) (American Academy of Sleep Medicine, 2014). In clinical scenarios, the former individuals are unlikely to present for care, precisely because "short sleepers" are, by definition, asymptomatic of either nighttime sleep disturbance or daytime sleepiness. Diagnosing an individual who does not present with DIMS or EMA with insomnia disorder because they have specific beliefs regarding their short sleep should never occur. Normal sleepers who are induced an objective sleep that mimics chronic insomnia, respond with a pattern characteristic of mild partial sleep deprivation (e.g., decreased tension, decreased vigor, decreased body temperature, and decreased MSLT) and not consistent with the clinical features found in those with chronic insomnia (Bonnet & Arand, 1996). "Insufficient sleep syndrome" has specific criteria that usually impedes an insomnia diagnosis, including daily periods of irrepressible need to sleep or daytime lapses into sleep, which are unlikely in most individuals with insomnia disorder, along with curtailed sleep because of sleep opportunity (e.g., alarm clock or being awakened by someone else), rather than DIMS or EMA; in addition, these individuals may sleep longer on weekends, days off or vacation, and such sleep extension is associated with resolution of daytime sleepiness (American Academy of Sleep Medicine, 2014). In summary, when the purpose is to identify the ISSD phenotype, an insomnia disorder diagnosis comes first and objective sleep measures second.

The evidence so far has not identified any clinical history data upon diagnostic interviewing that can reliably aid in differentiating the INSD and ISSD phenotypes. Despite some potential differences in associated features (e.g., NRS) (Fernandez-Mendoza, 2010) or reported duration of the disorder (Johann et al., 2017), these self-reports have not demonstrated enough reliability to distinguish the INSD and ISSD phenotypes. Fernandez-Mendoza and colleagues observed that a discriminant function of cognitive-emotional and subjective sleep measures showed that the strongest factor potentially discriminating the INSD and ISSD phenotypes was the degree of discrepancy between subjective and objective sleep duration, but not subjective (habitual or perceived) sleep duration alone; (Fernandez-Mendoza et al., 2011) in other words, "sleep misperception," a clinical feature of the INSD phenotype that requires objective sleep measures.

Another issue that remains unaddressed is whether there are specific demographic or social groups more likely to differentially experience the ISSD vs. INSD phenotypes. These data are important as they will help identify at-risk populations and develop targeted screening and preventative interventions at the population level. These social determinants of health should be thoroughly examined in large racially, socially and economically diverse samples in the near future, given that they may, or may not, be different from those observed so far for insomnia symptoms or subjective short sleep duration.

Patient-reported outcomes

Patient-reported outcomes are also essential in the routine evaluation of insomnia disorder, regardless of its phenotyping. This includes global insomnia measures able to provide cut-off scores for "caseness," subjective severity ranking, and sensitivity to treatment, such as the insomnia severity index (ISI), the consensus sleep diary as well as measures of behavioral, cognitive, and emotional perpetuating factors. As mentioned above, despite some differences in cognitive-emotional outcomes (Edinger et al., 2000; Fernandez-Mendoza et al., 2011) these patient reports, including sleep diary data (Bathgate et al., 2016; Bertisch et al., 2018; Jarrin, Ivers, et al., 2018), have not demonstrated to reliably distinguish the INSD vs. ISSD phenotypes in the absence of objective sleep testing.

Objective sleep measures

It may seem unnecessary to summarize herein the role of objective sleep measures when phenotyping INSD vs. ISSD at this point; however, a couple of concepts and theoretical issues may help practitioners for their clinical endeavors in the future. As shown in Table 1, PSG is currently not indicated for the routine assessment of insomnia disorder, unless there is a clinical suspicion of another sleep disorder for which it is indicated (e.g., sleep apnea); thus, its use would require nosology and practice guidelines changes indicating its need to assess the biological severity of insomnia and aid in its subtyping. If the practitioner has the ability to conduct in-lab or at-home PSG to estimate objective sleep duration and efficiency, it is recommended that in-lab PSG is conducted with a fixed-time recording (time in bed) of 8h; this allows the single-night PSG, as a measure of physiologic sleep ability, to conform with standard practices across labs and total sleep time and sleep efficiency estimates to be compared not only between labs but also between patients. Based on the previous extant evidence reviewed above, it is recommended to use a threshold of <6h in adults to identify the ISSD phenotype. Unfortunately, clinical sleep centers do not have the economic resources and insurance coverage to conduct at least two consecutive nights of in-lab PSG, which would be more optimal. If PSG studies are conducted at home with ad libitum time in bed, sleep efficiency thresholds may be used to account for individual differences in time in bed (e.g., <85%); however, there is no solid evidence to recommend this change over total sleep time < 6h yet.

In contrast to PSG, current practice guidelines do suggest (conditional recommendation) the use of ACT to estimate sleep parameters in

TABLE 1 Adaptations of clinical assessment for insomnia phenotyping.

Measure	Standard practice	Potential modifications/ adaptations
Polysomnography	Not indicated for the routine assessment of insomnia disorder, unless there is a suspicion of another sleep disorder for which it is indicated (e.g., sleep apnea)	– Indicated to assess the biological severity of insomnia and subtype (proposed modification) – Order in-lab or at-home polysomnography to estimate objective sleep duration and efficiency – If in-lab, request a fixed-time recording (time in bed), typically 8h in adults – Use a threshold of <6h to define ISSD in adults
Actigraphy	Suggested (conditional) to estimate sleep parameters in insomnia disorder, to estimate total sleep time in those with insufficient sleep syndrome or the assessment of circadian rhythm sleep-wake disorders, among others	– Indicated also to assess the biological severity of insomnia and subtype (proposed modification) – Order at-home actigraphy study to estimate objective sleep duration and efficiency – If using total sleep time, set a threshold of <6.5 or 7h to define ISSD in adults (needs validation) – If using sleep efficiency, set a threshold of <80% or 85% sleep efficiency in adults (needs validation)
Sleep diaries	Establish baseline sleep patterns	– As per standard practice – Concurrent with either polysomnography or actigraphy – Calculate the degree of sleep discrepancy based on concurrent and/or habitual (average) total sleep time either as an absolute difference (i.e., subjective – objective) or as a ratio [i.e., (subjective – objective/ objective) × 100] – Define "sleep misperception" as an absolute difference of −1h or greater or a ratio of −15% or greater

insomnia disorder, to estimate total sleep time in those with suspected sleep-disordered breathing or insufficient sleep syndrome, and in the assessment of circadian rhythm sleep-wake disorders, among other clinical uses (Smith et al., 2018). Thus, ACT is better positioned, from a practice guideline standpoint, to change nosology and introduce its use for insomnia phenotyping (Table 1). Moreover, more practitioners have access to ACT than PSG and, based on the previous evidence reviewed above, it appears that it may be useful in identifying the ISSD phenotype. While most practitioners may want to use the same threshold as for PSG to define the ISSD phenotype (i.e., < 6h in adults), ACT is known to significantly overestimate total sleep time; (Danzig et al., 2020; Withrow et al., 2019) thus, it is likely that a threshold of <6.5 or 7h in adults may be needed to reliably identify the ISSD phenotype. Alternatively, sleep efficiency thresholds may be used to account for individual and night-to-night differences in time in bed (e.g., <80% or 85%). This is an unresolved issue in the field that is similar to the measurement differences faced when estimating blood pressure levels from office (clinic) and out-of-office (home or ambulatory) monitoring, each of which has different recommended cut-offs to confirm office-based hypertension. In summary, this as an area of validation that is greatly needed, as it appears that ACT has a true potential to replace the expensive, inconvenient PSG for phenotyping insomnia based on objective sleep measures.

Finally, the question also remains open whether commercially available wearables (sleep trackers), mostly based on ACT, will become an objective sleep tool that can help practitioners to identify the ISSD phenotype. Given that physiologic hyperarousal is a pathophysiologic mechanism of the ISSD phenotype, it is likely that reliable, valid, and accurate wearables that include ACT and physiologic signals (e.g., HRV) to estimate arousal, sleep, and wake time will produce the best results for insomnia phenotyping. However, this has to be tested and wearables cannot be recommended for insomnia phenotyping yet.

Treatment of the ISSD phenotype

This section presents the approach to the ISSD phenotype initially proposed when it was first introduced. It also discusses the preliminary evidence on the response of the INSD and ISSD phenotypes to CBT-I in secondary analyses of existing randomized clinical trials (RCT). Thereafter, it discusses potential modifications or adaptations to CBT-I that need to be tested in the ISSD phenotype, including its combination or sequencing with sleep medication. This section should not be taken as recommendations ready to be implemented in routine clinical practice, rather as a guide that can foster new approaches in future clinical interventions.

Proposed approach

As extensively mentioned in this manual, cognitive-behavioral therapy for insomnia (CBT-I) is the recommended first-line treatment for the disorder in adults, with hypnotic medication suggested when CBT-I is unsuccessful (Edinger et al., 2020; Qaseem, Kansagara, Forciea, Cooke, & Denberg, 2016). We initially proposed that optimal treatment for the ISSD phenotype may differ from the INSD phenotype (Vgontzas et al., 2013). Specifically, while the INSD phenotype might respond better to CBT-I alone, medications that downregulate the underlying physiologic hyperarousal may be indicated for the ISSD phenotype. Of course, we also initially proposed that treatments that combine behavioral (i.e., CBT-I) and biological (i.e., medication) interventions may be the most effective for the ISSD phenotype, similar to what has been shown in other severe chronic conditions (Vgontzas et al., 2013). However, no prospective RCT designed to test the efficacy of CBT-I vs. inactive control, medication vs. placebo, CBT-I vs. medication, or their combination has been conducted to date in the INSD and ISSD phenotypes.

Treatment response

The current preliminary evidence on a potential differential response of the INSD and ISSD phenotypes to CBT-I comes from secondary analyses of existing RCTs that had objective sleep measures (PSG or ACT) at pretreatment and were able to stratify their sample of individuals with insomnia disorder according to this proposed phenotyping (e.g., ISSD defined as <6h of sleep). As shown in Table 2, four studies have found that subjects with the ISSD phenotype had a lower remission rate, as measured by patient-reported outcomes, to different forms of CBT-I (Bathgate, Edinger, & Krystal, 2017; Kalmbach, Cheng, Roth, Sagong, & Drake, 2020; Rochefort, Jarrin, Belanger, Ivers, & Morin, 2019; Troxel, Conrad, Germain, & Buysse, 2013), while three other studies report similar remission rates to CBT-I between subjects with the INSD vs. ISSD phenotypes (Cronlein, Wetter, Rupprecht, & Spiegelhalder, 2020; Lovato, Lack, & Kennaway, 2016; Miller et al., 2018). In one of these latter studies, however, Miller and colleagues showed that response rates were significantly lower in the ISSD phenotype (37%) than the INSD phenotype (70%) (Miller et al., 2018). A meta-analysis by the author using Neyeloff, Fuchs, and Moreira (2012) method of the remission data presented in Table 2 shows that the pooled remission rates across these seven studies are 23.7% higher in the 214 subjects with the INSD phenotype (53.5%, 95%CI = 42.9–64.2) than in the 196 subjects with the ISSD phenotype (29.8%, 95%CI = 13.5–46.2).

TABLE 2 Insomnia remission rates[a] in secondary analyses of clinical trials using pretreatment objective sleep to phenotype insomnia.

References	N (Men) Age	Type of treatment	Subjective criteria	Objective measure	ISSD criterion	Remission rate	
						INSD	ISSD
Troxel et al. (2013)	39 (33%) 72.5 ± 6.6	BBT-I	DSM-IV-TR & ICSD-2	PSG total sleep time	<6h	81.3%*	18.8%
Lovato et al. (2016)	91 (47%) 63.3 ± 6.4	Group CBT-I	Mod. DSM	PSG total sleep time	<6h	51.9%	55.6%
Bathgate et al. (2017)	60 (48%) 56.2 ± 10.1	Individual CBT-I	Mod. DSM-IV-TR	ACT total sleep time	<6h	88.0%*	2.9%
Miller et al. (2018)	39 (37%) 41.4 ± 11.8	Digital or Group CBT-I or SRT	DSM-5	PSG parameters	Clusters[b]	30.0%	32.0%
Rochefort et al. (2019)	159 (39%) 50.3 ± 10.1	Individual CBT-I	Mod. DSM-IV-TR & ICSD-2	PSG total sleep time	<6h	46.0%#	25.0%
Cronlein et al. (2020)	92 (22%) 50.8 ± 11.5	Inpatient CBT-I	DSM-5	PSG total sleep time	<6h	54.5%	51.7%
Kalmbach et al. (2020)	113 (0%) 56.4 ± 5.3	Individual CBT-I	Mod. DSM-5	PSG sleep efficiency	$<85\%$	61.8%*	37.8%

* $P < 0.05$.

$P = 0.09$.

[a] *Absence of clinically significant insomnia symptoms at posttreatment (Insomnia Severity Index < 8 in Lovato et al. (2016), Miller et al. (2018), Rochefort et al. (2019) and Kalmbach et al. (2020), Pittsburgh Sleep Quality Index < 5 in Troxel et al. (2013) and Regensburg Insomnia Scale < 12 in Cronlein et al. (2020)) or at 6-month follow-up (Insomnia Symptoms Questionnaire < 39.5 in Bathgate et al. (2017)).*

[b] *Miller et al. (2018) identified insomnia subtypes using cluster analysis of PSG total sleep time, sleep onset latency, and wake after sleep onset, and the resulting clusters were named ISSD and INSD commensurate with their total sleep time below and above 6h, respectively.*

All studies were retrospective analyses of existing randomized clinical trials. ACT = actigraphy. DMS = difficulty maintaining sleep. Mod. = modified diagnostic criteria, typically to include subjective reports of sleep onset latency or wake after sleep onset greater than 30 or 60 min or a duration criterion greater than 6 months. PSG = polysomnography. SRT = sleep restriction therapy.

These preliminary data support that the ISSD phenotype may be less likely to attain insomnia remission after CBT-I than the INSD phenotype. However, this meta-analysis of the data in Table 2 also shows that heterogeneity across studies is very large (>75%) for the ISSD phenotype ($Q=39.6$; $I^2=77.3$), while small (<10%) for the INSD phenotype ($Q=9.9$; $I^2=9.6$), which indicates that we still need well-designed, statistically powered, prospective RCTs to test the efficacy of CBT-I in those with INSD vs. ISSD phenotypes a priori before we can reach definitive conclusions regarding their differential treatment response to CBT-I.

No study to date has tested whether the ISSD phenotype responds better to medication than the INSD phenotype. A few studies have examined the effect of insomnia treatment on indices of physiologic hyperarousal. While CBT-I does not show meaningful changes in indices of physiologic hyperarousal (e.g., cortisol, HRV) (Jarrin et al., 2016; Miller, Kyle, Gordon, et al., 2015; Redeker, Conley, Anderson, et al., 2020), widely used sleep medications have been shown to lower cortisol levels and downregulate physiologic hyperarousal (Rodenbeck et al., 2003; Roehrs & Roth, 2019; Vgontzas et al., 2020). In a recent pilot study of the ISSD phenotype (i.e., ACT total sleep time < 7 h), trazodone significantly lengthened ACT total sleep time by about 50 min and decreased evening cortisol levels by about 21%–36%, while CBT-I did not improve any of these objective outcomes despite producing similar improvements on ISI scores as trazodone (Vgontzas et al., 2020). Out of the seven studies in Table 2, only one had an additional arm that included sleep medication. In their secondary analysis, Rochefort and colleagues showed that the 54 subjects with INSD who received CBT-I + zolpidem had a remission rate (48.0%), similar to the other 54 who received CBT-I alone (46%), while the 25 subjects with ISSD who received CBT-I + zolpidem had a remission rate 11.4% higher (36.4%) than the other 26 who received CBT-I alone (25.0%); however, these comparisons were not statistically significant (Rochefort et al., 2019). Furthermore, subjects with the ISSD phenotype who received CBT-I + zolpidem increased their sleep diary-derived sleep duration by about 22 min, while those with the INSD phenotype who received CBT-I + zolpidem increased their sleep duration only by about 5 min (p values were < 0.05 but not statistically significant after multiple comparisons) (Rochefort et al., 2019). Together, these data suggest that sleep medication may be a potential adjunct treatment in the ISSD phenotype, but this still needs to be tested in prospective, placebo-controlled RCTs.

Another set of studies have relied on subjective short sleep duration (as measured by sleep diary) and have provided mixed findings as it pertains to drop-out rates (Ong, Kuo, & Manber, 2008; Perlis, Aloia, Millikan, et al., 2000; Yeung, Chung, Ho, & Ho, 2015), and opposite findings as it pertains to treatment response to CBT-I (Galbiati, Sforza, Poletti, et al., 2020). However, this should not be surprising given that, unless a very low cut-off score is used (e.g., sleep diary total sleep time < 3.65 h in Ong et al., 2008), a subjective sleep duration <6 h is likely to misclassify many individuals with the INSD phenotype as reviewed above in the definition and health outcomes sections.

Potential CBT-I modifications or adaptations

As it pertains to the INSD phenotype, the overall approach should be to deliver CBT-I as per standard practice. However, the availability of objective sleep data after phenotyping posits some potential and interesting adaptations that are not currently available for the practitioner and that are presented in Table 3. For example, if a given patient does not present

TABLE 3 Potential, Untested Adaptations of CBT-I for the INSD Phenotype: Pending prospective randomized clinical trials.

CBT-I components	Standard practice	Potential modifications/ adaptations
Sleep education	3-P model, 2-process model of sleep regulation, sleep stages	– As per standard practice – Education about lack of increased risk of cardiometabolic and brain health outcomes by INSD itself (e.g., if not obese, poor diet, sedentary or other modifiable or fixed factors)
Sleep hygiene education	Address daytime habits and sleep environment interfering with sleep	– As per standard practice
Sleep restriction	Improve sleep efficiency by limiting time in bed to the amount of time sleeping then expanding slowly as long as sleep efficiency is preserved	– As per standard practice
Stimulus control	Associate bed/bedroom solely as a cue for sleep by eliminating nonsleep activities from the bedroom. Instruction to get out of bed at night if awake >15 min.	– As per standard practice
Napping/ daytime sleep	Discontinue or restrict daytime napping to 30 min	– As per standard practice – Discontinue daytime napping until remission is attained (untested adaptation)

Continued

TABLE 3 Potential, Untested Adaptations of CBT-I for the INSD Phenotype: Pending prospective randomized clinical trials—cont'd

CBT-I components	Standard practice	Potential modifications/ adaptations
Relaxation and meditation techniques	Relaxation can help reduce racing thoughts/tension that accompanies lying in bed awake and may include: deep breathing, progressive muscle relaxation, guided imagery, biofeedback, hypnosis, autogenic training, and meditation practices	– As per standard practice – Consider relaxation techniques focused on guided imagery and meditation (untested adaptation)
Cognitive therapy	Challenge patient's dysfunctional beliefs interfering with sleep and misconceptions about sleep. Replace/restructure to more helpful and realistic thoughts about sleep	– As per standard practice – Include sleep discrepancy data (see Table 1) to provide cognitive education, explain the role of cortical arousal, and conduct behavioral experiments to decrease the degree of sleep misperception (modification tested in trials of nonphenotyped insomnia) – Target maladaptive coping styles involved in increasing risk of or worsening adverse mental health outcomes (modification tested in noninsomnia trials)
Relapse Prevention	Discuss practicing less rigid sleep plan over time and what do to prevent sleep disturbance from turning into another episode of insomnia in the future	– As per standard practice
Sleep diaries	Establish baseline sleep patterns, track progress, reinforce appropriate behavior change, problem-solve obstacles to adherence	– As per standard practice – See also Table 1 and cognitive therapy above

with other fixed or modifiable risk factors, such as obesity, inadequate diet, sedentary behavior, or substance use or abuse, sleep education can expand to include reassuring information on lack of increased risk of specific morbidity (e.g., CMH, BH) in this INSD phenotype that is otherwise highly anxious and ruminative (Edinger et al., 2000; Fernandez-Mendoza et al., 2011) and holds greater sleep-related dysfunctional beliefs (Edinger et al., 2000), and may serve as a first introduction to upcoming cognitive therapy. This type of education would be similar to that currently conducted in other advanced fields in which risk stratification and prognosis is provided to the patient based on biomarkers, genotyping, or other types of objective measures of the disorder.

Although sleep restriction therapy has demonstrated good efficacy in reducing sleep misperception, cognitive therapy could also be boosted by the availability of data on the discrepancy between subjective and objective total sleep time, as suggested in Table 1. This can be used to provide cognitive education on the role of cortical arousal in sleep misperception and plan behavioral experiments to target perceived sleep ability. Cognitive therapy would also benefit from a more directed work on cognitive-emotional traits and coping styles, due to their known role in increasing the risk of or worsening the course of psychopathology, including panic, depression, and suicidal ideation and intent.

Finally, it is not recommended to use sleep medication in the INSD phenotype and other evidence-based, nonpharmacological treatment approaches may be needed if the response to CBT-I, as per standard practice, is not optimal (Lack, Scott, & Lovato, 2019; Ong, 2017). This may include a greater focus on relaxation techniques, which are not typically a standard in CBT-I protocols, and with a focus on imagery- or meditation-based therapies targeting cognitive arousal, rumination, and/or anticipatory anxiety.

As it pertains to the ISSD phenotype, the initial proposed approach and preliminary evidence reviewed above suggests a blunted response to CBT-I (Bathgate et al., 2017; Kalmbach et al., 2020; Rochefort et al., 2019; Troxel et al., 2013) and the potential need to combine CBT-I with sleep medication in this insomnia phenotype (Rochefort et al., 2019; Vgontzas et al., 2013; Vgontzas et al., 2020). Therefore, a critical modification in this scenario would be to introduce sleep medication if the response to behavioral therapy (i.e., sleep education, sleep hygiene education, sleep restriction, and stimulus control) is not optimal (see Table 4). This potential modification is also based on recent pilot data in the ISSD phenotype (Vgontzas et al., 2020) and on the relative impact of behavioral vs. pharmacological therapies on total sleep time in nonphenotyped chronic insomnia (Morin et al., 2020). Morin and colleagues have provided sequential evidence that CBT-I is most effective at increasing sleep efficiency (i.e., reducing sleep latency and wake time after sleep onset), while sleep medications show their strongest effect on increasing total sleep time (Morin et al., 2020). However, as mentioned above, this should not be our standard of practice for the ISSD phenotype until solid evidence from RCTs is obtained and we should continue to taper off sleep medications if patients respond well to CBT-I regardless of phenotype.

There are also potential modifications to CBT-I itself for the ISSD phenotype that could be tested in RCTs and that are presented in Table 4. For example, objective sleep measures such as ACT, instead of sleep diary, may be used to set the initial time in bed for sleep restriction, even if total

TABLE 4 Potential, untested adaptations of CBT-I for the ISSD phenotype: Pending prospective randomized clinical trials.

CBT-I components	Standard practice	Potential modifications/ adaptations
Sleep education	3-P model, 2-process model of sleep regulation, sleep stages	– As per standard practice – Education about ISSD and importance of CBT-I as first-line treatment (untested adaptation) – Education on the potential need to introduce sleep medication based on CBT-I response (untested adaptation)
Sleep hygiene education	Address daytime habits and sleep environment interfering with sleep	– As per standard practice
Sleep restriction	Improve sleep efficiency by limiting time in bed to the amount of time sleeping then expanding slowly as long as sleep efficiency is preserved	– As per standard practice – Set initial time in bed based on objective sleep duration, even if <5h (untested modification) – Consider intensive sleep restriction protocols (untested modification) – Consider sleep extension protocols if sleep ability is increased with behavioral therapy alone (untested modification)
Stimulus control	Associate bed/bedroom solely as a cue for sleep by eliminating nonsleep activities from the bedroom. Instruction to get out of bed at night if awake >15min.	– As per standard practice – Advise patient to not engage in wake-related or stimulating activities, foster dim lights, dearousal at night (untested adaptation)
Napping/ daytime sleep	Discontinue daytime napping to 30min, if any	– As per standard practice
Sleep medication	Decrease physiologic hyperarousal and increase physiologic sleep ability (total sleep time)	– Refer to a sleep physician for medication management after poor treatment response to behavioral therapy (untested modification, based on trials of nonphenotyped insomnia) – Consider sleep extension protocols if sleep ability is increased with sleep medication (untested modification)

TABLE 4 Potential, untested adaptations of CBT-I for the ISSD phenotype: Pending prospective randomized clinical trials—cont'd

CBT-I components	Standard practice	Potential modifications/ adaptations
		– Consider sleep medication discontinuation if sleep extension has been achieved (untested modification)
Relaxation and meditation techniques	Relaxation can help reduce racing thoughts/tension that accompanies lying in bed awake and may include: deep breathing, progressive muscle relaxation, guided imagery, biofeedback, hypnosis, autogenic training, and meditation practices	– As per standard practice – Consider relaxation techniques focused on somatic symptoms and deactivation (untested adaptation)
Cognitive therapy	Challenge patient's dysfunctional beliefs interfering with sleep and misconceptions about sleep. Replace/restructure to more helpful and realistic thoughts about sleep	– As per standard practice – Provide realistic expectations for sleep when comorbid conditions are present (untested adaptation) – Avoid wake-maintenance behavioral experiments or paradoxical intention (untested modification)
Relapse Prevention	Discuss practicing less rigid sleep plan over time and what do to prevent sleep disturbance from turning into another episode of insomnia in the future	– As per standard practice
Sleep diaries	Establish baseline sleep patterns, track progress, reinforce appropriate behavior change, problem-solve obstacles to adherence	– As per standard practice – Use objective sleep data, combined with sleep diaries, to titrate time in bed in sleep restriction protocols (untested modification)

sleep time is <5h, and, thereafter, titrate sleep opportunity based on objective total sleep time (or in combination with sleep diary data). This is a rather provocative modification that has a great potential for future RCTs, as the possibility exists that severe sleep restriction may be needed to increase sleep homeostasis and override physiologic hyperarousal in this more biologically severe phenotype of insomnia. Similarly, other intensive sleep restriction approaches could also be tested in the ISSD phenotype using similar logic (Lack et al., 2019). None of this has yet been done.

Another potential modification that remains untested in the ISSD phenotype is the implementation of sleep extension strategies either after sleep extension, if it has successfully led to increased sleep ability (i.e., nighttime and daytime sleep propensity), or after sleep medication, if it has achieved such goal. This is an important issue, as it is likely that individuals with the ISSD phenotype may benefit from evidence-based behavioral strategies on how to increase time in bed to achieve greater sleep duration without introducing sleep-incompatible or sleep-inhibitory behaviors.

Smaller-scale adaptations for CBT-I in the ISSD phenotype may include advising the patient to not engage in wake-related or stimulating activities, and foster dim lights and dearousal, while out of bed at night when implementing stimulus control, instead of allowing hobbies and engaging activities as some treatment manuals do. It is not clear, however, whether allowing restricted postprandial daytime napping (30 min), if significant physiologic sleep propensity arises with severe sleep restriction based on objective sleep, may be indicated (Bonnet & Arand, 1998b). From a cognitive therapy standpoint, identifying the ISSD phenotype may help the clinician provide realistic expectations for sleep, particularly when it is comorbid with medical conditions, and focus on specific dysfunctional beliefs that may sabotage recovery. Given the presence of physiologic hyperarousal, rather than anticipatory anxiety, wake-maintenance behavioral experiments such as paradoxical intention may not be indicated in the ISSD phenotype. Relaxation techniques may be indicated with a particular focus on somatic symptoms during the presleep and nighttime period. However, these proposed cognitive and relaxation therapy adaptations are based on theoretical grounds and not on evidence-based data from efficacy or effectiveness trials.

In summary, this proposed insomnia phenotyping has great potential not only for matching treatments to phenotypes, such as the INSD to CBT-I and the ISSD to sleep medication, but also to create more sophisticated forms of CBT-I that, alone or in combination with sleep medication, may help us achieve greater remission rates than the 50% currently observed in RCTs of individuals with insomnia disorder who have not been phenotyped. However, none of the modifications and adaptations of CBT-I suggested herein have been formally tested and should not be regarded as evidence-based recommendations.

Future directions

Although the ISSD phenotype has demonstrated the ability to predict adverse cardiovascular, metabolic and neurocognitive risk and to relate to specific pathophysiologic mechanisms, there is still a lot to be done to better support this insomnia phenotyping. There is a need for studies testing whether ACT or wearables can accurately identify these phenotypes and whether different thresholds for their estimated objective total sleep time or sleep efficiency are needed. Despite its greater risk of physical health disorders, there is still a need to understand the mechanisms underlying such risk in the ISSD phenotype, as well as those linking the INSD phenotype with mental health morbidity. Future RCTs need to identify the optimal therapies for each of these insomnia phenotypes, which may include CBT-I modifications, sleep medications, or both. Those future RCTs should not only focus on attaining remission of insomnia symptoms but also aim at modifying the pathophysiologic mechanisms, biological or behavioral, of each phenotype as well as their essential features, including lengthening sleep duration and improving health outcomes.

Summary

The ISSD phenotype represents a multidimensional, multimethod approach to better understand the pathophysiology, nature, and impact of insomnia as a heterogeneous disorder. The ISSD phenotype is linked to physiologic hyperarousal and adverse cardiometabolic and neurocognitive health outcomes and shares with the INSD phenotype its link with cortical arousal and adverse mental health outcomes. The INSD phenotype is also linked to sleep misperception, poor coping skills and is more likely to remit, while the ISSD phenotype has a persistent, unremitting natural course. These two insomnia phenotypes may require different treatment approaches, in which the possibility remains that modifications or adaptations to CBT-I may be needed. The latter, however, is an area in need of future research for which we do not currently have evidence-based recommendations.

References

American Academy of Sleep Medicine. (2014). *The international classification of sleep disorders (ICSD-3): Diagnostic and coding manual* (3rd ed.). Darien, IL: American Academy of Sleep Medicine. Academy of Sleep Medicine.

Bastien, C. H., Turcotte, I., St-Jean, G., Morin, C. M., & Carrier, J. (2013). Information processing varies between insomnia types: Measures of N1 and P2 during the night. *Behavioral Sleep Medicine, 11*(1), 56–72.

Bathgate, C. J., Edinger, J. D., & Krystal, A. D. (2017). Insomnia patients with objective short sleep duration have a blunted response to cognitive behavioral therapy for insomnia. *Sleep, 40*(1), zsw012.

Bathgate, C. J., Edinger, J. D., Wyatt, J. K., & Krystal, A. D. (2016). Objective but not subjective short sleep duration associated with increased risk for hypertension in individuals with insomnia. *Sleep, 39*(5), 1037–1045.

Bathgate, C. J., & Fernandez-Mendoza, J. (2018). Insomnia, short sleep duration, and high blood pressure: Recent evidence and future directions for the prevention and management of hypertension. *Current Hypertension Reports, 20*(6), 52.

Bertisch, S. M., Pollock, B. D., Mittleman, M. A., et al. (2018). Insomnia with objective short sleep duration and risk of incident cardiovascular disease and all-cause mortality: Sleep Heart Health Study. *Sleep, 41*(6), zsy047.

Biddle, D. J., Naismith, S. L., Griffiths, K. M., Christensen, H., Hickie, I. B., & Glozier, N. S. (2017). Associations of objective and subjective sleep disturbance with cognitive function in older men with comorbid depression and insomnia. *Sleep Health, 3*(3), 178–183.

Bonnet, M. H., & Arand, D. L. (1995). 24-hour metabolic rate in insomniacs and matched normal sleepers. *Sleep, 18*, 581–588.

Bonnet, M. H., & Arand, D. L. (1996). The consequences of a week of insomnia. *Sleep, 19*(6), 453–461.

Bonnet, M. H., & Arand, D. L. (1997a). Hyperarousal and insomnia. *Sleep Medicine Reviews, 1*(2), 97–108.

Bonnet, M. H., & Arand, D. L. (1997b). Physiological activation in patients with sleep state misperception. *Psychosomatic Medicine, 59*, 533–540.

Bonnet, M. H., & Arand, D. L. (1998a). Heart rate variability in insomniacs and matched normal sleepers. *Psychosomatic Medicine, 60*(5), 610–615.

Bonnet, M. H., & Arand, D. L. (1998b). The consequences of a week of insomnia. II: Patients with insomnia. *Sleep, 21*(4), 359–368.

Bonnet, M. H., & Arand, D. L. (2000). Activity, arousal, and the MSLT in patients with insomnia. *Sleep, 23*(2), 205–212.

Bonnet, M. H., Burton, G. G., & Arand, D. L. (2014). Physiological and medical findings in insomnia: Implications for diagnosis and care. *Sleep Medicine Reviews, 18*(2), 111–122.

Calhoun, S. L., Fernandez-Mendoza, J., Vgontzas, A. N., Mayes, S. D., Liao, D., & Bixler, E. O. (2017). Behavioral profiles associated with objective sleep duration in young children with insomnia symptoms. *Journal of Abnormal Child Psychology, 45*(2), 337–344.

Castro-Diehl, C., Diez Roux, A. V., Redline, S., Seeman, T., Shrager, S. E., & Shea, S. (2015). Association of sleep duration and quality with alterations in the hypothalamic-pituitary adrenocortical axis: The Multi-Ethnic Study of Atherosclerosis (MESA). *The Journal of Clinical Endocrinology and Metabolism, 100*(8), 3149–3158.

Castro-Diehl, C., Diez Roux, A. V., Redline, S., et al. (2016). Sleep duration and quality in relation to autonomic nervous system measures: The Multi-Ethnic Study of Atherosclerosis (MESA). *Sleep, 39*(11), 1927–1940.

Chouvarda, I., Grassi, A., Mendez, M. O., et al. (2013). Insomnia types and sleep microstructure dynamics. *Conference Proceedings: Annual International Conference of the IEEE Engineering in Medicine and Biology Society, 2013*, 6167–6170.

Cronlein, T., Wetter, T. C., Rupprecht, R., & Spiegelhalder, K. (2020). Cognitive behavioral treatment for insomnia is equally effective in insomnia patients with objective short and normal sleep duration. *Sleep Medicine, 66*, 271–275.

Danzig, R., Wang, M., Shah, A., & Trotti, L. M. (2020). The wrist is not the brain: Estimation of sleep by clinical and consumer wearable actigraphy devices is impacted by multiple patient- and device-specific factors. *Journal of Sleep Research, 29*(1), e12926.

D'Aurea, C., Poyares, D., Piovezan, R. D., Passos, G., Tufik, S., & de Mello, M. T. (2015). Objective short sleep duration is associated with the activity of the hypothalamic-pituitary-adrenal axis in insomnia. *Arquivos de Neuro-Psiquiatria, 73*(6), 516–519.

Dorsey, C. M., & Bootzin, R. R. (1997). Subjective and psychophysiologic insomnia: An examination of sleep tendency and personality. *Biological Psychiatry, 41*, 209–216.

Edinger, J. D., Arnedt, J. T., Bertisch, S. M., Carney, C. E., Harrington, J. J., Lichstein, K. L., et al. (2020). Behavioral and psychological treatments for chronic insomnia disorder in adults: An American Academy of Sleep Medicine clinical practice guideline. *Journal of Clinical Sleep Medicine*. https://doi.org/10.5664/jcsm.8986.

Edinger, J. D., Fins, A. I., Glenn, D. M., et al. (2000). Insomnia and the eye of the beholder: Are there clinical markers of objective sleep disturbances among adults with and without insomnia complaints? *Journal of Consulting and Clinical Psychology, 68*(4), 586–593.

Edinger, J. D., Fins, A. I., Goeke, J. M., McMillan, D. K., Gersh, T. L., Krystal, A. D., et al. (1996). The empirical identification of insomnia subtypes: A cluster analytic approach. *Sleep, 19*(5), 398–411.

Edinger, J. D., & Krystal, A. D. (2003). Subtyping primary insomnia: Is sleep state misperception a distinct clinical entity? *Sleep Medicine Reviews, 7*(3), 203–214.

Edinger, J. D., Means, M. K., & Krystal, A. D. (2013). Does physiological hyperarousal enhance error rates among insomnia sufferers? *Sleep, 36*(8), 1179–1186.

Edinger, J. D., Wyatt, J. K., Stepanski, E. J., Olsen, M. K., Stechuchak, K. M., Carney, C. E., et al. (2011). Testing the reliability and validity of DSM-IV-TR and ICSD-2 insomnia diagnoses. Results of a multitrait-multimethod analysis. *Archives of General Psychiatry, 68*(10), 992–1002.

Erwin, J. A., Buysse, D. J., Hall, M. H., Germain, A., & Kline, C. E. (2017). The insomnia short-sleep phenotype: Does one night of laboratory sleep accurately capture their habitual sleep? *Sleep, 40*(Suppl), A115–A116.

Fan, T. T., Chen, W. H., Shi, L., et al. (2019). Objective sleep duration is associated with cognitive deficits in primary insomnia: BDNF may play a role. *Sleep, 42*(1), zsy192.

Fernandez-Mendoza, J. (2010). *Insomnio crónico: Subtipos basados en hallazgos polisomnográficos, psicopatológicos y neuropsicológicos*. Doctoral dissertation Madrid: Spain: Universidad Complutense de Madrid. ISBN: 978-84-693-8335-3. Retrieved from http://eprints.ucm.es/11415/1/T32424.pdf.

Fernandez-Mendoza, J. (2017). The insomnia with short sleep duration phenotype: An update on its importance for health and prevention. *Current Opinion in Psychiatry, 30*(1), 56–63.

Fernandez-Mendoza, J., Baker, J. H., Vgontzas, A. N., Gaines, J., Liao, D., & Bixler, E. O. (2017). Insomnia symptoms with objective short sleep duration are associated with systemic inflammation in adolescents. *Brain, Behavior, and Immunity, 61*, 110–116.

Fernandez-Mendoza, J., Calhoun, S., Bixler, E. O., et al. (2010). Insomnia with objective short sleep duration is associated with deficits in neuropsychological performance: A general population study. *Sleep, 33*(4), 459–465.

Fernandez-Mendoza, J., Calhoun, S. L., Bixler, E. O., et al. (2011). Sleep misperception and chronic insomnia in the general population: The role of objective sleep duration and psychological profiles. *Psychosomatic Medicine, 73*(1), 88–91.

Fernandez-Mendoza, J., Calhoun, S. L., Vgontzas, A. N., et al. (2016). Insomnia phenotypes based on objective sleep duration in adolescents: Depression risk and differential behavioral profiles. *Brain Sciences, 6*(4), E59.

Fernandez-Mendoza, J., He, F., Liao, D., Vgontzas, A. N., & Bixler, E. O. (2018). Insomnia with objective short sleep duration is associated with an increased risk of cardiocerebrovascular disease. *Sleep, 41*(Suppl), A325.

Fernandez-Mendoza, J., He, F., Puzino, K., Amatrudo, G., Calhoun, S. L., Liao, D., et al. (2020). Insomnia with objective short sleep duration is associated with cognitive impairment: A first look at cardiometabolic contributors to brain health. *Sleep*. https://doi.org/10.1093/sleep/zsaa150.

Fernandez-Mendoza, J., Li, Y., Vgontzas, A. N., et al. (2016). Insomnia is associated with cortical hyperarousal as early as adolescence. *Sleep, 39*(5), 1029–1036.

Fernandez-Mendoza, J., Shea, S., Vgontzas, A. N., Calhoun, S. L., Liao, D., & Bixler, E. O. (2015). Insomnia and incident depression: Role of objective sleep duration and natural history. *Journal of Sleep Research, 24*(4), 390–398.

Fernandez-Mendoza, J., Vgontzas, A. N., Bixler, E. O., Singareddy, R., Shaffer, M. L., Calhoun, S. L., et al. (2012). Clinical and polysomnographic predictors of the natural history of poor sleep in the general population. *Sleep, 35*(5), 689–697.

Fernandez-Mendoza, J., Vgontzas, A. N., Calhoun, S. L., et al. (2014). Insomnia symptoms, objective sleep duration and hypothalamic-pituitary-adrenal activity in children. *European Journal of Clinical Investigation, 44*(5), 493–500.

Fernandez-Mendoza, J., Vgontzas, A. N., Liao, D., et al. (2012). Insomnia with objective short sleep duration and incident hypertension: The Penn State Cohort. *Hypertension, 60*(4), 929–935.

Floam, S., Simpson, N., Nemeth, E., Scott-Sutherland, J., Gautam, S., & Haack, M. (2015). Sleep characteristics as predictor variables of stress systems markers in insomnia disorder. *Journal of Sleep Research, 24*(3), 296–304.

Gaines, J., Vgontzas, A. N., Fernandez-Mendoza, J., et al. (2015). Short- and long-term sleep stability in insomniacs and healthy controls. *Sleep, 38*(11), 1727–1734.

Galbiati, A., Sforza, M., Poletti, M., et al. (2020). Insomnia patients with subjective short total sleep time have a boosted response to cognitive behavioral therapy for insomnia despite residual symptoms. *Behavioral Sleep Medicine, 18*(1), 58–67.

Hall, M. H., Fernandez-Mendoza, J., Kline, C. H., & Vgontzas, A. N. (2016). Insomnia and health. In M. H. Kryger, T. Roth, & W. C. Dement (Eds.), *Principles and practice of sleep medicine* (6th ed., pp. 794–803). New York: Elsevier Academic Press.

Hein, M., Lanquart, J. P., Loas, G., Hubain, P., & Linkowski, P. (2018). Prevalence and risk factors of type 2 diabetes in insomnia sufferers: A study on 1311 individuals referred for sleep examinations. *Sleep Medicine, 46*, 37–45.

Hein, M., Lanquart, J. P., Loas, G., Hubain, P., & Linkowski, P. (2019a). Risk of high blood pressure associated with objective insomnia and self-reported insomnia complaints in major depression: A study on 703 individuals. *Clinical and Experimental Hypertension, 41*(6), 538–547.

Hein, M., Lanquart, J. P., Loas, G., Hubain, P., & Linkowski, P. (2019b). Objective sleep alterations and long-term use of short or intermediate half-life benzodiazepine receptor agonists are risk factors for high blood pressure in individuals with insomnia: A study in 1272 individuals referred for sleep examinations. *Sleep Medicine, 53*, 115–123.

Hertenstein, E., Feige, B., Gmeiner, T., et al. (2019). Insomnia as a predictor of mental disorders: A systematic review and meta-analysis. *Sleep Medicine Reviews, 43*, 96–105.

Huang, Z., Goparaju, B., Chen, H., & Bianchi, M. T. (2018). Heart rate phenotypes and clinical correlates in a large cohort of adults without sleep apnea. *Nature and Science of Sleep, 10*, 111–125.

Jarrin, D. C., Alvaro, P. K., Bouchard, M.-A., Jarrin, S. D., Drake, C. L., & Morin, C. M. (2018). Insomnia and hypertension: A systematic review. *Sleep Medicine Reviews, 41*, 3–38.

Jarrin, D. C., Chen, I. Y., Ivers, H., Lamy, M., Vallieres, A., & Morin, C. M. (2016). Nocturnal heart rate variability in patients treated with cognitive-behavioral therapy for insomnia. *Health Psychology, 35*(6), 638–641.

Jarrin, D. C., Ivers, H., Lamy, M., Chen, I. Y., Harvey, A. G., & Morin, C. M. (2018). Cardiovascular autonomic dysfunction in insomnia patients with objective short sleep duration. *Journal of Sleep Research, 27*(3), e12663.

Johann, A. F., Hertenstein, E., Kyle, S. D., et al. (2017). Insomnia with objective short sleep duration is associated with longer duration of insomnia in the Freiburg Insomnia Cohort compared to insomnia with normal sleep duration, but not with hypertension. *PLoS One, 12*(7), e0180339.

Kalmbach, D. A., Cheng, P., Roth, T., Sagong, C., & Drake, C. L. (2020). Objective sleep disturbance is associated with poor response to cognitive and behavioral treatments for insomnia in postmenopausal women. *Sleep Medicine, 73*, 82–92.

Khassawneh, B. Y., Bathgate, C. J., Tsai, S. C., & Edinger, J. D. (2018). Neurocognitive performance in insomnia disorder: The impact of hyperarousal and short sleep duration. *Journal of Sleep Research, 27*(6), e12747.

Krystal, A. D., Edinger, J. D., Wohlgemuth, W. K., & Marsh, G. R. (2002). NREM sleep EEG frequency spectral correlates of sleep complaints in primary insomnia subtypes. *Sleep, 25*(6), 630–640.

Lack, L., Scott, H., & Lovato, N. (2019). Intensive sleep retraining treatment of insomnia. *Sleep Medicine Clinics, 14*(2), 245–252.

Li, Y., Vgontzas, A. N., Fernandez-Mendoza, J., et al. (2015). Insomnia with physiological hyperarousal is associated with hypertension. *Hypertension, 65*(3), 644–650.

Lovato, N., Lack, L., & Kennaway, D. J. (2016). Comparing and contrasting therapeutic effects of cognitive-behavior therapy for older adults suffering from insomnia with short and long objective sleep duration. *Sleep Medicine, 22*, 4–12.

Miller, C. B., Bartlett, D. J., Mullins, A. E., et al. (2016). Clusters of insomnia disorder: An exploratory cluster analysis of objective sleep parameters reveals differences in neurocognitive functioning, quantitative EEG, and heart rate variability. *Sleep, 39*(11), 1993–2004.

Miller, C. B., Espie, C. A., Bartlett, D. J., Marshall, N. S., Gordon, C. J., & Grunstein, R. R. (2018). Acceptability, tolerability, and potential efficacy of cognitive behavioural therapy for insomnia disorder subtypes defined by polysomnography: A retrospective cohort study. *Scientific Reports, 8*(1), 6664.

Miller, C. B., Kyle, S. D., Gordon, C. J., et al. (2015). Physiological markers of arousal change with psychological treatment for insomnia: A preliminary investigation. *PLoS One, 10*(12), e0145317.

Miller, C. B., Rae, C. D., Green, M. A., et al. (2017). An objective short sleep insomnia disorder subtype is associated with reduced brain metabolite concentrations in vivo: A preliminary magnetic resonance spectroscopy assessment. *Sleep, 40*(11), zsx148.

Mohammadi, H., Rezaei, M., Amiri, M. S., Rahimi, Z., Mansouri, K., & Khazaie, H. (2018). Sleep architecture and hypothalamic-pituitary-adrenal activity in paradoxical and psychophysiological insomnia. *Basic and Clinical Neuroscience, 9*(6), 397–407.

Morin, C. M., Bélanger, L., LeBlanc, M., Ivers, H., Savard, J., Espie, C. A., et al. (2009). The natural history of insomnia: A population-based 3-year longitudinal study. *Archives of Internal Medicine, 169*(5), 447–453.

Morin, C. M., Edinger, J. D., Beaulieu-Bonneau, S., Ivers, H., Krystal, A. D., Guay, B., et al. (2020). Effectiveness of sequential psychological and medication therapies for insomnia disorder: A randomized clinical trial. *JAMA Psychiatry, 77*(11), 1107–1115.

Nakazaki, C., Noda, A., Koike, Y., Yamada, S., Murohara, T., & Ozaki, N. (2012). Association of insomnia and short sleep duration with atherosclerosis risk in the elderly. *American Journal of Hypertension, 25*(11), 1149–1155.

Neyeloff, J. L., Fuchs, S. C., & Moreira, L. B. (2012). Meta-analyses and Forest plots using a Microsoft Excel spreadsheet: Step-by-step guide focusing on descriptive data analysis. *BMC Research Notes, 5*, 52.

Normand, M. P., St-Hilaire, P., & Bastien, C. H. (2016). Sleep spindles characteristics in insomnia sufferers and their relationship with sleep misperception. *Neural Plasticity, 2016*, 6413473.

Ong, J. (2017). *Mindfulness-based therapy for insomnia*. Washington: DC: American Psychological Association.

Ong, J. C., Kuo, T. F., & Manber, R. (2008). Who is at risk for dropout from group cognitive-behavior therapy for insomnia? *Journal of Psychosomatic Research, 64*(4), 419–425.

Parrino, L., Milioli, G., De Paolis, F., Grassi, A., & Terzano, M. G. (2009). Paradoxical insomnia: The role of CAP and arousals in sleep misperception. *Sleep Medicine, 10*(10), 1139–1145.

Perlis, M., Aloia, M., Millikan, A., et al. (2000). Behavioral treatment of insomnia: A clinical case series study. *Journal of Behavioral Medicine, 23*(2), 149–161.

Pérusse, A. D., Pedneault-Drolet, M., Rancourt, C., Turcotte, I., St-Jean, G., & Bastien, C. H. (2015). REM sleep as a potential indicator of hyperarousal in psychophysiological and paradoxical insomnia sufferers. *International Journal of Psychophysiology, 95*(3), 372–378.

Qaseem, A., Kansagara, D., Forciea, M. A., Cooke, M., & Denberg, T. D. (2016). Management of chronic insomnia disorder in adults: A clinical practice guideline from the American College of Physicians. *Annals of Internal Medicine, 165*(2), 125–133.

Redeker, N. S., Conley, S., Anderson, G., et al. (2020). Effects of cognitive behavioral therapy for insomnia on sleep, symptoms, stress, and autonomic function among patients with heart failure. *Behavioral Sleep Medicine, 18*(2), 190–202.

Regen, W., Kyle, S. D., Nissen, C., et al. (2016). Objective sleep disturbances are associated with greater waking resting-state connectivity between the retrosplenial cortex/ hippocampus and various nodes of the default mode network. *Journal of Psychiatry & Neuroscience, 41*(5), 295–303.

Riemann, D., Klein, T., Rodenbeck, A., Feige, B., Horny, A., Hummel, R., et al. (2002). Nocturnal cortisol and melatonin secretion in primary insomnia. *Psychiatry Research, 113*(1–2), 17–27.

Rochefort, A., Jarrin, D. C., Belanger, L., Ivers, H., & Morin, C. M. (2019). Insomnia treatment response as a function of objectively measured sleep duration. *Sleep Medicine, 56*, 135–144.

Rodenbeck, A., Cohrs, S., Jordan, W., Huether, G., Rüther, E., & Hajak, G. (2003). The sleep-improving effects of doxepin are paralleled by a normalized plasma cortisol secretion in primary insomnia. A placebo-controlled, double-blind, randomized, cross-over study followed by an open treatment over 3 weeks. *Psychopharmacology, 170*(4), 423–428.

Rodenbeck, A., Huether, G., Ruther, E., & Hajak, G. (2002). Interactions between evening and nocturnal cortisol secretion and sleep parameters in patients with severe chronic primary insomnia. *Neuroscience Letters, 324*(2), 159–163.

Roehrs, T. A., Randall, S., Harris, E., Maan, R., & Roth, T. (2011). MSLT in primary insomnia: Stability and relation to nocturnal sleep. *Sleep, 34*, 1647–1652.

Roehrs, T., & Roth, T. (2019). Hyperarousal in insomnia: Pre-sleep and diurnal cortisol levels in response to chronic zolpidem treatment. *Sleep Medicine, 61*, 52–56.

Smith, M. T., McCrae, C. S., Cheung, J., Martin, J. L., Harrod, C. G., Heald, J. L., et al. (2018). Use of actigraphy for the evaluation of sleep disorders and circadian rhythm sleep-wake disorders: An American Academy of Sleep Medicine clinical practice guideline. *Journal of Clinical Sleep Medicine, 14*(7), 1231–1237.

Spiegelhalder, K., Fuchs, L., Ladwig, J., et al. (2011). Heart rate and heart rate variability in subjectively reported insomnia. *Journal of Sleep Research, 20*(1 Pt. 2), 137–145.

Spiegelhalder, K., Regen, W., Feige, B., et al. (2012). Increased EEG sigma and beta power during NREM sleep in primary insomnia. *Biological Psychology, 91*(3), 329–333.

Spiegelhalder, K., Regen, W., Nissen, C., et al. (2016). Magnetic resonance spectroscopy in patients with insomnia: A repeated measurement study. *PLoS One, 11*, e0156771.

Stepanski, E., Zorick, F., Roehrs, T., Young, D., & Roth, T. (1988). Daytime alertness in patients with chronic insomnia compared with asymptomatic control subjects. *Sleep, 11*, 54–60.

St-Jean, G., Turcotte, I., & Bastien, C. H. (2012). Cerebral asymmetry in insomnia sufferers. *Frontiers in Neurology, 3*, 47.

St-Jean, G., Turcotte, I., Pérusse, A. D., & Bastien, C. H. (2013). REM and NREM power spectral analysis on two consecutive nights in psychophysiological and paradoxical insomnia sufferers. *International Journal of Psychophysiology, 89*(2), 181–194.

Sugerman, J. L., Stern, J. A., & Walsh, J. K. (1985). Daytime alertness in subjective and objective insomnia: Some preliminary findings. *Biological Psychiatry, 20*, 741–750.

Tempaku, P., Hirotsu, C., Mazzotti, D., et al. (2018). Long sleep duration, insomnia, and insomnia with short objective sleep duration are independently associated with short telomere length. *Journal of Clinical Sleep Medicine, 14*(12), 2037–2045.

Troxel, W. M., Conrad, T. S., Germain, A., & Buysse, D. J. (2013). Predictors of treatment response to brief behavioral treatment of insomnia (BBTI) in older adults. *Journal of Clinical Sleep Medicine, 9*(12), 1281–1289.

Turcotte, I., St-Jean, G., & Bastien, C. H. (2011). Are individuals with paradoxical insomnia more hyperaroused than individuals with psychophysiological insomnia? Event-related potentials measures at the peri-onset of sleep. *International Journal of Psychophysiology, 81*(3), 177–190.

Vasisht, K. P., Kessler, L. E., Booth, J. N., III, Imperial, J. G., & Penev, P. D. (2013). Changes in insulin secretion and sensitivity in short sleep insomnia. *Sleep, 36*(6), 955–957.

Vgontzas, A. N., Bixler, E. O., Lin, H. M., et al. (2001). Chronic insomnia is associated with nyctohemeral activation of the hypothalamic-pituitary-adrenal axis: Clinical implications. *The Journal of Clinical Endocrinology and Metabolism, 86*(8), 3787–3794.

Vgontzas, A. N., Fernandez-Mendoza, J., Bixler, E. O., Singareddy, R., Shaffer, M. L., Calhoun, S. L., et al. (2012). Persistent insomnia: The role of objective short sleep duration and mental health. *Sleep, 35*(1), 61–68.

Vgontzas, A. N., Fernandez-Mendoza, J., Liao, D., & Bixler, E. O. (2013). Insomnia with objective short sleep duration: The most biologically severe phenotype of the disorder. *Sleep Medicine Reviews, 17*(4), 241–254.

Vgontzas, A. N., Liao, D., Bixler, E. O., Chrousos, G. P., & Vela-Bueno, A. (2009). Insomnia with objective short sleep duration is associated with a high risk for hypertension. *Sleep, 32*(4), 491–497.

Vgontzas, A. N., Liao, D., Pejovic, S., Calhoun, S., Karataraki, M., & Bixler, E. O. (2009). Insomnia with objective short sleep duration is associated with type 2 diabetes: A population-based study. *Diabetes Care, 32*(11), 1980–1985.

Vgontzas, A. N., Liao, D., Pejovic, S., et al. (2010). Insomnia with short sleep duration and mortality: The Penn State cohort. *Sleep, 33*(9), 1159–1164.

Vgontzas, A. N., Puzino, K., Fernandez-Mendoza, J., Krishnamurthy, V. B., Basta, M., & Bixler, E. O. (2020). Effects of trazodone versus cognitive behavioral therapy in the insomnia with short sleep duration phenotype: A preliminary study. *Journal of Clinical Sleep Medicine*. https://doi.org/10.5664/jcsm.8740.

Vgontzas, A. N., Tsigos, C., Bixler, E. O., et al. (1998). Chronic insomnia and activity of the stress system: A preliminary study. *Journal of Psychosomatic Research, 45*(1), 21–31.

Vgontzas, A. N., Zoumakis, M., Papanicolaou, D. A., et al. (2002). Chronic insomnia is associated with a shift of interleukin-6 and tumor necrosis factor secretion from nighttime to daytime. *Metabolism, 51*(7), 887–892.

Withrow, D., Roth, T., Koshorek, G., & Roehrs, T. (2019). Relation between ambulatory actigraphy and laboratory polysomnography in insomnia practice and research. *Journal of Sleep Research, 28*(4), e12854.

Yeung, W. F., Chung, K. F., Ho, F. Y., & Ho, L. M. (2015). Predictors of dropout from internet-based self-help cognitive behavioral therapy for insomnia. *Behaviour Research and Therapy, 73*, 19–24.

CHAPTER

19

CBT-I for people who failed CBT-I

Michael A. Grandner[a,b], Denise Rodriguez Esquivel[a,b], and Spencer Dawson[c,d]

[a]Department of Psychiatry and Medicine, UA College of Medicine, Tucson, AZ, United States, [b]Behavioral Sleep Medicine Clinic, Banner—University Medical Center Tucson, Tucson, AZ, United States, [c]Department of Psychological and Brain Sciences, University of Indiana, Bloomington, IN, United States, [d]Better Sleep Bloomington, Bloomington, IN, United States

Introduction

Cognitive Behavioral Therapy for Insomnia (CBT-I) has been evaluated over the past several decades and demonstrated efficacy at treating insomnia alone (Brasure et al., 2016; Doghramji, 2010; Pigeon, 2010; Qaseem et al., 2016; Riemann & Perlis, 2009; Siebern, Suh, & Nowakowski, 2012) and within the context of other comorbid conditions (Grandner & Perlis, 2015; Taylor et al., 2018; Tubbs, Khader, Fernandez, & Grandner, 2020; Wu, Appleman, Salazar, & Ong, 2015). It has shown long-term efficacy (Brasure et al., 2016; Siebern & Manber, 2010; van der Zweerde, Bisdounis, Kyle, Lancee, & van Straten, 2019) and benefits compared to or better than prescription medications (Smith et al., 2002). It is a highly effective treatment. However, it is not universally beneficial to all insomnia patients. Some patients come to clinic after having already tried CBT-I (or a version of it) and failed. This chapter is meant to serve as a guide for clinicians who are working with patients who have already tried (and failed) CBT-I. Perhaps it was the case that the therapy was not done properly; it may be the case that the therapy was done properly but the specific needs of the patient required some modification; or the issue was with the relationship

Adapting Cognitive Behavioral Therapy for Insomnia
https://doi.org/10.1016/B978-0-12-822872-2.00020-7

between the therapist and the patient. This chapter addresses these and other issues.

When CBT-I fails

The limitations of CBT-I in a real-world setting

For better or worse, there is typically no external structure such as a study protocol enforcing specific therapeutic procedures in real-world settings where CBT-I is delivered. Individual clinicians may make their own decisions regarding how they implement CBT-I, adapting it to the individual, reordering the delivery of treatment components, incorporating elements of behavioral activation, problem solving focused on PAP adherence, etc. This is often necessary to match the needs of a diverse patient population that is sometimes not represented in clinical trials. Certain comorbidities, especially when unstable, are often excluded, as are environmental factors. Untreated obstructive sleep apnea (OSA), broken positive airway pressure (PAP) equipment, treatment-refractory seizures, undiagnosed nocturnal epilepsy, alerting maintenance drugs for cancer (e.g., Anastrozole), and other situations may complicate treatment.

Session frequency and number can vary considerably in real world practice as well. This sometimes occurs in clinical trials, but trials typically have staff who are tasked with keeping participants on track. While treatment in both the real-world and in clinical trials is voluntary, rather than compulsory, there is often a greater commitment made by patients in clinical trials. Patients have a different sort of freedom in the real world, where typically no formal agreement has been made to keep medications stable or hold off pursuing alternative treatment strategies. In some cases, this sort of information may be readily available in a patient's chart, such as in the number of notes pertaining to CBT-I or notes documenting changes in prescription or over the counter medications. A frank and direct conversation about the commitment required to benefit from CBT-I (e.g., minimum of 4 biweekly sessions) may be warranted.

People seeking help for insomnia in the real world may vary considerably in their familiarity with CBT-I, ranging from those whose hypnotic prescribers have given them an ultimatum to those who have spent weeks or months researching CBT-I and seeking a trained clinician. Even those who have done research on CBT-I may have misconceptions that need to be corrected. Finally, patients have often tried a plethora of treatments, which may include behavioral recommendations that may be regarded by the patient as CBT-I, whether or not this is accurate.

When is CBT-I not indicated in the first place?

Although CBT-I is considered the first-line and gold-standard intervention for insomnia and has broad applicability across different settings, there are circumstances in which it is inadvisable or may need significant alteration so as to not negatively impact patients' health and well-being. The core components of CBT-I are sleep restriction and stimulus control, and contraindications for each of these components have been identified. Sleep restriction is not recommended in situations in which it is known or suspected that sleep deprivation could worsen other co-occurring disorders. Similarly, stimulus control is not recommended in circumstances in which it is not possible or would pose a significant risk to the patient to leave the bed or for patients with diminished cognitive capacity. In each of these circumstances, modifications can be made to sleep restriction or stimulus control in order to still provide some relief of insomnia to patients presenting for treatment. These will be discussed later in this chapter.

When does CBT-I fail?

CBT-I can fail for many reasons. Some of these reasons may relate to characteristic of the patient, and some may be driven by characteristics of the provider. Perhaps the therapist did not apply techniques correctly or perhaps they focused on techniques that were not well-matched to the patient (e.g., focusing on cognitive rather than behavioral approaches). Perhaps the patient was taking medications that interfered with progress or refused to adhere to recommendations. Perhaps patients were unable to complete a sleep diary or had a medical condition that interfered with sleep consolidation efforts. There are many possible reasons why CBT-I may fail. Some may not even be the fault of CBT-I itself. This chapter will discuss some of the reasons that CBT-I may fail and some of the adaptations and modifications—and also just considerations—that can inform providing compassionate and helpful clinical care.

Approaching patients who failed CBT-I

Approaching patients who mistook sleep hygiene for CBT-I

Sleep hygiene certainly has its place in public health, and the recommendations typically made in sleep hygiene education are largely supported by sleep research. In nonclinical populations, individuals who generally adhere to sleep hygiene recommendations have been observed to have better sleep (Irish, Kline, Gunn, Buysse, & Hall, 2015). The accessibility of sleep hygiene recommendations often means that this is the default first-line "treatment" that patients struggling with insomnia might encounter, particularly if they bring sleep concerns to a primary care visit or look online for potential solutions. However, it is also largely well-known that sleep hygiene is not effective as a treatment for chronic insomnia, and in many clinical trials of CBT-I, sleep hygiene is typically what is offered in the control condition.

Given that many of the recommendations made in sleep hygiene recommendations can be behavioral in nature (e.g., setting a sleep schedule, avoiding caffeine), it is not unusual for patients to appear hesitant when presented with the option for CBT-I. Patients may feel that they have already engaged in behavioral change, and often have implemented new habits in order to improve sleep (e.g., cutting down or eliminating caffeine, avoiding "blue" light). Clinically, in these circumstances, it can be useful to review the definition of "hygiene" and draw a similarity between other hygiene practices; these are meant to promote health and prevent disease or a clinical disorder. However, hygiene is not medicine. Although handwashing is good practice in general, can prevent infections and transmission of disease, and can even reduce disease impact, handwashing will not cure an infection.

Patients who are presenting for or are considering CBT-I have typically crossed the line from an occasional problem with sleep to an acute problem that will now require more aggressive treatment. Acknowledging the need for a higher level of care can often be validating for patients, particularly if they may have been sent away from previous medical visits with a handout of general sleep recommendations.

Approaching patients who have tried and failed online CBT-I

There are currently a wide range of online CBT-I offerings, ranging from well-validated automated and interactive treatment programs (e.g., Sleepio, SHUTi) to series of readings/videos that present standard CBT-I information, similar to a bibliotherapy approach. Despite the encouraging findings that have been reported in large samples of people with insomnia undertaking these programs (Cheng et al., 2019; Erten Uyumaz, Feijs, & Hu, 2021; Werner-Seidler, Johnston, & Christensen, 2018), they are not a panacea.

Opportunities to capitalize on prior attempts at online CBT-I include existing knowledge of sleep regulation and rationale for CBT-I components, prior experience with tracking sleep, and of course the advantage of knowing how to avoid pitfalls. In cases where corrections or adjustments need to be made, these can be times to attribute prior treatment failure to extrinsic factors, rather than to the patient, thus instilling hope for improvement.

To understand how to approach a patient who has failed online CBT-I, it is helpful to discern the reason for that treatment failure. The primary weaknesses may stem from a lack of interaction with an expert. These interactions are helpful in a number of ways, including personalizing explanations of sleep regulation and the rationale for specific interventions. There is an opportunity to personalize and adjust interventions. The most helpful approach in this regard is to consider each recommendation, its intended effect, and whether it is actually functioning in that manner. From unabating anxiety produced from sleep logs to frustration and anger engendered by imagery and journaling, there are many occasions in which face-valid and broadly useful recommendations can backfire. Patients may freely volunteer this information, but in other cases, a few questions about past experiences may reveal this sort of problem. In these cases, the goal is simply to find an effective method for an individual patient to track their sleep, relax, or decrease cognitive arousal.

There is also personal accountability in the context of a therapeutic relationship that is difficult to duplicate. Having another person to whom a patient is socially, personally accountable may influence behavior and adherence.

Finally, the simple act of having another human express accurate empathy and convey hope for the patient can be a powerful experience as compared to similar reassurances that may be perceived as platitudes. Humans are also uniquely suited for discussions of past strengths, successes, and values. These can all be employed to increase patients' confidence and motivation.

Approaching patients who have attempted CBT-I with a prior therapist and did not see benefit

Occasionally, patients who present for CBT-I will report that they have already attempted this therapy and did not have their treatment goals met. In this instance, it is beneficial to review with patients why therapy can fail in general.

One of the most common reasons therapy fails can be lack of "fit." There are several reasons to use manualized psychotherapies like CBT-I. These allow for the scientific study and empirical validation of therapies, help facilitate targeted treatments, and allow for broad dissemination of therapies (Wilson, 1996). Yet, even well-versed practitioners sometimes find that standard delivery of CBT-I is insufficient. This may be attributable to problems with the therapeutic alliance, lack of individualization of therapy, inappropriate patient expectations, lack of therapist experience, or the patient's stage of change at the time of therapy.

Additionally, there may be other factors that interfered in previous treatment that may have gone unassessed and unaddressed. A thorough evaluation of other sleep, medical, and psychiatric disorders may be necessary to rule out other conditions that may impact sleep. This may necessitate coordinating care with other providers. Assessment tools that are available to behavioral sleep medicine providers will be reviewed later in this chapter.

It can be useful to take the time to explore with the patient what, if any, benefits they noticed in their previous therapy experience and what, if anything, could make therapy successful or more helpful for them. This can be an opportunity to discuss a patient's current motivation for change via motivational interviewing (Lane & Rollnick, 2009; Miller & Rollnick, 2013). Key to motivational interviewing is the perspective that patients are active participants in their own care, working together with their provider to come up with a plan that they feel that they can execute, rather than a purely directive approach where the provider tells the patient what to do. Because of the efficacy of sleep restriction and stimulus control, it can be difficult for some practitioners to veer away or soften these approaches, but a practitioner's willingness to meet a patient where they are can be immensely helpful in moving patients toward their identified goals.

Approaching patients who have completed CBT-I but relapsed

Many individuals who participate in therapy of any kind may find themselves encountering a relapse of symptoms, and theories of behavior change often include relapse or risk of relapse as part of the model (Prochaska & DiClemente, 1982; Prochaska, DiClemente, & Norcross, 1992). In many ways, the patient experiencing a relapse of symptoms can be the best case scenario for a patient who has "failed" CBT-I because they have previously had a period of success.

For these patients, it can be useful to review the techniques that they previously utilized in the past, if they can recall these. In doing so, this may allow patients to contrast current behavior with what they had done when successfully addressing their sleep. It can also be helpful for patients to conceptualize relapse as something that occurred over time rather than a sudden event (Brandon, Vidrine, & Litvin, 2007), and then identifying antecedents to full relapse. Use of behavior chain analysis (Lynch, Chapman, Rosenthal, Kuo, & Linehan, 2006) can lay out the roadmap of relapse with a patient and can also be used to identify multiple ways a relapse can be prevented. See Fig. 1 for an example of this concept. This experience can be reframed for patients as a new strength gained in treatment: they can now identify potential areas of future relapse, and these patients may be more readily able to identify and avoid or address these in the future.

Specific strategies for addressing patients who have failed CBT-I

Instilling confidence and building rapport

Many patients who have found themselves unable to successfully complete CBT-I may feel discouraged. Perhaps they believe that CBT-I is ineffective, perhaps they feel that their therapist was not able to successfully

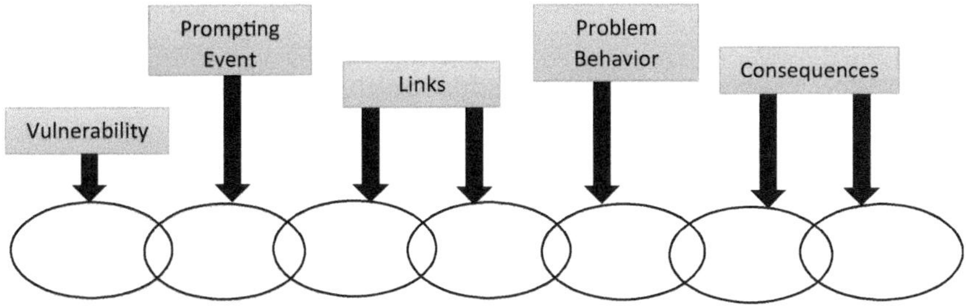

FIG. 1 A graphical representation of behavior chain analysis.

work with them or perhaps they did not think their needs were addressed. Frequently, when patients experience these uncomfortable situations, they face an uphill climb to therapeutic success because their expectations are aligned toward failure. For these patients, it is often advisable to eschew rapid initiation of treatment (even if the need may present as more urgent). In these situations, it is important to sacrifice some short-term efficiency in the service of overcoming some of these barriers. There is a well-established literature showing that rapport and therapeutic alliance are critically important to successful therapy (Baier, Kline, & Feeny, 2020). Although this is an important element of treatment, it is rather difficult to manualize. Still, there are some considerations that can facilitate the process. It is important to use the first session to listen to the patient describe not only their symptoms, but the emotional and cognitive reactions to their previous therapy experience. After listening to those experiences, the therapist can determine what needs the patient presents with and can reorient therapy in those directions.

For example, some patients who fail CBT-I believe that their sleep problems are special or unique or unusual and, more importantly, untreatable. These patients require reassurance that the therapist is skilled and will be able to navigate their complex presentation. These patients may be comforted by knowing that the therapist will be willing to get creative to solve their problems if the more obvious solutions (which were likely already tried) continue to fail. They may also be comforted by knowing that although their problems are certainly long-standing or "not a textbook case," the therapist has seen all these issues before and has helped people in similar situations.

For patients who have had unpleasant experiences within some aspect of the healthcare system, this is a good opportunity to empathize with the patient. The therapist can remind the patient that they themselves are a patient as well sometimes, and that they understand what it is like to be a patient at the mercy of the healthcare system. It can also be helpful to reassure the patient that you, the therapist, will fight for them on their behalf, be more flexible and understanding than they have experienced in the past, be more accessible than the system usually allows clinicians to be, etc. Whatever it is that was an important barrier, the therapist can take the empathic role and serve to reassure the patient that this relationship will be a partnership based on shared understanding, not hierarchical service delivery.

Some patients, on the other hand, would be reassured by a more concrete approach. Perhaps their previous experience was with a therapist that employed CBT-I in name but did not adhere to the treatment protocols. For these people, it may be comforting to know that this experience will be science-based, data-driven, and based on decades of peer-reviewed research. Often, patients who are wary of what they perceive to be a nonspecific or nondirected therapy are comforted to know that this approach is well-defined. For these people, introducing CBT-I as "less like psychotherapy and more like physical therapy" may help couch CBT-I in terms of a concrete, medically based processes where the body and brain learn to do a thing that cannot be taught except through shaping.

In addition to building confidence, the therapist should also focus specifically on building rapport with these patients. Since they have failed CBT-I in the past, the therapist will be asking the patient to trust them to do a thing that may not seem possible. And that trust requires a good working relationship that can withstand the likely obstacles and plateaus that arise with difficult patients. Wherever the patient is coming from, they should feel listened to, understood, and empathized with. They should believe that they are "in the right place" and are "being taken care of." This rapport will likely be tested, so the start of therapy is an important opportunity to build the working relationship and trust needed to persist through the difficult work of trying CBT-I again.

Considering additional assessment

Insomnia is an exceedingly heterogeneous condition. As it clinically presents as a subjective patient report, the underlying etiology can vary, and insomnia symptoms can coexist with a wide array of other clinical conditions (Grandner & Perlis, 2015). Fortunately, most of the time, CBT-I is well-equipped to handle this variability, even with relatively consistent methods (Wu et al., 2015). When the standard approach fails, however, there may be a need for additional assessment. Perhaps other sleep disorders are present, or there are behavioral, social, environmental, physiologic, or other contextual factors that are interfering with the ability of patients to successfully navigate treatment. For this reason, additional assessment may be warranted.

Typically, most CBT-I cases begin with an initial assessment that includes elements such as demographics, insomnia history, psychological/psychiatric history, medical and medication history, family and social history, and differential diagnosis (Perlis, Junquist, Smith, & Posner, 2005). Also, sleep diaries are standard for ongoing assessment (Abeln, Kleinert, Struder, & Schneider, 2014; Carney et al., 2012), and other self-report questionnaires such as the Insomnia Severity Index (Bastien, Vallieres, & Morin, 2001) are frequently used as tracking and outcome measures (Schutte-Rodin, Broch, Buysse, Dorsey, & Sateia, 2008). For patients with failed CBT-I, it may be useful to broaden this assessment approach to identify factors that need to be addressed prior to or during therapy.

First, consider otherwise unaddressed sleep disorders. This can be accomplished in a number of ways. For a broad overview of sleep disorders risk, several screening tools exist. The Sleep Disorders Symptom Checklist (SDSCL) is perhaps the briefest of these comprehensive assessments—it is a 25-item self-report questionnaire validated by Klingman, Jungquist, and Perlis (2017). It contains questions that address insufficient sleep, insomnia, daytime sleepiness, fatigue, circadian rhythm abnormalities, sleep apnea risk, restless legs syndrome, narcolepsy symptoms, bruxism, and daytime consequences. Other broad screening tools exist, including the General Sleep Assessment Questionnaire (Roth et al., 2002), SLEEP-50 (Spoormaker, Verbeek, van den Bout, & Klip, 2005), and the Structured Clinical Interview for Sleep Disorders (SCISD) (Taylor, Wilkerson, et al., 2018). The latter, in particular, is specifically designed for clinicians to administer and is similar to a sleep disorders version of the commonly used Structured Clinical Interview for the DSM (SCID) (First, Spitzer, Gibbon, & Williams, 1996).

When specific sleep disorders are suggested and a general clinical interview is too unclear, perhaps it would be useful to employ validated screening tools for suspected conditions. For example, the STOP-BANG questionnaire (Chung et al., 2012; Farney, Walker, Farney, Snow, & Walker, 2011; Silva, Vana, Goodwin, Sherrill, & Quan, 2011), Multivariable Apnea Prediction Index (MAPI) (Maislin et al., 1995), and Berlin Questionnaire (Netzer, Stoohs, Netzer, Clark, & Strohl, 1999) are useful for assessing risk of sleep apnea. The International Restless Legs Syndrome (IRLS) Scale (Allen, Kushida, Atkinson, & Consortium, 2003; Walters et al., 2003) is well-validated as are the Swiss Narcolepsy Scale (SNS) (Bargiotas et al., 2019) and the Ullanlinna Narcolepsy Scale (UNS) (Sarkanen, Alakuijala, & Partinen, 2019).

The Epworth Sleepiness Scale (ESS) (Johns, 1991, 1992, 1993; Smith et al., 2008) is a standard tool for quantifying daytime sleepiness, and scores can be differentiate from measures such as the Fatigue Severity Scale (FSS) (Krupp, LaRocca, Muir-Nash, & Steinberg, 1989) to discern sleepiness from fatigue. The impacts of sleep problems on quality of life can be assessed using the Functional Outcomes of Sleep Questionnaire (FOSQ) or the briefer FOSQ-10 (Chasens, Ratcliffe, & Weaver, 2009;

Weaver et al., 1997). For the assessment of general sleep habits and behaviors, the Sleep Timing Questionnaire (STQ) (Monk et al., 2003) may be useful for establishing the parameters of typical and atypical sleep schedules, and the Self-Assessment of Subjective Sleep (SASS) and companion weekday/weekend version (SASS-Y) may serve as helpful baseline measures of typical sleep patterns (Dietch, Sethi, Slavish, & Taylor, 2019).

Assessment of circadian factors can sometimes be accomplished using scales such as these, though other scales can capture circadian behavioral patterns and preferences, including the Munich Chronotype Questionnaire (MCQ) (Zavada, Gordijn, Beersma, Daan, & Roenneberg, 2005), which also has a brief version (uMCQ) (Ghotbi et al., 2020), the Horne-Ostberg Morningness-Eveningness Questionnaire (HOMEQ) (Horne & Ostberg, 1976), which also has a simpler version (Terman, Rifkin, Jacobs, & White, 2001), or the very brief Circadian Energy Scale (CIRENS) (Ottoni, Antoniolli, & Lara, 2011).

Contextual sleep factors may also be useful to assess. For example, sleep hygiene and other problematic beliefs and behaviors can be assessed using the Sleep Hygiene Index (SHI) (Mastin, Bryson, & Corwyn, 2006) and the Dysfunctional Beliefs About Sleep (DBAS) Scale (Morin, Vallieres, & Ivers, 2007). Other scales that assess sleep-related beliefs exist, including the Sleep Beliefs Scale (SBS) (Adan, Fabbri, Natale, & Prat, 2006) and the Pain-Related Beliefs and Attitudes About Sleep (PBAS) Scale (Afolalu, Moore, Ramlee, Goodchild, & Tang, 2016). Beliefs about an individual's ability to engage in healthy sleep behaviors (e.g., self-efficacy) can also be operationalized using the Brief Index of Sleep Control (BRISC) (Grandner et al., 2020), Self-Efficacy for Sleep Scale (SESS), Self-Efficacy Scale (SE Scale) for insomnia (Rutledge, La Guardia, & Bluestein, 2013), and the Sleep Locus of Control (SLOC) Scale (Vincent, Sande, Read, & Giannuzzi, 2004). Elements of the sleep environment that may be impacting sleep can be systematically assessed using the Assessment of Sleep Environment (ASE). The extensive Sleep Practices and Attitudes Questionnaire (SPAQ) (Grandner, Jackson, Gooneratne, & Patel, 2014) captures many of these elements and others, with subscales for sleep duration, sleep debt, sleep quality, sleepiness/tiredness, coping with sleepiness, coping with acute insomnia, coping with chronic insomnia, activities in bed, sleep environment, knowledge about sleep, importance of sleep, impact of external factors on Sleep, impact of sleep on daytime functioning, self-efficacy, sleep and health, and social norms.

Taken together, more assessment of habitual sleep-related symptoms, beliefs, practices, attitudes, consequences, barriers, facilitators, and context may be helpful in addressing elements that may have been previously missed. In summary, perhaps measures such as these can quantify aspects of the sleep experience that may be missed in a typical clinical interview and standard CBT-I approach. In addition to these self-report measures, it may be useful to also employ objective measures.

The use of objective sleep estimates in insomnia is a complex topic and is addressed to some degree in other chapters. However, it is worth mentioning that among patients who have failed CBT-I, there may be a reason to employ polysomnography and/or actigraphy. For these patients, these objective approaches may uncover otherwise undetected aspects of sleep and circadian physiology or behavior that may have been previously missed. Given the high rate of undiagnosed sleep disorders—especially sleep apnea (Peppard et al., 2013)—and the degree to which untreated sleep and circadian disorders may complicate CBT-I, this should be a consideration.

Regarding blood testing, a complete overview of blood measures that may be related to sleep problems is also outside the scope of this chapter. However, sometimes blood values can be helpful, including ferritin (for restless legs syndrome), thyroid measures, and measures suggestive of systemic inflammation.

In addition to these measures, clinicians may consider formal quantification of mental health conditions. This could include a more comprehensive assessment using a structured interview like the SCID (First et al., 1996) or the Mini International Neuropsychiatric Inventory (MINI) (Sheehan et al., 1998). It could also include screeners to detect clinically relevant psychiatric comorbidities, such as the PHQ9 depression scale (Spitzer, Kroenke, & Williams, 1999), GAD7 Anxiety Scale (Spitzer, Kroenke, Williams, & Lowe, 2006), Clinician-Administered PTSD Scale (CAPS) (Weathers et al., 2018), Yale-Brown Obsessive Compulsive Scale (YBOCS) (Goodman et al., 1989), or others. It may also be useful to capture subclinical symptoms using a measure such as the Positive and Negative Affect Scales (PANAS) (Watson, Clark, & Tellegen, 1988).

Assessment of physical health conditions may be outside the scope of practice of most CBT-I clinicians, but scales such as the Systematic Assessment of Treatment Emergent Effects (SAFTEE) (Clyde, 1986; Guy, Wilson, Brooking, & Fjetland, 1987; Guy, Wilson, Brooking, Manov, & Fjetland, 1986; Jacobson, Goldstein, Dominguez, & Steinbook, 1986, 1987; Levine, 1987; Levine & Schooler, 1984, 1986; Markowitz et al., 1987; Rabkin & Markowitz, 1986; Rabkin, Markowitz, Ocepek-Welikson, & Wager, 1992) could serve to quantify physical symptoms and a detailed medical history be useful for detecting conditions that may be related to sleep health that were overlooked. In cases where there are questions about accurate diagnoses, clinicians can differentiate where official diagnoses are made versus just suspected. In this vein, a detailed family medical history may also be useful.

Dealing with medications

Many patients come into the clinic with a history of using medications to ameliorate insomnia symptoms. In most cases, these attempts have been unsuccessful but sometimes medications are helping, but the patient still wishes to either more completely reduce symptoms or reduce reliance on medications. Prior medication use can complicate CBT-I, though the scope of this is outside the present chapter. Briefly, patients who have had some success with medications may be pessimistic about the benefits of a therapeutic approach that seems less immediate and concrete.

Also, medications can complicate treatment. Some medications may have side effects that conflict with therapy, and some may cause sedation during the night. Although sedation may be desired in these cases in general, pharmacologic sedation can interfere with stimulus control and maintenance of scheduled bedtimes. In any case, it is important to stay within scope of practice boundaries. Often, this may include collaboration with a prescribing physician. Often, this physician has little or no training in insomnia pharmacotherapy—they are often primary care, psychiatry, or other clinicians who are attempting to help patients who are very receptive to collaboration with a sleep specialist who has experience working with insomnia.

Developing and maintaining these relationships throughout treatment is important. As patients may have difficulty re-engaging with CBT-I, it is important to have an open line of communication with the prescribing physician, so that treatment can be coordinated.

Sometimes sedating medications can interfere with CBT-I. When patients are pharmacologically sedated, they may have difficulty staying awake until a prescribed bedtime. Also, they may have difficulty adhering to a scheduled wake time as well. Often, insomnia patients taking medication still experience awakenings. And sedated patients who experience awakenings may experience these events as especially disorienting and uncomfortable. This may make it difficult to follow stimulus control instructions, which involve awareness of time passing, getting out of bed, and engaging in alternative activities. In these cases, it is important to work with the prescribing physician to optimize the timing and dose of prescription medications so that one treatment is not sabotaging another. One specific suggestion for dealing with the morning sedation that remains after hypnotic use would be to reinforce healthy morning routines, including using light and movement to send a daytime signal to counteract the residual sleepiness.

Alerting medications can also complicate treatment. Many medications can cause sleep difficulties, especially among patients who already are predisposed to hyperarousal. Many patients, though, are taking alerting medications. Sometimes, these are antidepressants with known alerting effect, sometimes these are stimulants for attention deficit disorders, etc. In all of these cases, the timing of medication use is important to consider. Working with the patient and provider to strategically consider dose and administration time in terms of ability to initiate sleep may help facilitate sleep at night. For example, taking medications earlier, or having a cutoff time after which alerting medications should not be taken, could mitigate some of the insomnogenic effects of these medications.

When sleep restriction is not advisable

Although sleep restriction is a core component of traditional CBT-I, it cannot be applied equally in all patient presentations. In some instances, sleep restriction can be contraindicated. For example, for those with sleep disordered breathing (SDB) and other parasomnias, sleep restriction could increase the likelihood of breathing-related events and other sleep problems. It is well-documented that sleep deprivation can precipitate a manic episode among patients diagnosed with bipolar disorder. Other medical conditions, such as epilepsy, can be exacerbated by a reduction in sleep. Additionally, the presentation of a patient's insomnia may also lead a clinician to avoid use of sleep restriction. Among patients who experience consistent early morning awakenings, sleep restriction may be of limited benefit.

With these patients, it is often necessary to pivot to other techniques. One technique is sleep compression (Lichstein, Thomas, & McCurry, 2011; Riedel, Lichstein, & Dwyer, 1995). With sleep compression, rather than reducing a patient's time in bed to be closer to their subjective documentation of total sleep time from sleep diaries, a patient's time in bed is gradually reduced by 15–30 min increments until sleep efficiency meets or exceeds 85%–90% and then gradually increasing time in bed again if necessary. This approach is also often helpful with patients who express a great deal of concern or anxiety about a sleep restriction approach.

Sleep scheduling—that is, recommending a time for sleep and wake—can also be helpful in among patients who struggle with a disorganized sleep schedule. This approach does not intend to restrict or compress the sleep schedule, but simply to help a patient become more regular with their sleep. This is a technique that can be utilized for patients who do not have a regular sleep/wake time as is often found in patients who have a co-diagnosis of serious mental illness.

When patients have difficulty getting out of bed

Stimulus control is another core component of CBT-I (Bootzin & Epstein, 2000; Bootzin, Smith, Franzen, & Shapiro, 2010; Harsh & Badia, 1991) that may not be applicable to all patients presenting for therapy.

Stimulus control is not advised when a patient is disabled or cannot get out of bed unassisted. Similarly, it is not uncommon that patients presenting for CBT-I are currently on sleep or other sedating medications, and care must be taken as these patients are at higher risk for falls when leaving the bed during middle of the night awakenings. Additionally, among the elderly, particularly those taking these medications, stimulus control may be inadvisable because of risk of a fall or injury.

Stimulus control in CBT-I serves to reinforce the bed as a discriminative stimulus for sleep. This conditioning is built by using the bed only for sleep, and leaving the bed when a patient has extended periods (e.g., 30 min) of wakefulness. In counter control (Zwart & Lisman, 1979), the patient does not leave the bed but instead engages in a behavior that is not compatible with sleep (e.g., reading). Once the patient begins to feel sleepy, they can attempt to resume sleep. This technique has been found to be particularly helpful for sleep maintenance insomnia (Zwart & Lisman, 1979) as well as with older adults (Davies, Lacks, Storandt, & Bertelson, 1986).

When patients have difficulty adhering to a schedule

Some patients have difficulty adhering to a prescribed schedule. This can occur for many reasons. In some cases, patients' daily lives are disrupted by external forces that preclude regular schedules. For example, an individual may be "on call" for work or caregiving responsibilities that make reliable scheduling difficult. Or perhaps their schedule is reliable but variable—for example, perhaps someone needs to wake up extra early (like at 4:00 AM) a couple of days per week for work. It would probably not be feasible to keep this awakening time 7 days a week while also maintaining adherence and morale.

Adapting approaches to variable schedules out of the patient's control is possible. One approach would be to have a planned schedule that takes the expected variability into account. In the case of unplanned variability (such as someone "on call"), a planned nap that is not too long or too late on days where sleep is interrupted can help maintain regular bed and wake times. Or, if the interruption happens often enough, it could be treated as any other awakening and stimulus control (getting out of bed and not trying to sleep) could be followed. The main difference is that this awakening does not represent a failure of sleep ability. So the sleep opportunity could be artificially expanded to account for these times. As long as there is enough time budgeted for the patient to achieve adequate opportunity for sleep (within their ability), this could be planned for.

Another reason that people may have difficulty adhering to schedules is it may be a stressful experience. A sense of psychological independence may become threatened when an external force like a therapist imposes a set schedule. Some people will naturally rebel against any imposed restrictions; for some, it will be about control (e.g., feeling even less control of a situation that already feels out of control); for some, it will be about fear (e.g., fear of not getting enough sleep if recommendations are followed); and for some, it may be about an inability to organize time (e.g., making excuses for not adhering to the plan because other things need doing). Some patients have an extreme difficulty keeping a regular wake time in particular. Some patients are just unable to adhere to a fixed schedule. Either they do not have access to clocks or alarms, or they have a particular aversion to them, or they have difficulty with time. Some people have difficulty following a regular schedule because they do not understand the purpose of it. They may need additional education and explanation about why the regularity of schedules in CBT-I is important.

What patients have difficulty adhering to a schedule, CBT-I can be very difficult. The therapist should take steps to identify what the specific difficulties are, and whether they can be reasonably accommodated. For example, patients who have an unreliable schedule may be able to build a set of recommendations that accommodates this. Or patients that have psychological reasons why adhering is difficult can address those issues of fear and control. And those who just do not understand the purpose of this can learn more about the various ways in which a regular schedule helps promote sleep, by incorporating regularity, using time as a cue for sleep, and leveraging circadian rhythms and duration of wakefulness.

When nighttime awakenings persist

For some patients, sleep restriction, stimulus control, and other CBT-I techniques do not eliminate nighttime awakenings. Perhaps these patients do not have sufficient sleep pressure to maintain sleep across the night. Perhaps there is enough of an alerting signal that the homeostatic sleep pressure is not sufficient for maintaining sleep. Or perhaps a combination of these factors result in awakenings. There are many patients who, even after engaging in therapy, still experience extended awakenings at night. In these cases, perhaps attempts to eliminate the awakenings will not be successful. An alternative approach is to engage a form of paradoxical intention.

In the traditional paradoxical intention approach (Bootzin & Perlis, 1992; Espie, 2011), the therapist instructs the patient to stay awake as long as they can. This eliminates the performance anxiety associated with insomnia and replaces the feeling of not being able to sleep with the feeling of not being able to stay awake. It also serves to increase next-day homeostatic sleep pressure via sleep restriction. In the case of treatment-resistant nocturnal awakenings, a form of paradoxical intention can be helpful.

In the case when patients reliably have an extended awakening on the majority of nights, the therapist can instruct the patient to learn to identify which awakenings are going to result in quick return to sleep and which are not. Usually, this is consistent with stimulus control instructions (e.g., if awake for a certain amount of time, get out of bed). In many cases, though, patients will know very quickly (sometimes immediately) whether an awakening will be brief or extended. In some cases, patients will wake up to use the bathroom and have trouble returning to sleep. In any of these cases, patients should be instructed to get out of bad as soon as they know that the awakening will be prolonged. This could be immediately upon awakening or before returning to bed after using the bathroom. As soon as the patient knows they will not quickly return to sleep, they should get up.

Once out of bed, the patient is instructed to set a timer for the typical length of their awakenings, or, preferably, a longer time frame than is typical. For example, if the patient is usually awake for 1 h, they can set the alarm for 1 h, but it may be preferable to increase this to 90 min. The patient is then instructed that they are forbidden from returning to bed until the alarm goes off, even if they are very tired. Once they return to bed, preferably under higher than normal sleep pressure, they resume sleep quickly. Over time, the time window for the alarm can be gradually reduced until the least intrusive amount of time is identified that reliably ends with a quick return to sleep. Then, these awakenings can be planned for and budgeted for in bed and wake time schedules.

When sleep fragmentation limits progress

CBT-I is often very effective at treating insomnia, even in the context of comorbidities (Wu et al., 2015). This is also true when the comorbidities frequently accompany sleep fragmentation, such as sleep apnea, fibromyalgia, and chronic pain. However, CBT-I is often ineffective at eliminating sleep fragmentation. As a therapeutic modality, the increased sleep pressure and conditioned responses may help facilitate better sleep continuity, but it is often the case that patients still experience many awakenings during the night. CBT-I has limited efficacy at reducing these awakenings. For example, older adults will naturally wake up more during the night (Ohayon, Carskadon, Guilleminault, & Vitiello, 2004) for a wide range of reasons. Often, even after completing CBT-I, people with shallow, fragmented sleep may still experience too-frequent awakenings.

For these patients, perhaps a reframing of treatment goals away from limiting awakenings might be beneficial. For example, treatment could focus on reducing the impact of these awakenings, making them as brief and unobtrusive as possible. Perhaps the original cause of this fragmentation could be identified and ameliorated. Untreated sleep apnea is a common cause of sleep fragmentation (Moore, Bardwell, Ancoli-Israel, & Dimsdale, 2001). Other sleep disorders that cause sleep fragmentation might also be undiagnosed, such as narcolepsy, hypersomnia disorders, parasomnias, nocturnal movement disorders, and others. In addition, other medical conditions like chronic pain, autoimmune conditions, and other conditions can cause sleep fragmentation. Sometimes treating these conditions can alleviate the awakenings. Sleep fragmentation can also arise from external sources. External sounds (like a snoring bedpartner), movement (like from a pet in the bed), light (from streetlights), or other sensory input can interfere with sleep depth. From a patient perspective, sometimes patients are unable to even identify these environmental sources of disturbance. In the case of a light sleeper, it may aid treatment to insulate the sleeper with ear plugs or eye masks, or other barriers to these stimuli.

For patients who still experience too many awakenings during the night, treatment could focus on getting people back to sleep quickly, but in some cases even this is difficult. For these patients, it may be more beneficial to reorient treatment goals to improving daytime functioning and keeping the experience of nighttime awakenings as manageable as possible. The most common daytime effects of sleep fragmentation are daytime fatigue (Levy & Pepin, 2003; Stepanski, Lamphere, Badia, Zorick, & Roth, 1984). If the fragmentation itself cannot be reduced, perhaps the daytime symptoms can be mitigated.

Returning to first principles

Fundamental aspects of how insomnia is treated in CBT-I include increasing homeostatic sleep pressure, regularizing circadian rhythm, reducing conditioned arousal, addressing inaccurate/unhelpful beliefs about sleep, reducing arousal, and improving sleep hygiene. Manualized approaches often dictate a specific order in which to address these targets, as well as how to do so with specific interventions.

One of the main advantages of treatment provided by a behavioral sleep medicine expert is the ability to personalize and prioritize intervention components. These components should be chosen according to their ability to address key aspects of a case conceptualization. For example, a patient with rigid beliefs about a need for 8 h of sleep per night may benefit from cognitive therapy techniques before being able to even engage in standard behavioral interventions such as sleep restriction therapy and stimulus control instructions.

Keeping in mind the hypothesized mediators of CBT-I should be the foundation of any personalized application of CBT-I. The initial evaluation of a patient with insomnia should reveal some key contributing factors, such as excess time in bed, cognitive arousal, sleep-related worry, sleep effort, etc. These can be explained to the patient at the end of the evaluation to get buy-in and start explaining the rationale for treatment components. This is likely to be the first opportunity to begin to contrast prior CBT-I attempts with the current approach.

As previously mentioned, certain treatment components can have deleterious effects in isolated cases. For example, Kendall, Hudson, Gosch, Flannery-Schroeder, and Suveg (2008) discuss how in the case of CBT for anxiety in children, some children become very anxious in response to progressive muscle relaxation. In these cases, they recommend substituting imagery or breathing exercises. Each of these are distinctly different interventions, but all tap into the broader construct of relaxation, which consists of interconnected domains including both cognitive and somatic relaxation, as well as more specific subsets of these broad categories. The example of relaxation can be directly applied to past CBT-I failure, as prior CBT-I efforts may have included unpalatable relaxation exercises. The broader point Kendall and colleagues make is regarding multiple techniques that can evoke the intended effect.

An important counterpoint to the above is that excessive flexibility can lead to treatment bending so much in response to patients' anxiety that the treatment is broken. A common concern among CBT clinicians is avoiding colluding with avoidance, the tendency to want to slow down interventions that evoke anxiety in patients. Compassionately pushing through the anxiety can lead to more rapid improvements in symptoms and self-efficacy than may be obtained with slower progressive steps. However, this laudable goal should in turn be tempered by the maxim that perfect is the enemy of good. Making slow progress with a patient is universally preferable to making zero progress as a result of a patient simply dropping out of treatment because they find it terrifying. If dropping out because of treatment-related anxiety is the reason for past treatment failure, then clinicians would do well to avoid repeating the same doomed efforts.

Common examples of flexibility include relatively benign substitutions of one relaxation strategy for another, but also adjustments of behavioral components that are often considered to be critical to the success of CBT-I, such as sleep restriction and stimulus control. Both sleep restriction and stimulus control function to increase sleep drive, reduce time in bed, reduce sleep effort, and stabilize circadian rhythms through fixed wake time. Fortunately, there is evidence to suggest that sleep compression is effective intervention for insomnia (Lichstein et al., 2011; McCurry, Logsdon, Teri, & Vitiello, 2007; Riedel et al., 1995), and that both sleep restriction and stimulus control instructions are effective single-component interventions for insomnia (Chesson Jr. et al., 1999; Morin et al., 1999).

Other cases of paradoxical effects of face-valid recommendations or practices include anxiety-inducing evening prayers, avoiding electronic screens, and multistep evening wind down schedules that preclude valued or pleasurable activities. Sleep diaries deserve a special mention. Many clinicians and researchers regard sleep diaries as absolutely essential to CBT-I, and sleep diaries are recommended as a standard measure for assessment of insomnia and its response to treatment (Morin & Espie, 2003). Further, self-monitoring alone can help provide patients with a new, more functional view of their sleep. However, sleep diaries can also provoke significant anxiety and increased attention on sleep, essentially promoting clockwatching (with or without a timepiece). This is a common experience that often lasts only a few nights, but in other cases can continue without sign of remission.

Since sleep diaries have little intrinsic value and have little real purpose in the long term (except perhaps in the context of a return of insomnia symptoms), the pragmatic clinician may choose to substantially decrease the number of items tracked or rely solely on retrospective recollections of sleep in between sessions. Simplifications of a daily sleep diary may include tracking adherence (e.g., wake time) and more simplified measures of sleep initiation/maintenance problems (e.g., >30 min, or subjectively "too long"). While lower precision may prevent perfect calculation of sleep efficiency and thus prevent highly precise titration of time in bed, none of these are required for behavioral treatment of insomnia. For example, stimulus control instructions do not require a sleep diary, and decisions about time in bed titration in BBTI (another effective treatment for insomnia (Buysse et al., 2011)) are made based on the number of nights with SOL or WASO greater than 30 min.

Working with difficult patients

Why patients can be difficult

Difficult patients can take many forms. This can include rudeness directed at other staff and clinicians, timely arrival to appointments, frequent cancelations, excessive verbosity or minimal verbal interaction, distractions in session, direct treatment refusal, intoxication, insults, and even harassment, stalking, or physical violence. All of these can lead to failing CBT-I. The reasons for these sorts of behavior include high distress, complex or high demands on patients in their home or work lives, comorbid psychological or substance use disorders, seeking primary or secondary gains, or malintent.

The simplest, though not easiest problems to address are related to behaviors that violate the law or hospital/clinic policies. In these cases, treatment should be terminated and patients should be barred from the treatment facility. Sleep labs, rather than outpatient provision of CBT-I, may be a more common setting for certain problems due to fewer staff present, necessity of changing into bedclothes, and the stimulus value of the bed. Clinicians of any sort, including those providing CBT-I are under no obligation to be subjected to harassment, intimidation, or assault. Referrals may need to be provided to other clinicians should the patient wish to pursue continued treatment elsewhere. Legal remedies need not violate confidentiality in many circumstances, since the patient's behavior is at issue, and reporting these behaviors does not require disclosing that the individual was a patient or anything about their particular diagnoses or treatment. However, it may be beneficial to seek advice from a lawyer or liability insurance provider in these unpleasant and rare circumstances.

Another reason for difficulty behavior with a poor prognosis is seeking CBT-I (or any other treatment) for primary or secondary gains—assuming the sick role or in order to obtain some other benefit. In the case of seeking primary gains through assuming the sick role, this may not be a conscious effort on the part of the patient. In the case of secondary gains, it may be more likely that this is a conscious process. In either case, there is an incentive not to improve. While primary gains are relatively straightforward, being related to assumption of the sick role, secondary gains can be more varied. There may be certain accommodations being made for the patient because of their sleep problem (e.g., allowing late arrival to work or working from home) or lack of improvement during CBT-I may be a condition for accommodations or for pursuing pharmacotherapy for insomnia. In the case of secondary gains, there may be some benefit to discussion of the patient's personal values and whether improving their sleep may in fact bring them closer to their personal goals.

Comorbid psychological disorders can result in various problems, including canceling or arriving late to appointments, having a short temper, or arguing with staff. These often relate to an increased level of distress, low motivation, and anticipatory anxiety. Other chapters address how to modify CBT-I in these cases. In general, making patient feel heard and understood (see next section), along with instilling hope for the future and displaying confidence in the patient may be helpful.

Substance use disorders present unique challenges, since most commonly used recreational psychoactive substances have effects on sleep/wake systems during both intoxication and withdrawal. Intoxication in session is also likely to impair the patient's ability to engage in treatment. Setting boundaries regarding intoxication in session may help, though it is likely that patients who are intoxicated at outpatient visits need substance-focused treatment.

Factors related to the patient's home, social, educational, and occupational environment may significantly interfere with treatment and may not have been detected in previous CBT-I treatment, even in a one-on-one setting with a clinician. These can include to heating and air conditioning problems resulting in bedroom temperatures far outside the range of comfort, constant noise and interruptions by others in the home, nighttime communications with significant others in different time zones, daytime activities that extend late in the night and preclude adequate time to wind down before bed, frequent urgent deadlines, and acrimonious relationships with one's bedpartner, spouse, children, etc. These issues may not be readily apparent due to clinicians not asking and patients not volunteering this information. Patient motivations may range from not understanding the relevance of a problem (e.g., believing a hot bedroom is just a minor comfort consideration) or shame in discussing or revealing a problem (e.g., abuse by a family member). These patients may present as difficulty due to frustration in their lack of progress, which is not understandable by the clinician if the patient's full context is not clear. In some of these cases, the problem can be remedied (e.g., climate modifications), but in other cases referral may be warranted, such as in the case of significant acrimony in the patient's marriage or family.

Rigid thinking that interferes with acceptance of treatment interventions or their basic premises will no doubt impede CBT-I. In these cases, education about sleep/wake regulation, efficacy of CBT-I, and recommendations of CBT-I from prominent organizations may be of some help. In other cases, cognitive therapy techniques may be helpful in reducing all or nothing thinking. Examples include recollections of the frequency of obtaining 8 h of sleep in the patient's past coupled with presumably adequate functioning or engaging in behavioral experiments that directly test patients' rigid beliefs (Harvey & Talbot, 2011). While some patients may not be willing to engage in behavioral experiments, such an experiment can be unilaterally initiated by the clinician through abstaining from recommendations (allowing the patient to "test" their preferred method) or terminating treatment and referring the patient to a clinician more in line with their stated preferences. This type of intervention should be handled carefully and generally framed as a way to honor the patient's beliefs, rather than creating an opportunity for the patient to fail. Displaying genuine curiosity, interest, and hope for success of these experiments can decrease the likelihood that the patient perceives the clinician as not taking them seriously.

Patients who seek out CBT-I at the suggestion or demand of others may be relatively difficult to engage in treatment, particularly if they have failed CBT-I in the past. Like any patient who finds treatment foisted upon them, it is incumbent upon the clinician to build rapport, connect with the patient, and resolve ambivalence before moving forward with treatment. Past failure of CBT-I may be due to an overly hurried approach by a clinician that led to low adherence or lack of follow up. Attention to the stages of change and intervening with motivational interviewing in early stages is likely to be more helpful than providing directives to patient who is not ready to follow through on them.

When patients feel like they are not heard

In cognitive behavioral therapy generally, rapport is considered to be necessary, if not sufficient, for treatment to be effective. Feeling unheard is almost certain to negatively impact rapport, faith in the efficacy of treatment, and motivation to adhere to treatment recommendations including staying in treatment. For these reasons, it is critical to ensure that patients feel heard. Basic clinical skills such as reflections and summaries are helpful and should be used strategically to maintain rapport and demonstrate that we, as the clinicians, are hearing our patients. Probably the most important concepts to reflect are that the patient is miserable, nothing they have tried has worked, that there are very real consequences to their insomnia, and that CBT-I interventions can seem daunting and possibly hopeless. Beyond simply reflecting all the reasons to stay the same (sustain talk), it is important to evoke change talk in those patients who are especially demoralized.

Motivational Interviewing (Lane & Rollnick, 2009; Miller & Rollnick, 2013) provides clear guidance on how to do this. For example, "It's been a constant struggle for you to sleep so poorly at night, which fills your days with anxiety. Then, after your first attempt at CBT-I left you feeling even worse, it's hard to see how this time will be different. At the same time, you've come to the clinic today—which wasn't easy—because it's important to you to get better and you're not the sort of person who gives up." By reflecting the patient's difficulties and concerns, the patient is likely to feel heard. By ending with a statement that includes affirmations and reasons for change, the patient is more likely to continue speaking about those points.

Sometimes, however, feeling unheard can mean that a patient is feeling that they do not have a say in their treatment. If a patient voices a concern, but that concern has no effect on treatment, then a reflection may be insufficient. At this point, it may be helpful to explain rationale, explain alternatives and their drawbacks, and offer the patient an option. For example, in a discussion of sleep restriction, it may help to explain that, while the first weeks are most difficult, things subsequently become easier, which most people tend to prefer, and either offer alternatives behavioral approaches that can increase sleep drive such as stimulus control or sleep compression, or to ask the patient whether they have an idea of what sort of alternative may be better.

When patients do not believe in therapy

Some patients do not believe in therapy. There are many cultural barriers, unhelpful attitudes, or other sources of resistance. The complete list of reasons why some people do not believe in or trust therapy is beyond the scope of this chapter. However, fortunately, CBT-I can be very helpful for these patients. Some patients lost their optimism in the benefits of CBT-I because perhaps it was not applied well (e.g., focusing on unhelpful elements of insomnia treatment) or maybe it was applied well but was not flexible in the face of situational demands. Either way, this could lead to pessimism.

When approaching a patient who does not believe in therapy, there are two potential approaches that may help. First, for patients who do not believe in psychotherapy in general, therapists can emphasize the behavioral and "training" elements of CBT-I rather than the cognitive elements. Perhaps this focus on more concrete, tangible issues will assuage fears about something that is too much like their idea of psychotherapy for their comfort. Second, for patients who do not believe in therapy because of their past failures, therapists can emphasize how their approach will be different from what occurred in the past. For those who experienced a strict adherence to protocols, suggesting that this time will be more flexible may be comforting. For those who experienced an unhelpful therapist or had an unpleasant reaction to the therapeutic experience, the therapist can stress how, specifically, this therapeutic relationship will be different and will learn from what caused the previous attempt to be unsuccessful.

When patients feel like they are being taken advantage of

Some patients may feel like the therapist is taking advantage of them. This sometimes occurs with self-pay patients looking to minimize the amount they need to pay. Patients sometimes feel like they are treated more like billing codes than people. In these cases, it is especially important to take time to build rapport and trust. These patients need to feel heard and, most important, they need to feel like their needs are being met. It is the job of a therapist in this situation to identify what the needs and expectations of the patient are and help that patient see that their own goals are aligned with the therapist's goals.

When patients have trouble understanding therapy

While some patients presenting for CBT-I may be seeking therapy after doing their own research about addressing sleep concerns, many patients presenting for treatment may be referred by primary care providers, sleep medicine providers, other therapists, or other specialty care. Some patients may have difficulty understanding how CBT-I works or how it might apply to them. Often this can be attributable to low health literacy, the ability to seek out, think through, and understand health information. Low health literacy is particularly low among older adults, minority and immigrant populations, those of low socioeconomic status, and medically underserved populations. Thus, ensuring that patients understand CBT-I when they present for treatment can be an important way to address health disparities.

In order to make CBT-I accessible and understandable for as many patients who present for therapy, several steps can be taken. When providing psychoeducation and assisting patients with specific recommendations, it is important to use simple language and short sentences. Jargon should be avoided or defined when used. When available, supplemental materials should be used. These can include handouts, videos, pictures, and examples or metaphors to help convey information. When information is provided, a teach back method can be used in which patients are asked open ended questions to see if they retained the content conveyed. Important therapeutic points should be repeated. If possible, CBT-I psychoeducation and recommendations should be provided in the patient's primary language.

Summary and recommendations

Although CBT-I is an effective therapeutic modality, many patients do not benefit. Some of those patients return to clinic or seek out another provider. As a clinician, when approaching a patient who has previously failed CBT-I, consider the following:

1. CBT-I is not always indicated and perhaps this patient is not appropriate for CBT-I and should be considered for another treatment modality.
2. Patients sometimes believe that they have tried CBT-I in the past when, in fact, they only attempted other non-medication approaches like sleep hygiene. Perhaps they did not fail CBT-I after all.
3. Not all applications of CBT-I are performed correctly according to guidelines and/or the needs of the patient. It is possible that the previous provider either did not actually follow CBT-I guidelines (despite believing they did so, due perhaps to lack of proper training) or perhaps they did so too rigidly and the approach was not compatible with the patient in some way.
4. Further assessment may be warranted to identify other underlying sleep disorders, medical conditions, or other aspects of their condition that may have impacted treatment outcome.

5. Having previously failed CBT-I, patients may have unhelpful attitudes and beliefs about therapy in general, therapists in general, the healthcare system, and CBT-I in particular. Addressing these attitudes and beliefs should become part of the therapeutic approach.
6. Patients may have had previous experiences with healthcare providers that left them feeling unheard or unappreciated. They may also be feeling hopeless or at least apprehensive about initiating therapy. These and other sources of emotional resistance could be met by focusing on therapeutic alliance, rapport, and establishing a working relationship at the outset.
7. Sometimes minor modifications to CBT-I approaches can be highly beneficial to patients for whom previous approaches have had suboptimal success. To the degree to which these modifications are situational and not strictly evidence-based, adopting a collaborative approach with patients and communicating transparently about the likelihood that some of these modifications may not always work may help maintain therapeutic alliance (Table 1).
8. For patients who approach CBT-I with pessimism about the therapy, the provider, or the intractability of their sleep problems, it is critical to maintain an open, transparent, and communicative relationship with the patient, so that they are invested as a partner in their insomnia treatment. It is important that their concerns are heard and addressed, so that they are optimally prepared for doing the work required for treatment success.

TABLE 1 Adaptation of Cognitive Behavioral Therapy for Insomnia (CBT-I) for people who failed previous CBT-I.

CBT-I components	Standard practice	CBT-I adaptations for people who failed CBT-I
Sleep education	3-P model, 2-process model of sleep regulation, sleep stages	– Address misconceptions and gaps left by previous therapy – Focus on aspects of sleep physiology that concern their specific problem; expand information about aspects of sleep–wake regulation, circadian rhythms, or other areas that may pertain to their unique situation
Sleep restriction	Improve sleep efficiency by limiting time in bed to amount of time sleeping then expanding slowly as long as sleep efficiency is preserved	– Consider sleep compression or other modifications – Alternatively, consider a back-to-basic approach if previous modification attempts failed

Continued

TABLE 1 Adaptation of Cognitive Behavioral Therapy for Insomnia (CBT-I) for people who failed previous CBT-I—cont'd

CBT-I components	Standard practice	CBT-I adaptations for people who failed CBT-I
Stimulus control	Associate bed/bedroom solely as a cue for sleep by eliminating non-sleep activities from the bedroom. Instruction to get out of bed at night if awake >15 min	– Increase education and buy-in regarding stimulus control – Consider activities for what to do when out of bed – Consider planned awakenings or planned awakening durations – Consider counter-control for patients who are not able to leave the bed
Napping/ daytime sleep	Discontinue or restrict daytime napping to 30 min	– Consider allowing naps if not too long or too late
Sleep hygiene education	Address daytime habits and sleep environment interfering with sleep	– Address limitations of sleep hygiene – Consider alternative strategies for reducing barriers
Cognitive therapy	Challenge patient's dysfunctional beliefs interfering with sleep and misconceptions about sleep. Replace/restructure to more helpful and realistic thoughts about sleep	– Address dysfunctional beliefs and attitudes about CBT-I itself – Focus on building and nurturing a therapeutic alliance – Use empathy to identify worries and pessimistic beliefs – Use evidence from therapy to support helpful beliefs and attitudes about CBT-I
Relaxation and meditation techniques	Relaxation can help reduce racing thoughts/tension that accompany lying in bed awake, and may include: deep breathing, progressive muscle relaxation, guided imagery, biofeedback, hypnosis, autogenic training, and meditation practices	– Consider which previously used relaxation techniques have been unsuccessful and attempt alternatives – Consider whether to focus on mind, body, or mind–body techniques based on the presentation of arousal problems
Relapse prevention	Discuss practicing less rigid sleep plan over time and what do to prevent sleep disturbance from turning into another episode of insomnia in the future	– Reinforce realistic expectations – Recognize that some insomnia cases are difficult and problems may recur, and that the therapist will be there as a "safety net"
Sleep diaries	Establish baseline sleep patterns, track progress, reinforce appropriate behavior change, problem solve obstacles to adherence	– Consider modifying or adopting alternative strategies for sleep tracking – Provide additional support for completing sleep diaries if needed

References

Abeln, V., Kleinert, J., Struder, H. K., & Schneider, S. (2014). Brainwave entrainment for better sleep and post-sleep state of young elite soccer players—A pilot study. *European Journal of Sport Science, 14*(5), 393–402. https://doi.org/10.1080/17461391.2013.819384.

Adan, A., Fabbri, M., Natale, V., & Prat, G. (2006). Sleep beliefs scale (SBS) and circadian typology. *Journal of Sleep Research, 15*(2), 125–132. https://doi.org/10.1111/j.1365-2869.2006.00509.x.

Afolalu, E. F., Moore, C., Ramlee, F., Goodchild, C. E., & Tang, N. K. (2016). Development of the pain-related beliefs and attitudes about sleep (PBAS) scale for the assessment and treatment of insomnia comorbid with chronic pain. *Journal of Clinical Sleep Medicine, 12*(9), 1269–1277. https://doi.org/10.5664/jcsm.6130.

Allen, R. P., Kushida, C. A., Atkinson, M. J., & Consortium, R. L. S. Q. (2003). Factor analysis of the international restless legs syndrome study Group's scale for restless legs severity. *Sleep Medicine, 4*(2), 133–135. https://doi.org/10.1016/s1389-9457(02)00193-4.

Baier, A. L., Kline, A. C., & Feeny, N. C. (2020). Therapeutic alliance as a mediator of change: A systematic review and evaluation of research. *Clinical Psychology Review, 82*, 101921. https://doi.org/10.1016/j.cpr.2020.101921.

Bargiotas, P., Dietmann, A., Haynes, A. G., Kallweit, U., Calle, M. G., Schmidt, M., et al. (2019). The Swiss narcolepsy scale (SNS) and its short form (sSNS) for the discrimination of narcolepsy in patients with hypersomnolence: A cohort study based on the Bern sleep-wake database. *Journal of Neurology, 266*(9), 2137–2143. https://doi.org/10.1007/s00415-019-09365-2.

Bastien, C. H., Vallieres, A., & Morin, C. M. (2001). Validation of the insomnia severity index as an outcome measure for insomnia research. *Sleep Medicine, 2*(4), 297–307. https://doi.org/10.1016/s1389-9457(00)00065-4.

Bootzin, R. R., & Epstein, D. R. (2000). Stimulus control. In K. L. Lichstein, & C. M. Morin (Eds.), *Treatment of late-life insomnia* (pp. 167–184). Sage.

Bootzin, R. R., & Perlis, M. L. (1992). Nonpharmacologic treatments of insomnia. *The Journal of Clinical Psychiatry, 53*(Suppl), 37–41. http://www.ncbi.nlm.nih.gov/entrez/query.fcgi?cmd=Retrieve&db=PubMed&dopt=Citation&list_uids=1613018.

Bootzin, R. R., Smith, L. J., Franzen, P. L., & Shapiro, S. L. (2010). Stimulus control therapy. In M. J. Sateia, & D. J. Buysse (Eds.), *Insomnia: Diagnosis and treatment* (pp. 268–276). Informa.

Brandon, T. H., Vidrine, J. I., & Litvin, E. B. (2007). Relapse and relapse prevention. *Annual Review of Clinical Psychology, 3*, 257–284. https://doi.org/10.1146/annurev.clinpsy.3.022806.091455.

Brasure, M., Fuchs, E., MacDonald, R., Nelson, V. A., Koffel, E., Olson, C. M., et al. (2016). Psychological and behavioral interventions for managing insomnia disorder: An evidence report for a clinical practice guideline by the american college of physicians. *Annals of Internal Medicine*. https://doi.org/10.7326/M15-1782.

Buysse, D. J., Germain, A., Moul, D. E., Franzen, P. L., Brar, L. K., Fletcher, M. E., et al. (2011). Efficacy of brief behavioral treatment for chronic insomnia in older adults. *Archives of Internal Medicine, 171*(10), 887–895. https://doi.org/10.1001/archinternmed.2010.535.

Carney, C. E., Buysse, D. J., Ancoli-Israel, S., Edinger, J. D., Krystal, A. D., Lichstein, K. L., et al. (2012). The consensus sleep diary: Standardizing prospective sleep self-monitoring. *Sleep, 35*(2), 287–302. https://doi.org/10.5665/sleep.1642.

Chasens, E. R., Ratcliffe, S. J., & Weaver, T. E. (2009). Development of the FOSQ-10: A short version of the functional outcomes of sleep questionnaire. *Sleep, 32*(7), 915–919. http://www.ncbi.nlm.nih.gov/entrez/query.fcgi?cmd=Retrieve&db=PubMed&dopt=Citation&list_uids=19639754.

Cheng, P., Kalmbach, D. A., Tallent, G., Joseph, C. L., Espie, C. A., & Drake, C. L. (2019). Depression prevention via digital cognitive behavioral therapy for insomnia: A randomized controlled trial. *Sleep, 42*(10). https://doi.org/10.1093/sleep/zsz150.

Chesson, A. L., Jr., Anderson, W. M., Littner, M., Davila, D., Hartse, K., Johnson, S., et al. (1999). Practice parameters for the nonpharmacologic treatment of chronic insomnia. An American Academy of Sleep Medicine report. Standards of practice committee of the american academy of sleep medicine. *Sleep, 22*(8), 1128–1133. http://www.ncbi.nlm.nih.gov/entrez/query.fcgi?cmd=Retrieve&db=PubMed&dopt=Citation&list_uids=10617175.

Chung, F., Subramanyam, R., Liao, P., Sasaki, E., Shapiro, C., & Sun, Y. (2012). High STOP-Bang score indicates a high probability of obstructive sleep apnoea. *British Journal of Anaesthesia, 108*(5), 768–775. https://doi.org/10.1093/bja/aes022.

Clyde, D. J. (1986). SAFTEE: Data system for side effect assessment scale. *Psychopharmacology Bulletin, 22*(1), 287. http://www.ncbi.nlm.nih.gov/entrez/query.fcgi?cmd=Retrieve&db=PubMed&dopt=Citation&list_uids=3726074.

Davies, R., Lacks, P., Storandt, M., & Bertelson, A. D. (1986). Countercontrol treatment of sleep-maintenance insomnia in relation to age. *Psychology and Aging, 1*(3), 233–238. https://doi.org/10.1037//0882-7974.1.3.233.

Dietch, J. R., Sethi, K., Slavish, D. C., & Taylor, D. J. (2019). Validity of two retrospective questionnaire versions of the consensus sleep diary: The whole week and split week self-assessment of sleep surveys. *Sleep Medicine, 63*, 127–136. https://doi.org/10.1016/j.sleep.2019.05.015.

Doghramji, K. (2010). The evaluation and management of insomnia. *Clinics in Chest Medicine, 31*(2), 327–339. [pii] S0272-5231(10)00039-0 https://doi.org/10.1016/j.ccm.2010.03.001.

Erten Uyumaz, B., Feijs, L., & Hu, J. (2021). A review of digital cognitive behavioral therapy for insomnia (CBT-I apps): Are they designed for engagement? *International Journal of Environmental Research and Public Health, 18*(6). https://doi.org/10.3390/ijerph18062929.

Espie, C. (2011). Paradoxical intention therapy. In M. L. Perlis, M. Aloia, & B. R. Kuhn (Eds.), *Behavioral treatments for sleep disorders: A comprehensive primer of behavioral sleep medicine interventions* (pp. 61–70). Academic.

Farney, R. J., Walker, B. S., Farney, R. M., Snow, G. L., & Walker, J. M. (2011). The STOP-Bang equivalent model and prediction of severity of obstructive sleep apnea: Relation to polysomnographic measurements of the apnea/hypopnea index. *Journal of Clinical Sleep Medicine, 7*(5), 459–465B. https://doi.org/10.5664/JCSM.1306.

First, M. B., Spitzer, R. L., Gibbon, M., & Williams, J. B. W. (1996). *Structured clinical interview for DSM-IV axis I disorders*. non-patient edition Biometrics Research Department, New York State Psychiatric Institute.

Ghotbi, N., Pilz, L. K., Winnebeck, E. C., Vetter, C., Zerbini, G., Lenssen, D., et al. (2020). The micro MCTQ: An ultra-short version of the Munich ChronoType questionnaire. *Journal of Biological Rhythms, 35*(1), 98–110. https://doi.org/10.1177/0748730419886986.

Goodman, W. K., Price, L. H., Rasmussen, S. A., Mazure, C., Fleischmann, R. L., Hill, C. L., et al. (1989). The Yale-Brown obsessive compulsive scale. I. Development, use, and reliability. *Archives of General Psychiatry, 46*(11), 1006–1011. https://doi.org/10.1001/archpsyc.1989.01810110048007.

Grandner, M. A., Jackson, N., Gooneratne, N. S., & Patel, N. P. (2014). The development of a questionnaire to assess sleep-related practices, beliefs, and attitudes. *Behavioral Sleep Medicine, 12*(2), 123–142. https://doi.org/10.1080/15402002.2013.764530.

Grandner, M. A., Olivier, K., Gallagher, R. A., Hale, L., Barrett, M., Branas, C. C., et al. (2020). Quantifying impact of real-world barriers to sleep: The brief index of sleep control (BRISC). *Sleep Health, 6*, 587–593.

Grandner, M. A., & Perlis, M. L. (2015). Treating insomnia disorder in the context of medical and psychiatric comorbidities. *JAMA Internal Medicine, 175*(9), 1472–1473. https://doi.org/10.1001/jamainternmed.2015.3015.

Guy, W., Wilson, W. H., Brooking, B., & Fjetland, O. K. (1987). Intra-interrater reliability of SAFTEE using videotape interviews and clinical trial data. *Psychopharmacology Bulletin,*

23(1), 93–96. http://www.ncbi.nlm.nih.gov/entrez/query.fcgi?cmd=Retrieve&db=PubMed&dopt=Citation&list_uids=3299446.

Guy, W., Wilson, W. H., Brooking, B., Manov, G., & Fjetland, O. (1986). Reliability and validity of SAFTEE: Preliminar analyses. *Psychopharmacology Bulletin, 22*(2), 397–401. http://www.ncbi.nlm.nih.gov/entrez/query.fcgi?cmd=Retrieve&db=PubMed&dopt=Citation&list_uids=3774933.

Harsh, J., & Badia, P. (1991). Stimulus control and sleep. In R. R. Bootzin, J. F. Kihlstrom, & D. L. Schacter (Eds.), *Sleep and cognition* (pp. 58–66). APA.

Harvey, A. G., & Talbot, L. S. (2011). Behavioral experiments. In M. L. Perlis, M. Aloia, & B. R. Kuhn (Eds.), *Behavioral treatments for sleep Sisorders: A comprehensive primer of behavioral sleep medicine interventions* (pp. 71–77). Academic.

Horne, J. A., & Ostberg, O. (1976). A self-assessment questionnaire to determine morningness-eveningness in human circadian rhythms. *International Journal of Chronobiology, 4*(2), 97–110.

Irish, L. A., Kline, C. E., Gunn, H. E., Buysse, D. J., & Hall, M. H. (2015). The role of sleep hygiene in promoting public health: A review of empirical evidence. *Sleep Medicine Reviews, 22*, 23–36. https://doi.org/10.1016/j.smrv.2014.10.001.

Jacobson, A. F., Goldstein, B. J., Dominguez, R. A., & Steinbook, R. M. (1986). Interrater agreement and intraclass reliability measures of SAFTEE in psychopharmacologic clinical trials. *Psychopharmacology Bulletin, 22*(2), 382–388. http://www.ncbi.nlm.nih.gov/entrez/query.fcgi?cmd=Retrieve&db=PubMed&dopt=Citation&list_uids=3774931.

Jacobson, A. F., Goldstein, B. J., Dominguez, R. A., & Steinbook, R. M. (1987). Interrater agreement and reliability measures of SAFTEE: General inquiry vs. systematic inquiry. *Psychopharmacology Bulletin, 23*(1), 97–101. http://www.ncbi.nlm.nih.gov/entrez/query.fcgi?cmd=Retrieve&db=PubMed&dopt=Citation&list_uids=3299447.

Johns, M. W. (1991). A new method for measuring daytime sleepiness: The Epworth sleepiness scale. *Sleep, 14*(6), 540–545.

Johns, M. W. (1992). Reliability and factor analysis of the Epworth sleepiness scale. *Sleep, 15*(4), 376–381. http://www.ncbi.nlm.nih.gov/entrez/query.fcgi?cmd=Retrieve&db=PubMed&dopt=Citation&list_uids=1519015.

Johns, M. W. (1993). Daytime sleepiness, snoring, and obstructive sleep apnea. The Epworth sleepiness scale. *Chest, 103*(1), 30–36. http://www.ncbi.nlm.nih.gov/entrez/query.fcgi?cmd=Retrieve&db=PubMed&dopt=Citation&list_uids=8417909.

Kendall, P. C., Hudson, J. L., Gosch, E., Flannery-Schroeder, E., & Suveg, C. (2008). Cognitive-behavioral therapy for anxiety disordered youth: A randomized clinical trial evaluating child and family modalities. *Journal of Consulting and Clinical Psychology, 76*(2), 282–297. https://doi.org/10.1037/0022-006X.76.2.282.

Klingman, K. J., Jungquist, C. R., & Perlis, M. L. (2017). Introducing the sleep disorders symptom checklist-25: A primary care friendly and comprehensive screener for sleep disorders. *Sleep Medicine Research, 8*(1), 17–25.

Krupp, L. B., LaRocca, N. G., Muir-Nash, J., & Steinberg, A. D. (1989). The fatigue severity scale. Application to patients with multiple sclerosis and systemic lupus erythematosus. *Archives of Neurology, 46*(10), 1121–1123. http://www.ncbi.nlm.nih.gov/entrez/query.fcgi?cmd=Retrieve&db=PubMed&dopt=Citation&list_uids=2803071.

Lane, C. A., & Rollnick, S. (2009). Motivational interviewing. In S. A. Shumaker, J. K. Ockene, & K. A. Riekert (Eds.), *Handbook of health behavior change* (3rd ed., pp. 151–167). Springer.

Levine, J. (1987). Standardized techniques for side-effect assessment: Early results using SAFTEE. *Psychopharmacology Bulletin, 23*(1), 91–92.

Levine, J., & Schooler, N. R. (1984). SAFTEE (systematic assessment for treatment emergent events). A new technique for deteching side effects in clinical trials. *Clinical Neuropharmacology, 7*(Suppl 1), 856–857.

Levine, J., & Schooler, N. R. (1986). SAFTEE: A technique for the systematic assessment of side effects in clinical trials. *Psychopharmacology Bulletin*, *22*(2), 343–381. http://www.ncbi.nlm.nih.gov/entrez/query.fcgi?cmd=Retrieve&db=PubMed&dopt=Citation&list_uids=3774930.

Levy, P., & Pepin, J. L. (2003). Sleep fragmentation: Clinical usefulness of autonomic markers. *Sleep Medicine*, *4*(6), 489–491. S1389945703001977 [pii].

Lichstein, K. L., Thomas, S. J., & McCurry, S. M. (2011). Sleep compression. In M. L. Perlis, M. Aloia, & B. R. Kuhn (Eds.), *Behavioral treatments for sleep disorders: A comprehensive perimer of behavioral sleep medicine interventions* (pp. 55–59). Academic.

Lynch, T. R., Chapman, A. L., Rosenthal, M. Z., Kuo, J. R., & Linehan, M. M. (2006). Mechanisms of change in dialectical behavior therapy: Theoretical and empirical observations. *Journal of Clinical Psychology*, *62*(4), 459–480. https://doi.org/10.1002/jclp.20243.

Maislin, G., Pack, A. I., Kribbs, N. B., Smith, P. L., Schwartz, A. R., Kline, L. R., et al. (1995). A survey screen for prediction of apnea. *Sleep*, *18*(3), 158–166. http://www.ncbi.nlm.nih.gov/entrez/query.fcgi?cmd=Retrieve&db=PubMed&dopt=Citation&list_uids=7610311.

Markowitz, J. S., Rabkin, J. G., Stewart, J., Tricamo, E., McGrath, P. J., Harrison, W., et al. (1987). Validity assessment of SAFTEE: A preliminary report. *Psychopharmacology Bulletin*, *23*(1), 102–105. http://www.ncbi.nlm.nih.gov/entrez/query.fcgi?cmd=Retrieve&db=PubMed&dopt=Citation&list_uids=3299444.

Mastin, D. F., Bryson, J., & Corwyn, R. (2006). Assessment of sleep hygiene using the sleep hygiene index. *Journal of Behavioral Medicine*, *29*(3), 223–227. https://doi.org/10.1007/s10865-006-9047-6.

McCurry, S. M., Logsdon, R. G., Teri, L., & Vitiello, M. V. (2007). Evidence-based psychological treatments for insomnia in older adults. *Psychology and Aging*, *22*(1), 18–27. https://doi.org/2007-03358-004 [pii] https://doi.org/10.1037/0882-7974.22.1.18.

Miller, W. R., & Rollnick, S. (2013). *Motivational interviewing: Helping people change* (3rd ed.). Guilford Press.

Monk, T. H., Buysse, D. J., Kennedy, K. S., Pods, J. M., DeGrazia, J. M., & Miewald, J. M. (2003). Measuring sleep habits without using a diary: The sleep timing questionnaire. *Sleep*, *26*(2), 208–212. http://www.ncbi.nlm.nih.gov/entrez/query.fcgi?cmd=Retrieve&db=PubMed&dopt=Citation&list_uids=12683481.

Moore, P., Bardwell, W. A., Ancoli-Israel, S., & Dimsdale, J. E. (2001). Association between polysomnographic sleep measures and health-related quality of life in obstructive sleep apnea. *Journal of Sleep Research*, *10*(4), 303–308. https://doi.org/10.1046/j.1365-2869.2001.00264.x (pii).

Morin, C. M., & Espie, C. A. (2003). *Insomnia : A clinical guide to assessment and treatment*. Kluwer Academic/Plenum Publishers. http://www.loc.gov/catdir/enhancements/fy0819/2003051325-b.html. http://www.loc.gov/catdir/enhancements/fy0819/2003051325-d.html. http://www.loc.gov/catdir/enhancements/fy0819/2003051325-t.html.

Morin, C. M., Hauri, P. J., Espie, C. A., Spielman, A. J., Buysse, D. J., & Bootzin, R. R. (1999). Nonpharmacologic treatment of chronic insomnia. An American Academy of sleep medicine review. *Sleep*, *22*(8), 1134–1156. http://www.ncbi.nlm.nih.gov/entrez/query.fcgi?cmd=Retrieve&db=PubMed&dopt=Citation&list_uids=10617176.

Morin, C. M., Vallieres, A., & Ivers, H. (2007). Dysfunctional beliefs and attitudes about sleep (DBAS): Validation of a brief version (DBAS-16). *Sleep*, *30*(11), 1547–1554. http://www.ncbi.nlm.nih.gov/entrez/query.fcgi?cmd=Retrieve&db=PubMed&dopt=Citation&list_uids=18041487.

Netzer, N. C., Stoohs, R. A., Netzer, C. M., Clark, K., & Strohl, K. P. (1999). Using the Berlin questionnaire to identify patients at risk for the sleep apnea syndrome. *Annals of Internal*

Medicine, 131(7), 485–491. https://doi.org/10.7326/0003-4819-131-7-199910050-00002 (pii).

Ohayon, M. M., Carskadon, M. A., Guilleminault, C., & Vitiello, M. V. (2004). Meta-analysis of quantitative sleep parameters from childhood to old age in healthy individuals: Developing normative sleep values across the human lifespan. *Sleep, 27*(7), 1255–1273. http://www.ncbi.nlm.nih.gov/entrez/query.fcgi?cmd=Retrieve&db=PubMed&dopt=Citation&list_uids=15586779.

Ottoni, G. L., Antoniolli, E., & Lara, D. R. (2011). The circadian energy scale (CIRENS): Two simple questions for a reliable chronotype measurement based on energy. *Chronobiology International, 28*(3), 229–237. https://doi.org/10.3109/07420528.2011.553696.

Peppard, P. E., Young, T., Barnet, J. H., Palta, M., Hagen, E. W., & Hla, K. M. (2013). Increased prevalence of sleep-disordered breathing in adults. *American Journal of Epidemiology*. https://doi.org/10.1093/aje/kws342.

Perlis, M. L., Junquist, C., Smith, M. T., & Posner, D. (2005). *Cognitive behavioral treatment of insomnia: A session-by-session guide*. Springer.

Pigeon, W. R. (2010). Treatment of adult insomnia with cognitive-behavioral therapy. *Journal of Clinical Psychology, 66*(11), 1148–1160. https://doi.org/10.1002/jclp.20737.

Prochaska, J. O., & DiClemente, C. C. (1982). Transtheoretical therapy: Toward a more integrative model of change. *Psychotherapy: Theory, Research and Practice, 19*(3), 276–288.

Prochaska, J. O., DiClemente, C. C., & Norcross, J. C. (1992). In search of how people change. Applications to addictive behaviors. *The American Psychologist, 47*(9), 1102–1114. http://www.ncbi.nlm.nih.gov/pubmed/1329589.

Qaseem, A., Kansagara, D., Forciea, M. A., Cooke, M., Denberg, T. D., & Clinical Guidelines Committee of the American College of Physicians. (2016). Management of chronic insomnia disorder in adults: A clinical practice guideline from the American college of physicians. *Annals of Internal Medicine*. https://doi.org/10.7326/M15-2175.

Rabkin, J. G., & Markowitz, J. S. (1986). Side effect assessment with SAFTEE: Pilot study of the instrument. *Psychopharmacology Bulletin, 22*(2), 389–396. http://www.ncbi.nlm.nih.gov/entrez/query.fcgi?cmd=Retrieve&db=PubMed&dopt=Citation&list_uids=3774932.

Rabkin, J. G., Markowitz, J. S., Ocepek-Welikson, K., & Wager, S. S. (1992). General versus systematic inquiry about emergent clinical events with SAFTEE: Implications for clinical research. *Journal of Clinical Psychopharmacology, 12*(1), 3–10. http://www.ncbi.nlm.nih.gov/entrez/query.fcgi?cmd=Retrieve&db=PubMed&dopt=Citation&list_uids=1552037.

Riedel, B. W., Lichstein, K. L., & Dwyer, W. O. (1995). Sleep compression and sleep education for older insomniacs: Self-help versus therapist guidance. *Psychology and Aging, 10*(1), 54–63. http://www.ncbi.nlm.nih.gov/entrez/query.fcgi?cmd=Retrieve&db=PubMed&dopt=Citation&list_uids=7779317.

Riemann, D., & Perlis, M. L. (2009). The treatments of chronic insomnia: A review of benzodiazepine receptor agonists and psychological and behavioral therapies. *Sleep Medicine Reviews, 13*(3), 205–214. https://doi.org/S1087-0792(08)00056-7 [pii] https://doi.org/10.1016/j.smrv.2008.06.001.

Roth, T., Zammit, G., Kushida, C., Doghramji, K., Mathias, S. D., Wong, J. M., et al. (2002). A new questionnaire to detect sleep disorders. *Sleep Medicine, 3*(2), 99–108. https://doi.org/10.1016/s1389-9457(01)00131-9 (pii).

Rutledge, C. M., La Guardia, A. C., & Bluestein, D. (2013). Predictors of self-efficacy for sleep in primary care. *Journal of Clinical Nursing, 22*(9–10), 1254–1261. https://doi.org/10.1111/jocn.12005.

Sarkanen, T., Alakuijala, A., & Partinen, M. (2019). Ullanlinna narcolepsy scale in diagnosis of narcolepsy. *Sleep, 42*(3). https://doi.org/10.1093/sleep/zsy238.

Schutte-Rodin, S., Broch, L., Buysse, D., Dorsey, C., & Sateia, M. (2008). Clinical guideline for the evaluation and management of chronic insomnia in adults. *Journal of Clinical Sleep*

Medicine, 4(5), 487–504. http://www.ncbi.nlm.nih.gov/entrez/query.fcgi?cmd=Retrieve&db=PubMed&dopt=Citation&list_uids=18853708.

Sheehan, D. V., Lecrubier, Y., Sheehan, K. H., Amorim, P., Janavs, J., Weiller, E., et al. (1998). The mini-international neuropsychiatric interview (M.I.N.I.): The development and validation of a structured diagnostic psychiatric interview for DSM-IV and ICD-10. *The Journal of Clinical Psychiatry, 59*(Suppl 20), 22–33. quiz 34-57 http://www.ncbi.nlm.nih.gov/entrez/query.fcgi?cmd=Retrieve&db=PubMed&dopt=Citation&list_uids=9881538.

Siebern, A. T., & Manber, R. (2010). Insomnia and its effective non-pharmacologic treatment. *The Medical Clinics of North America, 94*(3), 581–591. https://doi.org/S0025-7125(10)00019-2 [pii] https://doi.org/10.1016/j.mcna.2010.02.005.

Siebern, A. T., Suh, S., & Nowakowski, S. (2012). Non-pharmacological treatment of insomnia. *Neurotherapeutics, 9*(4), 717–727. https://doi.org/10.1007/s13311-012-0142-9.

Silva, G. E., Vana, K. D., Goodwin, J. L., Sherrill, D. L., & Quan, S. F. (2011). Identification of patients with sleep disordered breathing: Comparing the four-variable screening tool, STOP, STOP-Bang, and Epworth sleepiness scales. *Journal of Clinical Sleep Medicine, 7*(5), 467–472. https://doi.org/10.5664/JCSM.1308.

Smith, S. S., Oei, T. P., Douglas, J. A., Brown, I., Jorgensen, G., & Andrews, J. (2008). Confirmatory factor analysis of the Epworth sleepiness scale (ESS) in patients with obstructive sleep apnoea. *Sleep Medicine, 9*(7), 739–744. https://doi.org/S1389-9457(07)00306-1 [pii] https://doi.org/10.1016/j.sleep.2007.08.004.

Smith, M. T., Perlis, M. L., Park, A., Smith, M. S., Pennington, J., Giles, D. E., et al. (2002). Comparative meta-analysis of pharmacotherapy and behavior therapy for persistent insomnia. *The American Journal of Psychiatry, 159*(1), 5–11. http://www.ncbi.nlm.nih.gov/entrez/query.fcgi?cmd=Retrieve&db=PubMed&dopt=Citation&list_uids=11772681.

Spitzer, R. L., Kroenke, K., & Williams, J. B. (1999). Validation and utility of a self-report version of PRIME-MD: The PHQ primary care study. Primary care evaluation of mental disorders. Patient Health Questionnaire. *JAMA, 282*(18), 1737–1744. https://doi.org/10.1001/jama.282.18.1737. https://doi.org/joc90770 (pii).

Spitzer, R. L., Kroenke, K., Williams, J. B., & Lowe, B. (2006). A brief measure for assessing generalized anxiety disorder: The GAD-7. *Archives of Internal Medicine, 166*(10), 1092–1097. https://doi.org/166/10/1092 [pii] https://doi.org/10.1001/archinte.166.10.1092.

Spoormaker, V. I., Verbeek, I., van den Bout, J., & Klip, E. C. (2005). Initial validation of the SLEEP-50 questionnaire. *Behavioral Sleep Medicine, 3*(4), 227–246. https://doi.org/10.1207/s15402010bsm0304_4.

Stepanski, E., Lamphere, J., Badia, P., Zorick, F., & Roth, T. (1984). Sleep fragmentation and daytime sleepiness. *Sleep, 7*(1), 18–26. http://www.ncbi.nlm.nih.gov/entrez/query.fcgi?cmd=Retrieve&db=PubMed&dopt=Citation&list_uids=6718922.

Taylor, D. J., Peterson, A. L., Pruiksma, K. E., Hale, W. J., Young-McCaughan, S., Wilkerson, A., et al. (2018). Impact of cognitive behavioral therapy for insomnia disorder on sleep and comorbid symptoms in military personnel: A randomized clinical trial. *Sleep, 41*(6). https://doi.org/10.1093/sleep/zsy069.

Taylor, D. J., Wilkerson, A. K., Pruiksma, K. E., Williams, J. M., Ruggero, C. J., Hale, W., et al. (2018). Reliability of the structured clinical interview for DSM-5 sleep disorders module. *Journal of Clinical Sleep Medicine, 14*(3), 459–464. https://doi.org/10.5664/jcsm.7000.

Terman, M., Rifkin, J. B., Jacobs, J., & White, T. M. (2001). *Morningness-Eveningness questionnaire (revised)*. New York State Psychiatric Institute.

Tubbs, A. S., Khader, W., Fernandez, F., & Grandner, M. A. (2020). The common denominators of sleep, obesity, and psychopathology. *Current Opinion in Psychology, 34*, 84–88. https://doi.org/10.1016/j.copsyc.2019.11.003.

van der Zweerde, T., Bisdounis, L., Kyle, S. D., Lancee, J., & van Straten, A. (2019). Cognitive behavioral therapy for insomnia: A meta-analysis of long-term effects in controlled studies. *Sleep Medicine Reviews, 48*, 101208. https://doi.org/10.1016/j.smrv.2019.08.002.

Vincent, N., Sande, G., Read, C., & Giannuzzi, T. (2004). Sleep locus of control: Report on a new scale. *Behavioral Sleep Medicine*, *2*(2), 79–93. http://www.ncbi.nlm.nih.gov/entrez/query.fcgi?cmd=Retrieve&db=PubMed&dopt=Citation&list_uids=15600226.

Walters, A. S., LeBrocq, C., Dhar, A., Hening, W., Rosen, R., Allen, R. P., et al. (2003). Validation of the international restless legs syndrome study group rating scale for restless legs syndrome. *Sleep Medicine*, *4*(2), 121–132. https://doi.org/10.1016/s1389-9457(02)00258-7 (pii).

Watson, D., Clark, L. A., & Tellegen, A. (1988). Development and validation of brief measures of positive and negative affect: The PANAS scales. *Journal of Personality and Social Psychology*, *54*(6), 1063–1070. http://www.ncbi.nlm.nih.gov/entrez/query.fcgi?cmd=Retrieve&db=PubMed&dopt=Citation&list_uids=3397865.

Weathers, F. W., Bovin, M. J., Lee, D. J., Sloan, D. M., Schnurr, P. P., Kaloupek, D. G., et al. (2018, Mar). The clinician-administered PTSD scale for DSM-5 (CAPS-5): Development and initial psychometric evaluation in military veterans. *Psychological Assessment*, *30*(3), 383–395. https://doi.org/10.1037/pas0000486.

Weaver, T. E., Laizner, A. M., Evans, L. K., Maislin, G., Chugh, D. K., Lyon, K., et al. (1997, Oct). An instrument to measure functional status outcomes for disorders of excessive sleepiness. *Sleep*, *20*(10), 835–843. http://www.ncbi.nlm.nih.gov/entrez/query.fcgi?cmd=Retrieve&db=PubMed&dopt=Citation&list_uids=9415942.

Werner-Seidler, A., Johnston, L., & Christensen, H. (2018). Digitally-delivered cognitive-behavioural therapy for youth insomnia: A systematic review. *Internet Interventions*, *11*, 71–78. https://doi.org/10.1016/j.invent.2018.01.007.

Wilson, G. T. (1996). Manual-based treatments: The clinical application of research findings. *Behaviour Research and Therapy*, *34*(4), 295–314. https://doi.org/10.1016/0005-7967(95)00084-4.

Wu, J. Q., Appleman, E. R., Salazar, R. D., & Ong, J. C. (2015, Sep). Cognitive behavioral therapy for insomnia comorbid with psychiatric and medical conditions: A meta-analysis. *JAMA Internal Medicine*, *175*(9), 1461–1472. https://doi.org/10.1001/jamainternmed.2015.3006.

Zavada, A., Gordijn, M. C., Beersma, D. G., Daan, S., & Roenneberg, T. (2005). Comparison of the Munich Chronotype questionnaire with the Horne-Ostberg's Morningness-Eveningness score. *Chronobiology International*, *22*(2), 267–278. http://www.ncbi.nlm.nih.gov/entrez/query.fcgi?cmd=Retrieve&db=PubMed&dopt=Citation&list_uids=16021843.

Zwart, C. A., & Lisman, S. A. (1979). Analysis of stimulus control treatment of sleep-onset insomnia. *Journal of Consulting and Clinical Psychology*, *47*(1), 113–118. http://www.ncbi.nlm.nih.gov/pubmed/429643.

CHAPTER

20

CBT-I in patients who wish to reduce use of hypnotic medication

Norah Simpson and Rachel Manber

Department of Psychiatry & Behavioral Sciences, Stanford University, Palo Alto, CA, United States

Introduction

In addition to being effective for reducing insomnia symptom severity, cognitive-behavioral therapy for insomnia (CBT-I) can be effective for reducing or eliminating hypnotic use. CBT-I providers are ideally positioned to promote and facilitate hypnotic medication tapers because of their knowledge of CBT-I, and because CBT-I treatment sessions are frequent and therefore allow for closer monitoring and troubleshooting of patient progress than typically is possible in medical clinics. Additionally, improvement of sleep with CBT-I treatment tends to increase sleep self-efficacy and thus can be a significant motivator to reduce hypnotic medication use. In this chapter, our focus is on medications that are FDA-approved for sleep, although the principles discussed in this chapter may be generalizable to use with other medications or supplements prescribed for sleep. It is important to note that sometimes benzodiazepine hypnotics are also prescribed for daytime use to manage anxiety. When such use is associated with medication dependencies, it is best addressed by an addiction specialist and remains outside the scope of this chapter.

In this chapter, we review patterns of hypnotic medication use among patients with insomnia and describe the effects of CBT-I on hypnotic medication use. We also describe best practices for collaborating a medication taper with prescribing providers, as well as approaches to the timing of medication and the schedule of medication reduction. We conclude with

Adapting Cognitive Behavioral Therapy for Insomnia
https://doi.org/10.1016/B978-0-12-822872-2.00014-1

a discussion of strategies for utilizing CBT-I to support successful hypnotic medication tapers, as well as the scientific rationale that informs them. As with all treatment provided in our clinic, we emphasize a flexible, patient-centered, case-conceptualization approach to treatment—one that is tailored to the specific patient presentation and anchored in the underlying processes that regulate sleep.

Hypnotic medication use

The use of hypnotic medications for sleep is common, with 16% of patients seen in general medical practice reporting hypnotic use (Bjorvatn, Meland, Flo, & Mildestvedt, 2017). The rate is higher among patients initiating CBT-I, with more than half of patients taking some type of medication for sleep (Adler, Carde, Kuo, Ong, & Manber, 2008). Once initiated, hypnotic use often becomes chronic. It is estimated that one in five new users of sedative-hypnotics will become a long-term user (Schonmann et al., 2018). A survey of 790 hypnotic users in a general practice suggests that 20% were interested in reducing use and nearly 50% had a failed prior attempt to do so (Siriwardena, Qureshi, Dyas, Middleton, & Orner, 2008).

These patterns of chronic hypnotic use help us understand the subsequent risk of dependence on medications, most of which are typically recommended only for acute (short-term) use. It is important to consider that dependence encompasses both psychological and physiological factors. Two studies suggest that psychological dependence might play a larger role in the experience of worsening insomnia following dose reduction and discontinuation than physiological dependence. The first study found that withdrawal symptoms were greater when measured subjectively, compared to objectively (Schneiderhelmert, 1988). In the second study, in which participants were assigned to receive either a hypnotic or placebo medication for a 12-month period, when placebo substitution was implemented during several 1-week periods, rebound insomnia was equivalent between the two groups (Roehrs, Randall, Harris, Maan, & Roth, 2012). These two studies underscore the importance of understanding and addressing the role of psychological dependence when helping patients successfully reduce medication use.

Effects of CBT-I on hypnotic medication use

Even when CBT-I protocols do not directly target hypnotic reduction, they can result in reductions of hypnotic medications. Two studies report roughly 50% reductions in hypnotic use (Morgan, Dixon, Mathers, Thompson, & Tomeny, 2003; Morin, Sonte, McDonald, & Jones, 1994), compared to only 17% reduction in a usual care control condition

(Morgan et al., 2003). It is possible that patients who improve their sleep with CBT-I may be more ready to experiment with dose reduction than before the start of CBT-I, potentially because they gained confidence that they can use tools from CBT-I to weather any transient sleep disruption associated with medication reduction. Increased sleep self-efficacy during CBT-I can also lead patients to spontaneously reduce or eliminate hypnotic medication use.

CBT-I principles can also be used to explicitly target hypnotic medication use. Several studies have examined the impact of adding a specific medication taper component to CBT-I on medication use outcomes. One meta-analysis of five studies concluded that CBT-I plus a gradual tapering plan was more effective than a gradual tapering plan alone for obtaining full discontinuation of hypnotic medication 2 weeks to 3 months after the intervention ended; hypnotic use rates were 45% in the taper only condition versus 27% in the CBT-I plus taper condition (Takaesu et al., 2019). The rates for discontinuation at the 1-year follow-up, reported in four of the studies, were 49% versus 30% and, although clinically meaningful, were not statistically significant (Takaesu et al., 2019). Effect sizes for a 50% reduction in medication were larger than for full discontinuation (Takaesu et al., 2019). In interpreting these results, it is important to consider that there was significant heterogeneity among the studies included in this analysis with respect to the CBT-I techniques included in treatment, whether CBT-I was used to directly target hypnotic medication use, and whether the CBT-I therapist was directly engaged in explicitly promoting and supporting the taper process (versus proceeding in parallel with a scheduled taper). There were also differences in sample characteristics relative to insomnia severity and patterns of medication use.

It is possible that a direct application of CBT-I to support a medication taper has longer-lasting effects on hypnotic medication use. This idea is supported by one study that was not included in the 2019 meta-analysis. This trial of internet-provided CBT-I reported that reduced levels of hypnotic medication use were evident 3 years following CBT-I treatment (Blom, Jernelov, Ruck, Lindefors, & Kaldo, 2016). In this study, participants assigned to the CBT-I condition received strategies for how to discontinue medication use and were encouraged to include reduction or elimination of hypnotic medication as a part of their CBT-I treatment. Forty-five percent were taking hypnotic medication at baseline. At the 3-year follow-up period, the active treatment and control groups did not differ in their insomnia severity but only 29% of participants who received CBT-I were taking hypnotic medication compared to 47% in the control group. This difference was both statistically significant and clinically meaningful (Blom et al., 2016). Collectively, these studies demonstrate that CBT-I can be used effectively to treat insomnia among hypnotic users as well as reduce or eliminate the use of hypnotic medication. Given the documented risks (e.g., falls, dementia) associated with hypnotic medication use, particularly in older adults (Bakken et al., 2014; Chen, Lee, Sun, Oyang, & Fuh, 2012), the ability to effectively leverage CBT-I to help motivated patients reduce hypnotic medication use and support them in this process is of critical importance for enhancing patient health and safety.

Collaboration with medication prescribers

Collaboration among clinicians treating the same patient for the same problem is always important for patient safety and best clinical care. Cognitive-behavioral therapy for insomnia is most often administered by a mental health provider without prescription privileges and limited medical knowledge. Hypnotic medications are prescribed by a medical provider, usually a physician, with limited knowledge about principles of behavior change and CBT-I. Collaboration of hypnotic discontinuation requires agreement between providers that hypnotic discontinuation (or reduction) is clinically indicated, a clear understanding of each provider's role, a discussion of a flexible taper plan that promotes patient safety and success of discontinuation, and continued communication as needed. In our experience, primary care physicians welcome collaboration with behavioral sleep medicine clinicians on hypnotic tapers. Consistent with guidelines by professional medical organizations, prescribers typically encourage their patients to reduce or discontinue the use of sleep medications. For example, the Beers Criteria for potentially inappropriate medication use in older adults includes hypnotic medications on the list (Radcliff et al., 2015). Further, the Evidence Report for a Clinical Practice Guideline by the American College of Physicians recommends that "physicians should be aware that many medications used regularly and long term for insomnia disorders have an FDA indication only for short-term" (Wilt et al., 2016). Even so, there are situations where discontinuation may not be advisable, such as when patients are in palliative or hospice care. Discontinuation of hypnotic medications might also not be clinically indicated for some patients in acute psychiatric care, such as those in inpatient treatment or recently discharged from an intensive care facility.

Prescribing providers are typically very open to discussions of hypnotic taper and, in fact, some refer hypnotic using patients for CBT-I with an explicit goal of reducing their hypnotic use. During discussions between a CBT-I therapist and a prescriber, the CBT-I provider brings expertise on issues related to psychological dependence and behavior change and the medical professional brings knowledge on relevant pharmacology and medical comorbidities. Consideration of both expertise areas promotes patient safety and success of discontinuation and sets the stage for determining the mutual roles of each provider. Usually, the prescribing provider will support any of the empirically supported gradual taper schedules discussed below because they reduce or eliminate safety concerns. Recognizing the challenges that patients often experience during hypnotic reduction, the medical professional readily understands the need for frequent check-ins and support to promote success, and is aware that CBT-I providers typically have more frequent and longer visits with patients than they do. As a result, the real-world role division between the two providers is such that the CBT-I provider takes the primary role of implementing the agreed-upon taper schedule. Even in some research protocols, which usually have a study physician manage the taper, the CBT-I therapist monitors withdrawal effects and may slow the withdrawal schedule as needed (Belleville, Guay, Guay, & Morin, 2007). Although in real life, most physicians are not as readily available as in research protocols, continued collaboration is in the best interest of the patient. It is advised that the CBT-I provider informs the physician about the results of the taper, particularly when a patient discontinues treatment before attaining their original hypnotic taper goal or when they have successfully discontinued hypnotics.

Timing of hypnotic medication reduction

As described above, the most successful taper plan will be one that is patient-guided and uses a collaborative approach. At the initial assessment, or when goal-setting is taking place, is an ideal time to ask patients if they would like their treatment to include reduction and/or elimination of hypnotic medication. This is true even when reducing/eliminating hypnotics is not a spontaneously identified goal by the patient. Many patients are unaware that a supported taper is a potential option for treatment, nor that CBT-I can help increase success in reducing or eliminating medication use. Occasionally, patients will be referred for treatment because the prescribing provider is no longer willing to prescribe hypnotics, but the patient would prefer to stay on their sleep medication. Treatment for patients in this situation requires discussion with the patient about readiness and commitment to change, using motivational enhancement strategies both at the initial visit and periodically throughout treatment. In this context, motivational enhancement begins with a discussion of the patient's personal medication goals in an empathic, nonjudgmental manner. The therapist then uses cost-benefit analysis to gain an understanding of factors contributing to the discrepancy between personal goals and referring physician discontinuation goals. Cost-benefit analysis involves the therapist eliciting, in a neutral manner, a list of the pros and cons of hypnotic reduction/discontinuation and assessing the emotional valence for each item on this elicited list, as well as of the overall pros and cons. As needed, the therapist can then help examine the validity and utility of each item on the list, avoiding arguments and supporting any sign of self-efficacy with respect to hypnotic reduction. The therapist encourages the patient to realize they are capable of many things, including an ability to sleep without medication, given that CBT-I will offer alternative tools in the process. Such cases also require discussion with the prescriber about willingness to support continued prescribing during the preparatory phase and throughout the gradual and supported taper process.

While the taper can be initiated at any point, patients might not be ready to do so early in the course of CBT-I, particularly when they have had unsuccessful past experiences with reducing medication use. Here too, it may be helpful to start with motivational enhancement strategies to address ambivalence about discontinuing hypnotics. If the patient is agreeable, we recommend integrating hypnotic taper into the time-in-bed restriction process. This involves initiating the taper after the time in bed was restricted but before it is fully expanded so that the strong homeostatic drive can support the taper. Specifically, a good time to initiate the taper is after sleep efficiency has sufficiently increased (e.g., to >85%), daytime sleepiness is within safe levels, and the patient is ready to start the taper. At that stage, sleep has started to improve and the patient has also developed confidence about applying CBT-I techniques and understands their rationale. Importantly, at this time, the patient's homeostatic sleep drive is likely still high and able to counter potential anticipatory arousal associated with the medication taper. Please see below for an additional discussion of this idea in, "Homeostatic sleep drive/time in bed restriction" section. If the patient is experiencing high levels of daytime sleepiness, the patient's time in bed window should be expanded to the point that daytime sleepiness is within safe levels before initiating the taper. This allows the patient to be in a sustainable and safe "time in bed maintenance phase" while they complete the gradual taper process, before proceeding to subsequent time in bed extension. When considering these individual factors mapped onto a standard CBT-I protocol, this means that most patients will be ready to begin a hypnotic taper no earlier than the third appointment (first appointment: intake, second appointment: initial time in bed restriction and stimulus control recommendations). However, for patients who have difficulty adhering to initial treatment recommendations or for whom are sleepy and need additional titration of the time in bed window to develop a sustainable "time in bed maintenance phase" for the taper, the first step of the hypnotic taper may occur in subsequent sessions. Hypnotic tapers will also begin later for patients who are ambivalent about medication reduction, as they will need additional cognitive therapy and motivational enhancement before they are ready to begin the taper.

Patients who do not identify a goal to reduce medication use at the start of treatment may be interested in a supported taper after other goals for CBT-I have been reached. Successful resolution of insomnia symptoms with CBT-I often increases self-efficacy surrounding sleep and, as described above, may be associated with some spontaneous hypnotic medication reduction. Indeed, even interventions that are designed to increase self-efficacy more broadly can increase success in a medication taper (Yang, Tseng, Lai, & Hsu, 2015). Thus, after the original treatment goals have been attained, the therapist can revisit the option of adding a goal of hypnotic medication reduction or discontinuation. Motivational enhancement strategies, as described above, can help address ambivalence or anxiety about embarking on a hypnotic medication reduction plan during this discussion and may result in more patients deciding to reduce medication use.

Schedule of reduction

There are multiple approaches to how quickly to reduce hypnotic medication use. We will first describe the most common reduction schedules described in research, followed by the protocol we utilize in our clinical work. The most common pace of reduction of hypnotic medications that has been implemented in research protocols is by a dose reduction of 25% per 1–2 weeks, with the goal of attaining 50% reduction in 4 weeks and discontinuation at 8 weeks (Belleville et al., 2007; Lichstein et al., 2013). These protocols describe the process in phases. The first phase of most taper protocols consists of a gradual dose reduction to a minimal available dose. When more than one hypnotic is used, some protocols, particularly those for tapering off of benzodiazepine hypnotics, first switch the patient to a single hypnotic, usually from a short to a longer-acting benzodiazepine hypnotic. (This benzodiazepine-focused approach to tapering differs from approaches to tapering nonbenzodiazepine hypnotics, which are more common in current clinical practice. These are discussed in the "Our protocol" section below.) The dose reduction has been implemented by cutting the dosage by 25% of the baseline dosage on all nights until the minimum dose is reached (consistent reduction approach (Belleville et al., 2007)) or on a preselected proportion of nights on which the dose taken is more than the minimal available (approximately every other night; intermittent reduction approach; (Lichstein et al., 2013)). One potential challenge with the intermittent reduction approach is the potential that coincidental worsening of sleep will be interpreted as causal and hence can increase psychological dependence. Another challenge with intermittent reduction is that high anticipatory anxiety about reducing a dose will interfere with sleep on the night of reduction. On the following night, which might be a night scheduled for a higher medication dose, sleep will be better for two reasons. One reason is that the higher dose promotes sleep, but another reason is that poor sleep on the previous night will lead to an increase in the homeostatic sleep drive that is likely to contribute to better sleep the next night. This leads to a missed opportunity for the patient to experience better sleep on the same reduced dose of medication the next night, an experience that can promote self-efficacy and encourage further reduction. The second phase of taper is an elimination phase. It consists of gradually increasing the number of hypnotic-free nights according to a set schedule. To promote success, elimination begins with nights that the patient predicts will be easier to do so. These multiphased approaches to medication reduction or discontinuation involve setting a realistic medication taper goal at each visit and providing a written plan indicating medication and dosage for each night. Goal setting and the taper schedule usually involve consideration of patients' readiness to discontinue medication and taking into account the presence or absence of withdrawal symptoms (Belleville et al., 2007). As a result, although a written plan at each session is provided, it is dynamically adjusted on a session-by-session basis based on patient progress. The most common withdrawal symptoms associated with gradual tapers are worsening of sleep in the context of anticipatory anxiety and/or dose reduction. Abrupt withdrawal symptoms for benzodiazepines may result in more significant and protracted side effects, such as benzodiazepine withdrawal syndrome (Petursson, 1994). For more information about benzodiazepines and approaches to reduce use, please refer to the Ashton Manual (Ashton, 2002). For patients taking high levels of benzodiazepines for sleep, collaboration with prescribing physicians is even more critical.

Other schedules of tapering have also been implemented. For instance, rather than reducing the dosage by 25% of the actual medication taken, Ayabe and colleagues implemented a reduction by 25% of baseline diazepam dose equivalent (Ayabe et al., 2018). Another novel approach to hypnotic medication reduction is to implement placebo substitution, which is intended to eliminate anticipatory anxiety on nights with reduced dosage. For example, an abstract using preliminary data from an ongoing clinical trial reports the success of a blinded taper where the medication dosage was reduced by 25% every 2 weeks over a period of 8 weeks or by or 10% every 2 weeks over 20 weeks (Edinger et al., 2019). Placebo substitution outside of a research context is more challenging and involves the additional cost of working with a compound pharmacy.

Our protocol

The protocol we use in our clinic is consistent with the general principles outlined in published taper protocols. We use a patient-centered approach that takes into account patient readiness for dose reduction and dynamically adjust the taper plan based on patients' goals and progress. Unlike research protocols where the protocol is time-limited, our real-life protocol has no such constraints, allowing for the option of a very slow pace, including pauses in the reduction process when needed. Similar to published protocols, our taper process proceeds in stages.

The first stage takes place even before the taper is initiated. During this stage, best described as the preparatory stage, we provide information about tolerance, psychological dependence, and the potential for transient worsening of sleep during dose reduction based on individual patient presentations or concerns. We do not present patients with a handout of potential "costs" of a hypnotic medication taper, as this can result in anticipatory arousal and affect expectations of success. Rather, this discussion is individually tailored to provide information to help reduce the patient's specific concerns about a hypnotic taper. Often this discussion will include basic information about the specific steps of the taper, the role of physiological vs psychological dependence (see discussion of placebo-blinded studies above), and psychoeducation about psychological dependence. To reduce psychological dependence, our first focus is on avoiding the use of medication as a rescue after trying to sleep without. (Also see, "Contingent reinforcement of beliefs" section.) In an effort to take as little medication as possible, many patients have had the experience in which they first try to sleep without taking medication, but then take it when they realize that they are still having difficulty falling asleep. This pattern reduces self-efficacy about sleep and about their ability to discontinue the medication. This manner of use may be nightly (taken every night after attempting sleep initiation without medication) or intermittently (only taken on nights when the patient has difficulty initiating or re-initiating sleep, in the case of middle-of-the-night awakenings). For nightly use, we recommend taking the medication nightly at bedtime, to avoid the self-reinforcing pattern of using the hypnotic medication as a safety net (i.e., when they cannot fall asleep independently). When patients are using hypnotic medication intermittently, we recommend continuing to take the medication on the same number of nights per week but work with them to determine a schedule with clear rules about which nights to take the medication. Most commonly, the developed plan is to take the sleep medications on specific days of the week. When a patient does not believe they can implement this type of plan, we work with them to identify clear rules for when to take it. For example, the clear plan may be based on life contingencies, such as the night before or after a specific event (e.g., the night before an important weekly meeting) or on a specific, limited frequency (e.g., to take medication no more than three nights a week).

When multiple sleep medications are taken, we identify which medication to start reducing first. To do this, we use input from the prescribing provider and the patient. In general, medications that are more likely to produce withdrawal symptoms, such as benzodiazepines, are targeted first, allowing the patient a sense of safety by still having some sleep medication on board. Alternatively, using a patient-centered approach, the taper begins with a medication that the patient believes will be the easiest to reduce. In the case of multiple medications, once one medication is eliminated, the second target of reduction is identified, and so on, until the patient has fully discontinued all sleep medications. When patients present on extended-release medications (e.g., Ambien CR), a medication dosage can gradually be reduced from extended-release to shorter-acting doses, which can then be reduced until full discontinuation is achieved. This type of taper requires the active collaboration of prescribing providers as different formulations of medications are prescribed as the taper progresses. For example, a patient who is taking 12.5 mg of Ambien CR at baseline may reduce to 6.25 mg Ambien CR plus 5 mg Ambien at the first step of the taper, then 10 mg Ambien as the second step. Subsequent steps may involve reductions to 7.5, 5, and 2 mg, and can require cutting the pill to achieve the desired dose. In rare cases, when a patient presents to the clinic taking high doses of multiple hypnotic medications, the full taper process may take a long time and may include pauses or longer time between taper steps. In these situations, patients are likely to increase self-efficacy around sleep during the taper process and will require less frequent appointments and treatment provider support during the second half of the taper.

When sleep medications are taken more than once per night, we recommend consolidating the doses and taking the total nightly dose at bedtime. As rationale, we provide information about medication half-life and carryover effects (Table 1), and how the use of hypnotic medications as a "rescue" for difficulty falling back asleep during the night can foster hypnotic dependence. However, sometimes the approach of consolidating doses is not acceptable to the patient. In such cases, we collaboratively agree on the time of night when the taper will begin (i.e., at bedtime or in the middle of the night) and how it will proceed. The key is to set the stage for success at each step to promote continued dose reduction. One challenge to the tapering middle-of-the-night hypnotics is establishing a rule about how soon after waking up to take the medication. This requires a balance between two problematic strategies that patients tend to use. One strategy is "wait and see if I can fall back asleep without it" and the other is to take it right away. As we discussed above, the first approach promotes psychological dependence. The second approach could deprive

TABLE 1 Adaptation of CBT-I for hypnotic dependence.

CBT-I components	Standard practice	Adaptations for hypnotic taper
Sleep education	3-P model, 2-process model of sleep regulation, sleep stages	– Education about the role of anxiety regarding the need for medication and potential taper as a perpetuating factor in the 3-P model – Education about the role of past negative experiences with rebound insomnia as a perpetuating factor in the 3-P model – Additional education about the distinction between psychological and physiological dependence on hypnotic medication and effects on sleep (e.g., placebo-blinded studies)
Sleep restriction	Improve sleep efficiency by limiting time in bed to the amount of time sleeping then expanding slowly as long as sleep efficiency is preserved	– Increase sleep efficiency before initiating hypnotic taper to improve access to sleep drive. This will also increase sleep self-efficacy and may further increase confidence in treatment – Option to leverage time in bed restriction during hypnotic taper if needed to help "smooth out" any transient disruption in sleep during the taper
Stimulus control	Associate bed/bedroom solely as a cue for sleep by eliminating nonsleep activities from the bedroom. Instruction to get out of bed at night if awake >15 min	– To reduce fall risk associated with sedating hypnotic use, consider counter-control (sitting up and engaging in pleasant activity while awake during the time in bed window) rather than full stimulus control
Napping/daytime sleep	Discontinue or restrict daytime napping to 30 min	– If a patient is using hypnotic medications during naps, discourage use. Consider eliminating use during naps as the first step of taper
Sleep hygiene education	Address daytime habits and sleep environment interfering with sleep	– If substances (e.g., alcohol, marijuana) are being used as hypnotic medication, use chapter guidelines to assist in taper (slow taper is particularly important when doses are high)

Continued

TABLE 1 Adaptation of CBT-I for hypnotic dependence—cont'd

CBT-I components	Standard practice	Adaptations for hypnotic taper
Cognitive therapy	Challenge patient's dysfunctional beliefs interfering with sleep and misconceptions about sleep. Replace/restructure to more helpful and realistic thoughts about sleep	– Provide realistic expectations for sleep without hypnotic medication – Identify and address beliefs reflecting: (1) low sleep self-efficacy ("I can't sleep without medication") (2) sleep effort (needing to work at sleep, "trying to sleep") (3) low tolerance of uncertainty ("I need to know I can get a good night's sleep") – Consider motivational enhancement and other third-wave therapy approaches if the patient is ambivalent about the taper (can be used before initiating taper or if the patient's commitment to tapering changes during the process)
Relapse prevention	Discuss practicing less rigid sleep plan over time and what do to prevent sleep disturbance from turning into another episode of insomnia in the future	– Discuss how to get sleep back on track after a transient disruption without hypnotic medication – Discuss how the patient would approach strategic brief use of hypnotics (e.g., planned using during international travel)
Sleep diaries	Establish baseline sleep patterns, track progress, reinforce appropriate behavior change, problem-solve obstacles to adherence	– Emphasize the importance of recording medication use, including dose and timing, in the diary – Modifications to the diary may be required to monitor the use of hypnotics multiple times during the night or for naps

the patient of the opportunity to learn that they indeed are able to fall back asleep without the hypnotic. Our recommendation is to use the same rule as we do for the stimulus control instruction to get out of bed if unable to fall back asleep. Rather than relying on the number of minutes that passed, we encourage patients to get out of bed when they first realize that they are in a state that is not conducive to sleep. Similarly, for the middle of the night hypnotic medication use, we advise patients to take the medication when they first realize that sleep is not easily within reach. Some patients present for treatment taking hypnotic medications to assist with sleep during daytime naps. In these situations, we provide psychoeducation about the detrimental impact of long daytime naps on nighttime sleep and potential hangover effects of the medication being taken. With few exceptions, we discourage the use of hypnotics for daytime naps and encourage eliminating this particular use of hypnotics before addressing nighttime use. (An example of an exception is a shift worker who needs to maintain an unusual sleep pattern to optimize safety and performance.)

At each step of the taper, we set the expectation that, once a reduction of the dose is initiated, the patient commits to avoiding dose escalation until the next session, usually a week or two later, based on clinical presentation. Patients are encouraged to reach out to their treatment provider if they are struggling with the taper between sessions to troubleshoot and receive support, rather than immediately return to a higher dose of medication. If the patient is not ready to make such a commitment, we may hold off or halt the taper and work through issues that hinder their commitment. We remind the patient that transient worsening of sleep during dose reduction may occur and that the homeostatic sleep drive after a night with poor sleep will be stronger the following night and will likely mean better sleep. We discuss the automaticity of the sleep process and how anxiety and apprehension about reducing the dose interfere with it.

As the taper proceeds and as the patient's self-efficacy and commitment increase, we may also provide guidance for an additional self-initiated dose reduction between sessions. To set the stage for success, we emphasize that the next dose reduction will be initiated only after sleep on the currently reduced dose is no worse than it was before the reduction. This is a dynamic, patient-centered process that further promotes self-efficacy and goal attainment. A patient's success in previous steps of reduction might change their self-efficacy and trust in their ability to continue the taper and, as described above, the later stages of the taper might be faster. Although less common, some patients experience increased difficulty on the last step of the taper (full discontinuation of medication), as this step represents a full reliance on the patient's own ability to sleep well and elimination of any perceived or actual support of the hypnotic medication in promoting good sleep. In these cases, a review of the patient's data (i.e., progress through earlier stages of the taper) and use of behavioral experiments may be helpful. During each treatment visit when a hypnotic taper is occurring, the written taper plan is documented in the patient's chart and provided to the patient as a concrete reminder of the plan and the patient's commitment to it. Taper plans are highly individualized, but typically include the specific plan for the timing and dose of medication use for the week. The plan specifies whether the use is nightly or, if not nightly, the conditions under which the medication is to be taken. The plan also includes self-statements that affirm and support the patient's commitment to the taper. If the interval for sessions is more than 1 week, the taper plan may also specify the conditions under which the patient can move to the next step of the taper.

Throughout the taper process, the therapist provides support and highlights progress, and promotes self-efficacy through attribution of progress to the changes that the patient has made. When setbacks arise, the therapist works with the patient to identify what may have hindered adherence with the taper schedule and plan how to proceed. This plan may involve ideas to address the hindering factors, such as worsening of sleep or increased level of anxiety about the taper, as well as slowing down or pausing the taper process, such as when stressful life events emerge and change the patient's priorities.

Use of CBT-I and behavioral principles

At its core, CBT-I is a skills-based treatment that leverages knowledge of the two-process models of sleep regulation as originally described by Borbély (1982) and arousal reduction strategies. Effective use of CBT-I to help patients reduce hypnotic medication use utilizes many of the standard components of CBT-I, albeit with a specific focus on issues relevant to hypnotic taper (Table 2). Examples, which are elaborated on below, are (1) leveraging a strong sleep drive during the time in bed restriction to offset potential increased arousal caused by anticipatory anxiety about reducing medication dose and (2) use of a range of cognitive therapy strategies to address factors that contribute to hypnotic dependence and promote sleep self-efficacy.

Homeostatic sleep drive/time in bed restriction

As described above, a good time to initiate the medication taper is during the implementation of time in bed restriction. This is because the reduced time in bed window increases the patient's homeostatic sleep to levels that can help counterbalance potential increases in sleep-interfering anticipatory arousal. If needed, due to increased sleep disturbances associated with the taper, patients can further reduce their time in bed window to leverage more sleep drive to smooth over increased anxiety and arousal associated with the taper. Psychoeducation about the role of homeostatic sleep drive and how limiting sleep opportunity can help the patient "tip the balance" toward good sleep over a period of several days can increase motivation and adherence to restricting time in bed. It can also increase self-efficacy for the patient to identify the time in bed restriction as a tool that they can use to allow their biology to help

TABLE 2 Commonly prescribed hypnotics.

Generic name	Brand name	Receptor binding specificity	Dose range (mg)	Elimination half life (h)
Doxepin	Silenor	5-HT, NE[a]	1–25 (1–6 most common for insomnia)	10–50
Eszopiclone	Lunesta	$GABA_A$, $\alpha_{1,2,3}$[b]	1–3	6
Lemborexant	Dayvigo	OX1R and OX2R receptors[c]	5–10	17–19
Ramelteon	Rozerum	MT1 and MT2 receptors[c,d]	8	0.8–2
Suvorexant	Belsomra	OX1R and OX2R receptors[b,c]	10–20	9–13
Temazepam	Restoril	Nonspecific	15–30	8–20
Zaleplon	Sonata	$GABA_A$, α_1	5–20	1
Zolpidem	Ambien	$GABA_A$, α_1	5–10	1.5–2.4
Zolpidem extended-release	Ambien CR	$GABA_A$, α_1	6.25–12.5	1.6–4.5

[a] *Serotonin, norepinephrine.*
[b] *$GABA_A$ (gamma-aminobutyric acid, type A receptor complex).*
[c] *Orexin receptors.*
[d] *Melatonin receptors.*
This table includes commonly prescribed hypnotics that are currently FDA approved for use in the treatment of chronic insomnia.

them adjust to any transient periods of sleep disturbance, including those associated with a medication taper.

It is important to emphasize the need for adherence to both the reduced medication dose and the recommended restricted time in bed window. It can be tempting for patients to relax their adherence to one or both of these if the first night of sleep on the new lower dose is worse than prior nights. For example, following a night of poor sleep (night 1), the patient may decide to either expand their sleep opportunity period or return to previous levels of medication use the next night (night 2). Both of these adjustments can result in increased sleep duration and an associated decrease in accumulated homeostatic sleep drive approaching the next night (night 3). If the patient attributes poor sleep on night 1 to the dose reduction they are particularly likely to increase the medication dosage back to the previous one. This in turn can reinforce beliefs that they are not able to sleep well without medication (see "Contingent reinforcement of beliefs/behavioral approaches" section below) and hence erode their sleep self-efficacy.

For patients who are using a hypnotic medication or are engaged in a hypnotic medication taper, when time in bed is restricted, the identified sleep opportunity window is often less than 8 h. This contradicts the written instructions that are included in the informational insert for many hypnotic medications. Such instructions are intended to promote safety. In these situations, it is still possible to promote safety with a more restricted time in bed that is consistent with CBT-I. This can be achieved by advising the patient to exercise caution during the 8h following the time the hypnotic dose is taken. For many patients, the critical period to be cautious about is a few hours after their recommended fixed rise time. Patients are therefore educated about carry-over risks and are encouraged to be cautious during this period about engaging in behaviors where alertness is critical (e.g., driving). Another modification to promote safety and adherence to the medication inset recommendation involves modifying the combined "time in bed restriction plus stimulus control" recommendations by asking that patients engage in counter-control (sitting up in bed and doing something pleasant while awake during the time in bed window) rather than to engage in full stimulus control (getting up and out of bed and bedroom).

Cognitive approaches/beliefs about sleep

The classic cognitive behavioral therapy cycle of thoughts influencing emotions, which in turn influences behavior choices that lead to reinforcement of maladaptive thinking plays a central role in maintaining patterns of hypnotic medication use. For example, if a patient decides to try not taking their dose of hypnotic medication on one night and then has difficulty initiating sleep, they may engage in a chain of thoughts illustrated in Fig. 1, which strengthens their belief about not being able to sleep without medication.

The utilization of cognitive approaches can play an important role in promoting the successful reduction of hypnotic medication. Patients' beliefs about their need to take hypnotic medication to sleep well, or

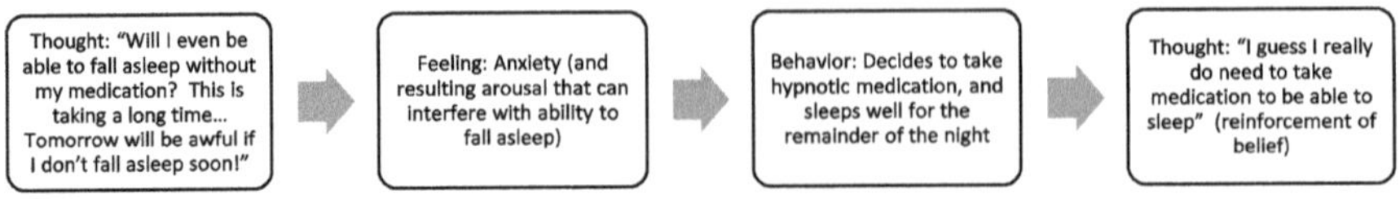

FIG. 1 Reinforcement of a patient's belief that they cannot sleep without medication.

uncertainty about their ability to function the next day following a night of poor sleep, often trap them into a cycle of relying on hypnotic medication to initiate or maintain sleep. Important domains to identify and address include themes reflecting low sleep self-efficacy ("I can't sleep without medication"), sleep effort (needing to work at sleep, "trying to sleep"), and an inability to tolerate uncertainty ("I need to know I can get a good night's sleep.").

Cognitive approaches, including cognitive restructuring, can be helpful in targeting unhelpful or inaccurate beliefs that can interfere with the patient's ease and ability to reduce sleep medication use. In this work, it may be more helpful to focus on how adaptive or helpful a thought is than on how accurate it is. This might be particularly important when working with patients who have had past negative experiences with single-night events where they intentionally or accidentally had a night without hypnotics and did not sleep well. These patients may have particularly strong beliefs that they are unable to sleep without medication:

> I've never slept well even with sleep medication, and when I've tried to stop using it before, I slept even worse. I'll always need to take it.

There are multiple points of discussion regarding accuracy/validity within these two sentences that could be explored. It can also be useful to examine the utility or adaptiveness of holding this belief, as well as to promote a beginner's mind stance and openness to change and potential willingness to engage in a medication taper. An example of an altered statement that reflects such openness is as follows:

> Well, my sleep is better now with this treatment than it has been. Maybe things are different now than when I tried stopping to take my medication before.

While the use of structured tools like cognitive restructuring worksheets can be helpful, adherence can be poor; this is particularly true when the patient perceives these treatment tools as "homework." In-session Socratic questioning and thoughtful discussion in session may be equally and potentially more effective in promoting patients' commitment to work toward their goal of reducing hypnotic use.

> Therapist: How do you think we could figure out if things are different now than they were before? And whether you might be more successful in reducing your medication use?
>
> Patient: I guess one thing would be to try reducing my sleep medication, but maybe just a little bit.
>
> Therapist: I agree. And how do you think you could use the things you've learned about sleep in this treatment to help you be successful?

Contingent reinforcement of beliefs/behavioral approaches

It is important for the CBT-I therapist to also be observant of behavior choices made by the patient that has the potential to reinforce beliefs that the patient is reliant on a hypnotic medication for good sleep. Such behaviors are can be classified as safety behaviors. A common example is the use of a hypnotic as a "rescue medication" taken only in situations when the patient has determined that they are unable to fall asleep. Taking the medication in this manner reinforces the patient's belief that they need the medication to sleep and prevents testing alternate, potentially more adaptive beliefs. Examples of alternative belief include beliefs that (a) they will be able to fall asleep eventually even if they do not take medication or take a reduced dose, (b) they can function adequately the next day even if they sleep poorly on a given night, and (c) they can use CBT-I tools they have already learned to help them overcome a setback while taking a lower dose of medication. In addition to taking rescue medications, there are also more subtle safety behaviors, such as keeping medication by the bedside to take "just in case," using medication following a night of poor sleep as a way to prevent another night with poor sleep, and taking the medication immediately when awakening in the middle of the night (note: this use strategy can be part of an intentional taper plan—see the "Schedule of reduction" section above). Understanding the role of contingent reinforcement informs choices for the schedule of hypnotic medication reduction.

General psychotherapy principles

As with all effective psychotherapies, the therapeutic alliance is another essential component of effective CBT-I. In our experience, the "T" in CBT-I is often underutilized and underemphasized. Genuine warmth and empathy, and the ability to meet the patient where they are with respect to their sleep difficulties are of critical importance. For instance, when a patient does not adhere to a particular treatment recommendation, it is better to become curious as to why the patient is having difficulty with implementing a particular treatment recommendation than to simply re-iterate the importance of adherence. A better understanding of obstacles to adherence helps the therapist identify with steps that allow the patient to be more successful in adhering to the original recommendation and to potentially modify the recommendation in a manner that will allow the patient to be successful. While CBT-I is a heavily technique-based treatment and can therefore become very prescriptive, we believe that approaching therapy with a flexible case-conceptualization-driven approach and creating an accepting and supportive clinical context can maximize the benefit for patients.

Conclusions

CBT-I is an effective therapy to improve sleep and help reduce or eliminate hypnotic medication use among patients with insomnia. In collaboration with prescribing providers, CBT-I therapists are uniquely placed to guide hypnotic medication tapers due to their therapeutic skill set, as well as their ability to meet with patients frequently, which together allows them to provide support and guidance through individualized recommendations. There is a critical need for CBT-I providers to develop the skills and knowledge to successfully guide patients through medication reductions; this chapter aims to provide basic knowledge and approaches to increase the effective use of CBT-I for hypnotic medication reduction. We also encourage providers who are interested in engaging in this type of work to also seek out additional knowledge about hypnotic medications, including their half-life and their potential for dependence, to deepen their knowledge in this area. By expanding their role to help address dependence on hypnotic medications, CBT-I providers have the potential to resolve insomnia, improve quality of life, and reduce health and safety risks associated with hypnotic medication use.

References

Adler, S., Carde, N., Kuo, T., Ong, J., & Manber, R. (2008). Use of and attitudes about sleep medications in a tertiary sleep clinic. *Sleep, 31*, A326–A327.

Ashton, C. (2002). *Benzodiazepines: How they work and how to withdraw*. https://www.benzo.org.uk/manual/.

Ayabe, N., Okajima, I., Nakajima, S., Inoue, Y., Watanabe, N., Yamadera, W., et al. (2018). Effectiveness of cognitive behavioral therapy for pharmacotherapy-resistant chronic insomnia: A multi-center randomized controlled trial in Japan. *Sleep Medicine, 50*, 105–112. https://doi.org/10.1016/j.sleep.2018.05.038.

Bakken, M. S., Engeland, A., Engesaeter, L. B., Ranhoff, A. H., Hunskaar, S., & Ruths, S. (2014). Risk of hip fracture among older people using anxiolytic and hypnotic drugs: A nationwide prospective cohort study. *European Journal of Clinical Pharmacology, 70*(7), 873–880. https://doi.org/10.1007/s00228-014-1684-z.

Belleville, G., Guay, C., Guay, B., & Morin, C. M. (2007). Hypnotic taper with or without self-help treatment of insomnia: A randomized clinical trial. *Journal of Consulting and Clinical Psychology, 75*(2), 325–335. https://doi.org/10.1037/0022-006x.75.2.325.

Bjorvatn, B., Meland, E., Flo, E., & Mildestvedt, T. (2017). High prevalence of insomnia and hypnotic use in patients visiting their general practitioner. *Family Practice, 34*(1), 20–24. https://doi.org/10.1093/fampra/cmw107.

Blom, K., Jernelov, S., Ruck, C., Lindefors, N., & Kaldo, V. (2016). Three-year follow-up of insomnia and hypnotics after controlled internet treatment for insomnia. *Sleep, 39*(6), 1267–1274. https://doi.org/10.5665/sleep.5850.

Borbély, A. (1982). A two process model of sleep regulation. *Human Neurobiology, 1*(13), 195–204.

Chen, P. L., Lee, W. J., Sun, W. Z., Oyang, Y. J., & Fuh, J. L. (2012). Risk of dementia in patients with insomnia and long-term use of hypnotics: A population-based retrospective cohort study. *PLoS One, 7*(11), 6. https://doi.org/10.1371/journal.pone.0049113.

Edinger, J. D., Wamboldt, F., Holm, K., Johnson, R. L., Simmons, B., Tsai, S., et al. (2019). A blinded hypnotic tapering approach for hypnotic discontinuation. *Sleep, 42*, 1.

Lichstein, K. L., Nau, S. D., Wilson, N. M., Aguillard, R. N., Lester, K. W., Bush, A. J., et al. (2013). Psychological treatment of hypnotic-dependent insomnia in a primarily older adult sample. *Behaviour Research and Therapy, 51*(12), 787–796. https://doi.org/10.1016/j.brat.2013.09.006.

Morgan, K., Dixon, S., Mathers, N., Thompson, J., & Tomeny, M. (2003). Psychological treatment for insomnia in the management of long-term hypnotic drug use: A pragmatic randomised controlled trial. *British Journal of General Practice, 53*(497), 923–928.

Morin, C. M., Sonte, J., McDonald, K., & Jones, S. (1994). Psychological management of insomnia—A clinical replication series with 100 patients. *Behavior Therapy, 25*(2), 291–309. https://doi.org/10.1016/s0005-7894(05)80289-8.

Petursson, E. (1994). The benzodiazepine withdrawal syndrome. *Addiction, 89*(11), 1455–1459.

Radcliff, S., Yue, J. R., Rocco, G., Aiello, S. E., Ickowicz, E., Hurd, Z., et al. (2015). American Geriatrics Society 2015 updated beers criteria for potentially inappropriate medication use in older adults. *Journal of the American Geriatrics Society, 63*(11), 2227–2246. https://doi.org/10.1111/jgs.13702.

Roehrs, T. A., Randall, S., Harris, E., Maan, R., & Roth, T. (2012). Twelve months of nightly zolpidem does not lead to rebound insomnia or withdrawal symptoms: A prospective placebo-controlled study. *Journal of Psychopharmacology, 26*(8), 1088–1095. https://doi.org/10.1177/0269881111424455.

Schneiderhelmert, D. (1988). Why low-dose benzodiazepine-dependent insomniacs cant escape their sleeping pills. *Acta Psychiatrica Scandinavica, 78*(6), 706–711. https://doi.org/10.1111/j.1600-0447.1988.tb06408.x.

Schonmann, Y., Goren, O., Bareket, R., Comaneshter, D., Cohen, A. D., & Vinker, S. (2018). Chronic hypnotic use at 10 yearsdoes the brand matter? *European Journal of Clinical Pharmacology, 74*(12), 1623–1631. https://doi.org/10.1007/s00228-018-2531-4.

Siriwardena, A. N., Qureshi, M. Z., Dyas, J. V., Middleton, H., & Orner, R. (2008). Magic bullets for insomnia? Patients' use and experiences of newer (Z drugs) versus older (benzodiazepine) hypnotics for sleep problems in primary care. *British Journal of General Practice, 58*(551), 417–422. https://doi.org/10.3399/bjgp08X299290.

Takaesu, Y., Utsumi, T., Okajima, I., Shimura, A., Kotorii, N., Kuriyama, K., et al. (2019). Psychosocial intervention for discontinuing benzodiazepine hypnotics in patients with chronic insomnia: A systematic review and meta-analysis. *Sleep Medicine Reviews, 48*, 12. https://doi.org/10.1016/j.smrv.2019.101214.

Wilt, T. J., MacDonald, R., Brasure, M., Olson, C. M., Carlyle, M., Fuchs, E., et al. (2016). Pharmacologic treatment of insomnia disorder: An evidence report for a clinical practice guideline by the American College of Physicians. *Annals of Internal Medicine, 165*(2), 103. https://doi.org/10.7326/m15-1781.

Yang, C. M., Tseng, C. H., Lai, Y. S., & Hsu, S. C. (2015). Self-efficacy enhancement can facilitate hypnotic tapering in patients with primary insomnia. *Sleep and Biological Rhythms, 13*(3), 242–251. https://doi.org/10.1111/sbr.12111.

Index

Note: Page numbers followed by *f* indicate figures, *t* indicate tables, *b* indicate boxes, and *np* indicate footnotes.

R

Kolibri 360 GmbH
Ferdinand-Jühlke-Straße 7
99095 Erfurt, Deutschland
produktsicherheit@kolibri360.de